"Posterity has bifurcated James Cowles Prichard's contributions: historians of anthropology rarely mention his ideas on alienism; psychiatrists know next to nothing about his ethnological work. At long last, these moieties have been brought together by Margaret M. Crump, who in a solid and sympathetic intellectual biography has regaled us with the first complete picture of this great Victorian mind."

    —GERMAN E. BERRIOS, emeritus professor of the epistemology of psychiatry at the University of Cambridge

"Margaret Crump rightly points out that for such an eminent Victorian, James Cowles Prichard has been strangely neglected. . . . Crump brings out the connections between Prichard's career as a physician and as an anthropologist and discusses the influences of his Quaker faith and Tory politics on his scientific thinking. . . . Her study is well written, carefully researched, and full of interesting information."

    —ADAM KUPER, fellow of the British Royal Society and author of *The Museum of Other People: From Colonial Acquisitions to Cosmopolitan Exhibitions*

"Margaret Crump has done a great service in writing this lively, informative, and meticulously researched biography of the remarkable James Cowles Prichard, the visionary and humane English physician and anthropologist whose landmark *Researches into the Physical History of Mankind* was read by both Charles Darwin and Alfred Russel Wallace. In telling the story of the eminent but often overlooked Prichard, Crump's wonderfully far-ranging book deftly interweaves the history of medicine, psychiatry, anthropology, linguistics, paleontology, evolution, and even a dash of Egyptology, illuminating the life and thought of this fascinating scientist in the context of his world-changing times."

    —JAMES T. COSTA, executive director and professor at Highlands Biological Station of Western Carolina University and author of *Radical by Nature: The Revolutionary Life of Alfred Russel Wallace*

"James Cowles Prichard achieved an international reputation for research on what he called the 'physical history of mankind,' publishing pioneering volumes on what is now called anthropology. He did this in the midst of a busy medical practice in Bristol, as well as dedicated participation in Bristol's civic and scientific life. Margaret Crump does Prichard proud in this fine study of such a multifaceted man and his times."
> —WILLIAM BYNUM, professor emeritus at the University College London and author of *Science and the Practice of Medicine in the Nineteenth Century*

"James Cowles Prichard was Britain's most significant nineteenth-century, pre-Darwinian anthropologist and brilliant polymath. At long last, Margaret Crump has provided us with a much-needed, comprehensive biography of this exceptional scientist and scholar. Her archival and bibliographical scholarship are second to none and cover such exciting topics as Prichard's Quaker background and his antiracist support for the notion of the unity of mankind. I wholeheartedly recommend this gem of first-rate academic learning that has implications for current affairs in race and equality."
> —NICOLAAS A. RUPKE, Johnson Professor of History at Washington and Lee University and author of *Richard Owen: Biology without Darwin*

"Like other famous Bristol figures, including Brunel, Elizabeth Blackwell, and Humphry Davy, Prichard finally has his definitive biography. In this exceedingly informative and engrossing account of the life and times of James Cowles Prichard, Margaret Crump expertly weaves together the life, medical career, and anthropological writings of one of Bristol's most interesting past inhabitants."
> —JONATHAN REINARZ, professor of the history of medicine at the University of Birmingham and editor of *A Cultural History of Medicine in the Age of Empire*

James Cowles Prichard of the Red Lodge

Critical Studies
in the History of
Anthropology
SERIES EDITORS
Regna Darnell
Robert Oppenheim

JAMES COWLES PRICHARD
of the Red Lodge

A Life of Science during the Age of Improvement

MARGARET M. CRUMP

UNIVERSITY OF NEBRASKA PRESS · LINCOLN

© 2025 by the Board of Regents of the University of Nebraska

All rights reserved

The University of Nebraska Press is part of a land-grant institution with campuses and programs on the past, present, and future homelands of the Pawnee, Ponca, Otoe-Missouria, Omaha, Dakota, Lakota, Kaw, Cheyenne, and Arapaho Peoples, as well as those of the relocated Ho-Chunk, Sac and Fox, and Iowa Peoples.

Publication of this work was assisted by the Murray-Hong Family Trust, to honor and sustain the distinguished legacy of Stephen O. Murray in the History of Anthropology at the University of Nebraska Press.

For customers in the EU with safety/GPSR concerns, contact:
gpsr@mare-nostrum.co.uk
Mare Nostrum Group BV
Mauritskade 21D
1091 GC Amsterdam
The Netherlands

Library of Congress Control Number: 2024024806

Set in Miller Text by A. Shahan.

Contents

List of Illustrations	vii
Preface	ix
Acknowledgments	xiii
Introduction	xv
Apologia	xxi

1. Time and Place: A Bristol Quaker Childhood in a Turbulent World — 1
2. "A Studious Turn of Mind": Preparatory Medical Education — 32
3. MD, Edin: *Lernfreiheit* in Scotland and Oxbridge — 51
4. Citizen, Husband, Gentleman, Physician, and Scientist: Getting Established in Bristol, 1810–16 — 90
5. "Sharpening Their Wits upon the Carcasses of the Poor": Working for Medical Charities — 118
6. The Single Origin and Unity of Humankind: Creating British Anthropology, 1805–26 — 153
7. Epidemics, History, and Mythology: Building a Reputation in Bristol, 1817–22 — 189
8. Nervous Diseases: Neurology and Psychiatry, 1822–47 — 212
9. "Irksome Things": Improving Bristol and Medical Practice, 1823–26 — 254
10. The Early Red Lodge Years: Improving Institutions and Publications, 1827–32 — 287
11. Life and Reputation at the Red Lodge: Family, Friends, and Science, 1833–39 — 330

12. New Scientists, New Organizations, New Ideas:
    Developing British Anthropology, 1833–48   367
13. Christian Humanitarian Anthropology:
    Publications, 1836–48, and Legacy   408
14. From the Red Lodge to Asylumdom:
    A New Career, 1839–45   443
15. Public Service and Private Misery:
    Living in London, 1845–48   462
    Conclusion   479

    Notes   483
    Bibliography   563
    Index   617

Illustrations

1. James Cowles Prichard in his forties	xv
2. "A Memoir of the late Thomas Prichard Esq. of Ross, Part 1, 1847"	xxiv
3. Young Prichard and Anna in silhouette	104
4. St. Peter's Hospital, Bristol	121
5. Bristol Infirmary	136
6. Bristol Institution	258
7. Advertisement for Dr. Prichard and Mr. Clark's lectures on Egypt, 1834	261
8. Red Lodge's facade and garden	289
9. The quay, with the tower of St. Stephen's, Bristol	310
10. Great Oak Room, Red Lodge	361
11. "A portrait of Rammohun Roy"	415
12. "Kooraï: A Fisherman's Family"	424
13. "The Last of the Charruas"	424

Preface

At the heart of this first comprehensive biography of James Cowles Prichard lies the conviction that he made substantial contributions to the science of his era, especially to the development of anthropology and psychiatry. After his death in 1848, however, his name gradually faded from history for more than one reason. For one thing, both anthropology and psychiatry entered a sort of Ice Age, a period of execrable notions some would wish forgotten. Eventually, these disciplines evolved into their modern forms—redefined and with new founders—leaving their origins in obscurity. A dearth of personal information about Prichard and the loss of his scientific archive have frustrated would-be biographers. Further, the very breadth of this early Victorian scientific celebrity's command of anthropology, psychology, psychiatry, physiology, medicine, linguistics, biology, and mythology has daunted specialist historians. From a modern perspective, Prichard's range of achievement is disconcerting; how could a provincial physician have strayed beyond bleeding and dosing his patients? This biography addresses these issues, revealing the scientist and his science in the context of the science and culture of his era.

Scores of obituaries were published, and in the decades following Prichard's death, some appreciative short memoirs came out, including a fuller one by his friend Thomas Hodgkin. It contains some tantalizing details, but without reference to their source. Biographical dictionaries and a more recent monograph on his anthropology present a smattering of Hodgkin's anecdotes.[1] Immensely proud of their famous father, Prichard's surviving children had dutifully preserved his certificates, mementos, copies of his publications, and a huge collection of personal and family material. They were planning to produce a typically Victorian "life and letters." But what happened? This biography draws on widely scattered and various types of resources. For instance, the Bristol Library has a record of the hundreds of books Prichard borrowed over four decades. Books from his own library appear on later donation lists, too, although his heirs disposed of many of his books to a Bristol book and manuscript dealer. The volumes still in stock there in 1854 are listed in the thirty-six-page *T. Kerslake's Catalogue of Books Including a Portion of the Library of the Learned James Cowles Prichard*

Esq. M.D. &c Author of the Physical History of Man ... and also that of Dr. Edward Jenner. Bristolians put Prichard before the hero of vaccination.

Kerslake's Catalogue lists eight of Prichard's own works, sixty-three other volumes inscribed to him, and others he had autographed. The proud teenager inscribed a popular book of French poetry "James Cowles Prichard—Staines—1804." In the inspiring *Decades craniorum* is written: "Given to me by Professor Blumenbach at Gottingen / J.C. Prichard." *The Pharmacopaeia of the Bristol Infirmary*, "interleaved with numerous Additions in the hand-writing of Dr. Prichard," and the *Reports of the Commissioners in Lunacy* (1844), similarly annotated, bookend his medical interests. Many of these titles appear in the footnotes to Prichard's own publications, such as Johann Christoph Adelung's *Mithridates oder allgemeine sprachenkunde*, an influential book he reviewed. His copy of Joseph Bush's *Evangelical Sermons at Long Ashton* (1842) points to more personal interests. The author of *Travels on the Continent* (1829) claimed Prichard as his friend, while his father-in-law presented him with his *Universal Restitution* (1813). He did purchase Carl Ritter's thirteen volumes of *Erdkunde von Asien* (1832–47) for 12 guineas, a considerable investment and invaluable for Prichard's third edition of *Physical History*. His annotated volume on numismatics and his autographed volume of notes on Professor Dugald Stewart's lectures signed "Edinburgh, 1806" promised much-needed biographical material.

The most enticing item in *Kerslake's Catalogue* has to be number 10498, "Manuscripts:—Eleven Thick Quarto Vols. and several smaller in the handwriting of the late Dr. Prichard, a large bundle, 2l 12s." Kerslake's warehouse was destroyed in a fire in 1860. His nephew in Birmingham sold the surviving stock to the dealer E. M. Lawson in 1926. Fifty years later, Lawson's descendants could offer no clue to the fate of Prichard's scientific manuscripts.[2] Had they been sold before 1860, destroyed by fire, or sold in Birmingham? The trail ran cold.

It was time for some genealogy. A canvas of hundreds of institutions around the world yielded many copies of Prichard's books and more than a hundred autographed letters, but no private papers. After combing the national registers of births, marriages, and deaths to trace his descendants with, and inconveniently without, his surname, their addresses were ascertained, and more letters of inquiry were dispatched throughout England and Wales. These yielded family jottings, a privately published Quaker family history, albums, letters, heirlooms, portraits, a diary, ephemera, books, and far too many genealogical charts. One elderly Prichard could recount a bit of family lore, some scandals, and a worrying account of his relatives' patriotic contribution of masses of old family documents to a World War II paper drive. Another recalled that "Constantine Innes Pocock is known to have family papers but is not interested and probably threw them away."[3]

One day, a North Wales descendant wrote, doubting whether a large old leatherbound manuscript would be of interest, especially as it was incomplete. It certainly was of interest. In Prichard's scrawl is the title page: "A Memoir of the late Thomas Prichard Esq. of Ross. By his Son. J. C. Prichard. 1847. (volume 2)." A few months later, a Bristolian descended from a different branch of the family regretted that he could provide only volume 1 of a manuscript biography of Thomas Prichard. The two volumes were reunited. From a somewhat tedious account of proud Quaker ancestry to Thomas Prichard's death in 1843, Prichard chronicles both his father's and his own life in 690 pages, drawing mostly on correspondence and his own reminiscences. His life was a reflection of his father's hopes, advice, admonitions, and injunctions.

Partway through the second volume of the memoir Prichard's handwriting ends and his son Constantine's begins. It was 1859, and Prichard's widow had just died. Con was looking forward to finishing his grandfather's biography and starting on his father's. But having to comprehend Prichard's science so overwhelmed this consumptive clergyman, he resorted to enlisting the aid of experts in several scientific disciplines. Con further complained: "The difficulty abt his life has always seemed to me that he wrote so few letters about private matters to us, but if there are earlier ones, they will afford materials for that time, or I daresay Aunt M. cd. supply some more." Much to Con's surprise, his brother Augustin and Aunt Mary Moline did have a lot of Prichard's private papers and correspondence. Things looked promising: "It will be very interesting to read the letters you have found. I am quite surprised, too, that my father kept so many—or wrote so many himself. I think my mother must have disliked the idea of their being examined in her lifetime, as she wd. have mentioned them." Con started writing Prichard's biography but died a few years later.[4] The materials were likely returned to Augustin, whose grandchildren contributed so generously to the World War II paper drive.

Two descendants of Prichard gathered some remaining material for his centenary celebration at the Royal Anthropological Institute, London, in 1948. They regretted the loss of the manuscript biography of Thomas Prichard, but the Rev. Edward Cowles Prichard exhibited some carefully preserved documents, Prichard's books, and the watch chain and seals depicted in his portrait. Theodore Pocock, son of Prichard's daughter Edith, contributed family lore, word of mouth linking more than a century and a quarter. The organizers of the seminar urged them to find a biographer for Prichard.[5] They never did. Elsewhere is a tantalizing sheet of notes for a grandson's 1912 lecture on Prichard, illustrated with a daguerreotype, an engraving, his Oxford MD diploma, some of his books, a letter from Robert Southey, an 1838 letter from New York, "notes of some of his medical cases," and "some of his manuscripts."[6] Of all these, only the diploma and New York letter were eventually deposited in the Bristol Archives. That grandson was the father of the paper drive family.

In his memoir of his father, Prichard describes his own late eighteenth-century childhood in the provincial English city of Bristol, the son of a prosperous, conservative, pious Quaker, educated at a time when education meant a thorough knowledge of the classics, theology, history, modern languages, and mathematics. His personality was formed by his father and his upbringing in a period of religious, political, and social upheaval strongly marked by a national urge to reform and improve society. Prichard chronicled family life and his career, reflecting on his efforts to contribute to knowledge in a changing, challenging world. "A Memoir of Thomas Prichard" scaffolds this biography.

Context is crucial. When considering Prichard's life and science, it has been beneficial to bear in mind the so-called emic approach to history: the analysis of past human behavior in terms meaningful to those doing the behaving rather than those doing the analyzing.[7] Continuing with more jargon, this approach can temper "presentist" and "progressivist" evaluations, for instance, when considering Prichard's focus on humankind's descent from a single original pair, his invasive treatments for mental illness and neuropsychiatric conditions, or even his copious bloodletting and purging for fever. By setting aside today's notions of valid science, it is possible to better appreciate the development of science and Prichard's place in its history.

Acknowledgments

A fuller list of the many institutions whose dedicated members of staff deserve my sincerest thanks can be found in the bibliography. Scores of libraries, archives offices, and other public and private organizations in Britian and beyond were exploited. Above all, staff members of the City of Bristol Central Library were invariably patient and helpful, as were their colleagues at the Bristol Archives. I am grateful to the staff of the University of Bristol Library, British Library, Museum of Mankind/RAI Library (London), National Archives (London), Wellcome Collections, Library of the Society of Friends (London), Royal Society, Royal College of Surgeons (London), University of Edinburgh Library, National Library of Scotland, Royal Medical Society (Edinburgh), National Library of Wales (Aberystwyth), University of Liverpool, University of Oxford, Boston Public Library, Countway Medical Library (Harvard University, Boston), University of Southampton, Niedersächsische Staats-und Universitätsbibliothek (Göttingen), American Philosophical Society (Philadelphia), New York Historical Society, the Peabody Essex Museum (Rowley, Massachusetts), Medical Reading Society (Bristol), Bundesarchiv (Koblenz), Staatsbibliothek Preussischer Kulturbesitz (Berlin), and many of Britain's county archives offices.

Scores of Prichard's descendants were variously puzzled or pleased to be traced and asked about an ancestor of whose significance or existence they were usually unaware. They generously allowed their heirlooms to be borrowed, photocopied, and cited. I am grateful to members of the Prichard, Pocock, Woods, Haines, Orton, Thomas, Fedden, and Gee families.

Several individuals contributed greatly appreciated observations on and corrections to my manuscript. Historians Nicolaas Rupke, Madge Dresser, Jonathan Barry, and Joan Leopold advised me while a band of knowledgeable Bristolians who rooted out inaccuracies include Peter Carpenter, Martin Crossley Evans, William Evans, Jon Stevens, and Michael Whitfield. Alex Baylis rigorously combed through several chapters. Crucial were the advice and encouragement of intellectual historian Ian Stewart and the unstinting kindness and patient support of David Page. I am sincerely grateful to Matthew Bokovoy and his colleagues at the University of Nebraska Press for believing in this project and helping me see it to completion. Any errors are my own. Finally, you are reading about James Cowles Prichard, the scientist and person, because John Osborn Crump (1935–2017) believed this subject merited our decades of effort. Memories of him are on every page of this book.

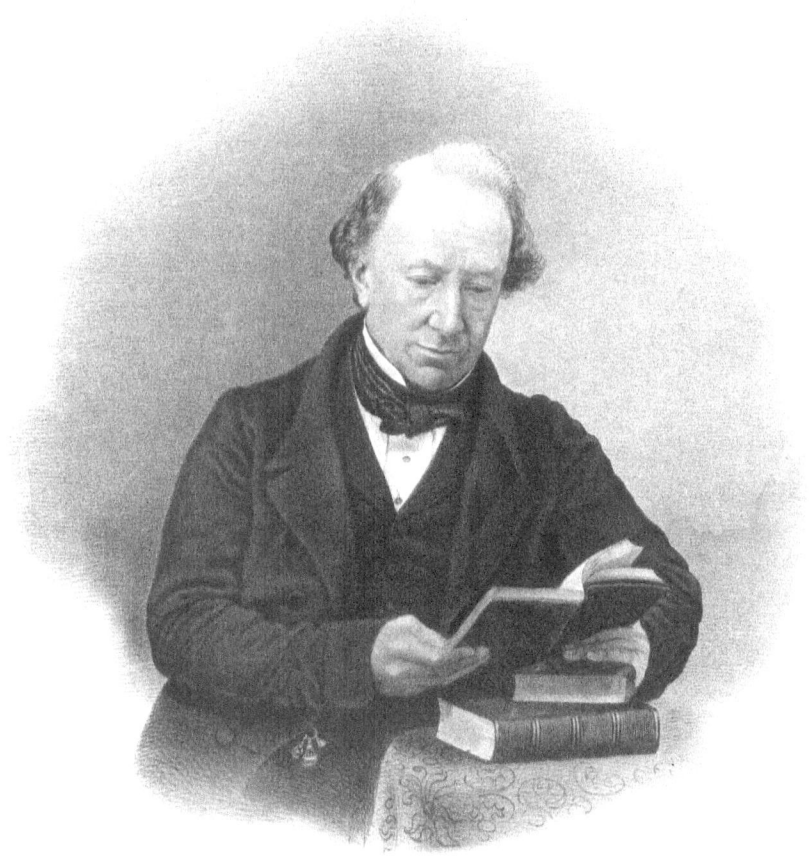

Introduction

The great breadth of James Cowles Prichard's scientific interests, his innovative research, and the sheer volume of his work astonished his fellow Victorians. Medicine, physiology, psychology, psychiatry, biological and cultural anthropology, linguistics, comparative anatomy, mythology, biblical criticism, and geology all came within his scope; his publications were widely read, translated, and reviewed. This humane physician-scientist's anthropological books were a resource for antislavery campaigners and later anthropologists. So respected was he and so greatly valued was his

1. ABOVE: Books and gold seals. James Cowles Prichard in his forties. Engraving from a portrait by Nathan Branwhite, c. 1827. Property of the author.

account of the specific unity and single origin of the human species that during his lifetime he managed to hold back a rising tide of proto-racialist theories among his fellow British scientists, if not among the general public. His treatises on psychological medicine and medical jurisprudence became landmarks in the history of psychiatry; they fostered understanding of insanity and sought to preserve the civil liberties of the insane. He was honored with election to many learned societies, including the Royal Society of London, the Institute of France, and the American Philosophical Society, and he received a rarely granted honorary MD from the University of Oxford.

Described as "of remarkable ability" and "one of the ablest men of our time," crucially during this era of religious orthodoxy, Prichard was an intellectual "in whose hands, science of *prime order* comes in as the handmaid and supporter of religion"; he was notably zealous in the "furtherance of the cause of true religion."[1] Historian and philosopher of science William Whewell considered Prichard

> a person of the highest talents and most profound and extensive erudition, and of a European reputation. . . . He is a man of genius. . . . His researches on the early history of nations, the affinities of races and the progress of civilization, have placed him very far at the head of our writers upon those subjects, or rather have placed him quite at a distance from all other English speculators on those matters, and have ranked him with the great German ethnographers, Niebuhr and Muller, and Ritter and the Schlegels and the Humboldts, with whose writings he is intimately acquainted; and perhaps he alone, among our English men of letters.[2]

When late Victorian novelist Anthony Trollope created a scholarly character in *Orley Farm* (1862), he gave him a taste for recondite German scholarship and a passion for the subjects of philology and the races of man. This earnest scholar pores over volumes of Prichard and his intellectual heir, Robert Gordon Latham. Prichard was no "gentlemen of leisure"; he had to juggle research with his professional obligations. Being a famous scientist, scholar, prolific author, and sought-after physician came with a price, however.

When Prichard took up his study of extra-Europeans, they were a subject of curiosity rather than denigration they would soon attract. Although deprecatory racial theorizing was not unknown among a few earlier philosophers and scientists, during Prichard's lifetime some writers started concocting and popularizing something later termed *scientific racialism* based on analyzing superficial human characteristics that conveniently found Europeans the superior "race." As attitudes began to harden, Prichard became alarmed, especially as the theory tended to justify exploitation of Britain's colonized peoples. While he evinced an occasional spark of modern cultural relativism, he was typical in believing in the superiority of Christian European culture—an attitude now discredited in theory, if not in practice. But as for the insidious notion of biologically defined, ranked races or even separate human species, Prichard was adamantly opposed. On the contrary, he wrote that he had

> for more than thirty years, desired to see established [the fact of] the unity of the human race, that is to say, that all men are descended from the same parents. This desire is not held for the love of a hypothesis but for the conviction that this doctrine is more consistent than the contrary with religion, simplicity of nature, and truth, and moreover with the voice of philanthropy and humanity, because if one succeeds in the claim of persuading the world that there are several races of men and that the Africans, for example are of an inferior species to ours, it would be exceedingly difficult to establish their just right of being treated as brothers of Europeans, and of possessing the liberty which the sentiments of enlightened nations have finally granted them.[3]

So how did Prichard's anthropology come to fall on hard times during the second half of the nineteenth century? The notion of the plurality of human races or species continued gaining ground in Britain as it had already done on the Continent and in American slave-owning states. Most anthropologists thus generally set aside the Prichardian holistic study of humankind and the search for human origins and created a post-Darwinian anthropology tainted with polygenetic theory and phrenology-inspired craniometry, stressing physical differences among peoples. New generations of biological anthropologists devised Eurocentric classifications and rankings, especially of intellectual capacity. During this sterile period, members of anthropological societies in France, England, and America asserted the notion of the physical and intellectual inferiority of some "races"; its counterpart, now termed *European exceptionalism*, is the belief that Europeans represent the apogee of physical and cultural achievement. This phase of anthropology fueled growing nationalism and helped rationalize colonial expansion, paving the way for later racialist, eugenicist, national socialist, and contemporary, ever-resurfacing supremacist delusions. It is no wonder historians have been tempted to expunge this discreditable phase of anthropology from its history. The Darwinian revolution, later nineteenth-century domination of biological anthropology, development of successive anthropological paradigms and methodologies, and increasing discomfort with his Christian bias alienated Prichard's name from the history of the discipline, leaving it to fade into a benighted sort of prehistory. His successors are generally considered the founders of British cultural and social anthropology, while other countries have their own anthropologies with their own founders.

Prichard's contributions to other disciplines occurred at the threshold of the modern Scientific Revolution of the later nineteenth century. In neurology he devised early and lasting descriptions of a variety of conditions such as the stages in an epileptic seizure and in senile dementia, the latter term he coined. In psychiatry he developed the concept of moral insanity, was considered psychiatry's authoritative English nosographer, and advocated the humane treatment of the insane in law and in asylums. In physiology he dealt a fatal blow to the traditional reasoning behind the concept of a "vital principle," advocating a scientific approach to researching the nature of biological development.

As for Prichard's contributions to medicine, in his day, ancient humoral medical theory reigned supreme. He had little choice but to cleave to it while predicting and welcoming a future scientific medicine founded on pathology, microscopy, and medical statistical analysis. He is credited with having introduced the modern form of linguistics into Britain, his being the first to demonstrate Celtic's membership of the Indo-European language family qualifies him as one of the three founders of Celtic linguistics. He also effectively classified some African languages.

By setting aside a how-did-we-get-here historiography of science, a fuller view of the history of science reveals Prichard's significant role in it. Although he did not "prove" the specific unity and single origin of humankind, create a humane and effective psychiatry, or cure epilepsy with turpentine, an account of his attempts to do such things enriches the understanding of the history of science during the Age of Improvement.

This biography sets Prichard and his science in cultural and intellectual context, among the people he loved, admired, and despised. His pious Quaker childhood ended in a period of medical training, following which he gained an MD at the University of Edinburgh, where he acquired skills in research and argument and some lasting friendships. His lifelong effort to improve the world through science is described in the context of his professional and personal life in Bristol and the medical, scientific, educational, professional, and charitable organizations he helped develop and supported, the appointments he held, the books he read, the clubs and learned societies he joined, the patients he treated, the friends he made, the religion he professed, how he lived, dressed, behaved, voted, and raised his children, and his all-important relationship with his father. For clarity, Prichard's anthropology and psychological medicine are explored in four chapters that interrupt the chronology of the text, while the mostly biographical chapters set these and his other work in personal, cultural, and historical contexts. An account of his careworn, final three years in London as a commissioner in lunacy completes the story of his life.

Apologia

Several terms used in early nineteenth-century science have evolved in meaning, confusing and offending unwary modern readers. To avoid misapprehension, terms are used anachronistically, including "psychological," "behavioral," "social," or "emotional" instead of "moral"; "depression" instead of "dejection"; "scientist" instead of "natural philosopher"; "archaeologist" instead of "antiquarian"; and "anthropology" rather than "ethnology" or "natural history of man." Before the 1830s a person studying chemistry or the digestion of earthworms would have been called a natural philosopher or natural historian, not a scientist. "Immaterial" meant "nonphysical," with spiritual connotations. Particularly misleading is "race," which still meant "group"; Prichard could describe a "race" or "tribe" of plants. If the term "ethnic group" had existed, he might not have used "races" as a synonym of "tribes" and "nations," misleading modern readers into thinking he believed there were biologically definable races or even more than one human race. He wrote about "African races" and "American races," meaning ethnic groups; the biological notion of race started developing gradually only during the final years of his life.

As for offense, "Negro," "savage," "native," and "Kaffir" were neutral terms. Prichard's neutral "savage races" became later anthropologists' "primitive peoples," "ethnic groups," and now "Indigenous peoples." The pitfalls of vocabulary extend to psychiatry. The psychiatric literature of Prichard's era bristles with nouns that have since become pejorative, like "mad-doctors," "madhouses," "lunatics," "imbeciles," "idiots," and so on. And while in this volume "humankind" replaces "mankind," all clergymen, doctors, scientists, and chairpersons are men; there were no recognized women among them. There is something to be learned by seeing the language of the time used authentically, but to obviate confusion or offense, synonyms and tiresome quotation marks are sometimes used.[1]

Prichard had a lively, creative, xenophobic interest in terminology. He wanted the new scientific approach to studying languages to be called "glottology" instead of Frenchified "linguistics." As for "psychiatry," no self-respecting English mad-doctor would deign to use that German term until the end of the nineteenth century. He employed the word "science" in its modern sense several times in his 1813 book, but "scientist" caught on only in the 1830s. Prichard gradually began to call his encompassing science of humankind "ethnology" because to him the equally foreign word "anthropology" meant German psychiatry, a contemporary Parisian physician's neologism for the study of the human brain relative to "race" and several other confusing and limiting fields of study. Only rarely did he use "anthropology" to denote the biological study of humankind. Prichard considered the "natural history of man" synonymous with "ethnology," and both meant the philosophical, historical, linguistic, cultural, biological, and eventually archaeological study of humankind. And as for "culture," the word in its anthropological sense had not yet come into existence in English; he therefore wrote about "society, customs, and habitudes," "political institutions," and so on. Prichard's ethnology was the science of anthropology in the Anglo-American four-fields sense, no matter what he called it.[2]

James Cowles Prichard of the Red Lodge

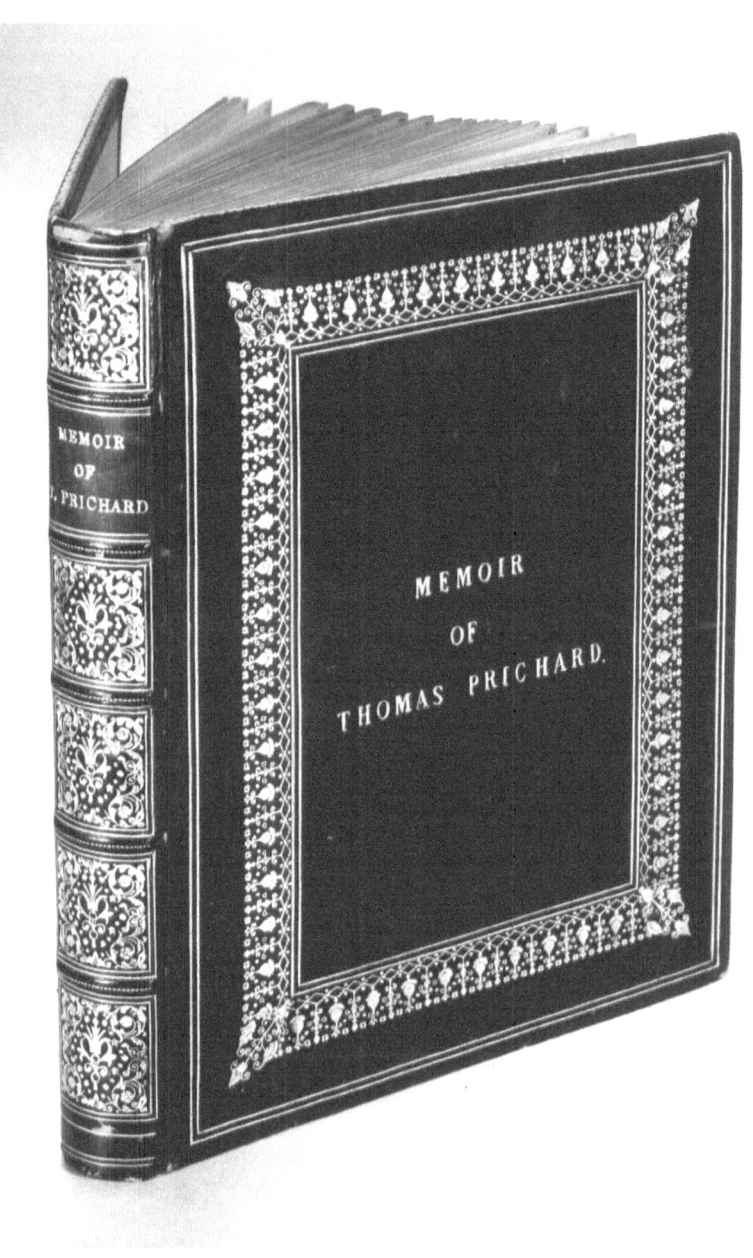

2. Filial duty. "A Memoir of the late Thomas Prichard Esq. of Ross, Part 1, 1847." Property of the Orton family.

1 · Time and Place

A Bristol Quaker Childhood in a Turbulent World

> There is nothing in their history which the most high-minded would wish to be forgotten or never to have happened.
> —James Cowles Prichard, "Memoir of Thomas Prichard, Part 1"

It was 1847 and high time to take a break from the misery of inspecting lunatic asylums and the drudgery of writing reports. Opening a fine new leatherbound volume of blank pages, Dr. James Cowles Prichard began: "I resolved long ago to employ the first opportunity of leisure that might fall to my lot in composing a short memoir of my Father's life. The many excellent and amiable qualities which rendered him esteemed and beloved by all who knew him have been since his death, even more strongly impressed on my mind than they were while he still lived and I have felt that they ought not to be left without some more lasting memorial than the recollection of those who will soon follow him."[1]

With Victorian filial piety, Prichard started writing a memoir of the long life of his father, Thomas Prichard. As he gathered family documents and correspondence for it, he found himself considering his own life as much as his father's. "A Memoir of the late Thomas Prichard Esq. of Ross" starts conventionally with an extensive genealogy; the Prichards were enormously proud of their long, prosperous Quaker heritage. Then into the scrawly lines creep Prichard's own upbringing, education, intense relationship with his father, the trials and triumphs of adulthood, the wider issues of the period that drove him in his life's work, and, of course, his opinions. Eventually, he filled two volumes with nearly seven hundred pages of personal history and Christian reflection.

A Bristol Childhood

James was born on February 11, 1786, in the quiet market town of Ross, Herefordshire, the eldest of Thomas and Mary Prichard's children. But when he was three the family moved from their comfortable home at the bottom of Brampton Street, looking up Over-Ross Street, to Somerset Street in the

Kingsdown suburb of the bustling cosmopolitan port of Bristol. The Ross home he vaguely remembered, but he vividly recalled his grandparents' visits to them in Bristol when Grandfather Prichard, lame with gout, could barely climb the steep garden steps.[2]

Kingsdown was a new development of mostly terraced houses clinging to the hillside above the city, built on fields once owned by St. James Priory. Its streets, tracing the contours of the hill, were intersected by precipitously stepped paths. The impressive homes on the south side of the street boasted long sloping gardens and distinctive bay windows providing panoramic views of distant hills. In their cellars were huge cisterns for collecting rainwater for cleaning purposes, and there were wells for drinking water—"two sorts of water," as newspaper advertisements boasted. Local rates funded street repairs and scavengers to collect rubbish and ashes. Of more interest to James and his younger siblings were the extensive fields stretching just beyond the brow of the hill where the famous Mother Pugsley's Well, a spring feeding ancient stone basins, was said to have curative powers.[3] Bristol might have been a magical place for childhood adventures, but it also opened a sad period for the Prichard family.

Thomas Prichard was not cut out to be a businessman. His daily grind at the Small Street countinghouse of Harford, Partridge & Company was barely tolerable. It had been unwise to move his family to Bristol to take up this inherited partnership. The Harfords themselves were a source of anxiety, those rich Quakers with fingers in the pies of many Bristol and South Wales businesses. They were Bristol industrialists and bankers well connected among captains of industry such as the Lloyds (banking), Wedgwoods (pottery), and Frys (chocolate and printing). Harfords manufactured a wide variety of metal products, including tin plate, bar, sheet and rod iron, steel products, tools, and utensils, and they handled similar products manufactured in the Midlands town of Coalbrookdale. The Harford and Bristol Brass Company had a brass wire and spelter factory in Keynsham, near Bristol, works in Swansea, and in Melingriffith, near Cardiff, a tinworks and shares in several Welsh iron companies.[4] But did Christian principles guide their wheeling and dealing as they engaged in the English habit of exploiting Welsh resources?

James's father would have been better pleased if his business associates had evinced a bit of Quaker altruism and restraint. Instead, they were exacting employers who relished the cut and thrust of competition. Worse still, their products supplied not just the domestic market and the colonies but the first leg of the Triangular Trade, the immorality of which Thomas

Prichard was acutely aware. His relative by marriage Richard Reynolds drew his great wealth from the South Wales iron industry but devoted it to philanthropic deeds. The Harfords, by contrast, plowed their profits into building a grand country estate—an ostentatious tourist attraction, in Thomas Prichard's opinion.

The modest, refined, pious Quaker longed to quit the unseemly strife and dubious ethics of business and devote himself to Christian reflection, hypochondria, and molding his children's lives. Prichard remembered:

> We were taught latin and arithmetic by an Irishman named John Barnes, and french by an emigrant, de Rosemond: at a later period Mordente, an Italian, or at least a man who said that he was a Roman, taught some of us Italian and Spanish. The Evenings were almost always spent by my Father in teaching us French, History &c. And it was his practice to read aloud in English from a French book (most frequently Rollin's history) and require that we should repeat what he read in French. This method was very serviceable in giving us a familiar use of the French language and an attachment to the study of history.[5]

Thomas Prichard's constant anxiety, sedulous instruction, and respect for learning and refinement soon manifested itself in James's strong inclination to scholarship. Each evening his father would escape from Harford's countinghouse to his four now motherless children and their private world of books and learning foreign languages. Tutors were employed only when necessary, and James attended Richard Durban's private school in College Green only briefly.[6] His upbringing stamped itself on his demeanor, for he "always seemed to bear with him some of the placid impress of his early bringing-up as a member of a serious Quaker family."[7] Thomas Prichard was intent on "unchilding" his children to create refined, pious companions for himself. He succeeded, at least with his firstborn, James.

In their insulated household, what his father valued, James valued. The "studies to which he most eagerly addicted himself were History and Languages," a friend later wrote. He was said to have "a knowledge of almost every European language, and a very considerable acquaintance with Arabic, Hebrew, and Sanskrit." His "most wonderful memory" extended to geography as well. Even James's childhood hobbies were scholarly: he was fond of tracing the genealogies of the kings of the most remote historic times, and he apparently collected coins. He described himself as sharing theologian John Wesley's "lust for finishing."[8] Notable aspects of his personality were his extraordinary memory and a passion for collecting and methodically arranging evidence, not just to accumulate but to analyze. With both parents of Welsh descent, learning about the language and culture of Wales was also an early, lasting passion.

The studious childhood of James and his younger siblings, Tom, Edward, and Mary, was also steeped in an atmosphere of gloom, anxiety, and Christian fervor, which affected them in different ways. It was wartime, with the imminent threat of French invasion plunging the country into economic instability. When James was seven years old, the death of his baby sister Anna brought on their mother's depression and a year later "proved her own path to the grave." Thomas Prichard never recovered from this double bereavement, just as Prichard himself would forever mourn the loss of his own baby Anna.[9] Frequently depressed, Thomas Prichard became obsessed over his and his children's health. If little Mary came down with a cough, it was a sign of the tuberculosis that had taken his dear wife. In 1795 he wrote to a friend that "apprehensions hang about me, which I have no strength to oppose, and it shudders with terror at my own gloomy images, suffering all that I could possibly suffer, if I were all at once deprived of all that is dear to me."[10]

From the time of his mother's death dissension grew amid the perpetual mourning and studious contemplative piety pervading the family home. Prichard bitterly recalled the aversion he developed toward the woman who was attempting to replace his deeply missed mother:

> My Father had only a house-keeper, Kitty Morgan a woman of disagreeable temper who gave him a great deal of trouble but who had a good deal of influence over him, principally through his confidence in the care that she took of my sister. She had some good qualities however, was very clever, and was considered to be a very religious quaker. She used to sit in the parlour, and therefore was in a manner a member of our family. There was a strong mutual dislike between her and me, and I used to listen with great disgust, when very young to what appeared to be the expressions of her spiritual pride, mixed with not a little moroseness. She lived at my Fathers house from the period of my Mothers death until 1801 or 1802 when she became intolerable. After her dismissal it was thought that she had been in the habit of drinking to intoxication.[11]

Although James had to be prized from his studies, he loved having fun; he could play with the best of them.[12] When the Prichard family moved to up-and-coming Park Street, he was just a minute's walk down the steep suburban hill to the Bristol docks near the confluence of the Rivers Frome and tidal Avon. The mile-long, hewn-stone quays backed with ancient premises served Bristol's international commerce. There he could watch raw materials being winched off the ships and Bristol products, Harford's included, being loaded for export to far-off places. James was drawn to the docks, with their casks and crates, rigging and repairs, working men and boys hustling for employment, orders shouted and obeyed in a multitude of languages, and all carried out to the screeches of large sledges being horse-drawn over the cobbles to and from the nearby warehouses. Visitors found this form of transport ludicrous.[13]

The cosmopolitan hubbub of the docks was magnetic. What wonderful features the seamen had, and what rich and fascinating languages they spoke! On Bristol Quay James "employed himself in finding out and examining the specimens of the natives of different countries who were to be met with amongst the shipping of that port; and he would occasionally bring a foreigner to his father's house." One time, on comprehending what a sailor was shouting, James hailed him in Romaic; the happy Greek caught the boy linguist up in his arms and gave him a hearty kiss. Decades later, the author of *Physical History* was described as a "philologist among philologists."[14]

When James was not hard at his studies at home, he sometimes accompanied his father on business trips and visits to relatives and a few family friends. As for leisure, in the summer he would ride out on horseback with his brothers and father around the beautiful surrounding countryside. Taking the Rownham horse ferry across the Avon, they could ride on the Somerset hills, or if it were a Thursday, there was always Blaise Castle, Mr. Harford's estate, where they could tour the grounds and the famous house with its battlements and eight cannons. Blaise was also on the Prichards' route to Wales and Ross, via the village of Henbury, past the Cribbs Causeway estate and to the horse ferry at Old Passage, Aust. They often went to Tockington on a Saturday evening to spend Sunday with their friends Daniel and Joan Holbrow.[15]

Being a member of the Society of Friends was a serious business. Thomas Prichard chose to wear distinctive "plain dress" and use expressions such as "thee" and "thou," "First Day" for Sunday and "First Month" for January. Quakers challenged the Establishment in several ways, for example, in dispensing with the need of a clergy and the rite of baptism and in allowing women's active participation in religious proceedings.[16] There were enough members of this influential sect in the 1790s to fill two Bristol meeting houses and host Society of Friends quarterly meetings. First-Day morning and evening meetings at Quakers' Friars Meeting House each lasted upward of two hours; there were Third-Day meetings and one on Sixth Day at the Temple Street Meeting House as well. Quarterly meetings meant more attendance and a lot of socializing.[17] Thomas Prichard's reserve did not fit him to "travel on the ministry" as some Quakers did, but he was devout and instilled in his children the religion of their forefathers.

Whether strict or lax, Quakers could not swear to uphold the tenets of the Established Church, thus practically barring themselves from English universities, the professions, and public office. Marrying out of the sect led to expulsion, a rule limiting family alliances. These restrictions did not bar Quakers from becoming rich, the Harfords being a case in point. Affluent and respected, as Protestant Dissenters their participation in civic life was nevertheless limited. Instead, they tended to be leaders in liberal and reformist causes such as the antislavery movement and prison, health, and asylum reform. As some Quakers tolerated radical thinkers' politically challenging views, they were open to charges of disloyalty. To be a "Dissenter" from the Church of England, the official state religion, was to be an outsider and object of suspicion that wealth could barely counter. Quakers drew attention to themselves for their religious and usually socially liberal beliefs and their distinctive dress and behavior—attention young James shrank from.

Thomas Prichard surrendered himself to the certainty of his pure Christian faith, a religiously conservative evangelical Quaker aloof from active participation in his sect's reformist causes. Only privately did he express concern for the plight of the poor, for instance. His views of society were generally negative, and Bristol and Britain offered plenty of examples of ills for him to lament. Civic life was founded on patronage and corruption, commercial life on graft and exploitation, while the spiritual life of the nation in the care of the Established Church reeked of neglect. The suffering of working people was all too apparent in wartime Bristol too.

James's homelife was shot through with gloom, tension, emotional intensity, studiousness, and Christian reflection. There were perpetual mourning for James's mother and fear of the diseases and insanity from which his family and their friends had little defense. In wider Britain, a social revolution was brewing. Christian values were increasingly expressed as a desire to improve society, from church and prison reform to the care of the mentally ill and the impoverished. Beyond subscribing to some medical and education charities, James's father admitted neglecting his civic duties; rather he urged his firstborn to dedicate himself to improving the world. James was groomed to become an evangelist in the Age of Improvement, but like his father, he would shrink from the public fray, choosing to contribute through scholarship, science, and medicine. While Thomas Prichard realized Bristol was no place to bring up his family, young James was fascinated by it.

Being a Bristolian

Bristol colored Prichard's childhood. Below his comfortable suburban home lay the ancient, cramped, paradoxically prosperous and depressed, attractive and repulsive, coherent and fragmented city. The erstwhile second city of England, by the 1790s this ancient West Country river port was a place of grinding poverty, festering with social and political strife. Its merchant elite's "glory days" of the slave trade were well behind them; desultorily, they cast about for new opportunities to bolster their wealth. Prichard would develop a love-hate relationship with Bristol, spending most of his life working to transform it into a city of which a citizen, scientist, and Christian could be proud. It was an uphill task.

Bristolian William Sturge wryly described Bristol's "peculiar characteristics." For some centuries it had boasted a lucrative foreign trade. The saying "ship-shape and Bristol fashion" indicated its enterprising approach to commerce, while "Bristol men sleep with one eye open" bespoke a vigilant and grasping spirit. Without serious competition from rival ports, Bristol merchants became complacent, but during the reign of George III, the technologically adaptable developing cities in the North surged ahead in manufacturing and trade. Having previously relied on the easy pickings of the slave trade, Bristol merchants neglected investing in new ventures. Even some technical improvements to the city's docks were negated by the heavy port dues levied by the Dock Company. As for prominent Bristolians, Sturge commented that "Bristol has not been prolific of great men[, being] somewhat narrow-minded, litigious, and stubborn in disposition; hard and close-fisted in money matters, brusque in manner, and careless in dress, but liberal in the support of public charities."[18]

Bristol had failed to produce great men and had little notable art, architecture, or inventions. Even the cathedral was something of an embarrassment. The reconstruction of its Norman nave had been halted by Henry VIII's suppression of the monasteries in 1538, and the dilapidated tenements built against its walls were known to house prostitutes. The Old City was a jumble of crooked, narrow streets crammed with ancient gabled, wood-framed buildings boasting projecting upper stories. The sluggish little River Frome threaded through it, taking the contents of the city's privies toward the tidal River Avon and washing it back again on the incoming tide. Were it not for the Great Fire, London would have been as filthy and wretched as Bristol, one visitor quipped. Another was disgusted when he "lodged in an ancient tavern at Bristol, where every *accommodation*, was under the same roof. . . . The pungent odour of ammonia mixed with some rather offensive effluvia, so completely pervaded the whole house, and especially the upper flats, where our bed chambers were, that tears were ready to start at every moment, although the people of the house seemed unaffected by it."[19] And Bristol's poor seemed no better off than their counterparts laboring on the outlying coalfields.

Bristol and the Triangular Trade

James and his father were acutely aware of the city's lingering role in the slave trade; local merchants and manufacturers such as the Harfords were still profiting from importing raw materials and exporting goods needed for the infamous Triangular Trade. While less than 10 percent of the British slave trade was Bristol based around the turn of the century,[20] other ships laden with slave-produced sugar, rum, and other products enriched the Bristol elite who, with the many absentee planters and merchants residing in the city, built mansions and supported some ostentatious charities. As the city's shipping, manufacturing and banking interests were so greatly overlapping, any attack on the slave trade was an attack on its general economy.

There had already been years of local and national agitation for and against the trade in human beings. Bristol's powerful Society of Merchant Venturers and its two local MPs were in favor of it, while Quakers, evangelical clergy, and some enlightened citizens were against. Conservative newspaper *Felix Farley's Bristol Journal* reprinted anti–slave trade articles from the American press, stimulated by the Society of Friends' steadfast campaign. In 1785 Bristol Quakers conducted a survey among its members to detect any who might be profiting from it; they found some families indirectly involved in that they supplied manufactured goods for the "Guinea trade"—uncomfortable findings for Thomas Prichard. The famous antislavery campaigner Thomas Clarkson gathered evidence from Bristol seamen. Members of the Bristol branch of the Society for Effecting the Abolition of the Slave Trade included Quaker Joseph Harford and Unitarian minister John Prior Estlin, Thomas Prichard's business associate and James's liberal future father-in-law, respectively.[21]

Bristol's pro-slave trade leaders brazenly and adeptly defended their interests, aided by the local MPs, one of whom distinguished himself by seconding a Parliamentary motion opposing legislation to regulate slave ship conditions. This powerful vocal faction predicted the collapse of the British economy and enrichment of enemy foreign rival slavers. In 1790, when the Prichard family was settling in Bristol, the city's elite entrepreneurs of the Society of Merchant Venturers got up a petition *against* national legislation to reduce the maximum number of enslaved people who could be carried in a vessel while Lord Sheffield, new Whig MP for Bristol, penned a pro-slave trade pamphlet.

Many other Bristolians, including clergymen of all faiths, signed successive abolitionist petitions and kept up the pressure while the number of slave voyages from Bristol continued to dwindle along with the defense of the trade.[22] This was less a matter of conscience than the result of a two-pronged attack on the city's economy: after a period of easy credit, the Napoleonic Wars sparked a full-scale financial crisis, causing many bankruptcies among Bristol's bankers, builders, and merchants, compounded by loss of international market share to rival Liverpool merchants. With dwindling profit in human cargo, Bristolians felt less need to defend it. One of its MPs did not oppose legislation against it, while another suggested "gradualism." When Parliament finally abolished the British slave trade in 1807, coverage in *Felix Farley's Bristol Journal* was muted.[23] This was more a symptom of Bristol's economic malaise than any triumph of humanitarianism. Evangelical Quakers had been at the heart of the campaign against the slave trade, even as Thomas Prichard continued to profit from his company's indirect involvement in it. With burdened conscience, he and his son would always deplore slavery. The shame of the slave trade underpins Prichard's development of anthropology.

Bristol Brass

The cosmopolitan port of Bristol that inspired James was losing position in general international trade as well. Its main colonial trading partner was the West Indies, which itself was becoming economically depressed by soil erosion and labor issues, while increasing Irish poverty and depopulation was taking its toll on another of its trading partners. Bristol had failed to build sizable post–Revolutionary War trading links with America, thereby missing out on a lucrative source of tobacco, cotton, and rice. Even the city's ambitious dock development scheme had limited benefit.[24]

Many Bristol manufacturers turned their attention to regional markets as the city was situated on strategic water and road routes. At high tide James could enjoy watching the Avon thronging with oceangoing ships, the profitable coastal trading craft called trows, river barges, market boats, pleasure boats, and ferries. As produce and raw materials flowed in from surrounding counties and abroad, regional and Bristol products flowed out on its three hundred or so ships. There was a thriving trade in Baltic timber, German linen, Mediterranean fruit and wine, Newfoundland fish, and limited American products. The road and water haulage industries prospered. Along the city's five major road routes to the surrounding region and beyond, Midlands grain, Devonshire cider, Gloucestershire vegetables, and Welsh, Somerset, Gloucestershire, and Wiltshire dairy products came into or through Bristol. Meat was supplied on the hoof to the city's rapidly growing population, with drovers ferrying animals across the Severn and fattening them up in the surrounding pastures before driving them into the city's central market. The brass foundries used Cornish tin and Anglesey copper; Bristol's major product, glass, required raw materials from Stourbridge; and the many soap boilers consumed factory ashes and kelp from Somerset ports. Ships brought in London or foreign pig and bar iron for local use or redistribution throughout the wider region. Bristol ironmasters dominated this trade nationally, the Harfords paramount among them, such that they became merchant-financiers,[25] playing a major role in the development of transport infrastructure in the region. Harford Bank also financed manufacturing and trade further afield. As for fuel, local coal supplies could not keep up with the voracious furnaces of Bristol, so by 1800 Newport had become its prime source of coal.[26]

As well as brassworks, major Bristol industries included iron foundries, leadworks, and soap boiling. Other quality products were the loaf and refined sugars produced in the city's more than twenty sugarhouses. The city was the country's greatest manufacturer of glass bottles for wine, cider, beer, liquors, and the famous Hotwells water for national trade, while its window glass supplied both the home market and the colonies. There were several distilleries, a large leatherworks, and all the manufacturing and services required of a port.[27] Bristol produced other goods such as textiles, pottery, toys, pins, japanware, and tobacco pipes, much of which was for export. Visitor Benjamin Silliman was particularly impressed with the pin-making process, in which Bristol children excelled. He found it amusing to see how exacting and complex the process was, describing the dexterity and speed of a row of little girls operating pin-making vices.[28] But all this manufacturing had its price.

In the bustling, polluted city of James's childhood, smoke and fume-belching factories sat cheek by jowl with blackened churches, counting-houses, and dwellings. Approaching the outskirts of Bristol, visitors' first impression was of smoke and filth. The Brislington road was lined with blazing furnaces and glasshouses and crowded with droves of overburdened coal horses. Arno's Vale contained nothing but smoking brick kilns and sooty furnaces: "The smoke issuing from the brass-works, glasshouses, &c. keeps the town in an almost impenetrable obscurity."[29] The coal mines of Kingswood, Brislington, and Bedminster were nearly exhausted, and its impoverished population "a wild race, whose countenances indicate wretchedness and affright. These are the wives and offspring of the labourers at copper and iron-works, glasshouses, and many other manufactories; where they are buried from the world, amidst fire, smoke, and dust; and when released, sufficient leisure is denied them to humanize themselves and families."[30] Thomas Prichard must have been aware of the wretched, uneducated, malnourished, unchristian state of his company's laborers.

Bristol Tourism and Leisure

A tourist industry thrived among all this trade, manufacturing, pollution, and poverty. Bristol's renowned hot springs and scenic surrounding countryside attracted wealthy visitors. Initially, they flocked to the riverside Hotwells spa, but the region's mild climate and the city's new elevated, airy Clifton accommodation allowed tourism to diversify. The playground of the rich and ill, the spa was fed by springs bubbling through the muddy banks of the Avon below the great cliff, topped by St. Vincent's Rock, on the threshold to magnificent scenery and rural delights. The Hotwells was a short walk from James's childhood Park Street home, along a route that jumbled modern and ancient architecture with industrial and slum chaos.

On the way to the Hotwells, James could make a short detour through fashionable College Green at the bottom of his street, a triangular-shaped park bordered by the cathedral, the parish church of St. Augustine's, an ancient carved stone gate, the Mayor's Chapel, and a terrace of modern homes. Enclosed by railings, College Green's graveled walk was shaded by lime trees, its two broader walks between stately elms lamplit at night. After Queen's Square, it was the pleasantest and largest open space in Bristol, frequented mostly on summer Sunday evenings like in London's

St. James's Park.[31] Having glimpsed the brilliant military uniforms and ladies' charming bonnets and hearing the band playing and the peripatetic fruit sellers calling out their wares, James would pass by the cathedral and the Bishop's Palace before starting along Limekiln Lane, near which wondrous feats of horsemanship were performed at the seductive Equestrian Theatre.

But just beyond this affluent neighborhood, the fog of fumes and snow of ashes from limekilns and enormous glassworks created an ethereal atmosphere. Above him sprang conical Brandon Hill, a place for a pleasant stroll when not in use as a venue for political rallies and radical protests. The road along the bank of the Avon was lined with the slum dwellings that would furnish the future Dr. Prichard with an abundance of patients at the charity Clifton Dispensary. In a sudden change of scenery appeared elegant Dowry Square, the Old and New Assembly Rooms, and a Tuscan-style shopping arcade clinging to the riverbank. The nearby Zigzag Path provided a stiff climb to the top of St. Vincent's Rock. There was an avenue leading to the Hotwells House, shaded by trees.[32] At nearby Rownham Passage, Welsh trading trows docked to offload their goods, and passengers boarded packets bound for Wales or Ireland. A movable walkway on the mud of the dramatically tidal river led down to a ferry to the Somersetshire bank, from which the rural landscape of Somersetshire undulates toward the landmark, long Dundry Hill.

Hotwells medicinal water was sadly tepid, but being low in mineral content it was soft and mild in taste. It attracted the ailing rich and created a lucrative trade in bottled water, which exceeded Bath water in volume of shipping, rivaled Continental brands, and could be found on the shelves of apothecary shops in London and elsewhere.[33] For those who could afford it, the water was pumped and dispensed by the licensee of the luxurious Pump Room and Baths. The nobility and gentry gathered there to drink and bathe, breakfast and promenade, listen to music and play cards, gossip and borrow books from the circulating library, eat soup made of "lively turtle" and take carriage rides. See and be seen. The funeral trade boomed too.[34] This was the Hotwells of James's childhood, but by the time he had returned to Bristol in 1810 as Dr. Prichard, its glory days were over. Price increases, the competition from other British and Continental establishments, the advent of artificial mineral waters, and a new craze for sea bathing were eroding its customer base. By 1816 it had "the silence of the grave." Where once there was opulence there were now desolation, desertion, and bankruptcies.[35]

A steep climb up the Zigzag Path would take James from the Hotwells to clifftop viewpoints, where he could watch the ships on the high tide being piloted along the treacherous River Avon far below; the view to the Bristol Channel and the purple smear of the distant Welsh hills was sublime. For James it held the romance of far-off places, while behind him there was a glimpse of the equally fascinating past. On the great crag just west of St. Vincent's Rock, near the derelict windmill, were the remains of an Iron Age fort, "evidently very ancient; the trench is still deep, and the rampart nearly entire; it appears to have enclosed two or three acres of ground, Roman coins, and other relics of the Roman people have been found on this hill."[36] From here the view opened over Durdham Down, breezy uplands that invited a refreshing walk and where James could ponder the past and the challenges of life that lay before him.

The opposite side of the Avon Gorge was just as attractive. Passing by an old sawmill, a steep climb through Nightingale Valley would take ramblers to the embankments of another ancient fort. Leigh Down was ideal for picnicking; here gentlemen might go shooting, hunt with the establishment at Ashton Court, or scour the exposed cliffs for specimens of minerals to add to their cabinet of curiosities. Of less interest to James and his father was the popular stroll to the village of Long Ashton, where exotic strawberry cream teas could be had in little alcoves behind its cottages. One resident effused: "Fair Nymphs more blooming than the flow'rs / In crowds, pass on to Ashton's Bower." It was that sort of place. Along the Avon, pleasure boats provided musical excursions to the picturesque little river port and former Roman military post of Sea Mills and nearby charming Shirehampton. A lengthier outing might take holidaymakers through the woods above Portishead, on a cruise around the little islands of Steep Holm and Flat Holm in the Bristol Channel or, tide permitting, over to marvel at the sublime ruins of Chepstow Castle.[37]

Bristol Culture

Some visitors found Bristolians less than attractive. They persisted in the outmoded habit of politely "giving the wall" when walking in the street, that is, both parties stepped toward the roadway, causing confusion, rather than stepping to the right as Londoners did. And Bristol women lacked the elegance of London nurse-maids. As for attitudes toward a very important subject: "Money is obtained with avidity, with eagerness, but is buried and lost in the hands of the possessor, through want of spirit to enjoy it; in short, the city is a mere sink of filth and smoke, and the best inn within it is the nastiest in England." Robert Southey generally agreed: "The people of Bristol seem to sell everything that can be sold. They sold their [High] [C]ross, by what species of weight or measurement I know not, they sold their [brass cathedral lectern] eagle by the pound, and here they are selling the sublime and beautiful [Avon Gorge stone] by the boat-load!"[38]

Another visitor less harshly described Bristol's "betters" as fleeing to the suburbs and emulating the London and Bath elite in dress, customs, pastimes, and domestic habits. Bristol homes were neat and commodious, and their servants decent.[39] When Bristol ladies were not visiting and drinking tea, they might engage in good works such as sewing infants' clothes, organizing bazaars or making charitable visits to the poor. Accompanied ladies could attend the more respectable public lecturers and entertainments, whereas gentlemen's wider scope included dining and socializing at coffee houses, taverns, and private clubs and networking at ubiquitous charity meetings. Drinking late into the night at public dinners was the norm.

For more formal occasions, the Assembly Rooms on nearby Prince's Street was a suitably imposing edifice boasting double Corinthian columns, with a drawing room and coffee room and a grand staircase leading to its large, chandeliered ballroom. To correct one's déclassé West Country accent, attention to the fine elocution of the Theatre Royal actors was recommended.[40] *Felix Farley's Bristol Journal* admiringly described one ball at the Mansion House that went on until 4:00 a.m.; perhaps the following day the guests refreshed themselves at Rennison's Baths.[41] More transient entertainment was on offer in the hired rooms of respectable inns where Bristolians could have their portraits drawn, listen to lectures, wonder at the marvels exhibited by the traveling museums of natural, mechanical, and artistic curiosities, or be astonished by chemistry experiments. The future Egyptologist Giovanni Belzoni conducted the optical "Phantascopia" and other experiments illustrative of what would later be called physics.[42] More sedate were James's teacher Dr. Thomas Pole's 1802–3 scientific and medical lectures.

Of appeal to James's less affluent fellow Bristolians was the rather rowdy annual fair in St. James's churchyard in the Old City. There one could bargain for clothes, leather, stockings from Tewkesbury, carpets from Kidderminster, hardware from Sheffield, and local shopkeepers' toys, sweets, trinkets, and millinery. The fair's two most popular products were entertainment and vice, however, blatantly pursued in the shadow of the church. "In some booths the tombs were made to serve as seats, and we were shocked with the gross indecorum of making the sanctuary of the dead a mart for fraud and vice."[43] A huge cattle and horse fair also filled the nearby street, still called the Horsefair, and spilled out over Broadmead. George Weare Braikenridge described St. James's Fair:

> For the amusement of the Populace, there is no deficiency in Flying Coaches, Ups & downs &c with exhibitions of wild beasts & birds, Equestrian Performers, Wax Work, wire dancers, tumblers, puppets, Punch & his Wife, Sea fights, conjuration hocus pocus, magic & mummery of all sorts, recommended by conjurors, Merry Andrews, Buffoons, Drums, Trumpets, French Horns, Fiddlers, Rattles & Vociferation. . . . Many laudable endeavours have lately been used to get these Fairs suppressed altogether as they are so productive of vice & ruin to many but considerable profit being derived by the Parishes of St James & Temple from the erection of the Rows of Standings which together with Houses situated in the Fairs rent at a high rate for the time, all attempts to put them down, have hitherto proved of no avail.[44]

Eventually, St. James's Fair's affront to morality was suppressed out of existence, to the Prichards' likely satisfaction.

While gentlemen drank claret, hock, and champagne to excess and decimated the turtle population, the "lower orders" did their best with cheaper fare while watching the more congenial amusements of bull, bear, and badger baiting and cockfighting; Bristol pugilism created long-remembered heroes.[45] There was a lot of vigorous firing of guns and letting-off of fireworks on Guy Fawkes Day in this strongly anti-Catholic city. Bristolians' fascination for more mystical phenomena was not limited to the working classes; in 1805 and 1806 Joanna Southcott's religious mysticism ran high in the city, with a special room hired to study the sacred teachings of this prophetess.[46]

Bristol Beliefs

More conventional religious affiliation was often linked to political party and limited some Bristol men from participating fully in civic life. Membership of the Established Church and being a man, a property owner, and a Tory were usually the ideal criteria for success in Tory-dominated Bristol.[47] The disadvantages of being a Dissenter or Roman Catholic could be addressed with wealth and party membership. For instance, "temporary" exemptions from taking the sacrament, a necessity in civic institutions, allowed some Dissenters to become members of Bristol Corporation. Although Protestant Dissenters were in the minority in Bristol, they made up a disproportionately large number of its prosperous and respectable citizens. They also added to Bristolian and national societal conflict by agitating for their civil rights, some on the basis of rational thinking and natural law, while others claimed their respectability and loyalty warranted it. Dissenter or not, all decent middle-class Bristolians attended a place of worship or risked scandal and social stigma.[48]

The Establishment's grip on social order did not go unchallenged. In the mid-1790s, poets Robert Southey and Samuel Taylor Coleridge fetched up in the city at the height of their radical political phase: the latter "in religion is a Unitarian, if not a Deist; in politics a Democrat, to the utmost extent of the word. Southey . . . is even more violent in his principles." Coleridge's well-attended Bristol lectures denounced the evils of the time and attacked government policies, a stance that encouraged a small group of Bristolians who dared to espouse republican leanings. He astutely managed to praise French principles while simultaneously upholding religion at lectures delivered under the auspices of the respectable Unitarian minister John Prior Estlin.[49] Neither Coleridge nor Estlin appealed to Thomas Prichard, and soon few such outlandish ideas were being aired in Bristol.

Bristolians were not noticeably devoted to the pursuit of science, and literature attracted moderate enthusiasm, unless interwoven with politics, religion, society, and scandal.[50] But one type of literature set the tone for the Victorian period to come, and its figurehead was a Bristol lady. The remarkable Hannah More dominated Bristol literary life for a generation, developing a conservative, evangelical and moralizing agenda and shaping and policing Bristolians' attitudes, the Prichards included. Hannah More was witty, pretty, an accomplished linguist, well read, and much admired for her amiability and early success as a playwright before she returned to Bristol to start a school for young ladies at 43 Park Street and turn her attention to the Christian education of the young.[51] During her long career as an evangelical moralist, she churned out enormously successful sacred dramas, pamphlets, tracts, and books that targeted the lamentable decay in domestic piety and even the decline in genuine religion among the ruling classes. Anything containing a trace of Enlightenment thought came in for her particular ire.

The scourge of working-class revolutionary tendencies, Miss More wrote an anonymous pamphlet countering the enormous popularity of Tom Paine's *Rights of Man*. Her *Village Politics* (1792), suitably penned in "the most vulgar of styles," hailed the British government as the best in the world, while French liberty, equality, politics, and philosophy were murderous, class-leveling, atheistic, and tyrannical.[52] More campaigned vigorously for Edmund Burke's election as MP for Bristol, for the abolition of the slave trade, and the Christianizing of the Somerset poor by lecturing and training them to be good servants. She was influential in her opinions that it was dangerous to teach them to write and, paradoxically, that women were unfit for public life. On the latter account, she refused to read Mary Wollstonecraft's *Rights of Woman*. She associated with the era's leading evangelicals, such as Zachary Macauley and William Wilberforce. The great, the good, the literary, and even the royal made pilgrimages to Hannah More's country home in Wrington to partake of healthy servings of literature, morality, and piety.

Mrs. Holbrow, a product of Hannah More's teachings and somehow associated with her, had influenced James's mother, and she found a like mind in Thomas Prichard, despite his being a Dissenter. Bristolians generally believed with Edmund Burke that the struggle against France was "just and necessary." Against a backdrop of war and economic hardship, support of the monarchy and defense of religion (particularly against "popery") united affluent Bristolians and excited the fervor of the working classes. Miss More informed Horace Walpole that she "had conceived an utter aversion to liberty according to the present idea of it in France";[53] and her *Strictures* (1799) warned the loyal British public against the revolutionary ideas permeating Continental literature. These typically Bristolian sentiments guided Thomas Prichard in educating his children.

Bristol Political and Civic Life

Bristol's merchants dominated civic life and looked after their own welfare keenly while failing to ensure stability and prosperity for its citizens. They served on the governing bodies of the city, acting more as associates than as rival businessmen and shaping policies to their own interests. These merchant-politicians were generally the rich sons of rich merchants who took few entrepreneurial risks and were averse to innovation, preferring to ape the landed gentry and aristocracy in building themselves mansions and in keeping their wealth in banks and property instead of investing in commercial development and infrastructure. Disastrously, the banks they founded took the short-term approach of lending to property developers who were rapidly throwing up mansions and terraces to cash in on the new fashion of suburban living. This inflation-stirring building frenzy had collapsed at the outbreak of war with France in 1793, along with general business confidence, the port improvement scheme, the banking system, and an associated mania for canal investment. Nineteen local finance houses failed, and at least five hundred unfinished houses still scarred the suburbs in 1798, giving James's Bristol a war-torn aspect.

Bristol's institutions of authority were interconnected. The Corporation, as local government was called, was an old, irresponsible oligarchy that had for centuries dominated Bristol.[54] Its aldermen chose the mayor, and the whole Corporation chose their successors, carefully excluding the minority political party. The status quo was a Whig Corporation in a Tory city. The measure of the Corporation's success seemed to be its members' personal wealth; they lobbied national government, defended Bristol's trading interests against those of more powerful London, and dispensed local justice at considerable cost and with considerable benefit to themselves. Moreover, Bristol's ancient status as a city and county gave it a degree of civic autonomy and a somewhat superior air that fostered a penchant for pomp. Beyond the Corporation, the institutions of authority included the Church, the Corporation of the Poor, and the Society of Merchant Venturers, with overlapping membership among them. As if to obscure its passion for money-making, Bristol's elite wished to be seen to use wealth wisely and demonstrate virtue palpably, particularly in ostentatious support of charities. But as Bristol's mercantile supremacy waned, the Corporation lost ground in the estimation of those Bristolians deprived of its sinecures and feasts.[55]

The civic life of James's Bristol childhood was thus rife with disputes, usually with blame justly laid at the door of the Corporation. While its members were carousing, the "lower orders" were suffering; 1790s newspapers, broadsides, and pamphlets attacked the Corporation roundly. Food inflation—116 percent for flour between 1789 and 1795—unmatched by wage rises, precipitated a tide of protests by artisans who were in turn suspected of organizing among themselves. Hannah More penned her warning pamphlets, and the Corporation readied the troops. Even though Bristol lacked Tom Paine followers, its alarmed citizens drew up loyalist declarations signed by the "Gentlemen, Clergy, Freeholders and Inhabitants of Bristol."

While middle-class Bristolians grumblingly tolerated the Corporation's inadequacies, the neglected "lower orders" expressed dissatisfaction by periodically rioting, as did their fellow sufferers around the country, both urban and rural. Nationally, the previous generation's infamous Gordon Riots against Catholic emancipation were seared into public imagination, and thanks to the development of the press, they could learn about grievances and riots. Wartime austerity throughout Prichard's youth spurred periodic riots extensively reported in the Bristol newspapers, conjuring images of diabolical French revolutionary urban insurrection.[56]

Not long after the Prichard family settled in the city, the Bristol Bridge Riot was sparked by the rumor that the Corporation was unjustly collecting crippling tolls. The toll gates were burned, the Riot Act read, the militia called in, eleven citizens were killed, and many were wounded. The Corporation's response was not conciliatory, nor would they admit to mishandling it. Rioting stopped only when four private citizens bought the toll contract and threw the bridge open, a measure condemned by the aldermen as encouraging future outrages.[57]

The Bristol Bridge Riot left a legacy of hostility among Bristolians. For instance, when the "gentlemen" of each parish were asked to serve as a kind of anti-riot militia, back came oblique condemnations of the Corporation's actions. Respectable Dr. Edward Long Fox led a group of citizens in an inquiry that criticized the Corporation's actions, but it was too wary of legal action to publish its findings. The Corporation remained intransigent, implying the riot had been seditious, thereby associating it with revolutionary francophobia. Fox, professionally damaged by his quest for justice, may have become part of a movement called the Bristol Society for Constitutional Information, providing a link to a later Bristol riot.[58]

The Bristol Bridge Riot was just one of several that took place throughout James's childhood in the city. While poor Bristolians rioted over food prices and squeezed wages, they more often did so in frustration with local government's failure to address local grievances and with unfair national elections. Not allowed to vote, they could riot. The food crises in 1795–96 sparked disturbances, followed by a price-fixing riot in Bristol Market and an election riot in 1796. The political riot of March 1797 exacerbated mistrust in local government, which had neglected to order the defense of members of the Constitutional Society during two days of rioting against them. Bristol riots, therefore, tended to be against the Corporation's unfairness and failure to accommodate the political and economic expectations of its citizens.[59] When Dr. Prichard hung out his shingle in Bristol in 1810, his fellow citizens were just as dissatisfied with the Corporation, and for the following two decades little changed.

There were further reasons why disadvantaged Bristolians rioted regularly. The streets and alleys of the city's slums were unpaved, unlit, and uncleansed, employment was uncertain, and health care barely existed. Smallpox could take anyone at short notice, and men could be taken even more quickly by roaming press-gangs. The 25 percent or so of working men who could read could not afford newspapers; crime was rife and punishment harsh. With Bristol's poor in a state of semistarvation, Dr. Thomas Beddoes reported a prodigious rise in the occurrence of fever among them.[60] The year 1800 was the fifth one of poor domestic crops, coinciding with a wartime virtual embargo on imported corn. Despite national legislation controlling the price of this commodity, a loaf of bread cost an unskilled laborer a day's wages. By the spring of 1801 there had been riotous attacks on market stalls, rises in burglary, highway robbery, and the inevitable executions.[61] While Thomas Prichard kept his family in comparative luxury, he nevertheless keenly regretted the "squalid and miserable aspect of a large proportion of our fellow creatures" and felt guilty under his "mantle of affluence."[62] Britain was evolving from the old moral economy to a harsh laissez-faire reality he considered essentially unchristian.

Bristol Environment

James could easily see the state of Bristol's economy in the city's buildings. The deteriorating homes of the poor had been thrown up on an ad hoc basis over the centuries in the Old City's confines, while the merchants started to abandon the custom of living "above the shop" among the populace; they migrated to the grand London-style terraces in more salubrious new suburbs. Development extended westward and northward up the hills to Kingsdown and to similarly elevated Clifton. Prichard's father and grandfather invested in this house-building boom. Running into Portland Square is Prichard (now Pritchard) Street; Thomas Prichard corresponded with his land agent Samuel Dyer, mentioning rent collecting from houses there.

The cityscape bristled with church towers, spires, and ships' masts jumbled together, intersected by polluted waterways. The enormous tidal reach of the Severn forced seawater up the Avon and into the River Frome along the Bristol quays. At high tide, ships made haste to enter or leave the port, for when the tide turned, the ships in Bristol were left, not high and dry, but low and embedded precariously upright at their moorings in soft, deep, filthy mud. All that remained in the center of the riverbed was the meager stream of the Frome coursing its fetid way.

When Prichard started life as a Bristol physician in 1810, the Merchant Venturers and Bristol Corporation's Dock Company had just completed a five-year, vastly over-budget project to adjust the course of the rivers, dig a linking channel called the New Cut, transform a meadow into the Cumberland Basin and build locks to retain the tide, creating the Floating Harbour. This sparked furious debate, particularly when the citizens realized that it would be partly financed by a property tax. The Dock Company's mismanagement, the Floating Harbour's technical faults, and the city's general economic stagnation did not bode well. The local press decried the poisonous pestilential miasma arising from the backed-up effluence in the silting-up Floating Harbour, and the Dock Company stonewalled for years, much to the detriment of its reputation.[63] Beyond the Floating Harbour, the serpentine river leading to the sea in just a couple of miles remained unnavigable at all but high tide. Those prohibitively high tides and port dues hampered local manufacturing for export. Bristol's economy stagnated and its waterways were polluted; the docks would be cited in sanitation surveys of the city's recurring epidemics.

Retreat to Ross, 1800

The conflicts and uncertainties in Britain and Bristol were reflected in adolescent James's personal life. The family's hated housekeeper Kitty Morgan had blighted his childhood, only temporarily lightened when Aunt Sarah Prichard came to live with the family in 1797. A cheerful girl with many friends, life became more pleasant, but after two short years, she married Francis Fisher, and James's feelings returned to not very quiet discontent.[64] Then, just after his eleventh birthday, his paternal grandfather's death brought grief and upheaval. When the family assembled in Ross for the reading of the will, Thomas Prichard learned he had inherited a considerable fortune that precipitated two momentous decisions. He could now afford to retire from active business and association with men of questionable character and principles. He would also flee to Ross.[65]

James's father decided to invest his new wealth in ventures further afield. One was an association with Nantucket Quakers Benjamin Rotch and Daniel Starbuck, refugees from the American Revolutionary War who had had plenty of adventures and acquired fortunes in whaling.[66] James was enthralled by Rotch's tales from far-off places. He had settled in France, became mayor of Dunkirk, and on one occasion was part of a delegation to Robespierre, but later he fled the country, narrowly escaping the guillotine. Rotch and James's tutor Mordente would regale the family with tales of revolutionary France until Thomas Prichard started to suspect Rotch of being an infidel, or at least not orthodox in his belief of the "great facts of Christian Revelation."[67] He dropped Rotch in favor of Daniel Starbuck's South Sea whaling concerns. James and younger brother Tom accompanied their father to meet his new partner in Swansea in February 1800, but it was the return journey from Wales that was so memorable:

We went on horseback and returned thro' Brecknockshire to Ross in very severe weather. I remember on this journey riding in a cold frosty day up the Neath Valley. We stopped to dine at a little public house at a place called Yrigs-y-collan and reached Pont-nedh-vychan[68] just before night-fall very much fatigued. There was the only tolerable hospitium in the whole way from Neath to Brecknock. The landlady, a saucy Welsh woman by some impertinence offended my Father, and he made us set out again on our ponies and ride on to a little village inn at Ysteud-vellty where we had been told that we might find a lodging. It proved to be a miserable hovel and we were obliged to lodge all night in a little room used for keeping cheeses where we were half starved. On the following day we rode on to Hay and thence to Ross, where my Father began to make some preparations for his intended removal to that place.[69]

Thomas Prichard's relationship with the unprincipled Harfords dragged on. He sought advice from Samuel Dyer, a Bristol Quaker elder celebrated for his piety and Christian humility. James must have been fascinated by this antiquarian who knew several languages and had a famous collection of ancient coins.[70] Dyer not only counseled Thomas Prichard on business matters, he also suspected that his plan to remove his family to Ross stemmed from a desire to shelter his children from the debased state of religion in Bristol. Dyer warned that they would be deprived of the educational advantages of city life, lecturing that "outward knowledge was better than none at all."[71] Perhaps Thomas Prichard had been alarmed by young James's desire for outward knowledge. Undeterred, in May 1800 he took James to Bridgwater to visit the widow of the Uncle Cowles from whom he had inherited his stake in Harford's. To his relief, she approved of his plan to break the partnership, as her late husband had also been troubled by similar concerns about the business. Now very wealthy, Thomas Prichard was in a position to condemn greed and the relentless pursuit of wealth.[72]

Samuel Dyer secured a tenant for the Prichards' 47 Park Street family home. Thomas Prichard was confident that his decision to flee Bristol had been wise.[73] But during the autumn of 1800, despite his near abstemious habits, he was fast becoming a martyr to gout as his father had been. It scourged him in every limb. James spent several weeks with him in Bath, that Georgian spa for the ailing rich, where he watched his father's gout-swollen limbs gradually recover.[74]

Erosion in Quaker Faith

When the Prichards arrived in Ross they found carpenters and masons still noisily building a large dining room for the entertainment of Quakers attending the Ross quarterly meetings. The project's "rustic" elderly architect Mr. Banks

> used to get his meals with our family and came into frequent collision with the housekeeper Kitty Morgan who was also a spiritualist of a high order. There was also another guest of a very different character. When my Father left Bristol he had engaged an old French Emigrant who had been educated at the Mazarin College in Paris and was believed to be a good scholar and a very respectable man, to follow him to Ross and to become our instructor not only in French, but in classics and Mathematics. De Rosemond (that was his name) died however soon after our removal and a friend of his was introduced to my Father as his successor. This person, Dr. Bonis a medical graduate of Montpelier was a most curious person. He had a good deal of humour and of the spirit of adventure and had lived in many scenes and witnessed many reverses of fortune. He was an excellent teacher of the French language, and had a very familiar though not altogether accurate knowledge of Latin. His society was very entertaining, and as he lived for sometime in our house he contributed to enliven our family circle.[75]

Quaker doctrine continued to lose James's respect as he watched housekeeper Kitty and Mr. Banks bicker and posture. While Dr. Bonis provided good instruction and pleasant diversion, James had another tutor, the Rev. James Mills. There had been no hesitation in exposing James to the opinions of this suitably pious local Church of England cleric.[76] These interesting tutors and lively discussions made for a pleasant, small-town adolescence.

Less pleasant was Thomas Prichard's implication in a schism then brewing among Quakers that further eroded fourteen-year-old James's opinion of the sect. His father had provided hospitality to American Quaker Hannah Barnard, traveling on her ministry and much admired for her powerful preaching. She arrived from Ireland, where a growing number of Friends had already been expressing shocking doubts of the authenticity, truth, and divine authority of the Holy Scriptures, the divinity of Christ, and the doctrine of atonement.[77] When Barnard published her explosive declaration that "the account of the miraculous conception & birth of Christ an imposture and that man's present state is the state designed him by his

Creator," a devastated Thomas Prichard denounced her: "I will make no comment on these sentiments but that to my mind they are full of horror [and] I would burn at the stake rather than lose hope which would be ill supplied by an exaltation of the Creature."[78]

British Quakerism was in turmoil; Barnard threatened the integrity of the sect, hardly inspiring James's faith. During the following decade, disgraceful expressions of apostasy spread among Quakers, such as the claim that the mystery of redemption by Christ was nothing but priestcraft designed to rob human nature of its glory. Writing in 1847, Prichard condemned this attempt to spread a "species of rationalism bordering on what is called Socinianism."[79] He pointed to his father's unprincipled Quaker partners; the vain religiosity of his housekeeper; Rotch's materialism; and this outbreak of Quaker irreligion. While he also cited the later reforms in the Established Church as obviating dissent, Prichard's disillusionment in Quakerism had these earlier roots.

Insanity

James's childhood was blighted by a family tragedy that would affect his choice of medical specialization. Thomas Prichard cherished his friendship with his late wife's intimate friend, Margaretta Cross, and James's schoolfellow during his short career at Mr. Durban's school in College Green had been her son John Brent. Just as their mothers had been close, the two boys became lifelong friends. Elder Mr. John Cross, well known and much respected as a man of strict integrity and uprightness of conduct, had been an accountant and prosperous oil and turpentine merchant on Small Street near the Bristol docks. Among the Crosses' relatives were several prosperous and pious medical men and Anglican clerics.[80] But Mrs. Cross was distraught. Her cherished son seemed at death's door; a fraudulent will had just deprived her of a huge fortune; and her husband had been seized by insanity.[81]

In November 1800 the Crosses visited Ross so the children could have a holiday together while James's uncle Dr. William Lewis treated Mr. Cross's insanity. En route at a Gloucester inn, Cross became so violent that he had to be locked in his room with the windows nailed shut. Dr. Lewis agreed with the renowned Dr. Edward Jenner that a counterirritating seton should be cut into the sufferer's neck.[82] For the following nine years his wife and daughter cared for him at their Bristol home, where James often stayed while studying medicine in the city. There he observed the course of Mr. Cross's insanity and later witnessed cases of mental illness among his own family. His mother's apparent breakdown and the social stigma of Mr. Cross's condition affected him greatly. When Prichard later became a mad-doctor, he was already on familiar ground.

The fine hot summer of 1801 should have been one of pleasure for the Prichards. The whole family jogged along in their large open carriage to the distant Welsh seaside resort of Tenby, accompanied by Aunt and Uncle Newman, Aunt Lewis, and her daughter Susannah. But tiresome Kitty Morgan and James's younger brother Edward were desperately ill the whole time. The party eventually returned via Swansea, Neath, the famous Aberdulais Waterfalls, Cardiff, and Pontypool, arriving at Ross toward the end of September. The holiday "was on many occasions highly interesting, yet the trouble preponderated against the pleasure."[83]

Prichard had some happy childhood memories, despite the family gloom, anxiety, and longing for better times not uncommon during this turbulent social, political, and economic period. It was also a time of family illnesses, mourning, and a new evangelical fervor that weighed heavily on the household. These shaped Prichard's life into one of respectability, religious orthodoxy, and boundless diligence. But even the more distant past affected him. Welsh blood coursed through his veins.

Welsh Roots

Prichard's "Memoir of Thomas Prichard" did more than just chronicle family life: "To these memoirs of my Father I have resolved to add whatever notices I have been able to obtain of the history of my ancestors. . . . None of them were very illustrious or highly distinguished. At the same time there is nothing in their history which the most high-minded would wish to be forgotten or never to have happened."[84] Prichard pored over ancient family archives, his father's correspondence, and the Society of Friends' registers to compile a history of the Prichard and Cowles families, enlivened with stories about his relatives in Ross, Bristol, Almeley, and Leominster. Letters from the Wabash in Illinois relay the adventures of Thomas Prichard's dear pioneering cousin Samuel Prichard. All of them were Quakers.

Prichard's immense pride in his Quaker and Welsh ancestry is apparent. He traced his ancestors back to the founding of the sect in the mid-seventeenth century. His need to justify their dissent from the Established Church illuminates his outlook:

> At that time there was no national church in the land, from which a good and wise man would be unlikely to separate himself. Cromwell's

soldiers as it is well known went about preaching and the pulpits were occupied in many instances by ranting Antinomians. Every man chose a religion for himself. Even after the Restoration, there was little inducement to persons who had formed religious attachments elsewhere, to return to a church, the ministers of which were too often men of worldly and irreligious character. These considerations will in the mind of every candid person suffice to defend my ancestors from the censure of having schismatised from a church, a separation from which in other times would have implied eccentricity or some perverseness.[85]

Prichard's forefathers' dissent was thus a legitimate reaction to the chaotic, corrupt Cromwellian past of an overturned monarchy and neglectful clergy. This passage explains his rejection of Quakerism: he now lived in those "other times" in which the reformed Church of England was an institution of upright moral and religious character representing the will of the State. No longer were there grounds for dissent.

The earliest known Prichard was seventeenth-century Roger Prichard of Almeley Wooton, Herefordshire. He appears to have been a merchant from, or trading with, Ireland and possibly from Llanfyllin in Montgomeryshire, Wales. After a temporary estrangement from the Society of Friends, he settled in Almeley, became rich, and built a meetinghouse that stands today. Prichard's paternal grandfather Thomas I of Ross (1722–97), was the son of Edward Prichard of Ross (1687–1739) and his wife, Elizabeth Sharman. That Edward was the grandson of Roger Prichard.[86]

Prichard's grandfather, like his father before him, was a prosperous tanner with his home and tannery in the Brookend of Ross. Prichard remembered him fondly as of gentlemanly, pleasing, lively, upright, benevolent character: "I have a distinct recollection of him, as he used to sit with his snuff-coloured clothes, white powdered bushy wig in a three cornered Chair on the point of which he would sometimes take me when a very young boy between his knees, and teach me nursery rhymes."[87]

Ann Cowles, James's paternal grandmother, was the daughter of wealthy glove manufacturer William Cowles of Worcester and niece of John Cowles, the owner of extensive properties in the Ross area. Ann, considered a person of "great mental cultivation and remarkable piety," died in childbirth. Thomas Prichard, a twelve-year-old at boarding school at that time, was traumatized by the loss of his mother. James remembered being taken to a particular garden that had been her favorite place, and forty years after her death, his father was still writing poetry to her memory.[88] Ann

Cowles Prichard's brother William Cowles II married the sister of the philanthropist Richard Reynolds and lived in Bristol, where he was in partnership with the iron-mining Harfords, the source of Thomas Prichard's inherited partnership in the firm.[89] One of Ann Cowles Prichard's aunts had a daughter

> who married Isaac Walker, a rich cockney merchant, who had an immense tumor at the end of his nose. I remember visiting Isaac Walker at Bath with my Father when a boy. He accumulated an immense property, and had a house at Southgate now belonging to his family. His son John Walker was a highly educated and accomplished man. He was a fellow of the Royal Society and had a house in Bedford Square but lived chiefly at Southgate. He was very kind to me when I was young, and I remember that I dedicated to him my Inaugural Essay, on taking a degree at Edinburgh. He was remarkably stiff and formal in his manners but was highly esteemed. And he associated with men of science.[90]

James's visits to Arnos Grove, John Walker's large country estate in Southgate, London, deeply impressed him. The house was famous for its painted ceilings and murals, museum of natural history, and lovely pleasure grounds full of exotic plants. Mr. Walker was a gentleman possessed of great taste in the arts, superior in mind, manner, and conduct. He had none of the spoiled habits of an extremely rich man, nor did he affect the dress and manner of a Quaker. This good taste and interest in science was complemented by considerable benevolence. Upon reading Robert Owen's essays "New Views of Society" (1812, 1813), he invested the huge sum of £30,000 in Owen's scheme for the utopian mill village New Lanark. Eventually, the entire ownership of New Lanark fell into the hands of Walker's two sons.[91] While Owen's pioneering socialist concern for the poor was not to Prichard's taste, he had great respect for his relative, an educated, kind, rich, cultured friend of scientists. Prichard had good reason to dedicate his MD thesis to his role model John Walker.

Another of Prichard's fond memories was that of his great-uncle James Cowles, a rich merchant of Bristol with connections in Charlestown and New York and who lived mostly abroad. The Prichard family often stayed at his home in Tockington, near Bristol, and Thomas Prichard inherited his other home in Gayton, near Ross:[92]

> In my younger days it was a place of pleasure and recreation to all the family. The house at Gayton was an old farm house of the most

primitive kind, situated at the bottom of a narrow valley, abounding in wood: the house itself was surrounded with gardens and orchards.... I remember it in my early days as a sort of paradise, particularly a beautiful flower garden of the oldest & most formal fashion, in which was a long fish-pond with a straight green terrace running along each side of it, and an alcove at either end—one the exact copy of the other; there was a formal painted chinese bridge over the middle of the pond at the top of which I used to stand when a child and throw bread into the water to feed the gold and silver fishes.[93]

Several other Cowles men had unusual histories: an eccentric one disappeared, possibly to India, while Joseph Cowles of Coed-y-Gric was said to have first been exceedingly pious but then an atheist before ending up a rich, eccentric, dissolute resident of Bath. Prichard thought he had been chosen as this Cowles's executor and residuary legatee merely because they shared the name Cowles. It was onerous, but he appreciated the fine library he inherited.[94]

Thomas Prichard's education at Quaker Thomas Huntley's school in Burford, Oxfordshire, finished when he was fourteen. In later years he taught himself Greek and Hebrew and attempted German in order to study German theology.[95] His four surviving sisters, James's aunts, were Elizabeth, who married tiresome Josiah Newman of Worcester, a shrewd businessman but a "man of mean capacity"; Ann, the wife of clever and sensible John Wilkins of Cirencester; younger sister Susannah, who married Dr. William Lewis; and Sarah, who became the wife of Francis Fisher.[96]

A very young Thomas Prichard fell in love with his sister-in-law Mary "Polly" Lewis. From some of her papers and an aunt's recollections, Prichard pieced together his mother's story. His parents' youthful courtship was the stuff of romance. Attempts to get Thomas to break it off and complete his apprenticeship under a nicely distant surveyor failed, especially as distraught Polly was threatening to "go into a decline." "Nothing would pacify [Polly] till Tommy arrived." Her parents were equally inconsolable.[97] Her father called in a Quaker elder to mediate and got Thomas released from his apprenticeship. The lovers could not be separated; they were married a few months later on March 30, 1785, but their married life was brief. She

died before I was nine years old. I well remember her as a most tender and affectionate parent wholly devoted to her family, and even more anxious about them than herself. Her health was always very delicate.

During the first years of my recollection, She was very cheerful and happy, but her mind sustained a severe shock, by the loss of her fifth and last infant. . . .[98] Early in 1793 my mother, who for some time before had been in very infirm health had a fifth child, a little girl who was named Anne. My mother appeared to recover her health after the birth of this child. When it was about a year old, it was inoculated for Small Pox and died under the consequent disease. On this event my father & Mother reproached themselves very severely for having by their own act given rise to a complaint which had proved fatal to the child. My mother never recovered her spirits and her health became gradually worse. During the summer of 1794 I remember being greatly shocked by hearing my Aunt who was then visiting my Father together with my Grandfather, say that she was certainly in a consumption and that her recovery was hopeless. She had gone two or three times in the earlier part of her illness to stay in the neighbourhood of Bristol for change of air, once to the Hotwells, once to the neighbourhood of Knowle Hill, when I had always been with her. In October 1794 my mother was fast sinking under Pulmonary Phthisis.[99] She died after an illness of several months under Pulmonary consumption. I have heard very little about my Mother from others, for my Father who was overwhelmed with grief at her death could never bear to speak of her, till within a very few years before he died and he then only mentioned her once or twice in a way that precluded any questions or conversation about her. . . . She was very clever and sensible. She was educated by Mrs Holbrow, a very superior and amiable woman who kept a school at Frenchay. . . . Mrs. Cross was her most intimate friend. Both of them were very much attached to my mother. After my Mothers death my Father had scarcely any other confidential friend for some years except these two old ladies and from his correspondence with them I shall obtain the best materials for this memoir up to the period when it terminated.[100]

Prichard's maternal grandfather, John Lewis, was living in Bristol where he married Mary Morgan of Ross at the Friends' Meeting House in 1759. Mary's family were Quakers who had moved from Worcestershire three generations earlier. The Lewises being an Abergavenny family, Prichard remembered attending his grandfather's burial at Pont-y-moel, Monmouthshire. A Morgan relative used to entertain James with tales of their forebears, like the story about the final battle of the English Civil War at Worcester where one of them distinguished himself, much to James's delight.[101] This ancestor had been both a Quaker pacifist and loyal to the king. One of his grandmother's stories concerned a James Morgan being led by divine guidance to Ross where he founded a dynasty of Morgans who feature in the archives of the Ross Society of Friends. A later James Morgan married Mary Reece, so through her family Richard Reece of Cardiff, Prichard's friend, was a distant relative as well.[102]

Prichard remembered Grandfather Lewis as mild in manner and short, "with a good deal of the Welchman about him" and rather henpecked by his shrewd, sensible, sharp-witted, very active wife who managed the family and kept a shop until she was ninety. There "she used to sit in a bee hive chair in a back-room or a sort of back-shop and always gave me half a crown when I went to call upon her. Her grandchildren often visited her, and we used to wander over her wilderness of a garden, in which there was a great deal of almost wild growing fruit."[103] Their son, James's uncle Dr. Lewis, inherited his father's considerable property and was another of James's role models.

Knowledgeable about and proud of all his Welsh ancestry, Prichard had an affection for all things Welsh; as a teenager he was fascinated by the language at a time when the English elite generally considered it inferior gibberish. He strove to please his father by diligently studying history, theology, and languages, by collecting and arranging data and by promising to benefit society. He would go on to gather information about the people and languages of the world to demonstrate the unity of humankind to defend the truth of Scripture and encourage the preservation of vulnerable colonized peoples.

Prichard had other influential childhood experiences, from the city of Bristol, the deaths of his mother and baby sister, and his father's preoccupation with illness, to the mental illnesses of relatives and friends. He observed the medical practice of his highly respected uncle and spent six weeks among the ailing rich in Bath. He would study medicine and do good in the world. Another of his childhood memories involved his father's entanglement in grasping commerce with unprincipled associates, and he wanted nothing to do with it. He valued respectability and shared his father's Tory views at a time when Dissenters with their socially liberal interests in reform, including their pressure to win the freedom to worship, usually placed them in the Whig party. He appreciated the respectability of devout members of the Church of England such as the Crosses and his tutor Mr. Mills. By contrast, while most of his relatives led exemplary Christian lives, all too many other Quakers were clearly shallow, egotistical, hypocritical, unprincipled, and downright subversively unchristian.

James's early years in Bristol had been both exacting and fascinating, and country life in Ross was idyllic. When he was fifteen and an obedient, pious, placid, self-effacing scholar smitten with collecting and analyzing facts, his father reluctantly chose a career for him.

2 · "A Studious Turn of Mind"

Preparatory Medical Education

> Regarding a profession as more favourable than commerce to those studies to which he was devoted, he rather accepted than chose medicine.
> —Thomas Hodgkin, "Obituary of Dr. Prichard"

Medicine Is Science, 1802

While Tom and Edward were in the countryside having adventures, caring for their livestock, and slaughtering every bird they could, their elder brother James was also learning about the natural world in the way he liked best—through books. He discovered how over the past three centuries travelers and explorers had been returning to Europe with shiploads of specimens of marvelous plants, animals, and minerals. The conquest of Mexico alone had revealed hundreds of new plant species, many taken from the botanical gardens where the Aztecs had studied them, devising a useful system of taxonomy and demonstrating an acute understanding of their medicinal qualities. But how could Europeans comprehend these plants and their uses when they were completely absent from the ancient Greek and Roman texts, Europeans' definitive source of knowledge? The Age of Exploration (fifteenth to seventeenth centuries) inspired a new, hands-on approach to gaining knowledge in, for example, studying plants. Botanical gardens started springing up in centers of European classical learning where the phenomena of nature were investigated. Historians have suggested that this contact with the extra-European world and its peoples' understanding of nature paved the way for a new European experimental approach to exploring the works of the Almighty. During the so-called Scientific Revolution (mid-sixteenth to seventeenth centuries) extra-European scientific ideas continued to be instrumental to the great discoveries of that period. Copernicus employed Arabic mathematics in his astronomy, to cite just one example.[1]

James was fascinated both by the world of science and the world beyond Britain that had stimulated it; he had been bitten early by the chemistry bug, especially popular since its laws had been fairly recently revolutionized.

And the study of anatomy, fundamental to medical knowledge, encouraged "philosophers," the term for scientists, to carry out comparative anatomical and embryological research. A few even dared to study and pronounce on the human species as if it were a mere animal. Continental scientists were famous and infamous for their unorthodox speculations; one had suggested that over an immense period of time all species had developed from a single simple aquatic ancestral organism, a theory of species' self-development first called transformism, then transmutation, and eventually evolution. Recent discoveries in geology casting doubt on the biblical account of the age of the world and the life it sustains lent credibility to transformism.[2]

It was a short step from applying new theories of nature in general to the history and structure of the human species itself. The resulting flowering of historical-scientific exploration of humankind reaching back into "deep time" can hardly be described as cross-disciplinary because boundaries between disciplines had not yet been drawn. Physicians, anatomists, natural historians, and moral philosophers studied nature, including humankind, drawing on evidence provided by travelers, explorers, missionaries, medical men, colonial administrators, colonists, abolitionists, philologists, geographers, and theologians. At the start of the nineteenth century, the ferment of ideas about the operations of nature and the nature of humankind whetted James's appetite for science.

James understood that only a complete body of facts could suggest and support a theory. Having a well-developed British philosophical disdain of empty theorizing, he wanted to see the proofs of transmutation and polygenism. Might he gather convincing evidence of the single origin and single species of humankind that would corroborate Scripture and refute the notion of polygenism, or would his passion for understanding the world lead him into Continental skepticism and irreligion?

Well aware of those unorthodox natural historians, philosophers, and other creatures of the Enlightenment, Thomas Prichard constantly monitored his son's commitment to Scripture. When one of James's Edinburgh professors later made unacceptable assertions about the development of variations among humankind, the scientific quest of his life was confirmed. James would plumb the natural history of the human species, at first just its physical and physiological characteristics, but soon all human history, culture, language, and eventually prehistoric remains would come within his scope. His proof of the specific unity and single origin of humankind would doubtless accord nature with Christian belief. Back in 1802, however, he almost missed his chance to do science at all. While James was enjoying his studies in Ross, his father made a most unwelcomed announcement. Prichard remembered:

> It had been his original intention to make me his successor in the house of the Harfords and to give me a share of his property in that establishment which he afterwards transferred to my second brother but finding that I had no aptitude for that undertaking, and was strongly attached to pursuits and habits incompatible with a commercial life, he determined, after some hesitation not to oppose my natural bent of mind and he proposed to me to devote myself to the profession of medicine. That was the only pursuit connected with scientific studies that was open to men brought up in the society of the Quakers, and I gladly embraced my Fathers proposal, more influenced as I believe by this consideration than by any particular predilection for the profession or study of physic. The next thing in my Fathers mind after determining this point was how to introduce me to the means & resources for acquiring medical knowledge. The University of Edinburgh contained the best then existing medical school and that most frequented especially by those who had not access to the English Universities. It was my destination.[3]

How could Thomas Prichard have imagined his studious son as a man of business unless he hoped to make him manager of his own considerable wealth and keep him close at hand? Far from being interested in commerce, James was aware of his father's dislike of commercial life, day in and day out in a countinghouse with men of dubious conscience, supplying goods for the Triangular Trade. James would have none of it. Rather, he chose medicine, not from a desire to cure the ills of and curry favor with rich patients, but from a passion for what medicine offered—the opportunity to study science at university. There courses in moral philosophy, physics, chemistry, anatomy, mathematics, and botany beckoned. Could he apply these subjects' methodology to studying the history of humankind and defeat that hateful notion of human pluralism? Even if it had been possible to gain a university degree in one of these scientific subjects, they offered little prospect of future respectable employment. While men of "independent means" might devote themselves to understanding nature, rarely could others scratch a living from science, for example, by lecturing. Physicians were respectable and financially secure, by contrast. Thomas Prichard wanted his son to earn his bread.

The Medical Profession

The development of the medical profession is just one aspect of the revolution in British society that affected and appealed to the Prichards. "Improving" had become a cultural imperative, so, for instance, apparent social problems could be tackled with education and reform. To the regret of conservative elements in society, including some property owners, manufacturers, and the clergy, reform became a common strand in British society during the first half of the nineteenth century, stimulated by the earlier anti–slave trade and church reform movements and the Evangelical Revival. As well as factory, penal, Poor Law, mental health care, and education reforms, medical reform became an ongoing concern at the very time James was considering entering the profession.

As the academic subject of science was yet to be developed in Britain, and as many of the men contributing to understanding the world were educated as physicians, James's choice of medicine was natural. An excellent example of a physician-scientist was Bristol's Dr. Thomas Beddoes. Although suspected of having associated with men holding unorthodox theories of nature, Beddoes was nevertheless a respectable doctor. He cared for and experimented on the Bristol poor while researching the curative properties of gasses. James's uncle Dr. Lewis was another respectable, affluent physician whom James admired. The Society of Friends was well represented in the medical profession in general.[4] There were other, more personal reasons for being attracted to medicine aside from its high social status and grounding in scientific method. The Prichard family had undergone one medical trial after another, and as a doctor he would be a benefit to society—just what his father desired. And medicine was not business.

In planning James's career, father and son understood that a future Dr. Prichard would need to settle in a city, as few country dwellers could afford a physician's fees. Bristol provided influential family connections and proximity to Ross. The city's wealthy and expanding suburb of Clifton would furnish enough patients for another physician. Bristol physicians had encouragingly high social standing and financial security. Formal and aloof, they drove fine carriages and lived in homes advertising their status. Some even possessed country estates, and several were nearing retirement. So Dr. Prichard would practice medicine in Bristol, but did he have a suitable personality for such a life? How did one succeed at it?

A recently published how-to book could assure Thomas Prichard of his son's suitability to the profession of medicine. James Parkinson's *The Hospital*

Pupil (1800) claimed that a medical man must be possessed of at least normal capacity, be able to accept the burden of medical duties, show empathy, and be highly educated, especially in Latin. The acquisition of French, German, shorthand, and drawing was also advantageous. So far, so good. But he then warned that scholarship alone was no guarantee of success; confidence and the manners of the world were vital.[5] These last two qualities were a challenge for the unassuming lad. He would just have to learn.

After denigrating the traditional apprenticeship pathway to medicine and lauding university education, Parkinson insisted that a university must provide anatomy and physics lectures as well as a clinical medicine course taught in cooperation with a hospital. In other words, the ideal curriculum was that of the University of Edinburgh Medical School. The only two English universities, Oxford and Cambridge, did not figure in the equation because not only was medical education there negligible, but requirements for admission excluded Dissenters like James. Parkinson concluded by warning would-be physicians' fathers that they would have to support their son's gentlemanly lifestyle during the several years it would take to build up a practice.[6] The Prichards followed Parkinson's advice. Unlike Oxbridge, Scottish universities welcomed Dissenters and foreigners. And unlike Oxbridge, Edinburgh and Continental institutions were famous for excellence in medical education. The Napoleonic Wars then raging prohibited Continental travel, and the Prichards' francophobia put the famous Paris medical schools out of bounds anyway. Bristol surgeon Francis Gold's long imprisonment in Paris testified to the foolhardiness of studying in France. Medicine had been the obvious choice of profession, and Edinburgh was the obvious choice of university.

The Prichards had chosen an up-and-coming profession. The Industrial Revolution had swelled the ranks of the middle classes, physicians' customer base. The provincial urban nouveaux riches were a magnet for physicians; not only could they afford physicians, but they began establishing their sons in this highly respected profession.[7] As opportunities for physicians increased, Continental and Scottish universities devised more efficient and effective curricula to cater to the growing student population.

A gradual process of medical professionalization got under way around the start of the nineteenth century, reflected in the formation of institutions for providing medical treatment, such as charity hospitals and dispensaries for the poor, at which medical training was often an acknowledged benefit. There was also some state involvement: the government strengthened the accreditation roles of the Royal Colleges and the Society of Apothecaries and funded the Royal Jennerian (vaccine) Institute in 1803, for instance. But medical reform and professionalization proceeded slowly; the Medical Act was not passed until 1858. James was entering a profession in transition.

At the start of the nineteenth century, the medical profession was multifarious, best defined in terms of social class. Medical men were ranked in Bristol's street directories according to prestige: physicians, surgeons (the most numerous), and apothecaries were men all acceptable to the middle classes and above. Physicians were more than a cut above other medical practitioners. Their professional body was the Royal College of Physicians, ruled by their strictly (and rare) Oxbridge MD fellows, who generally confined themselves to controlling London physicians, though they could also grant an "extra licence" to their provincial brothers. Next, the best qualified surgeons were members of the Royal College of Surgeons and licentiates of the Society of Apothecaries. They dealt with external conditions and diseases and, contrary to what their name now implies, carried out only the most superficial of surgical procedures. Importantly, surgeons and apothecaries' education through apprenticeship was more practical than theoretical. They were the family doctors, or the general practitioners of Britain today. Apothecaries, next in the hierarchy and ancestral to modern pharmacists, dispensed medicines and advice from their shops and visited the sick. Even the relatively well-off would head for the apothecary's shop for the treatment of a minor illness. There were also several other types of medical practitioner listed in the local directories such as herbalists. The poor might consult healers and "wise women" before resorting to charitable dispensaries, workhouse medical officers, or the gratis services of medical men.[8]

Following the strict medical professional etiquette of the time, physicians treated only the gentry and their servants and could direct the activities of the other medical practitioners of lower status. If a case was intractable, the family doctor would invite a physician into consultation, which involved his visiting the patient at home and directing the practitioner's conduct of the case accordingly. A patient's death was generally attributed to delay in calling in a physician. Disputes over protocol among the more elite classes of medical men were rife and steadily intensifying during this transformative period, when the medical qualifying bodies and education were the subjects of frequent reformist efforts. Dr. Prichard would be involved in such publicly aired quarrels, being something of a stickler for protocol.

Prichard did not actually need to attend university to obtain an MD. The more traditional and common, but somewhat less prestigious, route to a degree and status was to undergo a seven-year apprenticeship followed by licensing and years of doctoring to the middle classes as a surgeon or surgeon apothecary. Then, upon obtaining two physicians' testimonials, a practitioner could essentially purchase an MD from a Scottish or foreign university. Prichard would later sign testimonials on behalf of Bristol colleagues' applications for Aberdeen MDs. This type of degree was gradually losing credibility, however, so Thomas Prichard and his son would not have dreamed of this practical and less elite career path.

The mere possession of an MD was just the first step along the road to the respectable affluence James's father demanded, and in later describing the profession as "congenial," Prichard certainly did not mean he considered healing Bristolians a pleasant activity. Success and affluence were hard won, the fruits of diligence and more than a bit of self-promotion. Ahead of him were some cutthroat elections to the voluntary medical staffs of any Bristol medical institution that would have him. These charities provided medical and welfare services to the poor, funded mostly by the richer citizens directly through subscription or indirectly by local taxation. Subscribers' votes were like gold dust as posts were hotly contested on social and political grounds, with the victors' reputations established among the subscribers and their affluent friends. With his fine "MD, Edin," Dr. Prichard needed at least one of these posts. His father and uncles' voting rights at the Bristol Infirmary would come in handy.

Edinburgh's State-of-the-Art Medical Education

The year before James headed for Scotland, a visiting Austrian physician described the parlous state of English university medical education: it barely existed and was sadly unaffordable to those seeking to become hardworking military medics, for example. Not a single lecture had been delivered by the Cambridge Regius Professors of Medicine during the entire eighteenth century. Oxbridge medical professors considered their posts sinecures; only a handful of strictly "literary" medical degrees were awarded annually.[9] Although Edinburgh was a long and trying journey from James's home in Herefordshire, its education and diploma were worth the effort.

Modern university medical education had originated on the Continent, and by the mid-sixteenth century Paris and Padua were preeminent in it. Many English doctors flocked to Paris or later to the University of Leyden, where Herman Boerhaave shaped medical theory and founded the practice of clinical instruction. Thus the traditional, essentially classical literary approach to medical education became enlarged by the practical experience of dealing with real patients. Scottish students brought innovative Leyden medical education back to the University of Edinburgh which, in cooperation with the Infirmary, provided Britain's first university clinical lectures.[10] The two elite English universities, meanwhile, ignored this new form of medical education and science in general. So by 1800 Edinburgh had become the dominant producer of influential medical men, scientists, holders of public office, medical teachers, and British military and colonial medics. Uncle Lewis, MD, Edin, had not attained national eminence, but he ended his days as a gentleman in Bath. If James were intent on obtaining a university medical and scientific education of worth, Edinburgh was the place to go.

As highly prized an Edinburgh medical degree was around the world, it was not so among the elite of England. The matter of English social acceptability and the near impossibility of overcoming the lack of it is apparent in the disdain in which Oxbridge MDs held their more plentiful Edinburgh brothers. In an anonymous 1814 pamphlet, "Oxonian" opined Edinburgh unworthy of being called a university. Its medical men were fit only for colonial and military service, occupations disdained by English gentlemen. Oxonian considered this fortunate because the British Empire needed medical men for its dirty work: "For what highly accomplished physician would depart and sit down to be frozen in Newfoundland, Hudson's Bay, or the Orkneys, or broiled for a pittance in the West Indies, or starved in a little dirty Scotch, Irish, or Welsh Borough, or waste his health, his vigor, and his talents, amongst the out-casts and convicts of New Holland, &c. &c. [and] it is well known, also, that Scotch doctors often become surgeons in the army and navy. Now no such instance was ever known of an Oxford or Cambridge doctor, and indeed it would be a degradation."[11]

Crammed with classical Greek and Latin medical literature, the few Oxbridge MD candidates were tested without reference to any practical knowledge or experience of patients living or dead, and these gentlemen physicians did not intend to soil their hands with the untidy, demeaning aspects of common doctoring.[12] Sir Henry Halford would later testify to a Parliamentary Select Committee that only an Oxbridge MD denoted a proper gentleman of moral and intellectual experience who for reasons of pride and economics needed to earn a living in medicine. Edinburgh MDs, tainted by practical experience, were patently unfit to treat gentlemen and the nobility.[13]

Keener on doing science than memorizing Greek medical aphorisms, James understood he would be entering an elite profession that was in the process of transformation during this optimistic Age of Improvement. Ahead of him was a major challenge that would restrict the scope of his contributions to science and detract from his legacy, however. While he looked forward to being in the vanguard of progressive, scientific medicine and innovative science, he remained committed to preserving and illustrating the veracity of Christian belief. These tensions between past and future, belief and science, would be evident throughout his career. Back in 1802, Thomas Prichard reluctantly set him on his path to science through the study of medicine.

Pre-university Placements: Dr. Pole's, Bristol, Eighth Month 1802

Their summer seaside holiday in Tenby over, Thomas Prichard took James on a tour of his various business interests in South Wales, strengthening his son's choice of medicine. He dreaded losing James's companionship, but it was time to get the fifteen-year-old settled. How exactly was it to be managed? His friend Mrs. Holbrow's first husband had been a medical practitioner, so she might know what to do. He appealed to her in September 1801: "I feel so acutely on the subject of James' settlement that I hardly dare to take it up, but will you be so kind as to get the best information you can relative to T. Pole's place. It would be well to secure a preference as I do not doubt that the place for young men will be in request."[14] He procrastinated. Some months slipped by before he asked:

> My solicitude about James' destination daily encreases. Can you give me any information respecting the plan we have talked about? I wish to know in what manner youths are disposed of in the first steps towards a medical education. If it is undertaken at all, I should wish to have it done in the most effectual and extensive plan. If a temporary residence with any person in the line of an apothecary be needful, we must begin to look out. A Dr Owen, a very respectable friend in Merionethshire has been mentioned to me I have seen him in London, and perhaps you may be able to give some information about him from John Lucy. It is time James were disposed of, for Tommy is coming up after him pretty fast and I shall want some time to devote to him as I now do to James, and which I cannot well do, while both are with me, but alas! Heaven only knows how glad I should be to put the dreadful moment of separation at a distance.[15]

Mrs. Holbrow advised that James should prepare for university by first becoming a physician's private pupil, after which he needed to gain some clinical experience in a hospital as a physician's pupil. So Thomas Prichard arranged for a series of pre-Edinburgh placements with respectable Quaker medical men.

In James's last childhood summer in Ross, the peace of the Herefordshire town with its colonnaded Market Place, ancient shops and inns, the beautiful nearby River Wye, and farmland beyond was twice interrupted. The great naval hero Lord Nelson, his mistress Lady Hamilton, and her husband rolled into town one pleasant July day. The locals turned out to cheer them through the streets and down to a pleasure boat on the river to continue their journey into Wales. The citizens of Ross were better prepared for the celebrities' return visit on August 21, having erected an oak and laurel triumphal arch through which Nelson and his party smilingly passed.[16] Meanwhile, a negotiated period of study with Dr. Owen in the depths of Wales having fallen through, Thomas Prichard risked sending his son back to the corrupting atmosphere of Bristol.

As summer turned to autumn James prepared to leave home. Just before setting out for Bristol, he got a sleepless night, not from the prospect of parting from his father or from enthusiasm for his medical studies, but because he was so excited by the next day's visit by the Celtic scholar Rev. Edward Davies.[17] James looked forward to discussing the language of his ancestors with the poor curate. Thomas Prichard immediately started missing his serious young companion. His youngest son Tom's personality was completely different:

> It will be a good while before I shall be able to make Tommy a companion as James. His head and heart are so full of one pursuit or other, that if I did not know the power of habit, I should almost begin to despair of having much share in his mind. I know however the danger of attempting too much at a time, and must therefore bring him round by degrees. If I want him to sit down with me, his rabbits, his poultry or his birds claim his attention, and he is off directly. You must come and help me to unchild him. His heart is tender & of course I shall succeed with him one day or another.
>
> I have written to James and received a reply: His letter is a very agreeable one—no complaint of any kind, nor does he appear to suffer the least dissatisfaction in his allotment—it is a very manly letter

and though easy it is evident my interest in his heart is encouraged by distance—may the blessing of Heaven rest upon him.[18]

Continuing as he had started, Tommy became a lifelong headache to his father and brothers. Despite Uncle Lewis's expert care, Mrs. Holbrow died the following month, leaving Thomas Prichard with Margaretta Cross and his sister Elizabeth Newman as his remaining close friends. Mrs. Cross promised to keep an eye on James in Bristol.[19]

Now back in the heart of Bristol, ready to start studying medicine and hoping to spend his free time with the Crosses in nearby King Square, James promptly joined the Bristol Library Society and started borrowing books. Rather than choosing classical histories and religious commentaries as his father would have done, he started devouring the foreign travel books that fueled his life's work.[20] Prichard remembered his initial medical education with mixed feelings:

> In order to afford me this opportunity without exposing me to society not select and strict in morality and in full conformity with the manners and customs of the Quakers, my father entered into a most anxious correspondence with some of his friends. At length thro' the advice principally of Mrs Holbrow he determined to send me to Dr Pole . . . [,] a London apothecary who had gotten a diploma and had recently settled in Bristol as a physician & accoucheur. He had been born and bred in America and was originally a man quite uneducated, but got into some favour with /(some of)/ the Society of Friends, in London among whom he was a popular preacher/an accepted minister? Many of them supposed him to be a man of great talents and acquirements /not so others/ among whom was Mrs Holbrow, as well as several of my Fathers friends.[21]

Bristol had some scientific attractions for the young student. There were the inspirational chemical experiments being carried out by Dr. Beddoes. He had founded the Pneumatic Institute in 1798, a small infirmary with outpatients facilities, a lecture room, and a laboratory where he and his young researcher Humphry Davy could work on the therapeutic benefits of some newly discovered gasses. They experimented with nitrous oxide on their Bristol literary friends such as Robert Southey, Samuel Taylor Coleridge, and members of the Wedgwood family. Davy published his findings, pointing out that inhaled nitrous oxide had anesthetic properties; the medical world ignored it, but the hilarious effects of "laughing gas" became the talk of the town. Dr. Beddoes continued his experiments and became a tireless campaigner and publisher on hygiene and preventive medicine. In linking chemical knowledge to medicine, he made a valuable contribution to science—just the sort of thing James dreamed of doing.[22] First he had to serve his time with Dr. Pole, however.

Thomas Pole, pious descendant of Somersetshire Quakers, had been a London medical man of extensive practice, specializing in midwifery. He lectured and assembled a private anatomical museum, and his *Anatomical Instructor* (1790) was considered an excellent manual for the preservation of anatomical specimens. After obtaining an MD by testimonial from St. Andrew's University in 1801, Dr. Pole and his family settled at 14 St. James' Square, Bristol.[23] He was soon appointed one of the physicians to the Bristol Dispensary, and he published an impressive nineteen-page *Prospectus of a Course of Lectures, including the General Oeconomy of Nature; to Be Delivered in the City of Bristol*. The city had never seen such an ambitious educational undertaking. Lacking institutions of higher education, it was more reliant on occasional visits by itinerant lecturers.[24]

For 2 guineas, Pole's fifty-two weekly lectures promised to "enlarge the comprehension and improve the mind" of affluent Bristolians. The doctor pointed out that his course would especially benefit the young; reassuringly he undertook to use language appropriate for ladies, as well. He cleverly pitched to hard-nosed Bristolians his claim that the success of manufacturing depended on science. In stressing the importance of London's recently founded Royal Institution admitting all classes and both sexes, Pole correctly prophesized that its young professors would make the early nineteenth century "memorable in the annals of British history to distant posterity." The "light of science" will relieve the ignorance of the impoverished and the burdens of their labors, and reassuringly, scientists' "seeking to understand the truths of Nature as ordained by the Creator is a more worthy activity than the amusements that currently occupy men's minds." Dr. Pole's course highlighted the popular subject of chemistry but also included geography, botany, anatomy, first aid, basic surgical procedures, and natural philosophy (physics).[25] Fresh from associating with the London intelligentsia, he combined the Scottish Enlightenment philosophy of improvement and the contemporary Continental fervor for science, tempered by judicious reference to the Almighty's hand. His own scientific research involved making systematic meteorological observations.[26] Thomas Prichard was pleased with Pole's evangelical desire to improve the world and his son looked forward to studying in like-minded company.

James seemed to value his time at Dr. Pole's mostly for the friendship he developed with his son John, a most admirable fellow medical student. Father and son were quite a new experience in their own ways. Despite the doctor's glowing Quaker reputation, instead of remembering his teacher fondly, Prichard apparently added him to the list of several Quakers he distrusted.[27] Perhaps Dr. Pole was already evincing a liberalism later expressed in his dedication to the education of the poor: he was instrumental in starting a nonsectarian school dedicated to teaching working men, the second adult education institute in Britain.[28] This ostentatious Quakerism and Methodist-like fervor for the poor did not appeal to Prichard, boy or man. Pole's own recollection of James was unalloyed, by contrast:

> Soon after my settlement in Bristol, I took into my family, as a Pupil, a Youth about [my son John's] age, of extensive knowledge in the Languages and in History, who was of a very studious turn of mind. They became attached to each other as Companions, and united their efforts indefatigably, in the study of Languages, History, Medicine, Anatomy, Surgery, Chemistry, Botany, Natural Philosophy &c, in which they made very considerable progress. After continuing in my family one year [James] was removed to another place, in the county of Middlesex, to acquire the art of Pharmacy.

James and John Pole were inseparable. Only ten months older and considered already proficient in the art of pharmacy, John assisted in the surgery and at his father's lectures. As he was an excellent chemist, known for his love of literature and science, his friendship with James was understandable. Dr. Pole regretted his son's insistence on studying medicine because of its initial financial hardship, risk of corruption of the mind and faith, and, moreover, the obvious danger to his health.[29]

Dr. Pope and Mr. Tothill's, Staines, Middlesex, Autumn 1803

Mrs. Cross told James about a letter she had received from his father bearing excellent news. The abominable housekeeper Kitty Morgan was no more! Her replacement Joanna was

> quiet, yet very active, a little agreable woman of manners very pleasing even genteel, yet quite the consistent Friend, as far as I can yet judge I have gained much on the score of economy without the loss of a single comfort, and on the score of enjoyment let James judge, when I tell thee that my will is never rudely controverted (nor as yet even in the gentlest

manner opposed) that our family party is never intruded upon, that my ears are not at one time stunned with vociferation, nor at another my patience tried by obstinate tenacity. Never did a change in administration produce such an astonishing difference; quietness is the reigning character of the family—a character which it has had no pretensions to, for the last eight years. The children are delighted with Joanna, and behave to her with propriety, because she does the same to them. Mary was considerably affected by Kitty's departure during the first hour. I took care to lead on the conversation to pleasant subjects without any apparent design,—the clouds of anxiety soon dispersed, and ever since it has been one uniform scene of serenity and lively enjoyment.

—Yes I can indeed bear to hear our dear children spoken partially of-but I am almost afraid James intrudes upon you sometimes. I beg if he ever should come at an inconvenient time, that thou wilt not hesitate to tell him so. Dear John and he are so formed for companions, that I believe it is James' greatest delight to be in company with him. Please to inform James when thou seest him, that I have requested S. Prichard to commence a correspondence with Dr Pope of Staines, respecting his spending some time in the shop of himself and partners for the purpose of improvement in Pharmacy—it is a most desirable situation—if it can be obtained. Every advantage of his present one, and in addition the experience of the first country apothecary's shop in the Kingdom. I want to know whether James would have his removal deferred twelve months longer, or that it should take place in six. . . . A Fathers love to James—I long to see him.[30]

James reluctantly parted with John Pole and left Bristol to spend the blissful summer of 1803 in Ross with his family, reading books about far-off places.[31] Doting on his daughter, Mary, as usual, Thomas Prichard counted his blessings:

The dear children seem in possessing James to possess all that constitutes felicity, the affections of a sister are however distinguishable from the rest by a greater delicacy of fondness and by an artless freedom of expression that causes no blush in exposing the heart. The connexion between brother and sister is extremely delightful, and it doubtless derives its wonderful power of interesting from a participation in the joys of early youth; the countenance of each mutually reminds the other of the happiness that never accompanies an age of mature consciousness.

Of that blest age when no black cares annoy
And the heart dances to the song of joy.

And in them I live my youth over again.... I have been with James to Staines to pay a visit personally to the family with whom I am going to place him. It was a long journey, being within 16 miles of London, but I feel much satisfaction in having undertaken it because I have gained a knowledge not only of the family, but of the place. With the former I have reason to be particularly pleased, and I have contracted for his going there some time in the 8th Month (August). James has a droll story to tell thee about Black's lectures.[32]

In the early autumn James set off to spend eight months in Staines under Dr. Robert Pope and Mr. William Tothill's instruction in the arts of pharmacy, dispensing and treating patients. The doctor, apparently in the "expectant" wait-and-see camp of therapeutics, was the opposite of the "heroic" prescriber Prichard would become. A respected teacher with an impeccable Quaker reputation, Dr. Pope proved an excellent choice. He had recently been awarded the special distinction of a Lambeth MD by Archbishop Moore, which required his affirmation that he would practice honorably, abominate Roman Catholicism, and be loyal to the king. Quaker Elder Dr. Pope was famous for his piety, integrity, and benevolence; he treated the poor gratis, built two schools for them, supported the Bible Society and the Baptist Mission in India, gave the enormous sum of £500 to the York Quaker asylum, and still managed to leave a fabulous estate of almost £80,000 upon his death in 1827. His probity was such that on one memorable occasion, when he realized he had inadvertently neglected to hand over his valuable watch to a highwayman, it was with difficulty that he was dissuaded from chasing after the robber to rectify the omission. He was a friend of the poet Percy Bysshe Shelley and became highly regarded by the Royal Family, having treated the ailing, allegedly wayward Princess Amelia and the future obviously wayward George IV.[33] A highly respected, rich, and benevolent Quaker, Dr. Pope was all Thomas Prichard hoped his son would become. James lodged with Pope's partner, fellow Quaker apothecary William Tothill, where he applied himself to his various studies earnestly and diligently. He availed himself of the opportunity of acquiring much practical knowledge from William Tothill who had a very extensive practice. James liked Mr. Tothill and made a good impression on his family, conducting himself amiably and forming lasting friendships with the Tothill boys.[34]

While James was happily making progress in his medical education in Staines, he received the sad news of John Pole's death from typhus, aged nineteen. He kept a few of John's obstetrical illustrations for the rest of his life. Luckily, the three Tothill boys were companionable. William Tothill Jr. later settled in Bristol, married into the industrialist Darby family and became a highly successful businessman and fierce Liberal local politician.[35] Despite their different circumstances and political views, he remained one of Prichard's close friends.

After a rewarding period in Staines, it was back to Ross and Bristol for the summer to listen to his father's business concerns, read and spend time with his brothers and sister. Thomas Prichard dreaded "the temptation and dangers to which youth is exposed!" In other words, James would soon be off to the Sodom and Gomorrah of London, while Tom would work in the differently corrupting Harfords' Bristol countinghouse without being bound apprentice, a regrettable arrangement. Aware of the perils of overprotection, their father could only urge them to seek divine guidance through prayer.[36] In due course, James repaired to London and devoted himself to the study of anatomy in the school attached to St. Thomas's Hospital.[37]

St. Thomas's and Guy's Hospitals, London, Tenth Month 1804

James passed through Guy's Hospital's impressive wrought iron gates and forecourt graced by the statue of its benevolent founder and signed the student register on October 1, 1804. In the early nineteenth century, there were five main London teaching hospitals. Their Faculties were composed of elected, unremunerated medical men who had gained their coveted posts through a system of political and social patronage, nepotism and indirect purchase. There they commanded high tuition fees for themselves and built enviable reputations. Following a period of study, their students would sit examinations to qualify as an apothecary or surgeon, or enter university to study for an MD. Religion determined at which hospitals James would study: Dissenters and Whigs went to the united hospitals of St. Thomas's and Guy's, while St. Bartholomew's was Anglican and Tory. James paid 2 guineas to become a physician's pupil under Dr. John Haighton of Guy's on February 4, 1805, and he paid a further 5 shillings in May. This entitled him to attend the lectures and wards of both Guy's and St. Thomas's.[38]

It was an exciting time to be a medical student in London. The faculty did give lectures, but because there was no curriculum James was free to organize his own studies. He could also attend the capital's private anatomy schools for extra practice while he gained clinical experience in the hospitals.³⁹ London's several thriving medical societies were hubs of learning, and some newly founded specialized dispensaries had patients with interesting diseases to observe and sometimes experiment on. Medical reform was in the air too; the government was beginning to see the advantages of implementing public health measures such as vaccination; and there was a growing desire to reform medical education and practice.

Guy's had an excellent reputation for providing systematic instruction in medicine, medical therapeutics, and related sciences. It was founded in 1721 to treat the sick poor while training medical practitioners, the same aims expressed in the Rev. John Aylmer's sermon to the subscribers to the Bristol Infirmary in 1757. To gain clinical experience, James "walked the wards" during the academic term from October to May. He could also observe the dissections of the corpses of criminals and others obtained by the hospital as well as watch the routine "opening" of deceased patients to determine cause of death.⁴⁰ James was one of a very few physicians' pupils, some of whom already had MDs. Although he had some prestigious duties and many opportunities, he had no particular obligations; he observed, attended as he liked, and was rarely tested. Meanwhile, his fellow students variously serving as hospital apprentices, dressers, surgeon's private pupils, and house pupils were destined to become surgeons and apothecaries.

In Guy's Hospital's fine lecture theater, students studied physiology, medical pathology, materia medica, the practice of medicine, medical botany, and physics. Physiology seemed the most appealing to James. Then referred to as "animal economy" or "animal chemistry," it was considered a type of chemistry, stressed partly because chemistry was becoming increasingly used in medical diagnosis and treatment. "Animal chemistry," the study of the chemistry of animal substances and the vital functions, was growing in popularity, having been found useful in the analysis of urine for calculi and diabetes, for instance. The two physicians who lectured on physiology were Drs. Babbington and Haighton.

James's teacher William Babbington, MD, Aberdeen, FRS, was assisted by the Quaker pharmacist William Allen, a friend of Sir Astley Cooper and Humphry Davy who brought prestige to Guy's, and as a chemical manufacturer, personified the practical applications of the science. He was involved in the Royal Institution, antislavery activism, and other progressive movements. Their excellent lectures presented cutting-edge theories and illustrative experiments, complete with apparatus for students' use. Babbington, one of the founders of the science of geology, encouraged his fellow scientists.⁴¹ His colleague John Haighton, MD, Aberdeen, was an avid conductor of physiological experiments and a highly skilled obstetric operator who published widely on a variety of subjects. While a somewhat irritable, argumentative, and suspicious character, he was a good lecturer, generous and honest. Another of James's teachers at Guy's was James Curry, MD, Edin, a shrewd and observant doctor who stressed that the key to successful diagnosis was awareness of the structure and function of the parts in question. His attribution of so many conditions to disordered liver, for which he prescribed calomel (mercurous chloride), earned him the nickname "Calomel Curry," underscored by his fondness for sprinkling it on his sandwiches. His advocacy of mercury did much to establish its prevalence in therapeutics during the first half of the century.[42]

Guy's dynamic Physical Society ("physical" meaning the practice of physic) was modeled on the famous Edinburgh Medical Society. At their Saturday evening meetings James could learn about current cases and postmortems and participate in discussions attended by members of the faculty and visiting medical men. James's teachers at Guy's were actively involved in medical and scientific experimentation, carrying out clinical trials of medicines, experimenting with the therapeutic uses of gasses and identifying anatomical structures, for instance. The atmosphere was inspiring.[43]

James's fondness for anatomy was more than satisfied at St. Thomas's Hospital, with its excellent reputation for teaching both anatomy and surgery, but there were no separate clinical lectures. Instead, as the three surgeons and three physicians did the ward rounds of its 450 patients, they discussed cases and dictated their prescriptions in Latin, attended by all of the apprentices and pupils. James could attend the rounds of Drs. Wells, Turner, and Lister.

William Charles Wells, MD, Leyden, FRS, FRSE, was a man of two parts: the one James aspired to, the other he shrank from. Wells was an insightful, skillfully inductive scientist dedicated to scientific inquiry among a broad range of subjects. But lacking in prudence and self-control, to put it mildly, he was also notoriously stubborn, quarrelsome, easily offended, irritable, rude to staff and patients, and constantly in debt. His argumentativeness and violence twice landed him in prison.[44] One of Wells's publications, a model of inductive scientific method, earned him the Royal Society Rumford Medal, and his later Royal Society lecture touching on evolution through natural selection qualifies him as an anticipator of Darwinism. How gratified James must have been to sign the register as Dr. Wells's guest at a Royal Society lecture where he heard the famous astronomer Frederick William Herschel on May 23, 1805. Four years later, he also introduced Prichard to the celebrity scientist Humphry Davy's talk on electrochemistry. What lions of science![45]

James's other teachers were Thomas Turner, MD, FRCP, later one of his colleagues on the Lunacy Commission, and William Lister, FRSE, LRCP, a stickler for upholding the dignity of his profession. Surgeon John Birch was famous for his experiments and publications on the medical uses of electricity and for his vehement anti–smallpox vaccination stance. Surgeon Henry Cline managed to acquire patients of rank, despite being a notorious deist, supporter of the French Revolution, and associate of radicals, qualities to add to Thomas Prichard's list of London perils. Astley Cooper, the ultimate celebrity member of staff, was a highly skilled, informative lecturer, the maker of surgical and anatomical discoveries and founder of the Medico-Chirurgical Society. He further enhanced the fine reputation of St. Thomas's by his remarkably skillful bargaining with resurrection men for a generous supply of corpses for dissection.[46]

While in London, James's Aunt Elizabeth's relatives George and Ann Newman, prosperous Morocco leather manufacturers of nearby 58 Holborn Hill, kept a Quakerly eye on him, much to his father's relief. He was their welcome visitor, and they afterward remained keenly interested in his progress.[47] James was impressed by the talented medical men of St. Thomas's and Guys, members of the metropolitan scientific elite who gave him a foretaste of the contributions to science he longed to make. Although London offered a complete education for the average medical practitioner, he and his father had set their sights on three more years of scientific education and the prestigious university-earned qualification of MD. His London studies completed, he returned to Ross in the spring of 1805 for a long, studious holiday before setting out on the arduous journey to Scotland in October.[48] James was as thrilled and excited about this next phase of his life as his father was apprehensive.

3 · MD, Edin

Lernfreiheit *in Scotland and Oxbridge*

I hope thy ardour for Mathematics and natural philosophy will not prove them to be a knowledge that puffeth up.
—James Cowles Prichard, "Memoir of Thomas Prichard, Part 1"

Getting There, Tenth Month 1805

James was desperate to set out on his weeklong journey to Edinburgh and an independent life among an international group of men of various backgrounds, religious affiliations, and interests. He had three years to explore the sciences before the reality of medical practice began. A fellow student enthused about this intellectual mecca:

> In a town where learning is honoured and its votaries are very numerous, where public lectures are given in almost every department of human knowledge, and commerce and dissipation are comparatively in the background, a stranger almost necessarily inhales in the very atmosphere, the spirit of the place, and wishes to be, or at least to appear to be, a lover of knowledge. There is scarcely an hour in the day, that is not filled with a lecture on some subject, and the difficulty to a stranger who wishes to obtain as much information as possible is, not to know where to begin, but to know where to stop.[1]

James was not only looking forward to organizing his curriculum and learning from professors of international reputation; he realized he would no longer be monitored by his father and well-meaning Quakers. Thomas Prichard had insisted on accompanying James to Edinburgh to secure his son's safe and respectable accommodation, and carriage-sick sister Mary also managed to enjoy the trip.

The three travelers broke their journey northward from Ross to take in some natural and industrial marvels. The furnaces of Coalbrookdale presented a fiery spectacle after dark, inspiring James to "pour out his Latin & Greek descriptions of Phlegethon as he road along, & really there was some opportunity of applying them justly." They met with the usual tribulations of traveling in 1805. At the Tontine Inn in Ironbridge, they found themselves stranded for a time until they could secure fresh carriage horses for their onward journey, and Shrewsbury was so full of soldiers, Thomas Prichard had to spend the night in "one of the most wretched Beds that I ever stretched myself upon." Picturesque Lake Windermere inspired them to leave their comfortable chaise at Bowness and take a seven-mile boat ride up the lakes:

> It was a lovely day, and the scene novel to us all. As we approached the head of the lake we were astonished in contemplating the immense hills that enclose the extremity of this beautiful water. Our chaise met us at the Bank and took us to Ambleside to dine; where we went to see the cascades, the groves and Rydal water, a lovely little lake, and Grassmere, which for elegant scenery, and sweet tranquility of position has peculiar charms. Our next was Leathswater Lake with the majestic mountain Helvellyn on its side. It was from one of the crags of this hill that poor Gough, a Quaker lately fell and was dashed to pieces. He lay 3 months undiscovered and a faithful dog remained by his corpse.[2]

The scenery of Skiddaw and Borrowdale and the sublime cascade of Lowdore held the tourists in awe. From magnificent Derwent Water, they resumed their journey to Edinburgh through bleak hills punctuated by valleys through which ran mountain torrents worthy of the Scottish ballads that praise them.[3]

> We are at length arrived at the Scotch Metropolis: thus one half of a painful duty is fulfilled and so far I have satisfaction; but when I reflect that in accomplishing the other half, I leave my dear James behind me, then I feel it hard indeed that even to fulfill my duties, subject me to deep suffering. James has got many respectable introductions to characters of the first celebrity here, and when he has delivered them, I doubt not that he will find a circle of acquaintance that will much suit his taste.... For domestic accomodations I have been obliged to apply to a different set of men; Happily however I have found some valuable individuals of our society, who have recommended me to a lodging for James that I think will suit him very well, and such an one as they know to be safe with regard to manners &c. I dread however the moment when I shall leave him and though his raptures rose in proportion, as we approached this classical city, yet I plainly perceive

that his spirits are much tried at the thought of separating from us. It will indeed be dull, until the lectures begin, which will not be till the end of the month. However before we turn our backs upon him we shall get more acquainted with his hostess, and that will somewhat relieve us.[4]

Suffering from child separation anxiety even before they parted, the elder Prichard agonized to his friend:

> Reflect for a moment that I am going to place a beloved son at the immense distance of 400 miles from me. I am overwhelmed with the idea. It is indeed committing him to Providence in the circumstances perhaps even more trying than death! How continually present to my mind the impossibility of my going to see him in case of illness. It is an entire separation—a separation that, whatever may happen must continue to present insuperable obstacles to my personal intercourse. This is terrible. London seems next door to me when I think of Edinburgh; and yet I must sit and listen to the most rapturous delights the children promise themselves in this tremendous journey—thoughtless beings! What is a parents heart but a shuttlecock, thus continually agitated by contrary impulses! And yet I am best pleased to see them thus enjoying themselves in their future prospects. . . . James proposes coming home in the summer by the Edinburgh packet that sails for London and in which many passengers are generally found. The fare is but 2 guineas, bed and board found by the owners. This seems a little formidable but I daresay my desire of seeing him will reconcile me to it when the time comes.[5]

After tearing himself away from James on October 16, Thomas Prichard and Mary headed south to Carlisle, from where he wrote to warn his son of the cold weather in store for him, living so much more north than he was used to. Near Shap he described seeing something that would have thrilled James, "a Druidical Circle of very large stones, though none of them elevated from the ground."[6] He penned yet another epistle en route, repeating all his injunctions and demanding James write to him:

> Do frequent as much as propriety will allow, the families of the friends to whom I have introduced thee. I daresay thou wilt occasionally feel thyself dull and lonely, but it is much better to be so, than to be in hurtful company. I hope thy intentions to render thyself a useful member of society at large are full of integrity, and then I cannot doubt the

protection of Providence. . . . Do not omit to write me a letter with a full account of all thy introductions &c. Nothing thou canst communicate that concerns thyself will be indifferent to me. Mary has been merry and sad, and sad and merry. Ainsi va la jeunesse![7]

Thomas Prichard adopted a new tone in replying to James's first Edinburgh letter. Brother Edward looked forward to partridge shooting with James next summer. Was there any objection to their Park Street, Bristol home being sold? He assumed his son was diligently studying and drinking tea with only the most respectable citizens of Edinburgh, a credit to his family and the Society of Friends. But as he feared, Edinburgh would change James's life.

The Scottish Enlightenment and the University of Edinburgh

In a city famous for its culture, science, and medical education, James risked exposure to its undercurrent of impiety, a legacy of Scottish Enlightenment philosophy. How his loyalty to the Society of Friends might be safeguarded exercised his father greatly. The sect was notoriously weak in Scotland; its members were rumored to be lax. In fact, the English had long held all Scots under suspicion, as an American visitor observed of Edinburgh and its university:

> There existed in England, during the greatest part of the last century, a sort of jealous ill-will against the Scotch. It was the fashion to rail at their poverty, their rapacious industry, the proud servility of their manners, their uncleanliness, and, finally, their itch. . . . Edinburgh is the Birmingham of literature;—a new place, which has its fortune to make. The two great universities, Oxford and Cambridge, repose themselves under the shade of their laurels, while Edinburgh cultivates hers. The exterior of the establishment of education is very modest indeed. The professors are soldiers of fortune, who live by their sword,—that is to say, by their talents and reputation.[8]

Scottish universities embraced the future: English universities embraced the past. Then there was the country itself and the attitude of its citizens. Englishmen thought Scotland remote, foreign, and hostile, with alien customs and suspect Enlightenment freethinking. Its 1707 unification with England had led to Anglicization and increased prosperity, but one of the distinctive and vital qualities of Scottish culture that survived this process was its positive attitude toward education and progress. While in England attainment and status were based not on effort or ability but on breeding, Scotland had a tradition of encouraging progress through education. By contrast, the English elite tended to disdain interest in education beyond the study of the dead languages, theology, and mathematics; a tiny minority of its young gentlemen and aristocrats spent their time at England's two ancient universities mostly socializing in preparation to rule the country. Scotland had four and sometimes five thriving universities at which, in theory, any young man could obtain a beneficial education. The function and purpose of Scottish universities reflected Scottish society and beliefs.

The influence of the Scottish Enlightenment was apparent during James's years there. A chemistry of creative ideas permeated the country in an eighteenth-century philosophical movement influenced by, but distinct from, its Continental parent. Its two main schools of thought were Scottish common sense realism and utilitarianism, and into the mix, Scottish Calvinist ideals of moral and mental discipline were instrumental in stimulating this intellectual and cultural flowering. At universities, clubs, and societies professors, students, literati, publishers, and some members of the landed gentry espoused the broadly common values of civic virtue, commerce, agricultural reform, elitism, cosmopolitan refinement, and the desire to maintain a connection with England. Despite generally attempting to couch their ideas safely within the bounds of orthodoxy, Scottish Enlightenment figures were suspected and vilified by elements of the dominant Scottish Tory elite and by the Kirk. The practical outcomes of the movement were nevertheless recognized and appreciated, especially as so many were clearly money-spinners; for instance, discoveries in chemistry benefited agriculture and manufacturing.[9]

Among Scottish Enlightenment figures and their followers seeking to understand the world through science were William Cullen, who researched in chemistry, medicine, and agriculture; Joseph Black, who made remarkable discoveries in chemistry; James Hutton, the revolutionary geologist; and John Leslie, who studied and lectured on mathematics and physics. The Edinburgh Philosophical (meaning science) Society was thriving, while the members of the student Royal Medical Society emulated their elders by conducting scientific experiments and engaging in the wide-ranging debates of the day.[10] Scotland's intellectual atmosphere drew James to it like a magnet.

The conservative Scottish press and the Scottish Kirk were constantly on the lookout for signs of apostasy: the Enlightenment-tinged Edinburgh professors were suspected of atheism. Just before James arrived, there had been a campaign to block alleged freethinker John Leslie's appointment to the chair of mathematics. A local clergyman was set up as a rival candidate amid published accusations of skepticism, atheism, and heresy against Leslie. Professor Dugald Stewart and some of the students launched a pamphlet war. The Presbytery of Edinburgh, the local governing body of the Church of Scotland, was attempting to gain control of the religious integrity of the university's entire faculty in a bid to curb growing secularity, but the Town Council, in charge of university appointments, staved off this power grab. Leslie was eventually appointed, but endured unending harassment.[11]

The University of Edinburgh created professionals. Professor Stewart produced politicians, social reformers, economists, and educationalists while Professor Leslie educated engineers for new industries. Botanists, geologists, and explorers were educated there, as were leaders in the fields of medicine and mental and public health. A greatly disproportionate number of Britain's renowned scientists and government officeholders of the nineteenth century possessed degrees from Prichard's alma mater; for example, Prichard himself became one of four Edinburgh alumni serving on the Lunacy Commission in 1842. Edinburgh graduates led in the fields of public health, medicine, and science. In psychiatry, two experts of international reputation, Drs. John Conolly and Alexander Morison, were Edinburgh products. An Edinburgh medical degree was likewise beneficial in American science and academia. With the freedom to obtain both a broad, modern medical education and brandishing his "MD, Edin," Prichard could be confident of a successful future in medicine and science.

In the forefront of Scottish and Scottish Enlightenment–inspired liberal education aimed at improving all aspects of human endeavor, the university helped establish Victorian values of moral seriousness, commercial and industrial focus, inductive approach to research, and constant striving for improvement and reform.[12] Prichard's Edinburgh education made an impact on him evident in his contributions to the human sciences. "No place in the world can pretend to a competition with Edinburgh," Thomas Jefferson had claimed in 1789, and it was still true in 1805.[13]

Edinburgh Medical School and the University

The Medical School had long been preeminent in medical innovation and education although Napoleonic wartime insularity and the faculty's internal politics had started to take the shine off its reputation by the time James arrived in 1805. The faculty and the city's Royal Infirmary's adoption of the Continental method of medical education was just one factor in Edinburgh's success. Crucially, medical education itself was no longer based on the memorization of Latin classical texts but on actual observation of patients' and their histories, employing diagnosis, prognosis, and cure. During the previous century, the Edinburgh Medical Society published a journal that attracted contributions from physicians and surgeons all over Scotland, England, and Ireland; its sharing of information and promotion of debate became a paradigm for professional medical and scientific societies worldwide.[14] The Royal Colleges of Surgeons and Physicians of Edinburgh were open and positive in their relations with the Royal Infirmary and the Medical School, for example, with students allowed to attend each other's lectures. The city's government fostered the rapid development of an Edinburgh-centric medical education industry, which promoted research and standards of practice. The Medical School and Infirmary's faculties were inspired to develop inductive and experimental approaches to their research, a milestone in the history of medicine and medical education.

There were aspects of the organization of the university as a whole that accrued to its prosperity. Unlike its English counterparts, it was noncollegiate, nonsectarian, professorial in structure, and more centrally and coherently organized. It benefited the interests of commerce and the region's landed elite, and boosted Scottish nationalism and belief in accessible education throughout the country, fostered by the dominant Calvinistic ideals of education, progress, and effort. The university did not impose the Test Act's oath of allegiance to the Established Church; few of its professors were ordained; nor was religious dogma evident in their teaching, qualities that attracted Protestant Dissenters from the rest of Britain and abroad.[15] Among Edinburgh's foreign visitors and James's cosmopolitan cohort were also the sons of influential people deprived by war of the traditional Continental sojourn. All these men from different backgrounds delighted James. And as the cost of living was lower than at the English universities, his father had something to be pleased with too.

At the start of the nineteenth century about one thousand medical students boosted the economy of Edinburgh, aided by the wartime consumption of medical men. As the university prospered, so did the city, both financially and in international reputation. Soon half of the university's students were studying medicine under ten professors. But the Medical School's excellence also caused a decline in its student population as its international alumni established medical schools on Edinburgh principles back home. The Medical Colleges of New York and Philadelphia, University College, London, and several provincial medical schools are cases in point.

While it would become less imperative to travel to Edinburgh to obtain a progressive medical education, in 1805 it was a must.[16]

Edinburgh's Inspiring Science

Several Edinburgh exemplars of science inspired James. Passionate about chemistry, popular Professor Joseph Black's early abandonment of dead-end phlogiston theory in favor of Antoine Lavoisier's "reformed chemistry" and his research on carbon dioxide and latent heat were milestones in the science. Thomas Charles Hope followed in Black's footsteps; James diligently attended his lectures. Another Edinburgh giant of science was Dr. William Cullen, famed for his views on "rational physic," who stood at the transition from the dogma-led medical theory of the ancients to the recognition of the benefits of both experience and experimentation. He asserted that chemistry, anatomy, physiology, and pathology were all essential and blended aspects of medical diagnosis when used in relation to theory, a far cry from traditional medicine. He also laid great stress on a physician having an impeccable reputation and manners, a view Dr. Prichard would adopt.

Just as interesting to James as Edinburgh's scientific and medical achievements was the Scottish Enlightenment–inspired reputation for the study of humankind and human society, a discipline called moral philosophy. This broad science of human behavior would eventually comprise the modern social sciences of psychology, sociology, anthropology, political science, and economics. James's moral philosophy course explored the latest ideas about the nature of society as systematically as his natural philosophy courses tackled the rest of the natural world. His eventual anthropology and psychiatry would both reflect and challenge his moral philosophy professor's views. James avidly attended, took copious notes, and discussed controversial theories with his fellow students.

A long-rumbling contemporary Edinburgh controversy was the monumental issue of Scripture versus scientific evidence that would color much of Prichard's later efforts to prove the unity and single origin of humankind. Central to the early development of geology, for instance, was the struggle between two literally world-changing theories. James Hutton, University of Edinburgh student then professor of natural philosophy, devised a theory of the formation of the earth, qualifying him as the founder of geology. His so-called Plutonist theory that fire had been the agent of geological formation was purely speculative at the time, but its positing the formation of the earth through the natural process of heat scandalously threatened the integrity of Revelation.[17] All were taught that the Creator is reflected in nature, so how could Hutton's theory of self-sufficiency dispense with the hand of the superintending Deity? His famous quotation that "we find no vestige of a beginning, no prospect of an end" made matters even worse; he was undermining Genesis at a time when Godless, revolutionary, materialist Continental theories were gnawing at British Christian values. In stepped practically minded Abraham Gottlob Werner, mine inspector and teacher at the Freiburg Mining Academy. His "Neptunist" theory of the earth was based on water as the agent of change; there had been five flood-based stages of development, a notion congenially corroborating the Flood. Werner's former student, Robert Jameson, Regius Professor of Natural Philosophy at Edinburgh, staunchly defended Wernerianism against his opponent and colleague, the Rev. John Playfair, professor of mathematics and interpreter of Huttonian theory. James, firmly in the Wernerian camp, attended Jameson's lectures and joined his Wernerian Society in support of Scripture and against the dangerous views of the suspected materialist Playfair.[18]

The Professoriate

The structure of the university had some drawbacks that affected James's education. The professors, mostly middle-class Edinburgh-educated Scots, were rigidly independent, protectionist, and competitive. Crucially, their salaries were nearly nominal; they administered their courses themselves, directly employing assistants, purchasing materials, and collecting students' fees. With their income almost entirely dependent on the 2–3 guinea tuition fee per student, per course, there was fierce competition to be both popular and effective educators. Those who taught optional or less popular courses were financially disadvantaged.[19] While the professors controlled the finance and the content of their courses, their Oxbridge counterparts drew generous salaries irrespective of student numbers, pedagogical success, or whether they actually ever lectured.

The Edinburgh professors' productivity drive had its benefits. As publishing clearly enhanced one's reputation, they conducted research and published widely unless the popularity of their subjects rendered this unnecessary. This spurred the development of the Edinburgh academic publishing industry, producing both books and periodicals such as the *Encyclopaedia Britannica* that were circulated internationally and in which the discoveries of Edinburgh men were disseminated. A South Carolina or Jamaica planter reading about Edinburgh's scientific achievements might conclude his son's education under such eminent men would be a ticket to a successful career. As publishing fame thus attracted more and more students, those students consumed more and more textbooks. Black, for instance, earned a phenomenal £3,000 from a single book. The professors had ample leisure to do research and publish. They typically gave a one-hour lecture each weekday, though extra time might be spent preparing demonstrations or working with students, while some of the medical professors conducted daily clinical teaching at the Infirmary and saw their private patients too. They had very long holidays, participated in the prestigious Royal Society of Edinburgh lecture programs, and collected their students' fees. Most of them during this period were wealthy men.[20]

One detriment was that the professors' intense bias toward their own subject sapped their interest in the curriculum and standards of assessment. As a high proportion of students were military medical men on half-pay or those needing a short period of attendance to qualify as licentiates of the College of Surgeons, lectures were easily comprehensible to an audience of varied ability and maturity. Professors' popularity and income tended to reflect how little they tested their students and how exciting their demonstrations and lectures were. Some adopted a degree of showmanship.[21] As they did not receive pensions, they taught until they died, often hiring cheap assistants and aspiring successors to teach in their stead.

The professoriate also formed a powerful bulwark against the governing Town Council's attempts to entertain a wider pool of candidates for professorships. With their sons often their assistants and successors, veritable dynasties developed, the most famous being the three Alexander Monros (Primus, Secundus, and the incompetent Tertius), a regime spanning 1720 to 1846.[22] Such an employment structure spawned nepotism, resistance to progress, protectionism, and outright hostility. Not wanting to dilute their share of tuition fees, they succeeded in restricting the number of professorships, stymying the foundation of a chair of surgery until 1831, for instance. And as if nepotism and professorial conservatism were not detrimental enough, personal disputes were rife; one resulted in a pamphlet war, and in another Professor James Gregory was fined £100 for publicly thrashing a colleague.

Edinburgh's education industry certainly stimulated the local economy. New libraries, museums, laboratories, and lecture halls were demanded, the latter seating as many as six hundred. An imposing university building designed by the famous architect Robert Adam was under construction during James's time there, partly financed by one of the professors.[23] The university courses and their professors' research and publications were instrumental in the era's rapid industrial development. For instance, moral philosophy informed economics and government, while natural history's geology aided mining. The Town Council's investment in the student industry had paid off. Both the city and the nation benefited.

Student Life

James settled into his respectable lodgings, found his way around the city and university, and dutifully presented his letters of introduction to local Quaker families. Edinburgh in 1805 was a world away from uninspiring Bristol. Its architecture was striking, the city being the home of Scottish law, church, and ruling elite. There was Edinburgh's hilltop castle to explore, as well as the city's stepped passage "wynds" and the elegant Georgian New Town neighborhood and public buildings. The coast of the Firth of Forth stretched away in one direction and the imposing mountain Arthur's Seat loomed over the city in another. Soon he would be going on geological and natural history expeditions in the surrounding countryside as well. The city offered so much, from museums, societies, libraries, and institutions to a constant stream of ill or injured military men for medical students to practice on. The medical professors were not James's only role models; he also diligently attended lectures in the faculty of arts, such as the ones on natural history and moral philosophy. The university's ethos of progress through learning suited James to a tee.

Students were not insulated in colleges as at Oxbridge; James was free to live with whom he wished. The best lodgings were those provided in the homes of the professors or their relatives, where students could expect pastoral care, academic guidance, and access to the most beneficial and influential acquaintances in Edinburgh. But not all were so lucky. Contemporary student Benjamin Browne's domestic arrangements were as challenging as his spelling and grammar. He reported to his mother:

> Our Rooms (that is a sitting Room and a bed Room) is a very genteel looking place, forth door up stairs. The street that we live in is in general about 8 or 9 stories high and there is not a room but what is high as Mr Wilcock's great dancing room. We pay 12. 6d. A week for them and they find us fire, Cooks us anything we want an Cleans our shoes. We live well and cheap and is as happy as can be. . . . We get tea about 9 oClock and . . . dine about 4 afternoon and then has bread and Chese about 10 at night.

Happily, ale was 6 pence per bottle and porter 5. As to hygiene standards, he regretted that residents empty "there close stools out of the windows at Night, but it is all cleaned away in the Morning. We are very ill of that way. We are forsed to wait till Night and then when it is dark we go out into the street and obey the calls of nature in the Middle of the street."[24] Benjamin Silliman euphemistically completed this account: "There is a particular and most shameful deficiency in the accommodations of the town, which renders the environs at all times offensive; in the morning the nuisance exists in the streets, before the very doors of the houses. . . . I can hardly write upon the subject without offence, nor think of it without disgust."[25]

Lack of sanitation was just one of the disadvantages to lodging in Edinburgh. The landladies of the Old Town "are miserable wretches, even when they let their rooms, subsisting entirely on what they steal from their lodgers—half-starved, indolent—cruel and unfeeling towards their servants. . . . [Half] the immorality complained of, as said to proceed from Students, are entirely owing to them."[26] Scientist Humphry Davy's brother had additional domestic issues in his various lodgings close to the university: "In the first I remained only twenty-four hours, having been driven from them by bugs—one restless night sufficed." An annual allowance of £100 covered all John Davy's expenses, including tuition and board.[27]

Hard-studying Browne's daily routine was exacting:

> I get up as soon as it is light in the morning, gets breakfast, goes to the desecting room and stops there till 11 oClock and then attends Dr [John] Barclay on Anatomy and surgery from 11 to 12; attends the infermary from 12 to 1, the operating Room from 1 to 2; from 2 to 3 we have time to dine; from 3 to 4 I attend Dr Hamilton on Midwifery; from 4 to 7 I go to the College Liberary and reads; and then from 7 to 9 I go to the Hospital and write down Notes of different cases that happen to sick and lame people and then at 10 our people that we lodge with locks up the door and in general I write to near 12 oClock and sometimes later. . . . When we have nothing else to do we go and buy a sheeps head and desects it Brains and Eyes for they are the same as a Christians.[28]

Silliman corroborated less colorfully that he studied at least twelve hours a day, starting at 9 a.m. with two lectures, private study followed by a materia medica lecture at three, dinner at four, an anatomy lecture at six o'clock, tea at seven, a chemistry and mineralogy lecture until nine, "then I have three hours at my books and pen, and my rule is to stop at midnight, but not unfrequently I am up till one o'clock A.M."[29]

Edinburgh Societies and Institutions

Although a mere student, James could socialize with professional men at Edinburgh's broad range of clubs and societies. There were the elite scientific Royal Society of Edinburgh and the medical Harveian Society, as well as several serious student societies where members emulated the professionals, researching, writing, lecturing, and debating. Because the professors actively encouraged and occasionally attended these student societies, James could meet his otherwise remote teachers. At the meetings of these long-established prestigious societies, members read their essays and debated them into the night. As to the topics, unlike at the strictly controlled English and Continental universities, Edinburgh students were free to discuss whatever they wanted; their discussions were wide-ranging, often disputatious, and based on dialectic supported by evidence.[30] A few ephemeral student societies were occasionally somewhat daring. James immediately joined the most prestigious, exclusive, costly, exacting, and academically beneficial Royal Medical Society of Edinburgh.

Aside from attending lectures and society meetings, James could take advantage of the College of Surgeons' gradually expanding anatomical museum. There was a similar one at the university developed to supply preparations to illustrate the professors' lectures, access to fresh cadavers being limited and confined to the dissection rooms rather than the professors' lecture halls. Another valuable resource was the Old Town Dispensary, where innovative smallpox vaccination and other public health initiatives could be observed. Thanks to the Vaccine Institute established in 1801, by 1806 smallpox was rare in Edinburgh. With the later New Town Dispensary, the synergies among Edinburgh civic and educational institutions had a major impact on public health policy and knowledge, something Prichard would advocate in Bristol. For personal reasons, he was interested in vaccination, and he hoped to study mental illness in the Institutes of Medicine course. Edinburgh's Bedlam was inadequate; although Professor Duncan Sr. had started a campaign to establish a proper medically based lunatic asylum as early as 1792, it was not accomplished until James's last year in Edinburgh. His exposure to psychiatric theory was limited to the famous mathematician and philosopher Dugald Stewart's course on moral philosophy.[31]

James's *Lernfreiheit*

Conveniently for James, the faculty's resistance to control from above and its disregard for the curriculum resulted in a sort of *lernfreiheit*, the freedom to devise one's own curriculum that prevailed in some Continental universities. The vast majority of medical students did not intend to take degrees anyway, and the courses were all come, all served. But to qualify for a medical degree James found there were some requirements. The statute translated from the Latin specified that "no one shall be admitted into the number of candidates unless he shall have, for the space of three years, studied, in this or some other university, Medicine and the branches comprized in it, to wit, *Anatomy and Surgery, Chemistry, Botany, Materia Medica, and Pharmacy, and the Theory and Practice of Medicine*, and unless he shall have attended the Clinical Lectures, given by the Professors of Medicine, on the cases in the Infirmary." So there were some required courses that James had to take.[32] There were fees to pay, as well.

"The first week went very hard with my money, having to pay for Anatomy, surgery, Midwifery, Dissecting, Door Keepers &c." complained a student who had spent almost £57 just to get settled. An unforeseen expense was "buying dead bodies to desect."[33] On October 30 James and his 702 fellow students paid their course fees, while they dealt with the Infirmary and extra-collegiate expenses as they arose. James had to deposit a guinea for each book he borrowed from the university library's extensive collection. His first session soon started, each course beginning with the history of the subject. While the anatomy lectures lasted at least an hour and a half, others were one hour every weekday, with occasional catch-up lectures on Saturdays. Following an early interruption by a week of religious observance, James's lectures resumed the second week of November 1805.

Medical students' access to the Infirmary and its mandatory clinical lectures greatly enhanced their educational experience. After a period observing hospital practice, as a clinical student James was put in charge of a number of patients; he learned how to examine them, draw up a case history, and prescribe accordingly when on his almost-daily 8 p.m. rounds of the wards. One student's surviving case book includes 853 meticulous pages. The clinical professor and physicians visited each patient's bedside, where they dictated to their students the cause, prognosis, and remedy in English and then prescribed in Latin. Depending on their medical philosophy, they might prescribe a "full diet," including wine, porter, or gin; the opposing therapeutics demanded venesection, blisters, cathartics, emetics, or sudorifics.[34] The actual clinical lectures, held at 5 p.m. on Tuesdays and Fridays, were formal affairs, conducted on the most interesting cases separated into special wards. The clerk filled registers with the faculty's dictated account of each case and its daily progress, later pored over by the students. For an annual fee of 3 guineas James had access to all of the Infirmary's patients.[35]

James attended overcrowded lectures and took voluminous notes, but his progress was unmonitored; he had oral and written examinations only in the final weeks of his third year. Otherwise, he had to demonstrate his talents to his professors on the clinical rounds, or they could judge his performance at Royal Medical Society student lectures and discussions. He might have consulted Uncle Lewis about which courses to attend and in which order, and the library had a new copy of J. Johnson's *A Guide for Gentlemen Studying Medicine at the University of Edinburgh* (London, 1792), in which Professor James Hamilton Jr. pseudonymously provided a wealth of advice and unabashed self-promotion. He stressed taking courses in a logical succession from the foundation subjects to the more advanced or optional ones. For example, one should delay taking the Practice of Physic course until those in anatomy, the institutes of medicine (physiology), pathology, materia medica, and pharmacy had been completed. He considered the clinical lectures hugely beneficial and the extra-collegiate courses less so. The author went on to outline each course and even supplied a recommended reading list. He disapproved of students' comparing their lecture notes with what they found in textbooks, and he advised registering for supplementary dissection classes to view anatomical details at close quarters. Alas, the fury of the "low people of Scotland" required these dissections to be quite private, and hundreds of students were forced to share not more than twenty cadavers per year. Midwifery (Hamilton's subject) was unfortunately an optional course. "Mr. Johnson" warned his young readers that left to their own devices, they might "be led astray into the inticing fields of fancy and speculation, while they ought to be attending to other objects."[36]

The first course James chose was the foundational and wildly popular subject of chemistry.[37] The reputation of Dr. Thomas Charles Hope, professor of chemistry and of chemical pharmacy, could not have been higher. The son of a Glasgow professor, he was so popular and effective a lecturer, James found himself one of 342 students crowded into his lecture hall, fascinated by Hope's performance. In five one-hour lectures a week for six months he made chemistry accessible in clear exposition, covering the history of chemistry and its uses to pharmacy and manufacturing, chemistry in nature, light, heat, pneumatics, gasses, the production of acids and alkalis, the properties of the thirty known metals, and the chemical doctrines of organic and inorganic chemistry.[38] Even bored later student Charles

Darwin admitted to a flicker of interest. Professor Hope was inspirational in his fearless quest for scientific truth. However, students had to resort to extra-collegiate lecturers and even set up clubs in order to conduct their own experiments.[39] Hope was also admired as an oral examiner for asking clear and direct questions delivered in good Latin. James doubtless appreciated his politeness and kindness, his advocacy of science in general, and his staunch defense of the supremacy of medical etiquette and the medical profession.[40] He repeated Hope's course in 1807.

As well as grinding away at his medical studies, during his first year at Edinburgh James borrowed many volumes of classical literature from the library and attended lectures in the faculty of arts. He particularly admired his professor of humanities. From humble background and benefiting from his country's liberal attitude toward education and the patronage of talented boys, Alexander Christison had become eminent in his field. He "made his appeal to the sense of character, which the perception of worth, and the desire of approbation, so powerfully awaken in the youthful bosom. . . . Everything was solid without show, and useful without ornament." Christison fathomed the talent and character of all of his students, encouraging and supporting those who sought knowledge. A dedicated scholar, abstemious and severe in the exact distribution of his time, his profound knowledge of the classics matched that of history, but he also widened his interest to science, society, and the need to anchor education with religious instruction. He was known for his "perpetual habits of intense thinking, from which he seemed to have little pleasure in relaxation, which to ordinary minds must have been a fatigue."[41] James marked Christison as his role model by dedicating his MD thesis to him.

"The Gathering Place of All Zealous Students"

Anybody who was anybody was a member of the Royal Medical Society (RMS). Even before James attended his first university lecture, he had organized his six nominations and petition to join it. The society's membership registers list most of the university's medical professors, many future illustrious names in science, medicine, and government, and several of James's future Bristol colleagues. He took full advantage of the social and complex academic structure of the prestigious, costly, and demanding society. John Davy testified to the benefits of membership:

> The Royal Medical Society was the gathering place of all zealous students. There alone they had an opportunity of distinguishing

themselves. I entered it the first season, and at its weekly meetings formed many valuable acquaintances, and some lasting friendships. During my last year I was one of its four Presidents, my friend Dr Richard Bright was another. The animation with which discussions on medical matters was carried on then, was, as I now think of it, marvellous. Beginning about 8 o'clock p.m. they were often protracted beyond midnight. They were doubtless very serviceable in calling forth talent and inciting to exertion, and the excellent library belonging to the society was of great use.[42]

Founded in 1734, the RMS functioned more like a general department of the Medical School than a society, with a paid staff and its own premises at 11 Surgeons' Square. Most of its members intended to become elite physicians, while the 5 guinea entrance fee, another one for drawing up the membership certificate, and costly annual subscription further limited it to well-off young men. In the year of James's election less than 10 percent of students graduated MD, while under 5 percent were elected to the RMS. Applicants were required to have either an MD or at least six months' study at a respectable medical school. Starting on October 25, James had his application displayed in the library for a week; the required affirmative vote by three-quarters of the membership was secured on November 1; and he solemnly signed the society's laws four days later. Behavior was strictly regulated: fines were imposed for absence from meetings, and transgressors risked ejection. RMS meetings took place on Saturdays at 6 p.m. during the winter, with a business meeting followed by a public one at which a dissertation was read and discussed or a philosophical question or aphorism debated.

Students spent a lot of time at the RMS, studying in its library of several thousand books, a chemistry laboratory, and a museum of specimens. They took copious notes at their lectures and spent their evenings writing them up, along with taking notes from textbooks they bought or borrowed. The medical, scientific, and philosophical topics of the day were thoroughly discussed in the society's meeting room. By contrast, Oxford and Cambridge clubs and societies were devoted mostly to eating and drinking.

New Ordinary Members had to present a dissertation and a commentary on a case history and aphorism. The RMS provided a list of suitable topics to be drawn by lot, although they could be negotiated later. A professional scribe copied and circulated the dissertation in advance of its author reading and defending it before a meeting of the society likely attended by members of the faculty. This ordeal transformed an Ordinary into an Extraordinary Member, exempt from further such performances and absentee fines. This served to prepare students for writing and defending their MD thesis, James's being a good example of this. Another example of the serious educational ethos of the society was the requirement that members present and comment on clinical cases seen on their hospital rounds.

Members of the RMS vied in showing off their knowledge and facility of expression to bring themselves to the attention of the professors in the audience. A good performance could lead to an offer of a career-building assistantship, provision of a testimony, or letter of introduction. Membership provided grounding in the proper decorum of a physician; elegance of manner and ability to write, debate, and discourse learnedly, wittily, and with perhaps just a dash of arrogance on a wide variety of topics were de rigueur. James was learning to socialize, give lectures, and cultivate his manners to fit himself to enter the homes of the elite in a professional capacity. He valued the RMS and for the rest of his life preserved his membership certificate with his most precious documents.[43]

Independence and Advice

James's correspondence with his father chronicles his life in Edinburgh and acquisition of some alarming views, as his father had dreaded. After a short break on Christmas and New Year's Day, he began 1806 with customary diligence. Yet his letters seemed to bear the tone of a young man with new ideas and opinions to express, drawing Thomas Prichard's admonition. His son's spiritual welfare was at stake and he pulled no punches:

> I keep my belief as a Quaker, like a stronghold from which I would not be driven, for a thousand worlds [meaning the belief in immediate revelations in the present time] and I can venture to predict that if thou shouldst unfortunately take it into thy head to beat the bush for another way to happiness, the search will be vain, and thou will be glad to return to the way of thy ancestors. But I make great allowances for the cheerfulness of youth. . . . [I have] an affecting piece of intelligence, Chas Trusted Junr is very suddenly taken off by scarlet fever. He was at meeting on first day—complained on 3rd day morning of sore throat and died this morning. He has been visiting us once or twice since Tommy was at home. Let this, my dear James, be a lesson of profit to thee and indeed to us all.[44]

So happiness cannot be found by questioning pure faith and James should beware that his life might be snatched away when in a perilous state of disbelief. James attempted to qualify his previous expressions but in vain; his father considered such speculations shallow and lacking the weight of respectability:

> Ross 24th of 3rd month 1806
>
> I am not sorry thou hast felt a little compunction for the sentiments expressed in thy last, on the subject of Inspiration. Yet I endeavoured to make such allowances as saved my mind from distress. Grant only that man stands in absolute need of Divine Inspiration and is at times mercifully favoured with it and then I can bear with thee, although a great deal of abuse is thrown on the weakness of human nature, though that is perhaps best avoided. However it is happily not in thy power to exclude all the respectable names of those who have held these doctrines among the weak past of our species. On the contrary by far the greater number of justly revered Philosophers and scientific men of all ages appear in the cause of Revealed Religion. On this side is all the weight of respectability: on the other the pertness of flippant wit, abused ridicule and incorrigible vanity. I don't yet despair of thee—a few more years, especially if they are not spent like the present, in the cave of Trophonius, will sober thee a little.[45]

To Friends and Anglicans alike, a much-debated issue of revealed religion was the degree or directness of divine participation in the creation of Scripture in its various forms. James had undoubtedly been dabbling in dangerous Scottish Enlightenment philosophy, as popularized in Professor Stewart's moral philosophy lectures, which he was apparently attending at this time. There were Establishment attempts at this time to suppress overt skepticism expressed in science. Thomas Prichard could only hope his son's flirtation with Edinburgh skepticism was a passing phase.

James then had the temerity to take issue with the religious politics of the Edinburgh Society of Friends. He had made a firm friendship with Irish fellow Quaker Thomas Hancock, and the two young men were defending an old Quaker friend of Thomas Prichard from interference by Edinburgh Friends. His father was doubtful: "I am quite at a loss to conjecture under what circumstances George Millar could be placed to require the assistance of such champions as thyself and Hancock."⁴⁶ Prichard got his tendency to sarcasm from his father.

This same letter contains reproof of other of James's abhorrent tendencies: wanderlust, extravagance, and immoderation: "I am always glad to see thee write in good spirits, but I think thy two last letters contain rather more than the just modicum of the spirit of adventure. Be assured I shall never give my consent to thy Constantinpolitan expedition nor to thy return from Edinburgh by water. Therefore pray save money enough to pay thy way home by land. But enough in anticipation of thy return. Be assured we shall be glad to see thee and also very glad to entertain thy friend Hancock in the best manner we can."⁴⁷

Thomas Prichard was losing his grip on his son's mind even as he was beginning to show some respect for his medical knowledge; he asked him to recommend medical reference books for younger brother Tom, soon to be apprenticed to Bristol druggist Samuel Prichard. As for James's sad deterioration in faith, his father was a bit fed up: "I do not approve thy remarks on revelation—but I assure thee my housekeeper is no preacher. Pray don't talk of Freemasonry."⁴⁸

A Second-Year Student

Following a summer holiday back in Ross with his brothers and Thomas Hancock, James was Edinburgh bound again, this time breaking his journey in York to visit the famous Quaker lunatic asylum The Retreat. Only in its eleventh year, its reputation was already widespread; founder William Tuke was pioneering an innovative form of treatment based on the Quaker principles of compassion, respect, self-control, and recent Continental practice. James was able to reflect on this "moral treatment" (behavioral management) of the insane in the light of the subject as covered in his moral philosophy course. His father was keen to know James's opinion of The Retreat, being acquainted with its matron and one of the patients. It would not be Prichard's last visit to an asylum.

That autumn of 1806, James gained a Bristolian as a fellow medical student. John Bishop Estlin, son of the liberal, influential Bristol Unitarian minister John Prior Estlin, joined the RMS.⁴⁹ Thomas Prichard's reproving letters kept raining in as university course registration day approached. Nor was life in Edinburgh completely safe; in October Benjamin Browne reported that "a young Man was murdered, a Clarck to the Custom house at Lieth about a Mille from Edinburgh. He was going into the office and a man stabed him. He had with him £5000. There is a 500 Guineas reward."

Finding his lodgings unacceptable, James moved to the furnished ones of a Miss Fowlis at 15 Drummond Street.⁵⁰ His wanderlust was unabated, much to his father's regret:

> Ross 22 of 12 month 1806
>
> Thy last letter gave me a little surprize but I found its contents consolotary, and I hope thy removal will be an addition to thy comfort, but I think thou wilt also find it an addition to thy expenses. I do not feel myself capable of entering into the scheme thou hast unfolded of running over the North of Britain. My mind seems to have lost much of its elasticity lately. I believe I have carried into somewhat advanced years (my father was about 45 at this time) "the hope flushed enterer on the stage of life[.]" Therefore if what I lose in delight I can gain in repose, I must be content, not forgetting, when the infelicities of life press upon me "Dabet Deus his quoque fineum!"
>
> If thou wishest thy Uncle Lewis' advice respecting Hamilton, ask it in a latin letter.⁵¹

James decided to take the obstetrics course and with his friend Renn Hamden registered for Dr. James Gregory's all-important Practice of Medicine on November 21, 1806.⁵² Gregory, son of Professor John Gregory, was socially and medically well connected with the first names in science and among the aristocracy. His authoritative *Conspectus medicinae theoreticae*, a model of elegant classical latinity, was a standard textbook in Britain and Germany. In his dignified, eloquent, and captivating lectures he described the nature, symptoms, and treatment of diseases, following the nosology of his renowned predecessor William Cullen. So popular were his clinical lectures, some of the students in the packed ward had to perform the part of "repeaters," relaying Dr. Gregory's pronouncements to the more distant students. Sir Astley Cooper later reflected, "I do not think I acquired such substantial knowledge of practical medicine anywhere as from Dr. Gregory's clinical lectures."⁵³

Constantly feuding with his colleagues, Dr. Gregory "would not give up his point in argument, and would overwhelm his opponents with quotations, jests and satire." His celebrity as a medical theoretician was such that the term "Gregorian physic" was applied to the widespread practice of heroic bloodletting, cold affusions, brisk purging, frequent blistering, and the use of emetics. "His measures for the cure of disease were sharp and incisive.

In acute diseases there was no *medicine expectante* for Gregory. He somehow left us with the impression that we were to be masters over nature," wrote one of his former students. Gregory's initial literary, metaphysical, and philological education colored his impressive, well-illustrated lectures, attracting James's respect.[54] He became a lifelong adherent of Gregorian physic, publishing on the subject and promoting it even after it had started falling from fashion. Further, Gregory's 1805 reprint of his father's *Lectures on the Duties and Qualifications of a Physician* asserts the superiority of physicians—another view that Prichard would hold dear.[55] Gregory influenced his choice of medical therapeutics as much as Christison influenced his character.

James was among the nearly 250 students attending the course in obstetrics in the autumn of 1806, but he skipped its clinical lectures as he had apparently acquired practical experience in midwifery at Dr. Pole's. The lectures were divided into four parts: pregnancy, labor, child-bed, and the diseases of infants and children. In special sessions after hours, labor was helpfully illustrated using plaster casts and machinery imitating women and infants. Professor James Hamilton was the son of the previous professor of obstetrics and descendant of a great many other Scottish professors. He and his father founded a lying-in hospital for the poor where his students could gain experience, and he published respected textbooks and devised beneficial apparatus and procedures. "Summer and winter, fair day and foul, was Dr. Hamilton to be seen stepping along, with his thin-soled shoes, ornamented with large buckles, his black silk stockings, his formal, square-cut coat, and his redoubtable cocked hat—the whole in exquisite keeping with his upright elastic gait, and his expression of mingled shrewdness and eccentricity. He was the *beau ideal* of a physician of the last century."[56] Just as legendary as his obstetric knowledge was his permanent state of war with his colleagues.

At the turn of 1807, severe storms blew down trees and tiles from Edinburgh's roofs, killing three or four people in the streets. On the positive side as far as the medical students were concerned, a public hanging of a husband murderer and two horse thieves furnished some badly needed fresh corpses to dissect. Medical politics occupied the university's Senatus meetings, where there was stiff opposition to the medical reforms urged by some London physicians. As James continued his studies, his father's family news and reproofs also continued. His son's boasting and outrageous plans for the following summer appalled him. About the detestable French, however, they were in accord:

> There can be but one opinion in England and Scotland respecting the present state of Europe, and that is that peace is banished for the term of Buonaparte's natural life. However I do not think with thee on the subject of Russia. It is impossible from the situation of that country that its enmity can be so dangerous to us as that of France. Besides its commercial connections with England will always weigh in favour of alliance. However, savage may be the warriors of Russia, they are surely opposed to savages of still more detestable character. I wish thou wouldst read the life of Tallyrand in 2 vols 8vo I grant sufficient latitude for the opinions of the author, but the book interests amazingly, & that the public character of the hero is too true Bertrand and Barruel testify. . . . Enough of Frenchmen!
>
> Thy Grandmother has been very ill, one of her faithful maidens has brought forth a fine thumping boy. I profess to refrain from going to her house till she has dismissed Maria, for she is the Mother, but I shall not wonder if she keeps her long enough to bring her half a dozen such mamots.
>
> I hope thy ardour for Mathematics and natural philosophy will not prove them to be a knowledge that puffeth up. Surely it were to be wished that science were to be preserved from that perversion that too generally pervades almost all the gifts of heaven, when put into the hands of men, let it know its genuine effect humility—I shall certainly not insist on thy staying the summer at Edinburgh. This might possibly bring on me too heavy a responsibility, but I confess, I think of London and the employment thou hast mentioned with horror. However I hope not to anticipate evils.[57]

Instead of praising his son for diligently studying mathematics and natural philosophy and possibly spending the summer getting a bit of extra practice at a London anatomy school, Thomas Prichard lectured him on the evils of pride. His wariness of Edinburgh's skepticism and irreligion was understandable; after all, James's physics teacher was John Playfair, a minister in the Church of Scotland, former professor of mathematics, and member of the late Scottish Enlightenment group that included Adam Smith, Dugald Stewart, and Joseph Black. The very thought of Playfair, clarifier and promulgator of his friend James Hutton's geological theory, alarmed Thomas.

James continued honing his mathematical skills and looking for opportunities to learn more about Celtic history and languages. In July 1807 the Highland Society petitioned the University Senatus to institute Celtic studies. Although the university voted to propose the establishment of a Regius Professorship of Celtic Literature and Celtic and British Antiquities to the governing Town Council, the project foundered.[58] Had any courses on Celtic been offered, James certainly would have been the first student to register. Instead, as his final year at Edinburgh started, he had dissertations to write, presentations to make, and exams to face.

The Final Year at Edinburgh

James chose to repeat the anatomy and surgery course in the autumn of 1807 and obtain a certificate of attendance in order to qualify for his degree. Like the chemistry course, it was advisable to complete it early, when a student was "Prael. Clin" (pre-clinical).[59] The first part was taught by Professors Monro Secundus and Tertius, while a Mr. Fyfe delivered practical anatomy lectures and demonstrations under their supervision. The infamously indolent, eccentric, slovenly, indifferent, dull, digressive, and utterly disgusting Tertius lectured directly from his grandfather's notes, ignoring subsequent discoveries, Charles Darwin would later recall.[60] Monro Tertius is best remembered for holding back the progress of surgical education at the university for decades by tenaciously monopolizing its teaching and stressing the perfection of form and function in anatomy, an outmoded natural theological approach that suited the Edinburgh intelligentsia and physicians, but not so surgeons who needed practical anatomical knowledge to continue their progress in taking from physicians responsibility for internal bodily conditions.[61] James attended his lectures on anatomical structure and function, the diseased and injured states of the organs, treatments, all ordinary surgical operations, physiology, and comparative anatomy, illustrated with well-prepared specimens.[62] Tertius's incompetence fostered the popularity of the brilliant extra-collegiate anatomy teacher John Barclay's more successful course of lectures and dissections held every winter session, in nearby Surgeons' Square. His more modern Continental approach was founded on the "transcendental" doctrine of underlying unity within diversity of form. And he was much more generous in his provision of corpses.[63]

Ancient humoral theory had long held sway, but more recently some Continental theorists had attempted to formulate a monumentally new theory of medicine by which "the animal economy" (physiology) could be understood, diseases could be classified, and cures devised. They brought mathematics and metaphysics into their theories; Boerhaavian medicine was thought useful for a time, while the simplicity of Scottish Brunonian theory was attractive. At the start of the nineteenth century, Edinburgh medical theory was in disarray, with the professors combining a variety of often conflicting ideas.[64] The Scots' native distrust of empty theorizing led them to turn to the collection and arrangement of evidence from which theory was expected to emerge. A collector and arranger of evidence par excellence was Andrew Duncan, and it was evident in his teaching. James registered for his Practice of Physic course at the start of his last academic year.

Son of a St. Andrews merchant, Dr. Duncan studied medicine at Edinburgh, founded the charity Edinburgh Lunatic Asylum, published on therapeutics, and became professor of the theory of medicine (physiology) in 1790. His well-researched lectures were clear and candid.[65] He was erudite, organized, and industrious, if not a brilliant lecturer and a bit eccentric. Unencumbered by constraining theories, Professor Duncan's course started with pathological physiology and systematically described the fifteen fluids of the body, the vessels and organs and all solid parts such as the vascular, digestive, and reproductive systems, and there were many examples of their treatment. His book advocating heroic therapeutics for typhus reinforced James's belief in Gregorian physic. Prichard would mark his appreciation of his former professor in a fulsome testimonial on behalf of Duncan Jr.'s candidacy for the chair of materia medica.[66]

James studied botany and materia medica separately. He took Professor Daniel Rutherford's botany course in the spring of 1808 and would later apply what he had learned to considering the global distribution of plants and animals in his *Physical History*. Dr. Rutherford, son of an Edinburgh professor and an Infirmary physician, was a chemist at heart, publishing on that subject and inventing chemical apparatuses. His lectures were clear and praised for being full of condensed information delivered with barely a Scottish accent. Rutherford did not take his students on field trips, but under his superintendence the Botanical Gardens became one of the best in the world.[67] James's last course, materia medica, was taught daily at 8 a.m. by James Home, son of Professor Francis Home. It comprised pharmacology, dietetics, pharmacy, and the art of prescription, topics Home related to aspects of natural history, therapeutics, and the practice of physic, as his focus was on the practical application of medicines as opposed to the precise chemical understanding of them.[68]

James's raptures over being in Edinburgh seemed less about studying medicine under the guidance of these illustrious professors and more about attending courses among the university's other departments. Professor of Moral Philosophy Dugald Stewart's lectures on ethics, political philosophy, and the theory of government were famous.[69] His *Elements of the Philosophy of the Human Mind* deals with three matters that Prichard later explored: abnormal psychology, the therapeutics of mesmerism, and mass psychology. Stewart's research and contributions to original thought influenced Prichard's later scientific practice.

One of Professor Robert Jameson's natural history lectures inspired James's choice of the natural history of humankind as the topic of his dissertation. Jameson had enjoyed his childhood roaming of the Leith shoreline collecting and preserving plants and animals, and he later made a reputation for himself collecting and publishing on minerals. His time as a student of geologist Abraham Gottlob Werner instilled in him the value of scientific method based on systematically collecting, recording, and analyzing data, directly engaging with the actual materials of nature. Jameson, a deeply learned, diligent, and painstaking observer, was a desperately dull lecturer with a weak voice, serious manner, and disdain for colleagues' showmanship. One student likened his lectures to having a table of contents read aloud for an hour.[70] Jameson's earnest search for greater scientific truths inspired his many students to study natural history in all its forms. In this period before much differentiation among the sciences, his natural history course comprised mineralogy, geology, botany, zoology, meteorology, and hydrography, all concerned with the careful collection of facts from which conclusions are derived. Prichard adopted this fundamental tenet of the developing Scientific Revolution, starting with his inaugural dissertation for the Royal Medical Society.[71]

Remarkably for the time, Jameson was an educator who stepped outside the lecture hall to engage with students, inviting them to tea and examining fossil and mineral specimens with them at the University Museum. He was one of the earliest providers of field trips, conducting expeditions in the countryside around Edinburgh and even into the Western Isles. On his regular Saturday expeditions he made the personal acquaintance of every participant who displayed interest in natural history. Friendships arose that led to voluminous correspondence on scientific matters. His field trips were novel and memorable:

> Well do we remember his slender and wiry form erect on the summit of Arthur's Seat, his right hand grasping a hammer, and the crags and grassy spots around him covered with an admiring audience of

enthusiastic students, among whom might be seen often veterans of distinguished eminence and rising celebrities from all parts of the world. Then in perspicuous language he would expatiate on the structure of the beautiful and curious hill upon which he stood, and of the country far and wide spread out like a map before him. To those who heard him, that which at first seemed but a beautiful prospect, soon became a great geological chart and an index to the structure of the whole world.[72]

Enduring one of Jameson's field trips would make student Darwin vow never to study geology. James, by contrast, was inspired; he longed to roam over Scotland replicating his professor's expeditions. Some of his earliest publications were based on geological expeditions in Wales, and for some time he remained Jameson's anti-Huttonian ally. While Jameson helped amass a museum collection of minerals and fossils, advocating "first-hand contact with the materials of science," and coedited the *Edinburgh Philosophical Journal*, his greatest production was the many naturalists like Prichard he helped to form and encourage to publish, even when he did not agree with their findings.[73]

Training in Science at the RMS and Azygotic Club

James was not content with just learning about science; he wanted to become a scientist. So not only did he read extensively and attend lectures during his final year at university, but he threw himself into to the activities of the RMS and the private Azygotic Club, gaining experience central to his training as a scientist.

Public speaking was never his strong point, even after attending so many of his fellow RMS members' presentations. At the start of his third year of membership, it was time for him to get to grips with performing in public and fulfill his obligation. The case history topic he drew by lot was "virulent gonorrhoea," particularly appropriate considering how many of the Infirmary beds were occupied by war veterans. As luck would have it, "*cachexia syphloidia*" was the subject of his main RMS presentation, but no doubt feeling he was being made to do more research into venereal disease than was needed for the gentlefolk of Bristol, he traded it for another topic—one that had long been occupying his attention. He was allowed to have "What is the most rational theory of the varieties of the human race?" He researched it thoroughly, as a friend recalled: "His favourite topic was a frequent subject of discussion in a private debating society called the Azygotic. It consisted of six members, Charles and Patrick Mackenzie, Hampden, Estlin, Prichard and Arnould. We met at each other's houses one evening in the week for literary, scientific, and philosophical discussion. On the night of Prichard's paper, which was the basis of his thesis for his doctor's degree, we had a very long, animated, and interesting debate."[74]

James was ready for the RMS. His "Of the Varieties of the Human Race," presented on November 6, 1807, must have made for a very long meeting, as the text occupies forty-seven large manuscript pages in one of the society's volumes. It was followed by a discussion among the audience of members and visitors. His case history presentation on gonorrhea the following week was comparatively straightforward. Now an Extraordinary Member, during the 1808 session he was given the case "Hydrophobia" and the question "What are the moral and physical causes which produce difference of national character?"[75]

With these challenging public performances out of the way, James still regularly attended the RMS meetings and occasionally introduced a guest. He also continued his involvement in the day-to-day activities of the society. A member of the library committee, he reported on the society's acquisitions. He also joined the Apparatus Committee, where his friend Joseph Arnould was tasked with purchasing equipment for conducting the chemistry experiments its members were so keen on.[76] Now a senior member of the society with his university final examinations just a fortnight away, he joined the committee that chose topics for members' dissertations and questions. Not everything at the RMS ran amicably. James and his friends John Estlin and Renn Hamden got embroiled in a dispute over a rule depriving Extraordinary Members of more than two years the right to vote for the presidents of the society, bringing down a storm of protests and legal threats.[77]

The RMS's impact on James and his fellow members was considerable, and their loyalty strong, with one member reminiscing that membership benefited him more than his university lectures. The titles and content of its dissertations justify the society's reputation for openly debating general scientific and philosophical issues based on Scottish Enlightenment themes that were occasionally disputatious, challenging of authority, and dangerously skeptical in tone. Some of the first public discussions of groundbreaking theories in medicine and the natural and physical sciences were first aired there.[78] For James personally the RMS was invaluable; his "Of the Varieties" was the first draft of his MD dissertation submitted five months later, and its grueling public defense at the RMS trained him to survive his impending oral examinations.

RMS and Azygotic Club Friendships

Edinburgh brought James lifelong friendships. He and Thomas Hancock remained close, sharing some similar interests while differing in attitude, politics, and personality. Hancock, two years his senior, settled in the Quaker district of Finsbury Square, London, became an LRCP (licentiate of the Royal College of Physicians), joined professional organizations, and volunteered at and funded a host of mostly medical charities, such as the Finsbury Dispensary and the Guardian Society for the Preservation of Public Morals. He studied mental illness and epidemic diseases, but unlike Prichard, he was an active campaigner for asylum reform, the welfare of the poor, pacifism, and the abolition of the death penalty. Again unlike Prichard, Hancock was an orthodox Quaker and an elder of the sect.[79]

Dr. Hancock's publications were as various as his interests. In a series of articles in the *Belfast Monthly Magazine,* the young campaigner indirectly referred to the holiday of 1806 spent with Prichard during which they visited The Retreat and Dr. Fox's asylum near Bristol. Impressed by The Retreat's "moral treatment," he contrasted it with the less effective regimes found in public asylums, and called for Ireland to establish public asylums too. This was the first of his many sallies in the social reform revolution of the era. His *Researches into the Laws and Phenomena of Pestilence* (1821) referred to Prichard's evidence as to the contagious nature of typhus and erysipelas, and his *Laws and Progress of the Epidemic Cholera* (1832) is one of the Prichard family volumes donated to the Bristol Medical Library. After he published the *Principles of Peace* (1825), gaining Thomas Prichard's regard, Hancock began corresponding with the American reformer Samuel Joseph May on the topic of pacifism. Prichard's volume on nervous diseases refers to Hancock's *Essay on Instinct*. They remained friends, meeting on occasions such as a lecture at the Royal Society in 1829 and the 1835 British Association for the Advancement of Science meeting in Dublin. He was still paying visits to Prichard in the 1840s. Having retired to his native Lisburn, where he continued active in Quaker affairs and charities, Hancock died in 1849.[80]

John Estlin did not intend to gain an MD; instead he set up practice as a surgeon and ophthalmologist in Bristol and became Prichard's brother-in-law and closest friend.[81] Nearly four decades after leaving Edinburgh Prichard spent several days at Whitecross in Wallingford, Oxfordshire, with pillar of the community Joseph Arnould. Dr. Arnould originally practiced medicine in Camberwell, but by 1840 he was a magistrate and holding various other influential appointments, distinguished for his strict attention to duties impartially discharged.[82]

Renn Hamden's career could not have been more different. He dedicated his thesis to his father, John, a Barbadian planter. Dr. Hamden inherited three plantations in 1812 and was a prominent member of the Council of Barbados, where he gained notoriety and a place in the history of the island by publishing his council speech vigorously defending the institution of slavery and asserting the folly of banning the flogging of enslaved women. Returning to England, he failed to win the Lyme Regis seat at the parliamentary election of 1837 after a pamphlet labeled him a "woman flogger," but he later sat for Great Marlow as a Conservative until his retirement in 1847. Eventually, he returned to his debt-encumbered estates in Barbados and died on May 8, 1852.[83]

In Charles and Patrick Mackenzie, James associated with two young men who, like Renn, had lived abroad, an element of the exotic that was so attractive. Their Scottish lawyer father, Kenneth Francis Mackenzie, became acting governor of Grenada, owned three plantations in Demerara, and eventually retired to Wales and supported a charity called the Society for the Conversion and Religious Instruction and Education of the Negro Slaves in the British West India Islands. Prichard gave a copy of his MD dissertation to Mr. Mackenzie.[84]

Charles Mackenzie never lived in one place for very long. In London he began publishing articles on the geology of Scotland and failed to obtain a post as secretary on an ambassadorial mission to Constantinople. He became a member of the Wernerian, Linnean, Geological, and Royal Societies before leaving Britain for Haiti, where he was consul and then consul-general from 1823 to 1828. While there he contributed several articles to *Encyclopaedia Britannica*, mostly on botany and vegetable physiology. He handsomely dedicated his *Notes on Haiti, Made during a Residence in That Republic* (1830) to Prichard: "first to gratify my personal affections, and, secondly, to associate my name with that of a man whose profound research and accuracy of thought give him a high rank in the literature of the world. The largest portion of both our lives has passed away since it was my pride to be considered your friend; and it is now a subject of gratification, that neither separation nor diversity of pursuit has impaired our original feelings." After Havana, Charles Mackenzie practiced medicine, ran up some debts, and wrote for the Conservative newspapers in London until the 1850s, finally perishing in a New York hotel fire in 1862.⁸⁵

Charles's younger brother Patrick's *Practical Observations on the Medical Powers of Mineral Waters* advocated using mineral waters to treat a host of diseases, and he was as keen as Dr. Prichard on the extensive use of purgatives. He became assistant physician to the Institution for the Cure and Prevention of Contagious Fevers in the Metropolis, London, and died there three years later.⁸⁶ Prichard's Azygotic Club friends certainly had varying histories.

Final Exams, Spring 1808

His son's release from a corrupting university in the inclement North could not come soon enough, Thomas Prichard told a friend.⁸⁷ He expected James to stop dabbling in unorthodox beliefs and start writing up his dissertation on the unity of the human species. Toward the end of March 1808 James submitted an extended Latin translation of the RMS dissertation titled *De generis humani varietate* to the university. According to the rules, the most junior professor read, signed, and passed it on to the rest of the medical faculty for consideration. A series of examinations ensued.

While his friends Joseph Arnould and Renn Hamden were undergoing their ordeal at Dr. Gregory's, James's first and most important examination was taking place at Professor Monro's home on April 14. He was questioned by the six "facultas medica," with Dr. Monro taking the lead, starting with the circulation of the blood: "Mr Pritchard was examined De Sc / De Cord Fam et artm. / De Intestinis / De Entorit. / Hernia Ing. / Hydrary / ejus ppts. / Dyspepsia. Admitted."⁸⁸ That was that. It had lasted about an hour and included many questions on other topics such as the structure and physiology of the muscles, the symptoms and cure of various diseases, chemistry, and one requiring an example of "depraved sense of feeling."⁸⁹ A near contemporary, Henry Holland, considered himself unlucky in being sent to Dr. Monro's:

> I am to expect to be first questioned by young Monro; the old man being now utterly incapable of attending in cases of this nature. Young Monro, though deficient both in abilities & acquirements, has nevertheless contrived, by dint of hard application, to acquire a very minute knowledge, on a few particular points of natural & Morbid Anatomy— and these subjects he takes care to introduce whenever there is an opportunity. . . . This I should less regard, were he only to occupy

the same proportion of time as the other Professors; but it invariably the practice for the one who opens the examination, to continue his questions for ½ an hour—sometimes even during a still longer time. This of course will afford him the oppy of being very severe upon me, if he is so inclined. I have reason, however, to expect every thing that is fair & impartial both from him, & from all the other Professors.[90]

James's glad tidings of initial exam success were met with a lecture typical of his father:

My dear James. I have received thy letter of the 15th Instant which informs me that thou hast passed thy examinations. I am glad of this because I shall rejoice when the necessity of thy being at such a dreadful distance from us is at an end, and yet I confess I know not what may be real source for joy or what for grief: whether it is what thou art now, or what thou mayest in future be. This thou wilt think an odd sentiment: perhaps the sentiment of a fanatic. Be it so.—I hope I shall never more esteem any thing a real good that does not fix the hopes on the great concerns of a future life; rather than on the passing events of this. . . .

Thy Uncle and Aunt Fisher will be in Edinburgh sometime in the 6th month. Be sure to show them every thing worthy of their attention.[91]

On May 18 two professors grilled James in the presence of the entire faculty with questions based on the content of his courses, but there was actually not much to fear. "The public examn, which closes the whole business has relation to the Thesis, and is conducted with much form—but in point of fact the 1st private examn decides everything—and this is so completely understood that the day following it, the Dean of the university takes the [£13] graduation fees from each candidate."[92] James was then set an aphorism by Hippocrates on which an oral commentary was required, followed by a medical question demanding a properly argued answer. This was on May 30. On June 15 came the defense of his two written histories of diseases with appended questions, an examination generally considered quite reasonable. On the same day, the by now weary candidate had to submit six copies of his published dissertation without title pages to the dean for the faculty's approval. The final trial, entirely in Latin,[93] was on graduation day, June 24, 1808: "At a meeting of the University in the Library . . . after prayer by the Principal Thirty Seven Candidates for the Degree of Doctor of Medicine who had previously undergone their private Trials with the approbation of the Medical Faculty were now examined publicly by the Professors of Medicine on their printed Inaugural Dissertations, and being found duly qualified the said Degree was conferred on them with the usual solemnity."[94]

Henry Holland thought the Senatus Academicus's final public examination was little better than a farce; some candidates did not even attempt to answer the questions: "After each candidate had been examined for a few minutes, a sort of oath as to their future good behaviour was read, & signed by them all—& then after a few insignificant forms, the Principal put a black cap severally upon their heads, & dismissed the assemblage."[95] Dr. Prichard did not sign the oath recorded in the "Laureations & Degrees, 1585 to 1809." Instead, on a page set aside for the signatures of Dissenters is his name, dated June 24, 1808.[96] His was one of ten MDs awarded to Englishmen in Edinburgh that year, and the only dissertation unconnected with medicine.[97]

Ready to leave Edinburgh and thinking more of scholarly pursuits than practicing medicine, fledgling Dr. Prichard found his path daunting. His fellow Edinburgh MD Henry Holland had his doubts: "Doctors of Medicine are thus sent out to try their fortunes in the world; among which number I could mention some 6 or 8, to whom I should be sorry at present to trust the cure of a sore-throat, in the case either of myself, or of any one whose health I value."[98] The medical profession was rife with politics and contradictory theories and practices.

James had set out for Edinburgh a deferential son and left it a physician who could command the respect of his father and society in general. He had associated with intellectuals, developed valuable skills in scientific research, composition, and argument, and learned and adopted the form of medical therapeutics he would use in his medical and psychiatric practice. His clinical experience at the Edinburgh Infirmary prepared him to deal with his future patients and medical colleagues confidently. He was also influenced by his nonmedical professors Christison, Jameson, and Stewart, made several lasting friendships, had some adventures, traveled independently, and acquired a kinship with any fellow MD, Edin. He had, moreover, been free to entertain new views on the natural world and religion, although he left, as he had arrived, a member of the Society of Friends. His medical education was complete, but not his spiritual journey. Dr. Prichard was in no hurry to hang out his shingle.

Transition, 1808–10

Languishing in Ross that summer of 1808 and sorely in need of his son's support, Thomas Prichard was counting the days until his arrival. Residual involvement with his erstwhile business partners, the Harfords, had been dragging on for nearly eight years. Despite his complaints and resolutions, compromises had always been found. Now he had had enough. Harford's had been sustaining losses at home as well as those incurred owing to the ongoing war with France. It was hardly the best time for Thomas Prichard to set up a rival ironworks needing a capital of £100,000:[99]

> When I returned from Edinburgh [I found my father] much occupied with the two mercantile concerns in which my two brothers were to be engaged. He was planning with Joseph Reynolds, a son of Richard Reynolds the celebrated philanthropist, with whom he was connected by marriages between their families, a large iron company in which my brother Thomas was intended to take a principal management. My brother possessed talent of the highest order, but he and Richard Tomlinson who were to have acted together speedily disagreed. Tomlinson who was a relative of Blakemore & the confidential friend of Joseph Reynolds, got the better of my brother and my Father did not very decidedly support him, not knowing in reality on which side the fault lay. I believe they behaved harshly to him, but they had no intention of permanently superseding him in the management of the affairs of the concern. However he took umbrage against Tomlinson whom we regarded as his inferior, as he was infinitely in ability tho' not in attention to business.[100]

Younger brothers Tom and Edward could not settle down. Edward's situation with John Cross and Samuel Prichard's successful wholesale drugs business was insecure.[101] Even John Brent Cross and his sister Maggy's visit could not cheer Thomas Prichard. He fired off letter after letter to his friends along the lines of death, solitude, rewards in Heaven, and so on. In condoling with Mrs. Cross on the death of her insane husband the following December, he urged her "to reflect that his precious mind is now re-instated into a full capacity of adoring the author of his existence-perhaps of comprehending the dark mystery of that Providence that has led him thro' the paths of desolation: and that now in Glory liberated from the thraldom of an uncurable malady he is uniting in songs of praise with the spirits of all who have been redeemed thro' suffering."[102]

Prichard added to his father's anxiety with his scientific distractions, theological disputes, and reluctance to buckle down to medical practice. He resolved to take himself off to the University of Cambridge and its growing evangelical Anglican ferment. So traumatic were the following eighteen months that Prichard drew a veil over this period; in family records, lore, and in his obituary memoirs, it is unaccounted for.

Admitted pensioner at Trinity College, Cambridge, on October 13, 1808, Prichard matriculated Lent term 1809. There he had the elevated status and privileges of gentleman commoner, or fellow commoner, at higher tuition fees than those of commoners, or ordinary students without scholarships. "Commons," referring to dining and being eligible to dine with the college Fellows, was one such privilege. Cambridge, like Oxford, had well-established professorships in a variety of subjects, but their incumbents did not necessarily or regularly lecture or provide tuition. He could, however, attend what lectures there were and use the university's elegant and rapidly expanding library. He hardly needed access to the public tutors whose task was to translate from Greek and Latin. Evangelical fervor was then sweeping Cambridge, especially at his college, where his tutor, the Rev. John Hudson, was influential both in his piety and teaching of mathematics.[103] Oxbridge students lived in a communal setting and formed lasting social bonds. Their narrow and nonvocational curriculum comprised almost exclusively the classics, mathematics, and divinity. The tenets of the Church of England guided their studies, and there was little scope for more than casual exploration of other subjects, although there were already some stirrings of university educational reform to come. Prichard looked forward to steeping himself in these three subjects after all that medicine at Edinburgh; in later years his favorite pastime was reading, reciting, and translating from Greek, and he relied heavily upon the classical historians in his *Physical History*. Mathematics had a high profile at Cambridge, particularly in its degree examination, making it the possible source of Prichard's notable facility in it. The third subject, theology, would become central to his interests and future work.

Unlike most modern universities or, indeed, Edinburgh, Oxford and Cambridge were ecclesiastical institutions, dedicated to the interests of the Church of England. Chapel attendance was compulsory. Undergraduates swore allegiance to the Church and State, signing the Thirty-Nine Articles. This oath effectively excluded Dissenters from the university, although Cambridge permitted them to attend but not graduate. Almost two-thirds of loyal Anglican, Oxbridge graduates became Church of England clergymen. The universities were in full control of their own affairs, and their individual colleges made their own appointments, admissions, and development decisions, conforming to ancient university statutes. To these politically conservative and socially exclusive institutions, generations of the same families among the aristocracy, gentry, and clergy sent their sons to study at a cost beyond all but at least the upper middle class. The two English universities were not completely peaceful ivory towers, however.[104]

At such an elite institution, Prichard had the disadvantage of belonging to a minority—a graduate of "freethinking" Edinburgh and from a dissenting, commercial, and thus non-elite background. Studious Dr. Prichard must have found Oxbridge students' reputation for idleness and dissipation disappointing. In 1800, for instance, Oxford had found it expedient to pass a statute reforming and standardizing its examination rules to counter the criticism that it was possible to get a degree without actually doing any work. Sir James Stephen, a student at Trinity Hall in 1806, likened his time there to living in a pleasant hotel, a place that would have provided him with just as much intellectual discipline and knowledge as he had gained at Oxford. In 1807 another statute failed to address growing criticism of its narrow curriculum. Establishment Oxbridge attempted to defend their ancient curricula by insisting that the study of dead languages, mathematics, and religion was a form of mental training which matured the mind, preparing it to accomplish anything. They provided a beneficial atmosphere of discipline, order, method, and sustained application.[105]

Prichard decided to sample the atmosphere of Oxford. After several months at Cambridge, on June 3, 1809, he matriculated at St. John's College, but soon moved to more congenial Trinity College as a gentleman commoner.[106] During that summer holiday he returned to Bristol, where he resigned from the Society of Friends on August 4, 1809. On August 29, he presented himself at the ancient parish church of St. James, Bristol, for baptism into the Church of England by the Rev. Thomas Biddulph. The following month he was back at Oxford, a member of the Established Church.[107]

In later years friend, obituarist, and strict Quaker Thomas Hodgkin found himself reticent to press Prichard on his separation from the sect, nor in Prichard's personal papers could he find any reason for this monumental step. He could only stress that Prichard "retained in after life a most kind and amiable feeling and interest in relation to the Society and its members."[108] Prichard's family knew little about his time at Oxbridge and conversion to Anglicanism; nor did he discuss it in the memoir of his father, but nothing casts doubt upon the sincerity of his conversion.

Several factors would have contributed to this break with the faith of his ancestors. For one thing, individual Quakers had made a poor impression on his young mind. And as his childhood social circle had not been exclusively Quaker, he had been able to form close relationships with and admire members of the Church of England. His father had appeared to value evangelical fervor over sectarian loyalty, an example of which was his love of the Cross family, staunch members of the Church of England, while in Ross, he cooperated with the local Anglican parish priest on charitable projects and engaged him and other non-Quakers to tutor his sons. Prichard's childhood memories of Anglicans were positive: they were kind, modest, open, thoroughly respectable, pious, and loyal to king and country. Not so Quakers.

For all their pretentions to Christian piety, Quakers were suspect, as far as Prichard had experienced as a child. Take the interfering housekeeper Kitty Morgan, a posturing, hypocritical, secret inebriate, and stuff of childhood nightmares. Then there was the pretentious, repulsive, downright scandalous, treacherous American Quaker Hannah Barnard. The sect was rocked by schisms and scandals; apostates like Barnard and her ilk were making irreligious, materialist assertions. Membership was declining, and as for Quakers' place in society, even in their distinctive dress, speech, anti-oathtaking stance, and other controversial behavior they were uncomfortably ostentatious and demanding. Throughout Prichard's childhood, Quakers had come in for criticism, not only for their beliefs and behavior but for their involvement in reformist movements. During this period of long wars with the evil, revolution-tainted French, reformism implied criticism of civil society tantamount to disloyalty to king and country. Was not Thomas Prichard's erstwhile Quaker friend Benjamin Rotch suspected of being an atheist and known to have resided in revolutionary France? Amid national crisis and economic hardship, large, reactionary doses of distracting patriotism were the order of the day. This did not, however, stop Quakers from continuing to agitate for parliamentary, anti–slave trade, and other reforms as well as for their own civil rights. Unitarians, those other passionate reformers, were also and particularly loathed for more than just their supposed atheistic tendencies; famous Unitarian Joseph Priestly had been vilified for supporting the Americans during the Revolutionary War. So both reformism and Protestant dissent seemed to go hand-in-hand, associated with lack of patriotism.[109] Loyalist and conservative Prichard and his father generally avoided openly associating themselves with Quaker reformism and liberalism.

As for evidence of Prichard's mature sentiments toward Quakerism, he implied that his rejection of it had been on doctrinal grounds. He attributed his ancestors' original dissent from the Established Church to an excusable response to its corruption *at that time*, and his father's adherence to Quakerism sentimental. In other words, in the nineteenth century the integrity of the now-reformed Church of England rendered any continued dissent untenable. But that was not the whole story. At cosmopolitan, liberal Edinburgh, where Quakerism was in disarray, Prichard had been able to develop his own views and debate doctrinal issues, raising points that had alarmed and saddened his father. Doubts had set in even before Prichard left Edinburgh and entered those monuments of Anglicanism, the Universities of Cambridge and Oxford. For the rest of their lives father and son never stopped debating theological points such as the issue of divine inspiration and the need for a mediating priesthood. Prichard eventually implored his father to be baptized.

Prichard continued his Oxford studies until the summer of 1810. There had been few if any medical lectures to attend there, but his London friend Thomas Hancock did take him to a meeting of the Medical Society of London on December 5, 1809, also attended by his friend Dr. William Lawrence.[110] One of the last events of his Oxford career was the memorably lavish, four-day celebration marking the installation of Oxford's vice chancellor, the former Tory prime minister Lord Grenville. In the run-up to the ceremony the many carriages of the nobility pouring into the city caused traffic jams. On July 3 hundreds of ladies and gentlemen had to be turned away from the five-hour ceremony at the Radcliffe Camera. Processions, speeches, recitations, and awards of prizes and honorary degrees were complemented by days of religious services, ceremonies, and quite a few concerts, not to mention pioneering balloonist James Sadler's thrilling balloon ascent from Merton College. While all this was diverting, Prichard had his father's expectations weighing on him. In late July 1810 he settled in Bristol to earn his crust as a physician.[111]

Prichard had chosen to study medicine because it was the nearest thing to being a scientist. He might have deplored the Test Act that had barred him from obtaining an Oxbridge degree; on the contrary, as a member of the Established Church, he could not "imagine that it will ever be practicable to admit dissenters freely to the present Universities without completely subverting the system established and if at any time a great resort of such students to Oxford were to take place, you would have bands of Roman Catholic priests, and Unitarian & Independent ministers who would go to watch over their flocks & prevent them from being entered into the orthodox fold. I fancy that an interminable warfare would result."[112]

Having enjoyed a broad and varied education, Dr. Prichard turned his attention to establishing his medical practice and beginning scientific research in earnest. While the University of Edinburgh trained him to contribute to scientific knowledge, Oxford remained his intellectual home. Both stimulated a hunger for knowledge that he carried for the rest of his life.

4 · Citizen, Husband, Gentleman, Physician, and Scientist

Getting Established in Bristol, 1810–16

> I shall consider thy Anna and thyself as one and as claiming alike my affection and solicitude.
> —James Cowles Prichard, "Memoir of Thomas Prichard, Part 1"

Arriving in 1810 fresh from exciting Edinburgh and London and the academic luxury of Cambridge and Oxford, young Dr. Prichard would have preferred any of those places to "out of the way Bristol." Access to good libraries and opportunities to associate with like-minded men were what he longed for, but for professional advancement he needed to live in Bristol where his social connections would secure him a generous supply of rich patients. Aside from a few members of the library on King Street, learned men, their institutions, and opportunities to engage in science and scholarship were thin on the ground. Over the following thirty-five years Prichard would occasionally attempt to escape the city of his childhood by, for instance, applying for Oxford professorships. At least he knew Bristol well; his father still owned several properties there, his friends Estlin, Tothill, and Cross, and his brothers were all living there, and it was reasonably near his family home in Ross. As Dr. Prichard was financially dependent on his father, Thomas Prichard's wishes prevailed.

Bristol in the 1810s

Bristol's era of slave-trade-based wealth was long over. It had become a city of ill-fed laborers working in small factories, making products for distribution through its centrally located docks. The city's merchants were as famous for their charity and civility as their grasping commercial mindset, while local government was corrupt and self-serving. In a politically and economically volatile atmosphere and with little prospect of reform or improvement, Bristol's efforts at high culture, science, and scholarship were lackluster.

While Prichard was studying in Edinburgh, disadvantaged Bristolians were continuing their custom of rioting. In 1807 Radical Henry "Orator" Hunt was in his element; an incredibly handsome, charismatic, strident and popularist politician, he dared to campaign for annual parliamentary elections and universal suffrage, points that appealed to the disenfranchised while thoroughly disgusting local government, the Bristol Corporation, whose privileged members preferred the status quo. Not content with speechifying, Hunt established the reformist Bristol Patriotic and Constitutional Society, considered by Tories and Whigs alike just one step removed from French revolutionary insanity. That May, when Hunt's proposed parliamentary candidate was rejected, protests soon turned into riots, the MPs fled, and the Council House got its windows broken.[1] General shenanigans, excitement, corruption and violence continued to be a Bristol election tradition.

The year Prichard settled in Bristol, wartime blockades and successive poor domestic harvests led to huge inflation in food prices and semistarvation among the poor, sparking food riots. The April Assizes opened with a near riot at the arrival of the highly unpopular senior judge, Recorder Vicary Gibbs. Protestors showed their displeasure with the arrest in London of the reformer Sir Francis Burdett, MP, by breaking the Mansion House windows before proceeding to the Council House to do likewise.[2] At least glaziers were prospering. On the first of May, the costly engineering project the Floating Harbour was officially operational, but in financial, technical, and administrative disarray. The landscape surrounding the city was changing as well, the 1811 "enclosures" of common lands in Henbury and Westbury being just two of many such arbitrary transfers of property from public to private ownership. As for educational establishments, the charity Bristol Grammar School headmaster's post had become a nepotistic sinecure for aldermen's relatives who taught Greek and Latin to their private pupils while successfully excluding the city's poor boys.[3] The Hotwells health spa was dying as fast as its few visitors while opulent new homes were springing up in airy Clifton. But unattractive as Bristol appeared, it was the devil Prichard knew.

Year after year the Bristol Corporation took on more civic functions, such as cleansing and lighting the streets, fighting fires, providing a night watch, and administering prisons, the finance of which fell on householders. Overstaffed and nepotistic, local government was fond of staging a costly panoply of ceremonies involving parading and the purchasing of regalia. An example of its growing profligacy was its banquets, at one of which twenty guests managed to consume sixty-two bottles of sherry, port, hock, claret, and champagne.[4] The Corporation's reputation for avariciousness, unfairness, shortsightedness, and incompetence eroded its reputation among citizens of all classes. It seemed to set aside its obligation to foster the civic and economic welfare of the city as a whole, for instance, by failing to maintain law and order, vilifying migrants and the poor, and generally creating lasting animosity. Even calls for moderate reform were interpreted as threatened radicalism needing rooting out. Clever propaganda about the enemy French justified the harsh policing of rallies and prosecution of publishers and handlers of radical publications. By 1823 even some businessmen frustrated by Corporation inertia and greed formed a chamber of commerce to lobby for reform. Increasingly alienated from some of Bristol's reformist religious minorities and even some of its bourgeoisie, it became the butt of satire and negative contemporary histories.[5] Its reputation would be further tarnished when it bungled the famous Bristol Riot of 1831; rather than responding to its disaffected citizens' protest over political, religious, and other issues, the Corporation branded the rioters seditious revolutionaries.[6]

Political unrest and hardship led some poor, struggling Britons to take up American and French revolutionary ideals. The Establishment countered this by cultivating patriotism and piety, attempting to rehabilitate the dismal reputation of the monarchy and create new expressions of national culture. Everything British was aggrandized; patriotism was expressed in lavish national celebrations, ceremonies, displays such as tableaux, illuminations and the erection of triumphal arches and monumental statues, the painting of grand paintings, the composition of patriotic music and poetry, and so on. A prime example of these unifying expressions of loyalty was the king's lavish jubilee of 1809–10. The concurrent Evangelical Revival of religious fervor that fostered a trend toward doing good works to perfect society nicely complemented this ostentatious patriotism.[7] Prichard had also encountered the desire to "improve" society expressed in Scottish Enlightenment thought during his Edinburgh student years. It would motivate him throughout his life.

Bristol businessmen did attempt to reinvigorate manufacturing and trade. They were proud of the Exchange in Corn Street, the commercial heart of Bristol, but felt the addition of a coffee room would be conducive to prosperity. To this end they issued shares to finance the construction of the Bristol Commercial Rooms, a handsome, classically inspired veritable temple to commerce, complete with pedimented Ionic columns surmounted by statues personifying Bristol, Commerce, and Navigation, topped with an alto-relievo of Britannia with Neptune and Minerva receiving tributes from the four quarters of the globe. Opening soon after Prichard's arrival in the city, it demonstrated that the business of Bristol was business.[8] A few minutes' walk from the grandiosity of the Commercial Rooms, business was booming at the city's workhouse.

Looking the Part

The reluctant Bristolian found setting up as a physician costly. Prichard needed to reside in an affluent neighborhood, dress appropriately, subscribe to several rather costly charities, and engage in a good deal of socializing. He even joined the Commercial Rooms, where he could expect to come under the eye of the city's wealthy men, his uncle Fisher among them.[9] Nearly all of Bristol's eighteen physicians lived in the same neighborhood as their necessarily affluent patients. A Clifton house in 1810 typically cost 200 guineas a year, some taxes included. Taxation was an issue; instead of imposing income tax or property tax that would affect the more affluent, individual services were taxed, so that Prichard became responsible for separate land, window, security, pitch, light, sewer, and poor rates. The annual wages of a manservant were £35 and a woman cook £15, while meat was 6 to 8 pence a pound.[10] Householders shopped at the various specialist markets around the city held on particular days of the week, or more conveniently, any number of vendors of produce, bread, meat, fish, and butter would walk about the streets calling out their wares. In Napoleonic wartime Bristol, several staple foods such as bread, tea, and sugar were more than double the price they were sixty years later. Wheat, tea, and sugar were heavily taxed, as were windows and even cellar gratings, while newspapers were burdened with three separate paper, newspaper, and advertising duties that effectively put them beyond the budget of working people. The middle classes drank taxed port and sherry, two of Bristol's major imports.[11] Prichard's setting-up expenses were met by his father, while networking and developing a reputation were up to him. He rented a house in elevated and respectable Berkeley Square, Clifton, and set out his shingle.

Prichard needed to look the part. The powder tax had already relegated wigs to the attire of elderly gentlemen. Rather, as the young clean-shaven physician's silhouette shows, he wore his distinctively bushy hair cropped on top and with a short, tied queue. There had been recent great technical progress in the mechanization of textile and clothing production, leading to cheaper, lighter-weight, and more varied fabrics. His clothes would have been made by the artisan shopkeepers of Bristol, the more prosperous of whom invested in one of the newly invented stitching machines and advertised themselves in the local newspapers. Shops were usually open from 8 a.m. to 8 p.m., with dinner at 3, while office hours were 9 a.m. to 8 p.m.[12]

Prichard wrapped his fashionable, fine white starched cotton or linen stock several times around his neck and then knotted or tucked it in. His stand-up pointed collar was the era's equivalent of platform shoes in its extreme, stiff height, its little points protruding from his cheeks at nose level. "Bound in these fetters, the wearer could hardly turn his head to the right-hand or to the left, and the effect was a stiffness of manner, which added to his personal dignity, if not to his comfort," a fellow Bristolian reminisced.[13] Over his white linen shirt he could wear a plain white waistcoat and a closely fitted, single-breasted, lapelled tailcoat, cut short in front but long-tailed behind. Dr. Prichard's tightly tailored and beltless breeches showed silk stockings and a pair of fashionable Hessian boots. A long greatcoat and tall, slightly conical hat completed his winter wardrobe. No dandy, Prichard looked the part of a rising physician.

Reading, Reading, Reading

Prichard seemed keener on reading than attracting patients. He rejoined the Library Society in May 1810 and settled into serious research in late July, borrowing a new Gaelic dictionary, an ancient tome on even more ancient Italy, and for the first of many times, *Aristophanis comoediae undecim, Graece et Latine*. This last he memorized in Greek and enjoyed translating. As well as reading a few more histories and classical works, the autumn found him on armchair voyages to the Far East, North America, Germany, and India as he resumed his anthropological research. Medical books could wait. Lighter literature could be borrowed from local circulating libraries for an annual subscription of just 4 shillings whereas the Bristol Library's collection was of only the most serious, "improving" nature:[14]

> Novels, at least those of ambiguous character and ephemeral reputation, are excluded; but in History, Travels, Geography and Polite Literature, ancient and modern, the library is rich. The most approved reviews and periodical works are ordered and the Committee after laying in such supplies of standard works and books of reference, as are not likely to be found in private libraries, endeavours as far as

possible to comply with the wishes and accommodate the wants of the general body of subscribers.[15]

The Library Society's handsome premises on King Street, under the care of a clergymen librarian and his assistant, was open weekday mornings and evenings until 9 p.m. It did more than just house thousands of books; it was a resort of quiet, serious conversation. Young firebrands Coleridge and Southey had exploited it, and the librarian later boasted to William Wordsworth that one of its visitors was the famous essayist Walter Savage Landor, then resident in Clifton.[16] Only the well-off could afford this proprietary library's 4 guinea share investment, 1 guinea deposit, and 1 guinea annual subscription. Prichard's father, brothers, friends, and future medical colleagues were members.[17] Its subscription book a veritable *Who's Who* of Bristol, it was a rich source of private patients and patronage too. Literary lioness of the day Maria Edgeworth, author of educational novels and sister-in-law of Dr. Beddoes, wrote approvingly of the fine, exclusive library, "and what makes it appear ten times finer is that it is very difficult for strangers to get into. From thence he can get almost any book for us when he pleases, except a few of the most scarce, which are, by the laws of the library, immovable. No ladies go to the library."[18] As for Prichard, he preferred to have his library books delivered.

Unlike other Bristol charities and institutions, the Library Society was nonsectarian, banning volumes on theology, politics, and economics. Its governing committee was drawn from among Bristol's local merchants, manufacturers, councilmen, clergymen of all sects, a few gentlemen, and professional men. Some members donated "philosophical" collections such as apparatus and cabinets of minerals which later found their way to the Bristol Philosophical and Literary Society and eventually to the Bristol Museum.[19] From 1812, when the library held about twelve thousand volumes, until he left Bristol in 1845, committee member Prichard helped select books, made many special requests for extra privileges, attended thirteen to twenty of its fortnightly meetings each year, and went to its annual dinner. The hundreds of books that Prichard borrowed and which frequently appear as footnotes in his publications demonstrate his reliance on the Library Society.[20]

For many years the Library Society was controlled by Prichard's Berkeley Square neighbor, the Rev. Samuel Seyer. He shared with Prichard a commitment to scholarship and Tory principles. In one treatise this local historian patriotically demanded the French language expunged from

British life for its association with mischievous revolutionary principles, while his writing against clergy nonresidence marked him as an earnest church reformer.[21] The librarian Prichard knew best was John Peace, a most studious, shy bachelor who labored among his tomes near the library's beautiful fireplace, its elaborately carved overmantel said to be by the master Grinling Gibbons. So scholarly was this "fossil Tory," he famously forswore reading newspapers as a waste of precious study time. A devout churchman, Peace was also remembered for his outraged opposition to Catholic emancipation.[22]

The Library Society was not immune to the social change affecting Bristol. The building's upkeep became onerous and its location inconvenient to its members, who had mostly deserted the old city for the elevated new suburbs. Plans to relocate it were frustrated, as was an 1830s reformist bid to gain public access to the library on the grounds it contained some Corporation-owned collections.[23] Bristol lacked a university, so for Prichard the Library Society was the next best thing.

As well as mining the Bristol Library, Prichard bought, inherited, or was presented with many other volumes referred to in his publications.[24] Books were expensive, even for a young professional. Economy could be made in the quality of binding; until midcentury, books were usually sold unbound, the parts sewn into a sort of temporary paper or card wrapper. With a steep tax on paper, however, even the plainest bindings did not come cheap. The purchaser could then have the book properly bound in paper-covered card or quarter- or half-bound in leather as a cheaper alternative to full Morocco, half-calf, or other leather binding. Marbled endpapers and gold tooling were ordered according to individual taste.

Another way of gaining access to books was through subscription to the reviews, periodicals typically published quarterly and generally shared among several readers. These comprised long articles summarizing and reviewing one or more books on a particular topic that either satisfied readers or encouraged them to borrow or purchase them. Reviews had political or religious leanings that ensured reader loyalty. Prichard read them avidly, often sharing them with his father or recommending particular issues. He occasionally published articles in them and was concerned to learn how his own books fared in them. As for his own books, some later ones such as *The Natural History of Man* and the *Cyclopaedia of Practical Medicine* were published according to the trends of the developing industry: serially in parts and multivolume. In 1810 Prichard generally economized by exploiting the Bristol Library and a private medical book society.

Bristolians who could afford the heavily taxed, costly weekly newspapers had four to choose from according to political preference: *Felix Farley's Bristol Journal* (Tory), *Bristol Mercury* and *Bristol Gazette* (Liberal), and *Bristol Mirror* (neutral). Their front pages carried advertisements followed by three pages of international, national, and political news reprinted from other newspapers. Trials at the Assizes were well reported, as were sensational crimes and hideous accidents. There was also a page of Bristol and regional news, including local commodity prices, politics, births, marriages, and deaths and other notices, letters to the editor, poems, book reviews, and reports of the meetings of Bristol's many charities. Here Prichard advertised his candidacy for medical appointments and his courses of medical lectures, and he announced the publication of his books. His name appeared to his benefit in societies' and charities' reports and on their lists of subscribers. He occasionally engaged in the Bristol pastime of publicly quarreling in letters to the editor as well. Not only did newspapers provide Prichard with weekly news, but they aided his career development.

Communication

Even with the excellent library and the later Bristol Institution, science and high culture were muted in Bristol. Aspiring men of his class seemed keener to support the several thriving charities; with religion they were the city's main cultural activities. By and large, charity society membership was based on political and religious affiliation. There were some men's clubs and coffeehouses where the main topic of conversation was commerce rather than science. Another notable Bristol pastime was eating and drinking to excess. The city's thriving inns and taverns had long and complex bills of fare. When well-to-do Bristolians and visitors were not consuming boatloads of turtles, they could dine on bustards, cuckoos, hares, snipes, larks, and even swans. Byron quipped: "Too much in turtle Bristol's sons delight, / Too much o'er bowls of rack prolong the night."[25]

Prichard initially found it challenging to make contact with men of science beyond Bristol. The great expense, time, and discomfort involved in traveling limited opportunities for him to stray from the city, as did his need to be on hand for his precious patients. Travel to other cities was accomplished at eight to ten miles an hour by stagecoach with either three or four horses, depending on the importance of the route, at a fare of 6 pence per mile for inside passengers and about 3 per mile for cold, wet, and crowded outside seats. This was expensive even for middle-class travelers. A journey of one hundred miles took a very long, exhausting day. Servicing Bristol were six coaches to London daily and others to Birmingham and Exeter, while an hourly two-horse coach to Bath took ninety minutes. Alternatively, Prichard could hire a one-horse fly or two-horse carriage for local journeys or use his own for journeys to and from Ross. His father had a one-horse carriage that held six passengers, which he often drove himself, even for long distances, such as on the family's 1801 holiday to Tenby. The most expensive mode of transport was called traveling post chaise, in which a two- or four-horse carriage and driver could be hired, and at fifteen-mile intervals the horses exchanged at roadside inns or posting houses, at the phenomenal cost of £10 to £20 per day.[26] All this would change dramatically over the next few decades, however, when the communication revolution helped transform Prichard's later career.

Bristolians were keen on entertainingly innovative forms of transport. There had been intermittent enthusiasm for balloon flights since 1784; James Sadler, the first English balloonist, made a hydrogen-filled balloon assent from a field behind Stokes Croft, taking off on September 24, 1810, amid cannon-fire and the cheers of the astounded throng as it floated toward the Bristol Channel.[27] A more immediately practical form of transport was celebrated that same month with the opening of the Kennet and Avon Canal, which inefficiently linked Bristol and London; the average of seven days it took for goods to reach London meant that this major investment did not accrue to the wealth of Bristol.[28] With each decade, nevertheless, transport became more efficient.

Written communication was prohibitively expensive before the Penny Post's advent in 1840. A single-sheet letter to London cost the recipient 11 pence, and double that for two sheets, hence the custom of cross-writing over a previously filled page. The Prichards had post delivered three times a day, costing 1 penny or 2 pence for suburban delivery. Next-day delivery was expected, while post to Paris and return took a week or less, and India might take upward of a year. With no parcel post, the many books Prichard bought or borrowed from London learned societies were marked "by hand" and transported by stagecoach passengers.[29] The Bristol Post Office was next to the Exchange in Corn Street, opposite the Bush Tavern, where travelers could book tickets and obtain accommodation. It was a scene of constant bustle.

An Abundance of Religion and Charity

Bristol was rich in houses of worship, as religion was the glue of the city's social structure. The Test Act excluded all except communicants of the

Church of England from government appointments, the most overt discrimination against Nonconformists. The nation's Protestant state religion, known as Anglicanism, held sway in Bristol, but it was divided into two main camps, High Church and Low Church. In this period, High Church did not connote a leaning toward the doctrines and practices of Roman Catholicism but rather indicated its type of clergy. They were typically the younger sons of the aristocracy and gentry, Oxbridge products notorious for their perfunctory preaching, devotion to hunting and shooting, or even total absence. The "living" of a parish was usually the nepotistic gift of a local landowner, aristocrat, or institution. Prichard's son would fall foul of this corrupt system, so gleefully deplored by his Quaker grandfather.

High church complacency inspired the so-called Evangelical Movement, supported by elements among the Established Church, Moravians, and particularly Methodists. John Wesley, finding mid-eighteenth-century Bristol's poor ripe for Methodism, field preached and then established a meeting house in the Horsefair, leading Bristol to be claimed the birthplace of Methodism. Evangelical views spread rapidly among Bristolians, including some of the Anglican clergy and the more affluent.[30] Methodists and Quakers became highly active in many of the social issues of the day, such as education, prison reform, and abolition. Providing a bridge between evangelical clergy and the elite was the popular evangelical writer Hannah More. Bristolians could signal their evangelical leanings by the church they attended. Transcending sect, there was some unity among evangelicals in the causes they earnestly supported. They roundly criticized the High Church privileged old-guard clergy's lack of true piety—that corruption Prichard noted had been the cause of his ancestors' legitimate dissent.

Partly in reaction to the clergy's abuse of office, the Low Church, or evangelical party, prospered. Low Church clergy provided satisfyingly earnest preaching, Bible readings, prayer meetings in homes, and frequent church services. In their piety, dedication, and fervor, they could be doctrinaire, but they paradoxically shared with Dissenters a disgust of the laxity of High Churchmen. Prichard and his father subscribed to evangelical magazines and bought, read, and appreciated the books of the evangelical divines. In his reading and discussions with his father, close friendships with Bristol evangelicals, and the much later Tractarian movement lie the traces of Prichard's shifting religious views.

Bristol congregations of Quakers, Baptists, and Methodists could count among their numbers some of the city's affluent citizens. These Protestant Dissenters were exceptionally represented in local government and among the professions, with their names prominent on the donations and subscription lists of charities.[31] The Baptist community's strength was evident in its successful Bristol Baptist College and famous preachers such as the orientalist John Ryland and political and social reformer Robert Hall, both Prichard's later friends and patients.[32] In close sympathy with their evangelical qualities, Prichard and his father read Ryland, Hall, and other Baptists' works.

It must have been particularly challenging for Prichard to have anything to do with Unitarians, but at the nexus of Bristol's Unitarian elite was his university friend John Estlin and his father, Unitarian minister John Prior Estlin. Originating in Eastern Europe, the sect had become established in Britain in the second half of the eighteenth century. Unitarians stressed personal freedom in interpreting Scripture without priestly mediation and notoriously called into question the divinity of the Trinity. These anti-Trinitarians did not believe in the divine nature of Christ, original sin, or the damnation of souls, tenets cherished by other Protestants like Prichard. When Enlightenment thought was also influencing some educated Britons, Unitarians became known as "rational dissenters"—the word "rational" was no compliment.[33] Joseph Priestley, brilliant scientist and polemical writer, was instrumental in establishing Unitarianism, but as he was also famous for propounding theism, materialism, determinism, freedom of thought, and the principles of the French Revolution while abjuring the power of the Established Church, Unitarians became considered enemies of Church and State. When people like the Prichards decried Unitarianism, they conjured the specter of Joseph Priestly and his virtually Godless revolutionary ideas. There was a doctrinal gulf between the Prichards and Estlins.

Bristol's many charities' advertised their subscribers' generosity as well as political and religious affiliation. Their subscription and donation lists could be found in the columns of the local newspapers. This form of self-promotion benefited Prichard professionally. He was involved in serval charitable organizations whose members covered the spectrum of respectable citizens, his potential patients, from Dissenters associated with Liberal views such as Unitarians and many Quakers to evangelical Church of England Tories. Bristolians could consult these charities' membership lists and choose their family doctor accordingly. But the best way to put himself before the public was to be elected physician to a medical charity, a goal that exercised Prichard repeatedly. His actions were not solely careerist, however; he continued to support medical and reformist charities throughout his life.

Family Matters

Some responsibility for his brothers' welfare fell on Prichard's shoulders. Edward and Tom had finished their apprenticeships and were established in business in Bristol, but neither was happy with his lot. Edward distressed his father in 1810 by quitting the wholesale drug business he had been engaged in with family friend John Brent Cross. Prichard recalled this as "connected with circumstances which led to an estrangement between them, in which my father was involved and for some years before his death he ceased to have any friendly intercourse with his old correspondent Mrs Cross."[34] Edward returned to Ross and began his long career as manager of his father's and Uncle Newman's Ross Bank. Neither was Tom settling into his partnership, and he had been disowned by the Society of Friends for failing to attend meetings. Prichard diplomatically described his youngest brother as "possessed extraordinary talents, & particularly great powers of Calculation, and ability in business, but was of too adventurous a disposition for success in Commercial undertakings."[35] For "adventurous," read "reckless." Tom went on as he had started, a source of anxiety to his prudent brother and father; his adventurous disposition would lead him into danger, debt, and a premature end.

It is uncertain whether Prichard had known John Bishop Estlin when they were children in Bristol; it seems unlikely, given the Estlins' anathematic Unitarianism. But when he returned to Bristol in 1810, Prichard continued his Edinburgh friendship with Estlin, despite the Estlin household's liberal atmosphere. Their home was the headquarters and principal resort of Bristol's wealthy Nonconformists, and the Estlins had a reputation for welcoming the company of young literary men like Coleridge, Southey, and Charles Lamb.[36] Southey's early interest in Unitarianism apparently brought him and his friends there. Thomas Prichard would not have countenanced the company of these poets, who lived on their wits, spouted dangerous opinions, and accepted money from acquaintances. Unitarians and their literary dabbling were unconscionable. So why was his son socializing with the Estlins?

Lewin's Mead Unitarian Chapel was an impressive, state-of-the-art, neoclassical-style building. Far from being an insulated sect, Unitarians were prominent in business and in their protracted campaign for the repeal of the Test Act, the law barring them and other non-Anglicans from access to public office and other benefits. During the first half of the nineteenth century Bristol Unitarians collected funds for persecuted French Protestants and the starving Irish, petitioned against government discrimination against the Jews, and above all were dedicated to the abolition of American slavery.[37] John Bishop Estlin and his daughter Mary Anne would become the most prominent antislavery activists in Bristol. Estlin and Prichard had a common interest in science, abolition, and the career-building goal of getting elected to posts at the Bristol Infirmary. But perhaps what most attracted Prichard to the Estlin home was young Anna Maria.

Shipshape and Bristol Fashion?

As well as having a fondness for worship and charities, Bristolians relished occasional rousing patriotic celebrations and political strife. George III's lavish golden jubilee in 1809 had been commemorated with a statue of His Majesty erected in Portland Square, only for it to be toppled three years later after another of Orator Hunt's inspiring speeches.[38] The next, more exclusive celebration was even costlier: Lord Grenville, the new Whig high steward of Bristol, was feted at a Whig-only Corporation banquet. Local government's extravagant pomp and feasting allegedly consumed a quarter of the city's budget, and the generous salaries, pensions, and gifts the Corporation showered on its members continued unabated even as it consistently refused to allocate funds to public projects such as street repairs. Something of a protracted "velvet revolution" was under way, however. The Whig-dominated local government had become a public disgrace such that between 1810 and 1812 fourteen aldermen were fined for refusing to serve as common councillors. When two supposed Whigs were seated only to reveal themselves as Tory turncoats, the balance of power tipped to the Tories, who immediately set about lavishing the public wealth of Bristol just as liberally among their own kind, partly financing this with cripplingly high port dues. Even Tory merchants grumbled.[39]

During local political upheaval and stringencies of war, the elite of Bristol seemed relatively unaffected. A new Mall Assembly Room was opened in Clifton in the autumn of 1811 with the grandest ball ever held in the city.[40] Conservative as usual, Bristol reacted variously with indifference and hostility to one of its citizen's curious displays. In September, a mere dyer named John Breillat advertised his upcoming "Lecture and Exhibition of the Gas Lights" at his home, 56 Broadmead. Enterprising Mr. Breillat vainly attempted to interest investors in the production of piped coal-gas lighting. He next lit a few lamps in the street nearby, but investors were thin on the ground. It was not until 1816, amid admonitions from Peers and the sneers of scientist Sir Humphry Davy, that sufficient capital was raised to establish the Bristol Gas Company. After overcoming the objections of the Bristol Corporation, a gasholder was built near Temple Back, and the first few shops were lit in May 1817. Soon five streets had gas lights, and progressive Lewin's Mead Unitarian Chapel became the first public building in Bristol to adopt this innovation. The supply unmetered, customers had to arrange to use the lights during specified hours, with the company employing inspectors to check for infringements.[41] Some Clifton residents now had the further convenience of water piped from Sion Spring, but they were indifferent toward reestablishing the defunct Bristol Water Company.[42] Nor was sanitation yet of much concern. Richmond Hill, Clifton—laid out with one sewer pipe leading to a common cesspool—became the source of a future outbreak of cholera.[43]

Personal Circumstances

While Prichard was trying to establish his practice in Bristol, he kept in frequent contact with his father. Unworldly, introspective Thomas Prichard immersed himself in the classics and French and English historians, but without his children to educate or other pastimes, he spent his time reading mostly evangelical and theological tomes, some in Greek or Hebrew. Both father and son preferred reading sacred texts in their original idioms. A desire to access the German theologians inspired Thomas Prichard to attempt German as well. His correspondence continued redolent of gloom and anxiety for his soul. In his interests, habits, and constant ill health, he relied on frequent contact with his eldest son. At the threshold of Prichard's career in a city full of snares, his father provided constant guidance too. He must have been taken aback when Prichard "formed an attachment" to Estlin's sister.

On a chilly February Thursday in 1811, Prichard and Anna Maria Estlin were married at St. Michael's Church, Bristol, by the Rev. Griffith Williamson.[44] Thomas Prichard's congratulations arrived the following day: "Thou knowest that thy happiness in time and in Eternity, are dearer to me than my own, and in future I shall consider thy Anna and thyself as one and as claiming alike my affection and solicitude for these have been in my mind always inseparable."[45] Having disposed of that topic, he swiftly moved on to asking about using Eau Medicinale for his gout. As the years went by, he would send his daughter-in-law greetings and congratulations or condolences as the deliveries or deaths of her infants required. Anna subscribed to a charity school, wrote an account of family life in 1814, accompanied her husband to the Continent in 1823 and later often traveled with him,

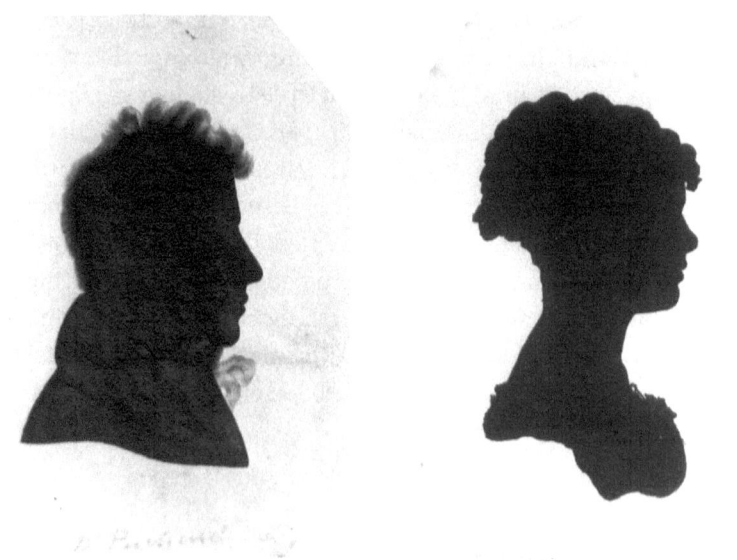

3. A respectable young couple. James and Anna, silhouettes. Property of the Orton family.

contributed a poem and her silhouette to a relative's album, and bore ten children. A beneficiary of Prichard's will, she outlived him by eleven years.[46] This was Anna Maria Prichard's life.

This family alliance of liberal Unitarians, evangelical Quakers, and Tory Anglican Prichard naturally required some tolerance on occasion. Soon after the young couple married, Anna's parents paid a visit to Ross, where they were received just a little too cordially for the groom's liking. Dr. Estlin and Thomas Prichard had earnest theological discussions, giving Prichard the unpleasant impression that his father had neglected to attack Unitarianism's abhorrent anti-trinitarianism. His father reassured him that he and Dr. Estlin had merely mitigated the sensitivity of the encounter by focusing on common beliefs. How could Prichard have called into question his father's pure faith in salvation through divine Christ? Actually, Thomas Prichard was becoming somewhat weary of doctrinal debates; he deeply regretted mankind's inability to simply surrender to pure faith. For the rest of his life, he never once deviated from absolute "faith in the doctrines of the Trinity & of that of the Atonement by Christ."[47]

The Estlins traveled from their Ross visit to Groes, their summer home at Southerndown on a beautiful, isolated stretch of the Glamorgan coast. The Prichard family would spend many happy summers there. Before Thomas

Prichard left for a summer tour of the Lake District, he wrote to Anna's mother approvingly about the young couple's start in married life and in praise of their new home in Berkeley Square, Bristol: "Their situation is a very pleasant one, and the house well furnished, if any room has my preference over the rest, it is the library: it is cool, silent, and has a sober and somewhat imposing effect on the mind. I felt myself very comfortable and much at home under Anna's kind care."[48]

The year 1812 brought the good news of the birth of the Prichards' first child, Anna Maria, on February 3.[49] It was also the year brother Edward sustained a compound fracture of the leg that the Ross surgeon could not set. Three Bristol surgeons were summoned; Mr. Hetling succeeded in opening the wound to retrieve a large fragment and realign the bone, saving Edward's leg and life. Prichard had to visit Ross several times during the latter part of the year, apparently to comfort his father in his anxiety over Edward.[50]

Bristol, as Ever

Bristol in 1812 continued to have its excitements. Long-standing economic depression and hardship had given rise to an alternative economy. The outlying parish of Bitton in the Kingswood colliery district had reached its peak of infamy for banditry of all kinds; the hereditary "Cock-road gangs" could not be entirely suppressed. Further up the social scale, but differently dubious were Bristol's elections—two in one year. On January 25 Prichard paid a fee and swore the oath of a burgess of Bristol, by virtue of his marriage to the daughter of a freeman of the city. Now he was entitled to vote.[51] That summer's parliamentary by-election for one of the city's two seats, Tory banker Richard Hart Davis versus Radical reformer Henry "Orator" Hunt, sparked the usual turmoil. The Tories were said to have spent a phenomenal £1,000 per week for the fortnight the poll was kept open, flooding Bristol with bribes and beer. Rival gangs fought and broke windows, as was their wont; there were casualties and one fatality while the Bristol Corporation lavishly entertained the officers of the troops brought in to quell the disturbances. Prichard, as conservative as his father, plumped for Davis and thereafter voted in the True Blue cause. Davis held the seat until his retirement in 1831, the year Bristol rioters planned to go up to Clifton to attack his mansion.[52]

As if that were not enough rowdiness for one year, October brought the general election. Two candidates formed a "West India interest" coalition comprising Tory Davis and Whig Edward Protheroe to thwart the third serious candidate, a reformist antislavery Whig. All three paid the fees of an estimated 1,700 burgesses to secure these Bristolians' votes; seventy-five of these burgesses were said to have been based on "marriages of convenience." Henchmen went about their marauding and club-wielding business, preventing rival candidates' voters from entering the poll. Beef, bread, booze, and cash were distributed openly and lavishly. The coalition defeated the progressive Whig, while a fourth candidate's legal claim of bribery was unsuccessful. It was a costly election year, with the Tories alone spending more than £29,000 on the elections and the extravagant "chairing" ceremonies that followed.[53]

Of potentially greater and lasting benefit to Bristolians than ceremonial chairings was the founding of the Prudent Man's Friend Society. Elsewhere these new "friendly societies" harbored radicalism, but the Bristol society's objectives illustrate four developments in Bristol's middle-class life: a passion for reform, a focus on charities that offered direct help, the formation of nonsectarian organizations, and the open participation of women. The Prudent Man's Friend Society managed to be both supportive and punitive in its dealings with the lower orders, and it was atypically nonpolitical and nonsectarian. Its driving force, Susanna Morgan, was backed by Prichard's relative philanthropist Richard Reynolds and businessman Thomas Sanders. At their inaugural meeting on December 22, 1812, Prichard joined its committee, with John Estlin and his brother Alfred also involved.

Morgan's pamphlet *Hints towards the Formation of a Society, for Promoting a Spirit of Independence among the Poor* began with a point that surely captured tight-fisted Bristolians' attention and approbation: parochial poor relief was a waste of money because it fostered idleness, improvidence, and dependence; its recipients became unashamed of begging, had no pride, and were rendered unable to plan for the future. Her threefold plan was to improve food supply, encourage moral restraint and sense of independence, and provide pecuniary aid for unforeseen needs. While nothing could be done about the food supply, the poor must learn it was not the obligation of the rich to provide. They also needed to acquire self-reliance and be taught to read improving moral tracts. "Lying-in" charities were pernicious because the poor should learn to have children only if they could afford to. Vagrancy, begging, and deception would be suppressed by handing out tokens instead of money to those providing proof of need. Finally, loans to the poor should replace alms. Financed by subscriptions, the Prudent Man's Friend Society's Savings Bank was the forerunner of the Bristol Savings Bank.[54]

Among Bristol's political ferment and charitable initiatives, religious revivalism was taking hold, inspiring the founding of even more charities. One fruit of the Great Awakening was an upsurge in the number of Anglican clergymen dedicated to evangelical principles of pure faith, personal redemption, and piety. Their vociferous spokesmen were the Reverends Thomas Biddulph, who had baptized Prichard, and James Vaughan. In 1813 the mayor and the city's MPs joined many other gentlemen in forming the Bristol branch of the highly popular Church Missionary Society for Africa and the East. It did not receive the support of the absentee bishop of Bristol, nor did it need it. Its well-organized national network of activists stimulated interest in the cause of global Christian evangelism, provided stirring sermons, and collected donations assiduously, making Bristol the most prominent and lucrative of its provincial branches.[55] Prichard joined it.

Family Matters and *Physical History* (1813)

Prichard's sister, Mary, wrote to Anna, "We have thought of you very frequently, and of your sad disappointment: it is however a great consolation to think that your little infant had he lived, would have lived only to suffer." The year 1813 thus started with bereavement and continued with disappointment and the threat of upheaval. The following month, Thomas Prichard and Anna's mother, Mrs. Estlin, commiserated over Prichard's negative attitude and poor prospects in Bristol. The young family had tried moving to the more prominent location of 39 College Green. Although the Doctor now held beneficial, but unremunerated, appointments to three medical charities, there had been no vacancies at prestigious Bristol Infirmary. Dr. Estlin attempted to encourage his disheartened son-in-law, and Thomas Prichard complained to Mrs. Estlin:

> I lament with you the change that has taken place in the Dr's views, and have repeatedly and very recently given him my opinions on this subject. The prospect at Guildford, even supposing the best can be made of it, is poor in comparison with what he may rationally promise himself by a few more years residence in Bristol. But all my representations are unavailing: it must of course be left with him, and I hope he has some foundations for his expectations, with which I am unacquainted.
>
> I confess the thing came upon me much by surprize, for it is not three weeks since he wrote in spirits respecting his residence in College

Green. I have pushed the subject as far as I can with him, I must therefore wait the event and whatever it be hope for the best.[56]

Prichard's plan to abandon Bristol and relocate in Guildford faded, and life in College Green settled down. Their stone-faced, modern home in an elite residential street on the foothills of suburban Clifton had an entrance leading into an impressive hall, off which were two parlors, a breakfast room, the principal staircase, and a separate staircase for their servants. The main kitchen (under separate roof) was fitted with an oven, hot-dresser, and every convenience, while a back kitchen, larder, and other offices were on the ground floor. On the first floor the Prichards had a drawing room to the front and a bedchamber and water closet, and there were four more bedrooms on the second floor and servants' quarters in the garrets. The two stone-arched cellars and an excellent laundry room served this large home. Prichard and Anna put down roots in Bristol.[57]

That summer the family had a happy holiday at the rural retreat of Pearhill, near Ross. Thomas Prichard devoted himself to spoiling little Anna and then joyfully admitted having done so. Tom, recently married to Jane Lawrence, and Edward were both working at the Ross Bank.[58] On returning to Bristol, the Prichards found their fellow citizens' mood upbeat. British victories over the French armies in Spain were celebrated for what the poor erroneously thought would be the end of hardship and what the merchants expected would be a return to unimpeded international trade and profit. The latter enjoyed their own exclusive, formal, and costly "grand gala fete" at a pleasure garden in nearby Stapleton.[59]

During his first few years in Bristol, Prichard had spent more time snug in his library researching and writing than an aspiring physician ought. He kept the Bristol Library clerk busy delivering books, and he bought, borrowed, and shared volumes. He would begin his day at about five in the morning to put in at least four hours of reading before breakfast and the start of his day as a physician. Although publishing on medical topics might have been more beneficial to his career at this point, he had gained little experience on which to base such a publication. Instead, he developed his MD thesis into his first book, the *Physical History of Man*. In the New Year of 1814 an advertisement in the Bristol newspapers announced, "This day are published, In Octavo, price 16s in boards, Researches into the Physical History of Man. By James Cowles Prichard, M.D F.L.S. &c. London: Printed for John and Arthur Arch, Cornhill; and Barry and Son, Bristol." Prichard waited for the all-important reviews that would promote his book and gradually help him make contacts with scholars in Britain and abroad. His mission to prove the unity of the human species had begun in earnest. *Physical History* not only established his reputation as a scholar; notoriety attracted paying patients, though Anna commented ruefully that after three years of being a physician, "Dr P. had no private practice."[60]

In war-weary Bristol as in the nation as a whole, 1814 started with weeks of such bitterly cold weather that the Floating Harbour froze solid along its whole polluted length, while drifting snow blocked the roads, cutting off contact with the outside world and disrupting trade. But March brought the capture of Paris, soon followed by the abdication of Napoleon. After two decades of almost constant warfare, Bristolians threw themselves into celebrating in almost every possible way. Illuminations turned the June nights into days, and there were proclamations, processions, triumphal arches, and allegorical displays, culminating in a spectacular bonfire at the top of Brandon Hill.[61] Anna recorded: "On the 3rd of June, at six oclock in the morning J.C.P was born: On the 27th peace was proclaimed and there was a general illumination." Father of two, loyalist Prichard nearly met his end celebrating: "Dr. P went to Portsmouth to see the allied Sovereigns and other celebrated foreigners. He had a very providential escape of being run over by one of the foreign carriages which was driven furiously down a narrow street. Dr P saw that by drawing himself up as close as possible to the wall that the wheel must touch him, he was accordingly knocked down, but by the mercy of God escaped with only a wound on the forehead."

Career-Building

After his close shave with death, a summer holiday in the countryside was in order. Anna and the children usually stayed either at her parents' summer home in South Wales or in Ross. Prichard joined them for part of the time when he had no professional obligations, but after a dutiful week in Ross he and his friend Dr. William Hall Gilby went geologizing around Malvern, Ledbury, and environs, gathering material for an article on the subject.

Prichard's recent appointments as physician to the Clifton Dispensary and St. Peter's Hospital gained him some publicity and occupied some of his time.[62] He also regularly debated at the fortnightly meeting of the Bear's Cub Club, some members of which were on the Infirmary's medical staff. There were the Library Society committee meetings to attend; with his friend John Cross, he enjoyed the society's annual dinner at Mangeon's Hotel, Clifton, on April 18.

Anna reviewed 1814 from her domestic perspective. Although her husband lacked paying patients, he kept himself busy doing things like translating *The Birds* from the Greek. There had just been a scathing review of a recent translation of Aristophanes's long and less popular work in the *British Review*, which might have inspired him to undertake this challenging project.[63] Anna did not, however, record where or whether he ever published it. As he was working on this he did try to drum up patients by getting himself noticed by his medical brethren and the general public; he proclaimed himself a medical educator.

Anna was so pleased and optimistic about her husband's new venture she carefully preserved one of the admission tickets for "Dr. PRICHARD's Lectures on Physiology, Pathology, and the Practice of Physic." Although she was soon to be "confined," she did not seem inconvenienced when her dining room was turned into a lecture hall for between twenty and thirty young men, three times a week for three months: "Dr P's library opened into the dining room, & unless reading any book of interest with Mrs. P. he sat writing in the library, as the lectures were written as they were wanted." He most likely based his course on his Edinburgh lecture notes and medical volumes, his medical experience still limited. That year and the following autumn Bristol's medical apprentices and Infirmary pupils got a taste of Edinburgh medical education.[64]

An excellent opportunity arose for Prichard to stake his claim as a scientist, stalwart of biblical truth, and active and humane citizen. In early June 1814 the terms of the Treaty of Paris were considered to have made inadequate provision for the suppression of the French slave trade. Britons expressed their great displeasure. Eighty-seven worthy Bristolians signed a letter requesting that the mayor convene a public meeting for the purpose of organizing a petition to Parliament urging the government to take steps to further the international suppression of the slave trade. Prichard was among the signatories, an early and rare example of his involvement in public life that was not of a learned, professional, or religious nature. It was a relatively safe, cross-party, nonsectarian affair.[65] The July 6 meeting was one of proposals, speeches, and handing over to Tory MP Richard Hart Davis a petition signed by thirteen thousand Bristolians, which he presented to Parliament the following week.[66] Prichard's opposition to the slave trade was clear and learned at his father's knee.

Anything more activist was not to Prichard's taste. Eventually, he would become an early supporter of the Aborigines' Protection Society, and one of his 1840s publications was forthright in condemning the slave trade. Not until 1841 would he openly engage in the antislavery movement by serving on the committee of a rather tepid society that hoped to obliterate the slave trade by civilizing and Christianizing Africans. Prichard's 1814 signing of the anti–slave trade letter indicated his humanitarian concern, nevertheless.

Participation in a specifically Anglican society was more typical of Prichard's interests in early life. Since at least the 1790s, Dissenters had been founding charitable schools for the general and religious education of children and adults, stealing the march on the Established Church. The archbishop of Canterbury chaired a meeting in 1811 to found the National Society for the Education of the Poor in the Principles of the Established Church, claiming it was the duty of the nation to educate its young in the national religion and that failure to do so would endanger the nation itself. All dioceses should set up local branches. The Bristol branch intended to raise sufficient funds to educate five hundred boys and three hundred girls in Scripture, writing, and arithmetic.[67] Their February 1814 meeting received the civic approbation of being held at the Guildhall under the chairmanship of the mayor. A Tory newspaper reported Prichard's enthusiasm: he had seconded a proposal made by the ubiquitous Reverend Biddulph, the fast-rising pillar of Bristol Anglican conservatism with whom Prichard would clash in later years, and he then proposed the vote of thanks to the treasurer, banker John Cave, who also served the Bristol Infirmary.[68] His active participation in a society fighting against Dissenters' influence over the lower orders and his support of Anglican religious education indicate Prichard's attitude on these matters as well as his effort to gain acceptance and status.

No sooner had Prichard published *Physical History* than he continued research for a new edition, but sorely needing access to German scholarship, he set about studying the language. His sister, Mary, was on a farewell visit to the Prichards before her marriage and decided to join Anna and her brother in taking lessons from a Mr. Drumpft. This did not go well. Mary's thoughts were elsewhere and Anna's were with her babies, so the ladies soon gave up their lessons. Prichard's friend from his Staines days, William Tothill, became his fellow student. They set themselves the exacting goal of translating a multivolume history book, which they published nearly four years later. By the following winter, Prichard was penning short letters to a relative in German.[69]

Throughout the year the Prichards had plenty to occupy themselves, even if there were few private patients to treat. They attended Mary's marriage at Ross Meeting House to the Godalming wool stapler Robert Moline.

Prichard then spent three autumn months tending the consumptive decline and death of one of his uncle Fisher's young nephews. More pleasurable was the visit of his Edinburgh friend Charles Mackenzie. Every Sunday evening Prichard and Anna dined at the Estlins' large home at the top of St. Michael's Hill, enjoying the stimulating conversation found there. The year ended with a family party at the Red Lodge, the Elizabethan mansion that would become the Prichards' home.

1815

With war at an end—including a short, trade-damaging war with America—instead of peace bringing a return to prosperity, it brought yet more hardship among the laboring poor. Once domestic production could no longer command wartime inflated prices, farmers who had secured land at inflated rentals could no longer profit from their harvests. The government's Corn Laws, concerned only with the welfare of rich farmers, attempted to maintain the high price of imported corn and other foods in order to keep domestic food prices from falling. Both skilled and unskilled workers, meanwhile, faced a series of wage cuts, while the wartime inflated cost of food did not decrease proportionately. Amid their protests and general unrest, the laboring classes' growing understanding of and involvement in political and economic processes alarmed the government, which responded repressively. Even the rise in newspaper tax was said to have been designed to further raise the price of reading the news beyond the means of working people.[70] Instead of peace and prosperity, the end of the wars brought dissention and distress. The medical charities Prichard was serving were busy.

Thomas Prichard desperately missed his daughter, Mary, now starting married life in distant Surrey; he developed the custom of residing with them for a few months every year. Edward, recently married to Rebecca Merrick, was living near him in Ross. Tom was his usual dissatisfied, restless self. He threw in his job at the bank and returned to Bristol, but the following year he decided to try his luck in America.[71]

Prichard kept his eye on the main prize, the post of physician to the Bristol Infirmary, but he would have to bide his time.[72] Meanwhile, not only because it would be useful to demonstrate to the Infirmary's voting subscribers his Tory allegiance, but because it was his inclination, he joined the Dolphin Society. Bristolian gentlemen were keen on commemorating the life of their early eighteenth-century paradoxically philanthropic slave trader Edward Colston, even as they signed anti–slave trade petitions. Three Colston societies were formed to do good works in his name and have convivial, alcohol-fueled annual partisan dinners. Prichard attended the (Tory) Dolphin Society's dinner in 1815 and several years thereafter. At their 1820 meeting one toast was a rousing "May the independence of Parliament never be shaken, either by the licentiousness of the Press, or the violence of the People."[73] This True Blue certification would stand Prichard in good stead for the next Infirmary election and among potential patients. His friend John King and the Unitarian Estlins were members of the (Whig) Anchor Society.

Medicine, Geology, and Philology

By the summer of 1815 Prichard had been able to put into practice a system of Edinburgh-inspired medical therapeutics supplemented by what he had learned from recent publications. He had been carefully recording the case histories of his St. Peter's Hospital pauper epileptic patients, using his observations to write an article for the respected *Edinburgh Medical and Surgical Journal*. He wanted to promote his name and champion heroic medical therapeutics by advocating Dr. Alexander Hamilton's use of evacuants as a treatment for epilepsy. Prichard cited several cases demonstrating the benefits of vigorous purging. With himself in mind, he assured his readers that physicians would inevitably make progress in understanding so-called nervous diseases. From this modest article on epilepsy stemmed his later work on neurology and mental illness.[74]

Anna was not exempt from Prichard and Estlin's heroic medicine; that summer at Ross her brother treated her ophthalmia and discomfort from pregnancy with bleeding, blistering, leeching, scarification, and "low" diet, but with little relief. While she endured this, Prichard and his relative George Fisher Jr. happily went mountain climbing and geologizing in Snowdonia, returning with some amusing tales of their adventures and keen to publish their new theory of the geological age of the mountain range. The Prichards' son Francis began his short life on November 5.[75]

Geology and Mosaic history occupied Prichard's attention and inspired him to write several reviews and articles in 1815. A member of the Wernerian Society, he was of course wary of the rival Huttonian unorthodox theory that rock formation occurred over an infinity of time. His "Remarks on the Older Floetz Strata of England," published in the *Annals of Philosophy*, sought to clear up an anomaly in the order of limestone strata associated with coal beds that would put the British coalfields in correct relative geological sequence. Prichard cited several authors' accounts, related what he had discovered in the Bristol area, and described a fossil in the possession of Bristol collector George Cumberland. He prefaced this with observations on the evidence of extinctions and evolution relative to geological dating: "A fossil which abounds in one formation is often seen more scantily dispersed through a second, in a third it is scarcely found, and at length withdraws itself altogether from our view. A continual progress seems to have been made from the more simple to the more complex forms. We observe no retrograde changes."[76]

Prichard shared his geological observations with future Clifton Dispensary medic and friend William Hall Gilby, who was similarly publishing on local and regional geology in another scientific periodical. Gilby described the relative positions of the red sandstone and limestone strata of Bristol and related these to what he had seen in and near Ross, citing Prichard's article and personal correspondence concerning other regional deposits.[77] Partly in response to Gilby's articles, an anonymous contributor "Homo" warned that geologists had better focus on establishing the veracity of Mosaic cosmogony instead. This inspired Prichard's next forays into print. He reviewed the Rev. Joseph Townsend's *The Character of Moses Established for Veracity as an Historian* (1813) in the August issue of the forcefully evangelical *British Review* and in the *London Critical Journal*.[78] Then came his article "On the Cosmogony of Moses" in the October 1815 issue of the *Philosophical Magazine*, where he nailed his colors to the mast of natural theology, the search for biblical truth through science. He professed himself surprised Homo wanted him to explain how Genesis is in accord with geology as the answer was strikingly obvious. But to oblige with concrete evidence, for example, that the word "day" in Genesis was synonymous with "an indefinite period of time," Prichard resorted to philological analysis. He then laid out the facts of the seven periods of Genesis before listing geological phenomena that supported each period. The first period of universal sea could be seen in strata in the highest mountains, which indicate formation in the presence of water. That there had been no life on Earth during the second period was apparent from the absence of organic remains in the oldest type of rock. To skip on to the seventh period: "That man was created at a later æra than all the above-mentioned beings, is proved by a similar method. The reason why no human bones are found even in the newest rocks, is, probably, that all the rock-formations were deposited before the creation of the human species." Prichard had made good use of Buffonian and Cuvierian paleontology to outline the progressive development of life, but without suggesting species transformation.[79]

Having successfully reconciled Genesis and geology, Prichard brought physiology to bear on the subject of Mosaic cosmogony but saved his ace card for last. Some people might be skeptical about the divine creation of humankind because there is evidence of the existence of life prior to that of human beings. On the contrary, this sequence of existence provides geological evidence of Creation. Prichard finished with a characteristic swipe at the fashion for materialist theorizing, stating that "all the metaphysical reasonings which have been essayed on this subject... appear to me to be as visionary as any piece of chimerical nonsense from the Cabbala, and to afford not the smallest presumptive proof that the world has not existed in its present state from all eternity." "Visionary" would become a favorite epithet.[80]

Prichard, the young biblical scholar, must have been taken aback when a few months later a highly critical riposte appeared in the same journal. "Francis E⸺s" (Francis Ellis of Bath) rounded on Prichard, accusing him of errors pertaining to the locomotive abilities of some of the animals created on the fifth day, for instance. Not taking this lying down, Prichard replied in the next issue, and then a Mr. Andrew Horn joined the fray. Prichard fielded "animadversions" with alacrity: any child knew that snails are possessed of locomotion. One or another of them had a letter in the *Philosophical Magazine*'s next seven issues. Prichard had the last word.[81]

It was not at all strange that a periodical devoted to discoveries in science such as the *Philosophical Magazine* should contain such a spirited defense of Genesis. On the Continent new theories on the nature of life were being aired openly in lectures and publications, posing a threat to Christian doctrine. These corrosive ideas were starting to seep into Britain, but Prichard did not waver; on the contrary, he was getting a taste for biblical scholarship. He reviewed Townsend's newly published continuation of his work on Moses, which deals with events subsequent to the Deluge, and grammarian Johann Christoph Adelung's *Mithridates oder allgemeine sprachenkunde* (1806–13), three volumes attempting to elucidate the history of the world's languages, tracing language to its most primitive origins.[82] Prichard's use of language as anthropological evidence would come to the fore in his later publications. He borrowed many relevant volumes from the Bristol Library on which to base these 1815 articles and reviews on the science of Creation through the exploration of geological, biblical-historical, and philological resources. Welsh studies also began to attract more and more of his interest.[83]

A celebrity in the increasingly popular field of Celtic studies was the poet and antiquarian Edward Williams, Bard Iolo Morganwg, collector, arranger, and publisher of ancient Welsh manuscripts. Active in preserving all things Welsh, he was lionized by the Romantic Movement's Gwyneddigion and Cymreigyddion Societies. Prichard wrote to him in the most respectful terms, expressing his appreciation of their friendship and inviting him and his son Taliesin ab Iolo to his home. On behalf of Bristol historian Samuel Seyer, Prichard sent Williams a list of questions in 1815 concerning the ancient relationship between Wales and Bristol.[84] His great ability as a student of Welsh would bear fruit in his *Eastern Origin of the Celtic Languages* and his appointment as adjudicator of the Eisteddfod competitions on Welsh linguistics.[85] Many years later, Iolo Morganwg's considerable number of literary forgeries were exposed, but in 1815 he inspired Prichard.

At the same time that Prichard was developing his interest in geology and philology, his library borrowing records and publications track his continuing work on the origin of humankind. In that evangelical periodical the *British Review*, he published a review of G. S. Faber's recent *The Origin of Pagan Idolatry* (1816) and Friedrich Schlegel's *Ueber die Sprache und Weisheit der Indier* (1808). Prichard condemned Faber but supported Schlegel for the evidence the latter supplied in support of the view that central to the history of religion was the matter of its origin in pure received monotheism and its subsequent degeneration into polytheism, idolatry, and the "licentious and atrocious rites of the worshippers of Nature."[86] This view suited Prichard's quest to demonstrate original human unity, original monotheism, and universal psychic unity, all vital to his anthropology. And this project helped him to master the German language.

As Prichard was evidently exploring the unity of the human mind, Anna noted that he was writing about the Dendera Zodiac, so he may have been the author of the review of C. G. Schwartz's three volumes on the subject that appeared in the February 1817 issue of his favorite *British Review*. This controversial Egyptian bas-relief had sparked a long-running astronomical-archaeological-theological debate: Did it prove that Egyptian civilization predated the Noachian Deluge or even the Creation? Certainly, the reviewer's derision of French thinking, of unsupported theorizing in general, and the claim of the greater antiquity of Scriptures are Prichardian. The Zodiac of Dendera was later taken to France, exhibited in London in 1825, and years later proven to be of recent date. Prichard had evidently started researching his *Egyptian Mythology*.[87]

As 1816 drew to a close, Prichard had cause to be better satisfied with his lot. Home and family life were pleasing; his scholarly breadth and output had benefited from access to German publications; peace, economic stability, and prosperity were on the horizon; his charity medical work was faring well; and most of his children were alive. While fee-paying patients were still sparse, at least he had finally secured the much-prized post of physician to the Bristol Infirmary. Things were looking up.

5 "Sharpening Their Wits upon the Carcasses of the Poor"

Working for Medical Charities

> Many men have wriggled themselves into notice by professions of charity, and have qualified themselves for genteel practice, by sharpening their wits upon the carcasses of the poor.
> —"Hints to Young Practitioners," *Edinburgh Medical and Surgical Journal*

Strategy

When Prichard settled in Bristol he needed to focus on earning his bread in a crowded field of physicians competing to win patients' confidence and fees. He got involved in local charities and made his religious and political party affiliation clear, but securing a post as physician to a medical charity was a must. Some sardonic tips for would-be physicians had just been published in the *Edinburgh Medical and Surgical Journal*:

> Do something that will make you conspicuous ... as it is well known no empiric ever reaches any degree of wealth and reputation till after he has been fairly convicted of homicide. Write a book with a taking title.... Quote as many cases as the alphabet will furnish initials for.... Write monthly reports of diseases in a newspaper or magazine; swell out the list according to your own fancy. Hire a chariot, and put a smart livery upon a bill-stick, to ride behind you ... for nobody in their senses, in London, will send for a walking physician. Endeavour to establish a hospital or dispensary by the voluntary subscriptions of your friends; for many men have wriggled themselves into notice by professions of charity, and have qualified themselves for genteel practice, by sharpening their wits upon the carcasses of the poor.[1]

Prichard was ready to try all but hiring a liveried bill-stick. Bristolians in need of a physician valued religious and party allegiance, status as a gentleman, and the endorsement of influential citizens more than actual medical skill and experience; it was who you knew and what you were rather than what you knew that mattered. This made building a career in a sectarian city tricky. Campaigning for the opportunity to sharpen his wits on the poor in medical charity service was time-consuming. These charities were controlled by Bristol's elite, who demonstrated their social status by subscribing to them, serving on their committees, or being elected one of their unremunerated medical men. During his first five years in Bristol, Prichard attempted to establish his own medical charity, was elected physician to four charitable medical institutions, became involved in several nonmedical charities, and gave medical lectures in his dining room. Once he had established his career, he continued to serve two of these charities for many years.

An anonymous 1825 pamphlet pointing out that a Bristol medical man's top career-enhancing prize was election to the staff of the Bristol Infirmary cited Dr. Prichard as a prime example. The writer asserted that members of the faculty derived advantages in their private practice from their charity appointment. The effects,

> like professional stilts, suddenly lift them to eminence and extensive practice.... The splendid literary attainments of Dr. Prichard reflect honour on the City, whilst the mildness and urbanity of his disposition have endeared him to an extensive circle of his fellow-citizens; but I defy even Dr. Prichard, whom no man more respects than myself, to say that his appointment to the Infirmary did not assist in extending his professional practice; and, if so, who will deny that this is an adequate return for the services he renders to the Charity; it is at least such a one as will always make the office an object of eager solicitation to the most eminent professional men.[2]

Undeniable as this was, Prichard would have wanted the author to mention how dog-eat-dog the election process could be; another candidate would call his competitors "young sharks." Prichard had to cultivate the patronage of hundreds of subscribers, assemble a phalanx of canvassers, and be ready to swing into action as soon as a vacancy occurred—or better still, when rumors of one started to swirl. While waiting for an opening he got involved with Dr. John Edmonds Stock and medical practitioner Mr. John King in Dr. Beddoes' Medical Institution in Little Tower Court, but it soon closed.[3] Impatient and with a humanitarian point to make, he decided to establish his own medical charity, just as the Scottish article had advised.

Castle Green Dispensary

Prichard circulated an appropriately anonymous leaflet pointing out that the abject poor could not obtain the required subscribers' sponsorship for treatment at the Infirmary or the Bristol Dispensaries. He believed a medical charity that would examine and prescribe for needy patients gratis without discrimination or qualification would address this lacuna in medical services, so he rented rooms in Castle Green and tested the viability of his innovation. During the first six months of 1811, patient numbers increased steadily to almost five hundred. It looked promising on paper. This trial had had the crucial support of three respectable citizens: prominent Quaker chocolate manufacturer Joseph Storrs Fry, druggist friend John Brent Cross, and businessman relative George Fisher Jr., signatories to Prichard's circular canvassing for donations.[4] His efforts on behalf of the indigent must have come to the attention of Bristol's Guardians of the Poor, for when they increased the number of physicians in the service of the city's workhouse, St. Peter's Hospital, they appointed Prichard one of them.

Rather than dropping his dispensary project upon starting at St. Peter's, Prichard and his supporters gained more publicity for it in the local newspapers in early 1812. There were flaws in the scheme, however. His backers were, perplexingly, two Dissenters and one Anglican in a city of sectarian charities. Perhaps the charitable citizens of Bristol preferred to bestow their treatment vouchers on their more respectable, deserving servants and factory workers through the usual ostentatious patronage of the existing medical charities. At any rate, as he settled into curing the ills of the incarcerated paupers of St. Peter's and heard rumors of a medical post in another proposed dispensary, he abandoned the Castle Green Dispensary.[5]

St. Peter's Hospital

Joining the medical staff of St. Peter's Hospital greatly enhanced Prichard's reputation. There he gained twenty-one years' experience that would shape him as a medical and psychiatric theorist focusing on the etiology, nosology, and therapeutics of fevers, epilepsy, and insanity. St. Peter's was not only the city's poorhouse or workhouse but the receptacle of its lunatics and idiots, as they were called. He had a captive set of patients—literally.

For centuries religious institutions and charities had cared for the destitute and insane, but the dissolution of the monasteries led to this being succeeded by the poor rate, a tax financing parish "relief" to the poor. To avoid this expense, parishes policed their borders to keep out or eject vagrants not "of the parish." Parliament enacted a law in 1696 allowing Bristol to establish the nation's first Board of Guardians, a watershed in the history of British welfare. These elected worthy citizens were empowered to pool a tax from surrounding parishes not only to maintain the poor efficiently

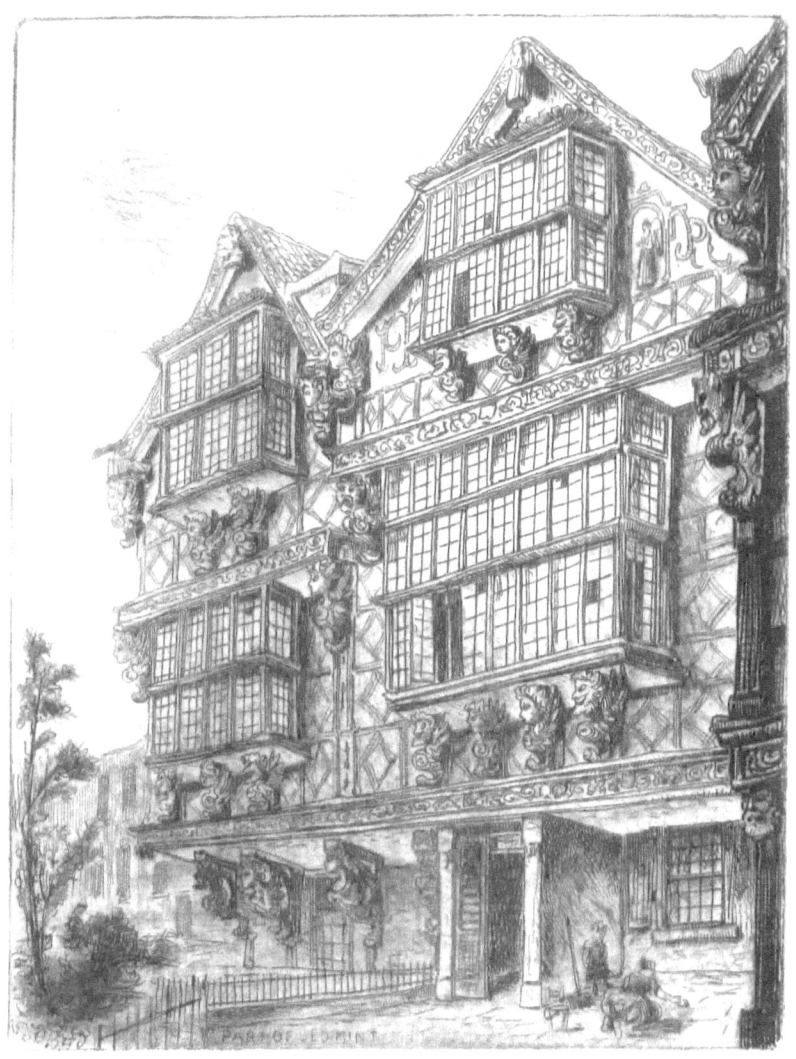

4. Storing the poor and insane. St. Peter's Hospital, Bristol. Etching by Charles Bird. Courtesy of Bristol Libraries.

but to ensure that all who were able worked.[6] In 1698 they transformed a sugar refiner's ancient mansion on Peter Street in the heart of the Old City into St. Peter's Hospital—a general depository of pauper Bristolians. There the Guardians ensured "the regulation, management, maintenance, and employment of the poor of the city." At the time of Prichard's appointment, St. Peter's was thought relatively humane, though corporal punishment was administered; its lunatics were restrained with straps only when necessary. The apothecary and midwife were paid members of the medical staff while the surgeons and physicians were not. Dr. Colin Chisholm painted an idyllic picture in 1817:

> The house is calculated for the comfortable accommodation of 400 paupers of all descriptions. It is always full; and the unfortunate, the superannuated, and the orphan poor, are perpetual inmates. The males and females have distinct wards; and such is the attention to feelings of delicacy and decorum, the superannuated, the decayed, and the children, have their respective wards separated from the rest, the latter with suitable superintending matrons. There are also distinct wards for male and female lunatics, with attached and appropriate cells for the worst cases. The sick, more especially cases of fever, are placed in wards, spacious, clean, and well ventilated, which have no interference with other parts of the house.[7]

When two vacancies for physicians occurred, Prichard made his interest known. He soon complained to his father about one supporter's neglect, but his father fired back a reprimand reminding him that an indication of moral perfection is the ability to be indulgent in judging the failings in others.[8] The Incorporation of the Poor's Governor Daniel Wait, Esq., an influential Tory alderman and former high sheriff and mayor, appointed him physician to St. Peter's on August 8, 1811. Prichard and fellow appointee Henry Hawes Fox, son of the famous alienist Edward Long Fox, joined Dr. Edward Kentish, while the newly appointed surgeon was Dr. Pole's son-in-law, Nehemiah Duck—two Anglicans and two Dissenters.[9]

Business was booming at St. Peter's. The city's manufacturing, trade, and building industries were suffering severe wartime depression, exacerbated by ill-fated speculative investments and government financial incompetence. The unemployment and wage deflation among Bristol laborers and increase in the number of incoming vagrants plunged the poorhouse into crisis. The Bristol Mendicity Society founded for the purpose of scooping up vagrants and returning them to their parishes or to Ireland had its work cut out for it. Prichard attended the sick at St. Peter's on a weekly rota, taking on responsibility for those admitted on his shift. He visited them at least once a week, kept precise records, and attended in emergencies at the apothecary's request. A rule enjoined all members of the medical staff to pay special attention "to all Lunatic Paupers, and that their cases shall be noticed in a separate Book."[10] Prichard described the inmates, then averaging 420, as of three classes of persons; the most numerous are of the same description as the inmates of other poor-houses; viz. The aged and infirm, who have a parochial right in Bristol, together with orphan children and all other persons possessed of the same claim, who on account of sickness or other circumstances are unable to maintain themselves, and do not receive pay out of doors. The second class includes all the vagrants and beggars who are found in Bristol, except such as the magistrates immediately expel from the city. . . . Of this description of persons there is always a considerable number, Bristol being the port at which Irish paupers are embarked from all the neighbouring parts of England, on their way to their native country; and during the late period of distress among the lower orders of people, there has been an unusual overflow of such visitors. The third class of inmates in St. Peter's hospital, are the idiots and lunatics of the lower orders, who are sent to the house, under warrants, from all parts of the city, and are received, under particular circumstances, from the towns and villages in its vicinity.[11]

Most of St. Peter's inmates were incapable of performing any tasks, but some worked as its servants, cooks, and brewers, and a few dozen elderly paupers were employed in picking oakum and hair. The boys were taught to read and write before being apprenticed, while the girls learned to read and sew. Food and clothing were the institution's main expenses; meat and vegetables were provided twice a week. As the population of Bristol increased, so did the pressure on St. Peter's, especially as it also had to provide maintenance payments and medical care to more and more nonresident paupers. In 1820 a James Johnson began publishing pamphlets urging St. Peter's expansion. He also wanted it reformed so that the indolent could be excluded; Ireland's custom of shipping its wandering vagrants to Bristol was becoming intolerable.[12]

The new appointees had a lot in common: Prichard and Fox were former Quakers and Edinburgh trained. They would be elected physicians to the Bristol Infirmary on the same day, specialize in psychiatric medicine, and produce medical sons and grandsons. Fox had been a member and one of the presidents of the Royal Medical Society, but he left Edinburgh without taking a degree, instead proceeding to Cambridge, where he obtained an MB in 1811 and a rare, career-enhancing MD in 1826. Fox's key to success was his eminent father, Bristol Infirmary's long-serving physician and proprietor of an elite asylum in nearby Brislington. The elder Dr. Fox had confidently proposed his son as physician to the Infirmary even before the young man had settled in Bristol.[13] Fox père had managed to build a large, lucrative medical practice, and his son soon did the same. Fortunately for Prichard, there had been two vacancies to fill.

By 1820 Prichard was bravely campaigning for the improvement of St. Peter's Hospital's care of the destitute, orphaned, sick, and insane of Bristol's nineteen parishes and of any transients to the city. The few attempts made to meliorate conditions there only highlighted the building's total inadequacy, to Prichard's mind:

> Its construction is as awkward and inconvenient as it is possible to imagine. It is a confused heap of buildings, appended one to the other, without symmetry or plan, each part having been raised to answer some occasional purpose, as the original edifice, which is very old, was found inadequate to the exigencies which from time to time arose. Accordingly there are many parts of this hospital which it is impossible by any care sufficiently to ventilate, or to render decent and comfortable. During the last eight years it has undergone many improvements, among which is the establishment of medical wards, or distinct apartments for the sick, who previously to that time had no separate station, but were scattered through the whole house. Some of the wards, in their former state, particularly those appropriated to passengers, that is, to vagrants who are brought into the Hospital, and remain until they can be sent forward to their homes or parishes, were fitter receptacles for wild beasts than for human beings. There is still great room for improvement, though it would perhaps be difficult to devise a means of effecting it, without pulling down the whole building to its foundations.[14]

Provision for the insane earned Prichard's barbed observation: "The accommodation provided for these afflicted beings consists of an airy and spacious ward for the female lunatics, and a row of pens for the temporary confinement of those patients who are violent and intractable, not unlike the domiciles of the royal lions and tigers in the menagerie of the Tower, though by no means so respectable in their appearance, or so commodious. . . . The male lunatics and idiots in the house have been generally stationed in the medical wards."[15]

The local government was required to shelter and maintain the mentally ill and disabled, but not to treat or rehabilitate them. Not only was

St. Peter's appallingly overcrowded; it was situated on the bank of a polluted river detrimental to its inmates' health. Dr. Chisholm suggested that since the river had been dammed in 1810 to create a nontidal harbor, the resulting trapped sewerage could be linked to the poorhouse's high rate of disease. The number of "outdoor" (nonresident) destitute sick paupers rose inexorably. Overcrowding continued unabated until the 1832 cholera epidemic ravaged its six hundred inmates. Although the national lunacy commissioners, Prichard among them, found St. Peter's unfit to house the insane in 1844, the City Asylum was not established for another twelve years.[16] Care of the poor and the insane became two of the nineteenth century's growth industries.

Volunteering at St. Peter's kept Fox's and Prichard's names before the public and furnished them with a generous supply of the mentally ill to study. Even after both had been elected to the more prestigious Bristol Infirmary, they continued serving St. Peter's, resigning only during the 1832 cholera epidemic when it was alleged that Fox had not attended his duties for three years. He promptly opened his own asylum in Northwoods, Gloucestershire, and Prichard later committed patients to the Foxes' asylums and inspected Northwoods in his capacity as a commissioner in lunacy.[17]

The Clifton Dispensary

Below the high, airy limestone plateau of the affluent suburb of Clifton, a slum scarred a thirty- to fifty-yard-wide stretch of low land along the riverbank, home to three thousand or so Bristolians, mostly sailors, tradesmen, laborers, superannuated servants, washerwomen, and their children. Overcrowding, poor ventilation, malnourishment, and lack of sanitation made this impoverished part of Clifton a hotbed of contagion; epidemic and endemic diseases such as typhus, cholera, and consumption were rife. The Bristol Infirmary, only a twenty-minute walk away, was generally not for the likes of them, however. One of Britain's relatively few large charity hospitals, it dealt mainly with accidents, emergencies, and some fevers but excluded the contagious, consumptive, pediatric, obstetric, and terminal cases.[18] Although the Bristol Infirmary did have an outpatient department, it failed to cope with rising demand. A newer, smaller charity medical service would help fill this gap in the care of the poor, economically dealing with those who could not travel or be treated at other dispensaries or the Infirmary. As Infirmary cases were more likely curable, its reputation was higher, and its larger staff and more elaborate and complex premises were impressive, making a Bristol Infirmary post a safer and more prestigious appointment for professional advancement. Prichard could actually learn more about disease as a dispensary physician, however. The poor down by the river near Hotwells were in dire need of medical care.

Most dispensaries were financed by subscribers and governed by a committee. They elected unremunerated physicians and surgeons to serve on a rota six days a week. Subscribers were entitled to recommend a given number of "deserving poor" for treatment either as outpatients or for home visits. Because the sick poor applied directly to them, these benefactors saw for themselves that their money was well spent on suitably grateful objects.[19]

Working for the Clifton Dispensary provided Prichard with opportunities to network among its subscribers, study diseases, and risk catching them too. He could learn how to treat diseases and describe and classify them in the fashion of the eighteenth-century natural historians, a scientific practice reinforced in Scottish Enlightenment thinking.

The Clifton Dispensary got off to a surprisingly rocky start. When some altruistic citizens met at Hotwells School-Room on October 29, 1812, for the purpose of "establishing a DISPENSARY or some other mode of Medical Relief, for the Indigent Sick in the Parish," their plans sparked public outrage. The local newspapers printed letters protesting that there was no need for medical assistance; the already appointed parish doctor was all that was needed; the dispensary would attract the poor into the area; it would encourage sloth; it would be uneconomical; the Infirmary met the need adequately; and medical men were just trying to create employment for themselves.

The Clifton Dispensary came into existence anyway. Two doctors and a committee of gentlemen drew up rules, astutely securing the participation of the local clergy, churchwardens, and overseers of the poor. It was generally organized and controlled by Tory Anglicans and a few Unitarians and included a vice admiral, two clergymen, a physician, and several gentlemen. Within a fortnight, 144 of Bristol's elite and their wives and daughters, Prichard's potential private patients, rallied with 1 or half-guinea annual subscriptions. The higher rate entitled one to recommend four sick poor and one lying-in patient, while the half guinea bought patronage for three sick patients. Drs. Chisholm and Prichard and surgeons Thomas Roblyn and Peter De Jersey were appointed on December 1. From the dispensary's opening on New Year's Day 1813, the medical staff carefully recorded the diseases they encountered, pursuing what his colleague Dr. Chisholm termed "statistical pathology," an element of future public health practice.[20]

Prichard would eventually adopt this methodology to compile a nosology of mental illness.

Prichard's new colleagues were from very different backgrounds. A generation older, Dr. Colin Chisholm had the social disadvantage of having begun his career in military medical service, but he made up for it by publishing a huge number of articles and some books on medicine and natural history. He had already acquired an international reputation for his assertion that fever was essentially contagious. Like Prichard, he was a data collector, especially on typhus, which allowed him to claim that if the disease were merely the result of squalor, the Clifton slum should have been devastated. In fact, the relative mildness of the disease there and other factors "proved that the infection of typhus is a specific virus ... and regulated by the same laws." The medical world would remain generally indifferent to this notion for decades.

Prichard was also interested in Chisholm's articles on bloodletting and the use of calomel in fever and mercury for cerebral disorders. He belonged to several prestigious learned societies such as the Royal Society of London, something Prichard aspired to. Chisholm had also recently published a defense of the specific unity of the human species based upon the necessary and authentic principles of divine law at the very time Prichard was writing his *Researches into the Physical History of Man*. Respected and experienced Dr. Chisholm had views Prichard could support.[21]

Prichard's other two Clifton Dispensary colleagues were a surgeon and man-midwife and an apothecary. As the only medical member of its governing committee, Dr. William Gilby was perhaps instrumental in Prichard's initial appointment. His son, Prichard's geologizing friend William Hall Gilby, MD, Edin, eventually succeeded Prichard.[22]

The Clifton Dispensary's first annual *Medical Report* sparked a row played out in the columns of the local newspapers. As Prichard's senior, Dr. Chisholm put his name to an extensive statistical table of diseases dealt with by the dispensary staff in which he indulged not only in using impressive Latin terminology but in applying the Linnaean device of genus and species, with disease genera having one or more species.[23] This was too good an opportunity for "Junius," claiming to be on the faculty of the (rival) Bristol Infirmary, who penned a long letter to the editor ridiculing the pomposity and doubting the validity of the report.

Prichard, deeply offended by Junius's imputations and nicely keeping his name before the public as a properly university-educated physician, carefully signed his letter to the editor from prestigious College Green. He explained he had considered the aspersions unworthy of notice until he realized some readers might have thought Junius a genuine, authoritative faculty member of the Bristol Infirmary. Impossible. The scurrilous, naive author was undoubtedly a young pupil, nor could he have attended a London medical school. At any rate, those London institutions could not hold a candle to the University of Edinburgh Medical School. Prichard seized this opportunity:

> The School of Physic in London has never indeed made high pretensions. It is a very good preparatory school, where the first rudiments of medical knowledge are taught in very short courses of lectures [suitable for those] destitute of any previous knowledge of their future profession, except some acquaintance with the manipulations of pharmacy. But if the author of the criticism had acquired even a slight tincture of the science he claims, he would have spared me the irksome task of commenting upon remarks which originate in the grossest ignorance. . . . If the critic had even entered the precincts of a Medical school, he must have heard of the nosological writers, and would have acquired more or less acquaintance with the most distinguished of them, namely Sauvages.

Warming to his task, Prichard accused Junius of blunders in logic, being more ignorant than even the youngest pupil and "not a giant in the disguise of a dwarf, but is yet a more puny personage than he professes to be." He finished by announcing he would spare himself the trouble of making any further comment.[24] Dr. Prichard, not yet twenty-eight, brooked no criticism in defending his august status in the medical world. Bristol medical men spilled a lot of ink on skirmishes like this over the years.

The Clifton Dispensary continued its work among the Hotwells poor, smoothing their passage from privation to the grave. Its medical men tackled diseases before the advent of medical microbiology, and they introduced generally beneficial vaccination and midwifery services. Chisholm and Prichard attributed the district's huge mortality rate mostly to appalling diet and living conditions, and decades later the denizens of the dispensary's catchment area were just as miserable.[25] The Clifton Dispensary furnished young Dr. Prichard with medical experience, good publicity, and access to its well-to-do subscribers for the four years he volunteered there. It continued to serve the district's needy residents for more than a century.

The Bristol Dispensaries

Not long after starting at the Clifton Dispensary, a similar post at the Bristol Dispensaries came up. Founded in 1775 by Methodists renowned for their concern for the poor, this charity treated the sick poor in their homes and provided midwifery services to certified married women. Its large staff comprised a secretary and two apothecaries/men-midwives who were paid about £450 annually, while less than £150 was sufficient to employ five women-midwives. Additionally, six volunteer men-midwives and two physicians were consulted in difficult cases. Prichard first appeared in its 1814 *State of the Bristol Dispensaries*, when the charity proudly recorded having treated 1,897 patients and delivered 802 babies.[26] This charity ran a highly successful weekly clinic for cowpox inoculation, the revolutionary prophylactic introduced there in October 1801 "to extirpate the small pox with its fatal consequences from this city."[27]

Prichard was among the Dispensaries' nearly five hundred subscribers comprising medical men, clergymen, many ladies, and some businesses, another *Who's Who?* of Bristol and source of fee-paying patients. Its ladies' auxiliary committee monitored the work of the midwives and their cases. For every guinea subscribed, benefactors could recommend one midwifery and four sick patients, thus providing cheap medical treatments for their servants and employees while marking their own charitable worth in the community. The Dispensaries also attracted legacies like the one for £100 from John Scandrett Harford Sr., and it benefited from a proportion of fines received from the Customs House and for offenses such as indecent behavior.[28]

Prichard valued his association with his Dispensaries and St. Peter's senior colleague Dr. Edward Kentish, then at the height of his career. Kentish published widely on the treatment of burns and scalds, gout, cancer, vapor baths, and other topics such as electoral reform. He owned the Madeira House for warm and vapor bath treatments and, a typical Unitarian, was a forthright and active reforming Whig, as well as president of the Anchor Society, the Whig Colston charity. As a non-Tory Dissenter, he was socially ineligible for election to the Bristol Infirmary; rather he would be instrumental in founding the rival (Whig and Dissenter) Bristol General Hospital. Prichard and Kentish would serve on the Bristol Board of Health, founded to deal with the cholera epidemic of 1831–32.[29]

"Charity Universal"

The Bristol (later Royal) Infirmary was a medical charity conducted on a much larger scale than the dispensaries Prichard was serving. Founded to supplement the meager medical service provided by St. Peter's Hospital, it admitted its first inpatients to adapted premises on Maudlin Street in 1737. It was expected that it would help stave off Bristol's social unrest and allow Bristol to match ever-dominant London in civic pride.[30] The Infirmary was a complex organization governed by subscribers who were supposed to cooperate with its elected medical faculty. This cooperation frequently broke down, and among the faculty there were conflicting theories of treatment. The Infirmary's huge archive documents its rich history.

A contest for the post of physician to the Infirmary had all the hallmarks of a general election campaign, apparently minus the corruption. Succeeding on his third attempt, Prichard spent the following twenty-seven years conscientiously fulfilling his obligations, working to improve the Infirmary's service, developing his medical experience and reputation, publishing medical books and articles, forming professional and personal relationships, and regularly quarreling with colleagues and the governing committee. He held on to this unremunerated post even after he no longer needed it to further his career.

Nine trustees, the so-called House Visitors, oversaw the hospital's administration and reported to the House Committee, and any of the more than a thousand subscribers could get involved in the management of the Infirmary by attending its weekly meetings. The Infirmary's byline, "Charity Universal," advertised Bristolians' munificence more than the universal access to health care. For a few guineas annually, subscribers could issue tickets of admission to those sick poor who applied to them directly. They were thus able to send their sick and injured employees, servants, and parishioners for free out- or inpatient treatment, which otherwise would require the paid services of practitioners such as apothecaries and bonesetters. The Infirmary's *respectable* sick poor patients found themselves closely controlled by its rules as they had their wounds tended and diseases cured so they could be promptly returned to work. It was no place for the truly destitute or vagrant.

By the time Prichard settled in Bristol, the Infirmary had become essentially an Anglican Tory institution: the overwhelming majority of the committee as well as the faculty were Tories, even though the subscribers were of all persuasions. As with the other medical charities, being a subscriber confirmed high social standing. The Infirmary's published reports and subscription lists ensured public recognition of all contributions, whether of money or expertise. Its several honorary and remunerated administrative posts also afforded opportunities for subscribers' sons' professional advancement. In 1832, when it could no longer cope with increasing patient numbers, Dissenters and Whigs would establish the Bristol General Hospital.[31]

The Infirmary Election Campaigns, 1810 and 1811

Another benefit of the Infirmary was the excitement of its staff elections. There were religious and party affiliations to discriminate, candidates' leaflets to read, campaign visits to make, gossip to share, patronage to bestow, scores to settle, and deals to do. Candidates' advertisements and sometimes anonymous, insinuating letters to the editor spiced up the newspapers and furnished a few weeks of debate and intrigue. Finally came the gala election day at the Guildhall, when the most prestigious patrons floridly proposed and seconded their candidate. The ballots were then handed in and counted, and grudges were formed and held.

So highly prized was an Infirmary post, multiple attempts at it were not uncommon—like Prichard's three and Estlin's unsuccessful four. Even losing was good publicity. Prichard's first opportunity came just a few months after he had settled in Bristol, too soon for him to have established his Tory credentials and sufficient patronage. His rather halfhearted advertisement of August 31, 1810, was published along with those of six rivals, most of whom already had established careers and posts at other medical charities.[32] By election day there were just three remaining. Dr. Andrew Carrick received 448 votes, while Dr. Stock came second with 216. Prichard, proposed by Alterman Daniel Wait (a St. Peter's connection) and seconded by Uncle Francis Fisher, attracted only 81 votes, a creditable first attempt. Stock conceded with praise of the victor, while Prichard earnestly announced he did not despair of success on a future occasion. Rather than being motivated by private interests, he wished to render himself useful to his fellow creatures, promote their well-being and alleviate their sufferings.[33] Hopefuls had to go to the polls regularly, gradually accumulating votes, and that is what Stock and Prichard did. The losing candidate of today was the successful one of tomorrow.

The following year there was another resignation. In the ensuing race Drs. Stock, Charles Edward Bernard, and Prichard were joined by Thomas Webb Dyer, MD Aberdeen, a practicing physician but tainted by his position as the erstwhile, socially inferior Infirmary house apothecary. Dr. Dyer rather rashly considered the board's approbation of his twenty years' service a recommendation,[34] and he would have won but for an eleventh-hour plot: instead of splitting the Unitarian vote between Prichard, son-in-law of the Unitarian minister, and Unitarian Stock, Prichard strategically resigned in his friend's favor.[35] He would have to bide his time.

A Brief Career as a Medical Lecturer

While waiting for another shot at the Infirmary, Prichard volunteered at his three other medical charities and devised another plan. Immensely proud of his Edinburgh medical degree, he found himself in a city where medical education could be had only through lowly apprenticeships to surgeons and apothecaries, attending private anatomy classes, or becoming a Bristol Infirmary pupil. Prichard's "MD, Edin" put him a cut above his rival physicians, especially as many had essentially bought their degrees rather than attended university. He would play this card to the hilt. Inexperienced as he was, his degree qualified him as a medical lecturer, and becoming one would remind Bristolians how well educated he was. He advertised on February 26, 1814: "Dr. PRICHARD proposes to commence, early in the month of March, a COURSE OF MEDICAL LECTURES, comprising Physiology, Pathology, and the Practice of Physic. For particulars apply to Dr. P. College-Green."[36] When the Infirmary subscribers next saw his name on their ballot paper, they would recognize him as a physician and medical educator.

Prichard gave his successful course of lectures at his home, 39 College Green, in a neighborhood not yet scarred by shops. There had been some eighteenth-century public medical lectures in Bristol, and by 1813 two private schools of anatomy and medicine had been established. In 1815 Prichard's second annual course began on November 6 and lasted for about six months. His neighbor Mr. Francis Gold offered a course in anatomy and physiology, and the following year a Mr. Rolfe announced his series of lectures on obstetrics "illustrated by an ingenious machine and apparatus contrived for the purpose."[37] But all lacked the added dimension of clinical lectures such as Prichard hoped to introduce. Meanwhile, without access to the Infirmary wards, anatomical specimens, or apparatus, his course was necessarily theoretical. He did not have to wait for long; in early 1816 another vacancy occurred, and once again Prichard, now the successful medical lecturer and charity physician, threw his hat in the ring.

The 1816 Infirmary Contest

The Infirmary's Dr. Fox began canvassing on behalf of his son, Henry Hawes Fox, Prichard's St. Peter's colleague. Learning that subscribers seemed to object to a father and son on the faculty at the same time, Fox Sr. obligingly resigned.[38] As in the St. Peter's appointment, there being two vacancies greatly improved Prichard's chances of success. He threw himself into securing pledges, and the newspapers splashed gossip and even some verse about this election. The Infirmary had to advertise its rule barring subscribers of less than six months from voting.[39]

The 1816 contest opened with some negative campaigning and went downhill from there. The third candidate in the field, Dr. Thomas Dyer, could not shake off his reputation for being a jumped-up apothecary, even though he affected the supercilious demeanor of an eighteenth-century physician. His colleague Richard Smith unkindly observed that he "walked as if he shit himself—& looked as if he smelled it." Dyer could boast positive testimonials from his physician colleagues and the Infirmary Board. On February 7 "A Subscriber" appealed to readers of *Felix Farley's Bristol Journal* to set partiality, amiability, and "other causes" aside and choose the best physicians for the posts. "Best" in this case meant properly qualified, as in having attended a medical course leading to an MD rather than having obtained a "diploma purchased from one of those degraded universities," which even street corner quacks could boast of. The waspish writer considered a British MD based on a university course of study the best medical qualification in the world. For the sake of the Infirmary's reputation, therefore, only regularly and properly educated candidates should be considered. A Subscriber was none other than Dr. Stock, Infirmary physician and proud possessor of a university MD; he anonymously and effectively undermined Dyer's credibility.[40] His own supporters did not take these aspersions lying down. "Fair Play" (Infirmary Surgeon Richard Smith) proclaimed A Subscriber's arguments specious and illiberal.[41]

Everyone had an opinion. "Another Subscriber" (Dr. Stock again) enlarged upon the inferior status of any physician "irregularly educated"—all very beneficial to Drs. Prichard and Fox. Other physicians anonymously joined the fray, one observing Dyer had never furthered medical knowledge by a single publication and another countering by pointing out that there was a precedent for electing "irregularly educated" physicians and that Fox's exact medical education was something of a mystery anyway. This was strong stuff. Prichard sent out special cards and a very polite printed letter to his supporters, reminding them to attend and cast their ballots on his behalf.[42]

Prichard insisted on having the last word. Writing as "Candidus" in the *Bristol Mirror*, he defended his alma mater "from the foul aspersions which have been so abundantly cast on her." Safely anonymous, he attempted wit, promising not to throw "peristaltic motions," and then a bit of hyperbolizing in his outrage at Edinburgh's fine MD being compared to one purchased from "those pestilent nurseries of Quackery, in the North of Scotland, those head quarters of imposture, whence issue all the venders of Enchanted Beds, Balms of Gilead, Solar Tinctures, Balsams of Life, Magic Girdles,—all the Casters of Nativities, and the whole tribe of Mountebanks, licensed to kill hundreds of his Majesty's liege subjects, that a few pounds may accrue annually to the Treasury." He then pointed out that a medical degree examination was as exacting as the classical and mathematical ones at Oxford and Cambridge. Clearly, Edinburgh and perhaps Glasgow had the only medical schools worthy of the name. While Oxford and Cambridge were excellent in what they did teach, "as for a medical School in either, no such thing exists; and it is well known that the Students of both resort to Edinburgh and to Foreign Universities, for Medical Instruction." Prichard then treated his patient readers to an outline of Edinburgh's curriculum, its illustrious professors, and its grueling private and public examinations. As for the accusation that "Grinders" were employed to school candidates in pat Latin responses, they were merely tutors of spoken Latin to those students who needed it for their examinations. In sum, the University of Edinburgh was everything it should be and not what its vile calumniators insinuated. Prichard ended his diatribe by congratulating those Infirmary subscribers who wisely valued proper medical education.

Another candidate then withdrew, narrowing the field. Prichard advertised again, entreating his supporters to arrive at the Guildhall at an early hour to ensure victory.[43] The whipped-up disdain for MDs granted on testimonial worked to Prichard's favor. The poll commenced at 11 a.m. on Leap Day 1816, Sir Richard Vaughan presiding, and there was a supplementary polling station in St. George's Chapel doorway where invalids, medical gentlemen, and ladies could submit their ballots. John Estlin was Prichard's special steward, while artist Edward Bird and the Rev. John Eagles attended the door on his behalf, personifying nonconformism, fame, and Anglicanism, respectively. Sir Abraham Elton nominated Dr. Fox in a grandiloquent speech decrying the letter to the editor's scurrilous imputations concerning the validity of his candidate's Cambridge degree. The influential Rev. Thomas Biddulph seconded Fox's nomination, the stamp of Establishment approval.

Alderman Thomas Stock, governor of St. Peter's Hospital, liberal supporter of religious and educational institutions, and a cultivator of the society of literary and well-informed men, nominated Prichard. Prichard was covering the vote-winning bases. After Mr. Stock dealt with the medical qualification issue, he praised Prichard for his "ardour of mind, the love of science, [and] the laudable ambition after excellence," which had uniformly characterized his pursuits. He stressed Prichard's "professional skill, humane consideration, and assiduous attention" in his service to St. Peter's, where his conduct was "unvariably attentive and satisfactory." In an appeal to civic pride, Stock promised that if Prichard was elected, he and Dr. Stock would provide courses of medical and surgical lectures that would further science and put Bristol on a par with London as a city with a teaching hospital fit for the nineteenth century. Prichard would be a credit to the Infirmary and the city. The nomination was seconded by another well-selected local figure, philanthropic businessman Thomas Sanders, a citizen in sympathy with the Society of Friends.[44]

The turnout was high. At 7:00 p.m. it was announced that Fox had come in first with 968 votes; Prichard received 670 and Dyer 515. *Felix Farley's Bristol Journal* proclaimed that Dyer's failure was a vote for the advantages of a regular and classical education. In short, his twenty years of experience could not compare to three years at university.[45] Prichard resigned from the Clifton Dispensary and started juggling St. Peter's Hospital's, Bristol Dispensaries', and the Infirmary's weekly rotas. His father was pleased with the victory; Dr. Prichard's career was set to flourish.

Infirmary Staff and Students

With the defeat of the 1782 plan to move to the salubrious site of the Red Lodge, the Infirmary's patchwork of old, makeshift, overcrowded and unventilated wards on its original Maudlin Street site was redeveloped in stages. Progress on this state-of-the-art temple to civic beneficence was less than rapid; in June 1814 the proceeds of a fundraising music festival at the Theatre Royal allowed the West Wing to be furnished for use.[46] It accommodated fifty patients and nurses and had cold, warm, and vapor baths designed by Prichard's Dispensaries colleague Dr. Kentish. Large windows ensured health-promoting ventilation.

The Infirmary's 180 beds were divided into wards of twelve or thirteen beds, roughly equally divided between medical patients on the first floor and surgical patients on the upper ones. Strong metal gates separated the male and female wards.[47] The year of Prichard's election, 2,870 outpatients were treated and 1,576 inpatients admitted, with a daily average population of 192. These figures steadily rose until patients often had to be put two in a

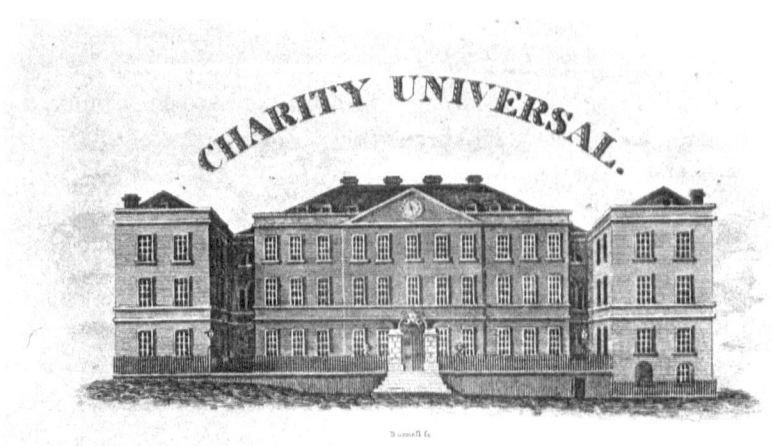

5. Charity Universal. Bristol Infirmary, 1816. Engraving. Property of the author.

bed.[48] Overcrowding and the turning away of patients went on throughout Prichard's time there, even though pediatric, maternity, and venereal cases and those suffering from itch and fits were excluded, and fever cases were immediately removed to special lodgings elsewhere.[49]

Among the several paid members of the Infirmary staff were a dispenser, laboratory man, and shop boy, assisted by the "house pupils." For an annual salary of £20, the matron was responsible for making all household purchases, inspecting the wards daily, seeing to security, and supervising the nurses who were treated as domestic servants. The secretary, a post for a young respectable man, was paid £63 a year for keeping the ledgers and records of the committee and conducting its correspondence. An Anglican chaplain served the spiritual needs of the Infirmary, but to assuage sectarian objections, his stipend was not derived from general funds.[50]

Interaction between the four physicians and five surgeons was guided by custom. The physicians' superior social and financial standing perpetually offended the surgeons, however. The students had to cooperate among themselves, sharing duties unofficially and broadening their experience in a hostile atmosphere. The apothecary, supervised by the physicians, was responsible for the medical patients. He and his apprentices could have nothing officially to do with the surgical patients, as the surgeons resented any interference.[51] Attended by his two senior pupils, he went around all the medical wards daily, seeing every patient, and for an extra fee the surgeons' pupils were allowed to observe. During this daily round, the respect of the patients and pupils was assured and marked by a convention: the faculty wore hats. Prichard's grandson reminisced that this was still the case in the 1870s when the pupils longed for the day they could don their silk "toppers" in the wards.[52]

The fees the pupils paid for the much sought-after privilege of hospital experience were split between the Infirmary and their masters. In 1818 sixteen Infirmary students studied medicine, surgery, and anatomy by attending the medical officer on duty during the daily outpatient session and on his ward rounds; they processed prescriptions, performed triage duties, and either carried out basic emergency care or fetched the duty surgeon of the week. They were also not above creating occasional disturbances with their quarrels and neglect, despite the many rules forbidding impertinence and impropriety.[53] Students played a vital role in the function of the Infirmary while learning on the job.

One of the periodic crises among the faculty involving students unfolded in 1824. Officially, the physicians were not allowed to have their own pupils or apprentices, partly for historical reasons, but mostly owing to the hostility of the surgeons constantly vying for supremacy with both the physicians and the committee. For some years this ban on physicians' having pupils had been subverted by students' paying a small fee to the apothecary, which would allow them to observe both his and the physicians' practice, but the fee was not shared with the physicians. This state of affairs became intolerable to the physicians, who were striving for the same prestige, satisfaction, and pupils' fees their London counterparts enjoyed. Besides, there was a demand for this new type of medical education that prepared men for the recently liberalized system of certification. But supported by the rival surgeons, the committee held firm against this until the physicians resorted to citing the 1743 rule that the charity had been founded to treat the poor and provide instruction to medical practitioners, presumably of both sorts.[54] The Physicians' Pupils War won, they were allowed three pupils at 3 guineas each for a fifteen-month term. This was increased to six pupils per physician in 1838, while the surgeons were allowed three "dressers," or assistants, and three non-assistant pupils. Over the years, Prichard had at least twenty-one such pupils, adding moderately to his income and more substantially to his reputation beyond the Infirmary.[55]

As soon as Prichard gained his Infirmary post, he underscored his commitment to improving medical education in Bristol, and the Infirmary would be instrumental to his plans. He discontinued lecturing from his home and planned a new course with Dr. Stock. This time it would have the prestige of its Infirmary location and include clinical lectures with examples from the wards, just like those of the Edinburgh Medical School. They advertised their course on the "INSTITUTES and PRACTICE of MEDICINE" for the ensuing academic term.[56] The fee for Stock and Prichard's course of sixty lectures on physiology, pathology, therapeutics, and the practice of physic was 3 guineas, while another 2 guineas bought daily attendance of the clinical wards with either physician. They printed an eight-page syllabus for their physiology lectures and asked permission to use one of the Infirmary's rooms. Importantly, they informed the committee they intended their course to be the foundation of a hospital medical school, so they formally requested the approbation of all the members of the faculty, inviting the surgeons to contribute surgical lectures in the future.

After a good start, attendance dwindled. One member of the committee suggested the surgical pupils had too many different lectures to attend, while Prichard himself complained that he could not fix a time for the lectures that suited the pupils. There was some opposition from the committee, and the pupils seemed apathetic. Eventually it was claimed that students could gain sufficient clinical instruction during the course of their ward rounds anyway; formal lectures were superfluous. Notwithstanding, both Stock and Prichard's reputations were bolstered by their concern for medical education in Bristol.[57]

Although the medical lectures were discontinued, the Infirmary gradually became more of a teaching hospital in other ways. The faculty increased students' access to wards and developed the Reading Room on the ground floor next to the Museum, overseen by the house surgeon with a pupil as the acting librarian.[58] Almost in the span of Prichard's lifetime, the medical profession and medical education evolved from apprenticeship-based training for the vast majority to more formally organized programs delivered at hospitals and medical schools. More medical lecture and anatomy courses would spring up in the city, the latter obtaining recognition by the London authorities as early as 1818. Prichard consistently called for the foundation of a much-needed organized medical school. He was delighted when a prospectus for a school of medicine based on the amalgamation of the private Bristol Medical and Surgical School and the School of Anatomy and Medicine was published in 1832.[59] In Prichard's support of it, his other Bristol educational initiatives, and even his call to found a local university, his dedication to making Bristol a provincial seat of learning is apparent.

Infirmary Practice: Snatching, Bleeding, and Feeding

The Infirmary naturally played a central role in public health care in Bristol. It became apparent, however, that while the practice of surgery was making great strides, medicine was not. Physicians employed various and clearly contradictory forms of therapeutics usually with similar outcomes; there was hardly any preventive medicine and only the most tentative steps toward developing a theory of contagion had been taken. By contrast, surgery was progressing, even without anesthesia or antisepsis. Both surgeons and physicians could agree that medical and surgical progress depended on sound knowledge of anatomy and physiology, achievable only through human dissection. They set about this enthusiastically.

The faculty regularly "opened" diseased patients in the face of their families' entrenched ignorance and prejudice, or justifiable outrage, depending on point of view. Human dissection was illegal on all but executed criminals, so blatant infringements drew public wrath. The not-unfounded belief among many poor Bristolians was that this desecration of the human body practiced mainly on their relatives ultimately benefited the rich. The Infirmary responded by generally turning a blind eye to the rampant practice while stonewalling complaints about the routine dissection of the dead.

Infirmary patients and Bristol's executed failed to supply enough of their unclaimed corpses to satisfy the Infirmary and local anatomy lecturers, so the medical students took the matter into their own hands by taking to body snatching. Bristol magistrates were complicit in this illegal business: for while they would sentence a poor boy to transportation or even death for the theft of a shirt, they might punish Infirmary students who stole bodies with a small fine, if that. The situation was similar at St. Peter's Hospital, where the routine dissection of its deceased paupers was the medical staff's perk. This could usually be done with impunity, as the body was destined for the hospital's graveyard, but when relatives did arrive to collect what turned out to be a mutilated corpse, there would be a fuss. This happened so frequently that the board had to put new rules in place to control and limit dissection.

The faculty and Infirmary pupils engaged in trading "subjects." Possessing the key to the deadhouse, they had free run of its contents such that one former pupil recalled he had had more opportunity for dissection at the Infirmary than he later got at the London hospitals.[60] The students of the independent anatomy schools took it in turn to provide corpses, either from the Infirmary's deadhouse by swapping them from their coffins for objects of similar weight, or from a graveyard; one anatomy teacher boasted of having keys to every churchyard in and around Bristol. Nor were students averse to depredating outlying villages for particularly interesting bodies. In one episode, an inconvenient breakdown of their hired coach resulted in two Infirmary pupils being left holding the bag, literally, when they were caught red-handed with a body in a sack. Their only punishment was having to bear the cost of reburial.[61] Bristol's body snatchers were regularly exposed, but unlike Edinburgh's infamous lowlife Burke and Hare, the city's resurrection men were generally middle class; they cut out the middlemen and did the deed themselves.

Accounts of some of these incidents appeared in the local newspapers. In 1819 a mob stormed the dissecting room of the anatomy school in Lower College Green to retrieve the mutilated body of the wife of one of their number. Body snatching was not an exclusively student avocation. In 1828 two men caught red-handed with telltale equipment in the dead of night in Brislington Churchyard were fined by the magistrate. Three weeks later the same magistrate proposed one of the foiled "resurrection men" for election to the Infirmary. Dr. George Wallis and his co-conspirator, Dr. Henry Riley, became Infirmary physicians. The Infirmary's surgeon Richard Smith, with his passion for macabre tales, even drew up a body-snatching league table of the students, with Prichard's young brother-in-law Edward Rochemont Estlin achieving the top score of thirty.[62] Despite the gallows' generous supply, body snatching continued. No wonder Prichard would sign the national petition calling for legislation liberalizing dissection.

For the Infirmary's living subjects, Prichard was on duty in the Out-Patients' Room or visited the wards two days per week from noon until one o'clock on a rota with his fellow physicians. The House Visitors, volunteers from among the subscribers, first checked patients' eligibility for treatment before sending successive batches of them into the dirty and overcrowded Admissions Room, where the physician and surgeon of the week sat at a table with the apothecary opposite and a few pupils looking on. The patients were sorted into medical and surgical cases before being stood before the staff to be examined without privacy.[63]

Prichard was responsible for patients admitted during his duty week, which meant he had to attend more often if a case required or when there was an emergency. On Saturdays he and the duty surgeon examined and reviewed all of the inpatients. Prichard had a form that he could fill in to request a special consultation with a colleague, and he wrote to charities on patients' behalf. If unavailable to carry out his duties for the week, he could arrange for a colleague to substitute.[64] As members of the faculty aged and became incompetent or unable to attend, it became necessary to make do with fewer medical men, for these were lifetime appointments they seemed loath to relinquish; successive attempts to institute fixed tenure were vigorously contested.[65] The revised Rules of 1832 allowed one physician and one surgeon on annual rotation to serve on the committee. Another innovation that year was the new role of Female Visitors, who saw to the welfare of the female patients and supervised the nurses.[66]

One Infirmary pupil found Prichard impressive:

Dr. J. C. Prichard, although the junior physician at the Infirmary in my time, was far in advance of the others in culture, in general and professional knowledge, and in literary reputation, which was not limited to Bristol or to England, but was European. He was a small, spare man, with a short, quick decided step; sharp and somewhat curt in his speech, but kind and very attentive to his hospital patients. He generally wore a large, loose overcoat, with roomy side-pockets, large enough to hold a quarto or small folio case-book; and he generally carried other books with him on the seat of his carriage. He took notes of the cases of his patients in the Infirmary, in short, terse Latin sentences, in his case-book, which he always carried himself, and brought to the Infirmary and took away with him. He was a great linguist, and would talk to his patients, when necessary, in their own language, French, German, and especially Welsh, from which country we had many in the Infirmary, some of whom could hardly understand English. (I have heard that Dr. Prichard considered the Welsh the most musical and melodious of languages.) It was said that he had talked Hebrew with a Jew. . . .

Dr. Prichard's treatment of the cases under his care was, even then, considered heroic. He did not bleed so much as Dr. Carrick; but counter-irritation in every form he pushed to an extreme degree. Blisters, often very large ones, setons, issues made by caustics or the knife [were frequently prescribed]. Dr. Prichard's heroic treatment extended to the use of drugs. Mercury, digitalis (generally given in the form of infusion and in large doses), colchicum, and other potent drugs were often pushed to the extreme limit of safety in the treatment of acute diseases. I may give an account of the treatment of myself, as a fair example of his usual mode of practice. Shortly before the end of my apprenticeship, in my twenty-first year, I had an attack of continued fever of some form, not very severe, principally affecting the head, but without delirium. Dr. Prichard attended me with Mr. Morgan, the then resident surgeon. He directed me to be bled to twenty ounces one forenoon; the same evening he ordered twenty leeches to be applied to my temples; and the following morning ten grains of calomel to be taken in one dose. This last acted as an emetic, and I brought it up.... However, I recovered well, and without any continued drawbacks, except some prolonged weakness.

Dr. Prichard was in great general esteem as a man of wide knowledge and high literary accomplishments. He had a large consulting practice; not, I believe, an extensive private one. He drove a carriage and pair, like all the other physicians. He appeared to be always reading in his carriage, and had generally a heap of books with him.[67]

Some of the Infirmary physicians were, like Prichard, "bleeders," while others were "feeders." "Heroic," anti-inflammatory treatment was the more popular medical practice at that time. The patient was usually prescribed venesection, or leeches for localized bloodletting. One method of abstracting blood was wet-cupping, the creation of a vacuum by a hot glass cup applied to an area of pierced skin. For this Prichard was able to endorse the services of a professional cupper. The Infirmary's annual accounts show considerable expenditure on leeches. These useful little creatures swam actively about their large glass tank until they were fished out when the nurses brought down their order papers with the number prescribed.[68] Venesection, however, was more economical and efficient; most of Carrick and Prichard's patients were bled twelve ounces at a time from the temporal artery, the jugular, or a vein in the forearm.

The students considered "blooding" drudge work to be delegated to their most junior colleagues, some of whom stropped their lancets on their boots to avoid the expense of getting them sharpened. They treated the patients just as roughly. The procedure was efficient: five or six patients at a time were sat on a long bench in the special Bleeding Room, each holding a pewter bleeding bowl for catching their own blood; the pupil went along the row opening each patient's vein; and by the time he had finished lancing the last patient, it was time to return to the start of the row to bind the wound of the first one. Occasionally, some inconvenience arose from patients falling off the bench in a faint, spilling their blood. Luckily, the room had a red floor cloth. When both Prichard and Carrick were on duty, the room was awash with blood. Gallons were taken away.[69]

Bloodletting, the mainstay of traditional, humoral-based, evacuant heroic therapeutics, was experiencing a resurgence in popularity during Prichard's university years. It can be contrasted with the alternative "expectant" therapeutics of the feeders, who administered nourishment, warmth, and stimulants. It was obvious which of these diametrically opposed methods was more efficacious. For acute diseases and inflammations, a former Infirmary student reported no apparent difference between these treatments, whether in recovery or mortality. If anything, the recovery rate seemed to depend on the constitution of the patient. In chronic or terminal diseases such as tuberculosis, however, the difference was remarkable: "Many of these were admitted into the Infirmary, and a large proportion remained there till the fatal termination. Of these Dr. Fox's patients especially, who had no medical treatment but mild opiates and placebos, with warm comfortable quarters and a suitable diet, lingered on from week to week and month to month, as if they set death at defiance. But those who were subjected to active treatment of any kind, whether by drugs or counter-irritants or any experimental management, soon gave us an opportunity of studying the morbid effects of the disease in the dead-house."[70]

The pupils' noses were kept to the grindstone filling and administering prescriptions, especially for all that bleeding. Young apothecary William Swayne had only just been appointed after his predecessor's acrimonious resignation owing to overwork. Although Prichard and his colleagues thought highly of cultured and professional Mr. Swayne, the pupils found him quiet and sedate to the point of being uncommunicative; walking the wards with him could be tedious. The matron, apothecary, and the apothecary's pupils had bedrooms on the ground floor, and they all dined together in the matron's sitting room, but without much conversation on the part of quiet Mr. Swayne, who was actually in a protracted consumptive "decline" that ended him in 1825.[71]

Membership of the faculty conferred eminence beyond the Infirmary. In 1813 the four physicians had written a public address pointing out the shocking conditions prevalent in Bristol Gaol.[72] In 1827 they petitioned the committee to set guidelines for the training and duties of the nurses to improve the quality of care.[73] The faculty served on the Bristol Board of Health during the 1832 cholera epidemic. In the same year they managed to get the committee to deal with the growing scandal of turning away hundreds of sick poor every year; they agreed to construct an extension to the Infirmary. Other calls upon Prichard's time involved writing testimonial letters for his pupils and for the candidates for various Infirmary posts such as matron. He occasionally testified in court, in one case as an expert witness in a case of child neglect, and on one uncomfortable day in December 1839 he testified on the cause of death at the inquest of an Infirmary patient.[74]

Infirmary Colleagues

Prichard formed alliances with his fellow physicians, especially when it involved asserting their superior status. Quarrels erupted among the faculty such that they were sometimes not on speaking terms. Prichard's senior, Andrew Carrick, MD, Edin, was a tall, grave, dutiful, kind and gentle, gentlemanly Scot who published a notable paper on the Hotwells and was a stalwart supporter of several Bristol organizations such as the Bristol College and the Bear's Cub Club. So painstaking was Carrick, he took an inordinately long time to examine his patients, trying the patience of the serving pupils. Yet his treatments were anything but gentle; acute cases were sure to be bled copiously and repeatedly, dramatically purged, administered saline antimonial mixtures, and put on a "low slop diet." There seemed to be little variation in his prescriptions, no matter the ailment. The friend and physician of much-admired conservative and evangelical author Hannah More, Carrick was very well read and pious, occasionally supplementing his prescriptions with words of spiritual comfort and advice.[75]

Cooperation with his colleague Dr. Stock must have been at some sacrifice of scruples on Prichard's part. No stranger to controversy, he had had as disreputable a past as anybody could, to Prichard's mind; there once had been a bounty for high treason on young Stock's Radical head. A product of John Prior Estlin's liberal school, he had had to leave Oxford upon his conversion to Unitarianism. When studying medicine at Edinburgh, he became so vociferous in defending that sect, Protestant dissent in general, and Republicanism that he was indicted and narrowly escaped capture and execution by taking passage on a ship bound for America. There he gained a medical degree, obtained a pardon for his youthful indiscretions, and returned to Bristol to settle into practice and work with the once-Radical Dr. Beddoes at his new Medical Institute for the Sick and Drooping Poor in Broad Quay. This short, slight, squinting doctor with a shambling gait and indecisive manner was unenhanced by his habit of constantly having pockets full of food, which he munched as he did his ward rounds. In fact, this habit was reflected in his medical practice, as he seemed to attribute all deviations from health to want of vital power or deficiency of food. He rarely prescribed anything other than tonics and stimulants, supplemented by a full, nutritious diet. Stock's expectant therapeutics were diametrically opposed to Prichard and Carrick's.

Far from being a typical Infirmary Tory, Stock was president of the (Whig) Anchor Society in 1816 and mixed in literary and intellectual circles. Prichard did approve of Stock's sensational renunciation of Unitarianism around the time they were promoting and conducting their medical lecture course. In 1816 Dr. Stock's bombshell of a resignation letter to his Unitarian minister claimed his new belief in the divinity of Christ. All Bristol was agog over "Dr. Stock's Conversion," as the newspapers, pamphlets, and handbills called it. Evangelicals were still celebrating this major coup against dissent more than two decades later. Although Stock remained a Dissenter instead of joining the Established Church, at least he was an evangelical Trinitarian rather than a Unitarian, and being a member of the Bear's Cub Club, he was Prichard's friend as well as colleague.[76]

The third Infirmary physician, St. Peter's colleague Henry Hawes Fox, acted the part to perfection. This stout, handsome, dapper doctor with the manner of a courtier processed around Bristol in enviable equipage. A physician of the old school, he wore shiny Hessian boots with silk side-tassels, conspicuous white shirt frills, a cravat, and black garments. Of languid gait and speech, Fox was gracious to staff and patients alike in a kind and insinuating manner. Like Stock, he favored expectant therapeutics. But for all his polite and leisurely demeanor, nobody could get through his duties faster than Fox; he could examine and prescribe for upward of fifty outpatients in twenty minutes compared to Carrick's usual two hours. One at a time the patients would stand before the charming physician, who would courteously ask, "How-do-you-do, my friend?" Whatever the reply, he would tell the attendant "Repeat" or "Continue," unless it were a new case; then "Next, if you please." The prescription scribe could hardly keep up with him. Fox resigned from the Infirmary in 1829 but continued to live near the Prichards; their boys were the best of friends.[77]

Prichard had three more physician colleagues. One was sometime body snatcher George Wallis, MD, Edin (1812), BA, Camb, member of the Royal Medical Society, and Bristol lecturer on anatomy. He was elected in the place of Dr. Stock in the tumultuous Saints vs. Sinners election of 1828, in which Wallis was the Sinner. The "Evangelical or Pious People" opposed to Wallis included Prichard and Fox. Wallis qualified as a sinner by having misrepresented the award of his Cambridge degree and by being often seen in the company of a lady not his wife.[78] The Saint, John Howell, MD, Edin, was elected the following year upon Fox's resignation. He had had a distinguished career as a military surgeon and sported a Napoleonic War wound. Like Prichard, Howell was active in medical and Anglican societies, the Bristol Institution, and Bristol College.[79] In 1834 Henry Riley, MD, Edin, succeeded Dr. Carrick. Formerly physician to St. Peter's Hospital and the Clifton Dispensary, he was a founder of the Bristol Zoological Gardens, published papers on archaeology and natural history, and was the first to introduce the use of the stethoscope in Bristol. As great a bleeder as Prichard, when both happened to be on duty at the Infirmary, there would be blood.[80]

Prichard's several surgeon colleagues were just as varying in character as the physicians. The most colorful was the senior surgeon, Richard Smith Jr., son of a former Infirmary surgeon. Prichard must have found Dick Smith overwhelming, a burly, florid, bewhiskered, popular, jovial, extremely gregarious, loud, brusque man with a well-developed taste for coarse stories and jokes and for anything gory. An ardent Freemason and Tory, Smith had a particular fondness for hearty Bristol drinking and glee-singing too. Amicably married to a stalwart of the evangelical church and childless, he took no noticeable interest in either his wife or her religion. Instead, his mornings started with what was coyly described as a surgery mostly for young men who would enter his house from a back door and be provided with powders, pills, and ointments in a rough and ready way. After that, Smith would repair to the Infirmary Museum, the home of one of the finest collections of anatomical and forensic specimens, the spoils of dissections and body snatching.[81] Here he curated specimens, whether medically relevant or entertainingly gruesome. Prichard was the third person to sign the register "Visitors to Mr. Richard Smith's Museum" in December 1828, the many signatures following demonstrating its popularity among medical and nonmedical visitors from Bristol and beyond. A connoisseur of fine gossip, Smith assembled a huge archive of the Infirmary and everyone connected with it.[82] He was a bold, skilled operator, but rather slapdash and reckless—not at all mindful of the feelings or state of his patients, but solicitous of his students. He remained surgeon to the Infirmary well into his incompetency, dying suddenly at a Phil & Lit meeting, surrounded by his friends. Prichard was one of his pallbearers.[83]

Infirmary-educated William Hetling was a slight, thin, uncommunicative, but reliable member of the faculty. A slow, methodical, and clumsy operator, his results still seemed good.[84] Richard Lowe, the son and apprentice of an Infirmary surgeon, was a tall, spare, good-looking, proud man, rather cynical and extremely fond of sneeringly sharing any piece of gossip or scandal with his great friend Dick Smith. He was greatly admired for his bold and dexterous operating style.[85]

Two other surgeons were Nathaniel Smith and his former pupil Henry Daniel. Stout, good-looking Daniel was a loud and opinionated man who gradually developed the largest and most lucrative practice in Bristol and lived in some style. A gregarious member of the Dolphin Society and a Freemason, Tory Daniel was famed for aiding the rescue of the mayor during the Bristol riots. A bleeder like Prichard, he was notably bolder and more confident than skilled in his use of the scalpel. His singular piece of professional advice was that "a man might write illegibly without losing caste; but no gentleman spells badly."[86] Having publicly fallen out with Daniel, Prichard refused to speak to him thereafter. Nat Smith, formerly indentured to Dick Smith, managed to get elected to the faculty not long after Prichard despite his Baptist connections. He had a busy Bristol midwifery practice and offered smallpox vaccinations at a weekly surgery. This short, bright, pleasant surgeon was as neglectful of his Infirmary duties as he famously was of his finances. When he did operate, he was remarkably precise, clean, steady, and prudent, keeping his presence of mind even in the most arduous of cases.[87]

Prichard briefly had another colleague whose history further illustrates the times. Thomas Shute, after declining to fight a duel over an affair of the heart and having arranged to marry the lady in question, experienced discomfort and a pain in his side. He had himself bled on two successive days, the second time until he fainted. Despite the warning of his physician, he sat up—and died. While his Infirmary colleagues were shocked and saddened, their immediate reaction belied other feelings. Dick Smith was seated at the Admissions Room table beside Prichard, the physician for the week, and opposite the apothecary Mr. Swayne when the news of Shute's death was brought in. The three medical men looked at each other and had the same thought. Swayne had a brother, Prichard a brother-in-law, and Smith a friend, all anxious to gain the now-vacant post, so each dispatched a messenger and returned to his occupation. Within an hour the city was filled with the bustle of a canvass.[88]

Bristol Infirmary Sturm und Drang

Prichard gained excellent experience at the Infirmary and formed useful professional relationships, but it was never a place of peace and harmony. Disagreements and ill will among the faculty and administration were the norm. The former's views were generally ignored, and they bridled against being dictated to by nonmedical men. The press enjoyed reporting the conflicts, scandals, accusations, demands, and threatened and actual resignations, usually in the form of the combatants' letters to the editor. A quarrel among the surgeons a few years before Prichard joined the Infirmary had resulted in the committee's taking control of the pupils and excluding the faculty from its meetings for the next twenty-two years, negatively affecting the administration and progress of the charity.[89]

Recruiting subscribers to the Infirmary was a constant struggle, especially during the frequent periods of the nation's economic instability and social unrest. While the number of inpatients rose substantially during Prichard's first ten years there, the number of subscribers dropped dramatically to 972. Those dedicated enough to serve on the committee were strict in their control of finances and resistant to the faculty's attempts to get the rules of the Infirmary modified. Dealing with the committee must have given Prichard and his colleagues plenty to discuss at their own private quarterly meetings held at the Montague Tavern in Kingsdown. There they reviewed recent Infirmary events and statistics, considered recommendations for improvements, and no doubt complained and plotted, before finishing with a good dinner of the Bristol staple—turtle soup washed down with wine and punch.[90]

By 1824 the Infirmary was in dire financial straits. Rumors circulating about internal dissent inhibited subscribers' willingness to serve on the committee. The situation came to a boil that winter when it proposed a set of new rules. The two major bones of contention were the aforementioned continued exclusion of the faculty from the Infirmary's administration and the question of allowing physicians to have pupils. The committee did not even acknowledge the faculty's suggestions, made only a few minor revisions, and then added some completely new rules for good measure. Prichard informed the surgeons that the physicians had decided to resign; all but one surgeon followed suit. After some crisis meetings, the superior Infirmary Board intervened with a month's cooling-off period. A pro-faculty faction mustered subscribers' support, meanwhile, and conducted a comparative study among twenty-seven hospitals. Prichard drafted a statement titled "Reasons Why the Faculty Ought Not to Be Entirely Excluded from the Committee," and subscribers started packing the weekly board meetings, causing administrative chaos.[91]

Dr. Carrick took up his polite, but gall-dipped, pen. His lengthy pamphlet *Observations* stressed the impropriety of administering a medical institution without the aid of the experts involved in it. He applied the effective, negatively charged term "Exclusionists" to those committee men who had so insulted, degraded, disrespected, and misrepresented the expert and selfless medical volunteers, treating them like servants. Calumnious publications were circulated, accusing the faculty of selfishness, negligence, and tyranny.[92] An eventual compromise allowed the faculty limited membership on the committee.

Despite their differing personalities and therapeutics, the members of the faculty had much in common. They were mostly Bristol Infirmary educated, True Blue, Church of England, subscribers to the Bristol Library Society, members of the Dolphin Society, and highly respected and tenacious holders of their posts. Some became active in establishing the Bristol Medical School and the later Bristol branch of the Provincial Medical and Surgical Association, the forerunner of the British Medical Association. Many were members of the Bear's Cub Club, the later Bristol Philosophical and Literary Society, and the Bristol Institution and supporters of Bristol College, all dear to Prichard's heart. His post at the Bristol Infirmary helped him establish his medical standing in Bristol and provided him with thousands of patients whose diseases he could study and on whom he could carry out the form of medical therapeutics he believed most efficacious. While Infirmary politics and relationships were frustrating at times, his colleagues and the subscribers helped broaden his social network. In his twenty-seven years' service, his increasing fame gave some luster to it in return. Among the archives of the Bristol Infirmary there is hardly any reference to its patients' experiences. One, however, described Prichard:

> Dr. Prichard do appear
> With his attendance and his care.
> He fills his patients full of sorrow,
> "You must be bled to-day and cupped to-morrow."[93]

Bristol, Rich in Medical Charities and Societies

Prichard's brother-in-law took a different path to building his career. John Estlin's background should have smoothed his road, having an influential Unitarian father and a Guy's and St. Thomas's Hospitals and Edinburgh education. He chose the challenge of practicing as a surgeon and starting his own charity, setting up the Bristol Eye Dispensary in 1812 in an ancient house on the corner of Frogmore Street and Pipe Lane, near the central Bristol docks. His dispensary operated without the interference of subscribers because his charity was not governed by them as other Bristol medical charities were, and it accomplished a lot of good on a small budget. Two surgeons examined its many patients by the light of a window, carrying out on-the-spot surgical procedures such as unanesthetized cataract removal. Estlin also ran a highly successful smallpox vaccination program, being particularly concerned to prevent the blindness this disease could cause. Even without the benefit of election to the Bristol Infirmary Prichard's brother-in-law went on to enjoy a successful career as an ophthalmologist among both the rich and poor. The fame of his clinic extended beyond Bristol, and it served the city for 140 years.[94]

Prichard's former teacher Dr. Pole was a physician to a less prominent Quaker charity serving poor Bristol women. The Bristol Refuge Society for the restoration of females unhappily fallen from virtue transformed them into servants. Its first report published in 1815 lists Prichard as a subscriber.[95]

Bristol medical men seemed particularly fond of forming societies, and Prichard benefited from membership in them. The Medical Book Society was attractively patterned on Edinburgh's Royal Society of Medicine. Its members took turns delivering lectures at their meetings and dined together, and they purchased and shared books and periodicals. The group was superseded by the Medical Reading Society, several members of which were on the staff of the Bristol Infirmary. This society brought Infirmary and other medical men together for the purpose of "promoting a friendly intercourse among its members, and purchasing medical books." Prichard was elected on March 20, 1812, and John Estlin was a fellow member. By limiting membership to twelve, the Medical Reading Society remained selective and exclusive, even instituting elitist rules banning lowly druggists and requiring elections to be unanimous. He took his turn hosting meetings at his home, and he served as secretary in 1819 and 1833.[96]

Members of the Medical Reading Society met to discuss medical subjects and drink tea, and they enjoyed an annual dinner. They proudly promulgated professional standards, printed a book of rules, and kept detailed archives. Each member had to bring his own "Green Register" of book borrowings to every meeting; the society's ledgers and minute books chart Prichard's medical and general reading and attendance. He complained about the fines he frequently had to pay for failing to attend meetings, but when he did, he was always forthcoming with requests for the purchase of natural history and travel books rather than medical tomes, more than sixty in all over the years.

At the Medical Reading Society's annual auction of these books among themselves, those failing to meet half their original price fell to the lot of their original proposer. Not only medical books but very popular and informative journals such as the *Quarterly*, *Edinburgh*, *British*, and *Westminster*

Reviews were circulated to a strict schedule at the risk of further fines. On occasion, there were disagreements, for example, for and against subscribing to the reformist *Lancet*. This new medical weekly was as sharp as its name, full of gossip and medical exposés—its editor reveled in taking the medical elite down a peg or two. The Medical Reading Society discontinued its *Lancet* subscription on the grounds of its being "a publication injurious to the respectability and best interests of the profession and disgraceful to the medical men who conduct it," an indication of the society's conservative leanings. On August 20, 1825, after the society voted to resume subscribing to *The Lancet*, Prichard resigned; he rejoined in 1832 and again resigned seven years later. The Medical Reading Society has continued to exist into the twenty-first century, its records tracking the reading habits of generations of Bristol physicians and surgeons. Prichard valued his membership for the books, the company, and the status it conferred.[97]

When Prichard joined the Bristol Medical and Surgical Association in 1818, he might have anticipated a society similar to the Medical Society of London, which he once attended and of which he had been corresponding member since 1815. But while the Bristol society circulated books, it stressed "friendly intercourse." At a meeting at Prichard's house in 1819, members decided to dine twice a year at the Montague Hotel. The association attempted to deal with the rivalry and occasional outright hostility between physicians and surgeons and to extend cooperation and influence beyond the city. To promote the interests of the profession, members formulated a tariff of fees for professional visits according to distance traveled, strongly advising that all their members should charge the same fees, for example, from half a guinea to Clifton to 5 guineas to much more distant Wrington. Importantly, night visits should never cost less than a guinea. This association was a departure from the other book societies in that its prime interests were professional and ethical, but once it set professional standards, it lapsed into a mere dining club. Estlin resigned, citing neither leisure nor inclination to be involved in a society that had little object other than dining.[98] In 1832 Prichard would become involved in a medical association of national standing.

Prichard continued to hold several voluntary medical posts in Bristol even after he had gained a large consulting practice, was publishing widely, and was a member of several societies and charities. He even held the post of examining physician for two insurance companies at 1 guinea per examination and served as Medical Visitor to Gloucestershire private madhouses before becoming a metropolitan commissioner in lunacy. This last appointment required frequent travel outside of Bristol. Prichard had so many irons in the fire, they distracted him from doing the research he most valued. Amid some disagreement among his Infirmary colleagues and yet more quarrels thrashed out in the newspapers, he resigned on June 7, 1843, and was appointed to the newly created post of honorary and consulting physician.[99] He discouraged his sons from studying medicine, just as his teacher Dr. Pole had discouraged his.

6 · The Single Origin and Unity of Humankind

Creating British Anthropology, 1805–26

> Thomas Prichard "expressed his desire that his son would maintain the orthodox side of the question with respect to the unity of our race."
> —Thomas Hodgkin, "Obituary of Dr. Prichard"

Prichard's earliest and lifelong scholarly endeavor was founded on a childhood curiosity about foreigners, love of books about travel, exploration, and history, identification with the Welsh, passion for learning languages and ordering and analyzing information, fascination with geology and archaeological remains, abhorrence of the mistreatment of extra-Europeans, and desire to preserve scriptural integrity. He was raised a Quaker in a period of national religious and moral revival and zealous social reform that reinforced his commitment to Christian doctrine and doing good. A friend later explained that Prichard had always "maintained a correspondence with his father on the subject of his investigations, and that the good man not only took a lively interest in the inquiry, but expressed his desire that his son would maintain the orthodox side of the question with respect to the unity of our race. Judging from the uniform tenor of Dr. Prichard's mind, I am induced to believe that to this side his own views were always disposed to incline, although he has collected and stated the arguments on both sides with perfect fairness and impartiality."[1]

Early Life in Anthropology

> My attention was strongly excited to this inquiry many years ago by happening to hear the truth of the Mosaic records implicated in it and denied on the alleged impossibility of reconciling the history contained in them with the phaenomena of Nature, and particularly with the diversified characters of the several races of men. The arguments of those who assert that these races constitute distinct species appeared to me at first irresistible, and I found no satisfactory proof in the vague and conjectural reasonings by which the opposite opinion has generally been defended. I was at least convinced that most

of the theories current concerning the effects of climate and other modifying causes, are in great part hypothetical and irreconcilable with facts that cannot be disputed.²

Perhaps it was for dramatic effect that Prichard claimed initially to have taken the easy option of believing in the plurality of the human species; in contrast to accepting facile "arguments," his exacting research had led him to the opposite and scientifically sound conclusion. When he explained in 1813 his inspiration to study humankind, he did not exaggerate the incredulity with which he and his fellow Britons considered anything that might undermine Christian doctrine.³ Being a Christian was a matter not of individual choice but of reality; the facts of Holy Scripture were undebatable. Studying the human species as one would an animal or plant challenged humanity's status, humankind being God's special creation. Those few Britons who might have felt unfettered by religion for the most part wisely kept it to themselves. Religious and social order were as one, as it is in some countries today.

The question of the plurality of the human race was linked to a burning topic of Prichard's youth—the abolition of the slave trade. The Society of Friends prohibited their members from engaging directly or indirectly in the heinous business. After publicly expressing his anti–slave trade position early in his career, however, Prichard left overt campaigning to his antislavery friends and relatives. Rather, he would focus his efforts on protecting the rights of Britain's colonized peoples through his research and writing.

Other currents in society informed Prichard's outlook. His childhood had been blighted by the threat of Continental revolution spreading into Britain, bringing dangerous ideas such as materialism, anticlericalism, and various heterodox theories, not just about the unity of the human species, but about the origin and development of the earth and all life on it. Challenging the long tradition of Christian thought on nature and humankind threatened Christianity's tenets, political and social stability, and the English scientific status quo.⁴ Nevertheless, belief in the divine creation of a single human species begged the question: by what natural law had the single original human species acquired such global spread and huge variation in form since the time of Adam and Eve?

By 1800 the orthodox understanding of the unity of the single, divinely created human species as expressed in Genesis was being questioned by a variety of naturalists, such as Briton Charles White and Frenchman Julien-Joseph Virey, who asserted humankind comprised several distinct species. While this view did at least allow these separate species to have been divinely created, it still contradicted Scripture, an offense to James, his father, and every right-thinking Christian Briton. Had not Saint Paul pronounced that God "hath made of one blood all nations of men?" Polygenism, as this notion became called, was in opposition to the scripturally compatible doctrine of monogenism. Scripture provided no evidence of multiple human creations. Clearly, instead of separate creations, varieties *within* the single human species had gradually and naturally arisen somehow among the descendants of divinely created Adam and Eve as they had among other forms of life. Superficial variation did not indicate the plurality of the human species any more than it did among dogkind.[5]

Theorizing on the human species and its diversity was a popular activity in Edinburgh lecture halls and student society debates, inspired by Scottish Enlightenment philosophy. Prichard chose it for the topic of his Royal Medical Society student essay and then expanded it into his MD dissertation. In the latter he broadened his research to consideration of language. As history did not reach back deeply enough in time, he thought that analyzing languages might help in this quest, believing they were the most reliable marker of relationships among peoples and over time. He had been gathering descriptions of cultures from accounts of travel and exploration, but such material was not appropriate to use at this point. Biology, geography, history, language, and culture would eventually scaffold his anthropology.

The Plurality of Anthropological and Evolutionary Thought

Anthropology has several interrelated origin myths. Nowadays, anthropologists studying the history of their discipline tend to trace it to this or that relatively recent "inciting incident," often depending on their nationality or subdisciplinary interest. They point to the founding of anthropological organizations, development of sociological theory, impetus of abolitionism, advent of archaeology, expediencies of colonialism, establishment of anthropology's first professorship, and even the granting of the first degree in anthropology. For the most part, the nineteenth-century British science of humankind is either ignored or dismissed for being an outdated, Prichardian, monogenetic Christian, historical linguistic terra incognita succeeded by a later nineteenth-century, race-fixated, biological anthropological terra best forgotten.

Histories of anthropology also reflect what the discipline is thought to comprise. Intellectual historians conceiving of it as the study of human culture may give a nod to the classical historians; indeed, Strabo, Tacitus, and Herodotus generously populate Prichard's footnotes. Others note the activities of explorers, merchants, and missionaries of more recent centuries who considered minor differences among foreigners a matter of adaptation to local conditions: humans are of a single origin, despite ancient historians' fondness for sensationalizing their ethnographies. Late medieval Christian doctrine held that degeneration or divine intervention after the Tower of Babel had caused human populations to diverge, and the notion of the Great Chain of Being's arrangement of the entire universe in an immutable hierarchy would seed the idea of racial hierarchy. Renaissance scholars' desire to fathom human diversity paved the way to gathering cultural data during this so-called Age of Discovery, a period of world exploration, particularly of the New World. So, for instance, when the Conquistadors returned to Spain with evidence of Incan civilization, the classical notion that the extra-European distant world was peopled with monsters and freaks gave way to curiosity about these peoples and their achievements that classical historians had somehow failed to describe. How had Indigenous peoples gotten from the Garden of Eden to such far-flung places?[6]

When the Age of Discovery gave rise to more questions than answers about the peoples and peopling of the world, new theories were concocted. As to why human populations varied in superficial appearance and in their beliefs, there was initially general agreement: humankind was God's single divine creation, so any deviation from Adam and Eve's state of original perfection must be a matter of unfortunate degeneration, perhaps brought about by the environment in which they lived. Fascinating specimens of natural history arriving in Europe included captured human beings, stimulating the study of extra-European peoples. Early anthropological literature generally took a natural historical approach to the subject, describing human beings as biological specimens.[7]

In an era of theorizing on the nature of humankind, French philosopher Montesquieu insisted that climate was responsible for physical or cultural differences among humankind, daringly leaving God out of the equation. The seventeenth-century race theory of Isaac La Peyrère, termed "pre-Adamism," qualifies him as founder of racialist polygenism. His hypothesis that human beings had existed before Adam spawned the notion of a "non-Adamic" race—in other words, that there is more than one human species. Applying Linnaean taxonomy, the philosopher Immanuel Kant created the first definition of "race" as a stable, irreversible conglomeration of hereditary differences among members of a single "stock," first suggesting and then rejecting the idea of racial hierarchies.[8]

The histories of the peoples of Europe were studied more deeply as well. Several encyclopedias published in the decades around the turn of the nineteenth century contain comparative histories and descriptions of the various nations of Europe and the affinities among them. The notion of "race" was gradually taking shape. Complementary to this is an attitude now referred to as "European exceptionalism," a notion developed among eighteenth-century philosophers like Voltaire—a sort of "superiority complex" characterized by the belief that European physique, language, religion, and general culture represented the apotheosis of human existence.[9] This idea did not go completely unquestioned, as awareness of the ills of civilization and a comparison of primitive life to that of the Garden of Eden engendered the perplexing notion of the "noble savage," for instance. Could civilization itself be a degenerated form of culture? As discomforting as it was useful was the Scottish Enlightenment view that all cultures went through stages of development, from savagery to barbarism to civilization; this meant that the study of contemporary "savages" could illuminate the prehistory of civilized Europeans.

The later eighteenth-century French anatomist and natural historian Georges-Louis Leclerc, Comte de Buffon, as well as suggesting the vast age of the earth, devised extensive criteria to account for environmentally caused variation. His strict empirical research implied the unity of the human species. Supporting his anatomical observations with explorers' and travelers' descriptions of Indigenous peoples, Buffon concluded there was no demonstrably logical category of "race." Instead, a myriad of physical nuances could be found among the "kinds," "varieties," "races," "nations," and "peoples" composing the single human species. Not all race theorists were French. Reinhold and Georg Forster's various accounts of South Seas populations make use of these interchangeable terms in holding their monogenetic position, irrespective of their denigratory descriptions. Gottfried Herder's *Ideen zur philosophie der geschichte der menschheit* (1784–91) also upholds the unity of the human species and dismisses "race" for its implication of different origins. Prichard found these views acceptable.[10]

Prichard lamented that at the start of the nineteenth century few English scientists risked studying the history and development of the human species, but those who did publish on the subject were, for the most part, polygenists. They relied on claims such as that the short span of biblical history was insufficient to produce such variation among human groups, and that diffusion of a single species around the globe could not have been accomplished so rapidly. Tweaking Genesis, they asserted God had created several human species, each suited to a particular habitat. While it seemed unnecessary for polygenists to prove this, monogenists were taxed with demonstrating how human diversity and world diffusion had come about during the mere six thousand years since Creation. They could conveniently hark back to the views of the notorious polemical, slave-owning historian of Jamaica Edward Long, who, having no truck with the environment as a cause of variation in humankind, claimed there were several different human species.

A generation of well-known European polygenists went beyond mere speculating; they conducted research. Englishman Charles White assembled anthropometric data, citing Dutchman Petrus Camper and the Great Chain of Being in aid of his views, while Prussian Samuel Thomas von Sömmerring based his on comparative dissections of Europeans and Africans. In opposition, American Samuel Stanhope Smith's *An Essay on the Causes of the Variety of Complexion and Figure in the Human Species* (1787, 1789) considered baseless polygenetic claims contemptible and strongly advocated human specific unity.[11]

The study of variation among humankind was naturally associated with biological evolutionary thought. Linnaeus's contemporary Pierre Louis Maupertuis entertained ideas approaching the theory of natural selection, suggesting that naturally occurring changes during reproduction accumulate to form new species. Another view held existing life was just what was left over after all things had been created but some had become extinct. Then there was what Buffon had explained as spontaneous generation in his *Histoire naturelle* (1749).[12]

Claiming authority to determine the age and origin of the human species, British theologians were in the vanguard of attacks on notions of evolution, human or otherwise. During this same period, discoveries in geology made it obvious that the span of Christian European existence occupied a mere fragment of history, a blow to the delusion of Christian European primacy. In 1802, when James was dreaming of a life in science, the English clergyman and "Christian apologist" William Paley tackled Continental notions of evolution head-on, setting out an alternative approach to understanding nature: biological change is evidence of divine design, not species' self-development. Natural theologians brandished their pens in defense of the Established Church's authority over science, education and civil life, vigorously condemning transformism; one species could not evolve into another. At the Universities of Cambridge and Oxford, where science was in the safe hands of ordained professors, one studied the natural world as an illustration of God's work. Students were closely examined on their understanding of Paley.[13]

Central to early nineteenth-century British science was Paley's doctrine of God's laws governing the operation of the universe, a principle known as First Cause. Questioning the validity of the First Cause risked accusation of heretical "materialism" and could precipitate personal and professional condemnation, not to mention the ire of loyal "Church and King" mobs. God's will kept all organisms constant and upheld the status quo. This was good theology; applied to society, it was good Tory politics too. Theories were elaborated. John Bird Sumner, the archbishop of Canterbury, in his *Treatise on the Records of Creation* (1816) interpreted Thomas Malthus's principle of population, a theory that would later influence evolutionist Charles Darwin.[14]

The British Establishment at that time thought suggesting life's independence from First Cause not only undermined religious doctrine but potentially threatened social order. If the Revolutionary French could imbibe these Godless theories, abolish the Church, and move on to confiscating the property of their aristocracy in pursuit of a perfect society, why should this poison not spread to Britain and pervert the poor into rising up to improve their lot? There was overt hostility to unorthodox speculation about the origin and development of life, whether Continental or homegrown. English physician and freethinker Erasmus Darwin risked censure when he insinuated into the text of his incendiary *Zoonomia* (1794) the idea of evolution from a single original primitive filament, and he mooted the mechanism of sexual selection, an idea that would later interest Prichard and eventually Darwin's grandson Charles. A host of detractors derogatorily dubbed transformism "transmutation."[15]

As Prichard started researching his topic at the University of Edinburgh, there was an array of past and contemporary natural historians' racial and biological theories to sift through and the pronouncements of natural theologians and his own firm Christian faith to guide him. How might he reconcile Genesis and science? No wonder Thomas Prichard had been wary of sending his son out into this world of new and challenging ideas.

Initial Research into the Origin and Unity of Humankind

At university, Prichard tackled the question of human origin and diversity by adopting the natural historical methodology of collecting, arranging, analyzing, and presenting information systematically. In his human anatomy and physiology courses he gained observational skills useful in describing and comparing human groups. Lacking extra-Europeans to study physically, his research was essentially literary.

Among earlier scientists of humankind, he most appreciated the work of German naturalist and comparative anatomist Johann Friedrich Blumenbach. Even during the late nineteenth-century's deplorable decades of race science, Blumenbach was referred to with respect. Reasoning by analogy was central in his methodology, a practice Prichard wholeheartedly adopted. Both Blumenbach and Prichard were greatly exercised by the desire to accommodate human physical diversity within the bounds of a single human species, yet there was the expectation that this involved framing a descriptive taxonomy of humankind as was done for all species. Blumenbach had taken up Kant's idea of "race," dividing the single human species into five varieties, Caucasian, Mongul, American, Malay, and Ethiopian, based on a broad range of features rather than solely on skin color. He produced convincing, unranked illustrations of human varieties. Prichard agreed with Blumenbach that the characteristics of these varieties were overlapping, the boundaries unclear and criteria merely superficial rather than indicative of the existence of multiple human species. Neither tolerated the Great Chain of Being's ranking of everything from simple minerals to the most advanced priests, kings, and then God. That might have been useful in ordering society and inspiring Linnaean taxonomy, but it was unsupported by Scripture and disturbingly placed all humans on a continuum from apes to superior white Europeans. They both avoided hierarchical arrangements of human varieties and stressed their equal intellectual capacity. Prichard did not follow Blumenbach slavishly; rather he would contradict the German's degeneration notion of vaguely defined environmental influences having caused the original white stock of humans to darken gradually. He also objected to Blumenbach's adoption of the term "Caucasian" for lending itself to polygenist arguments that sparked decades of controversy.

Prichard acknowledged Blumenbach as the father of anthropology. Prichard's visit to him in Germany in 1829 had the air of pilgrimage and inspired him to begin studying crania in earnest. Like his mentor, he attempted to group human varieties according to the shape of the skull, variations Blumenbach had attributed to "art" and "mode of life." Prichard later carefully explained his ordering the human species into seven "races" instead of Blumenbach's previous five, and he added geographical distribution to their description. Soon he would progress to observing that "races" (a word then closer in meaning to ethnic groups) could only be described properly in terms of cultural factors. Other men with quite different motives were busy devising racial categories, however. Prichard complained that Blumenbach's five varieties of humankind were being misrepresented as permanent and indelible races, which was neither Blumenbach's nor Prichard's intention.[16]

University student Prichard not only read Blumenbach closely; at Edinburgh he took full advantage of the relative freedom to study whatever he wanted in a stimulating and challenging atmosphere. His fellow student Joseph Arnould was struck by his passion for learning about humankind and Celtic culture, in particular:

> From the year 1807 we were very much together, and from that time, during our stay in Edinburgh, the history of his book is the history of his life, for it was the continual occupation of his mind. In our daily walks it was always uppermost: a shade of complexion—a singularity of physiognomy—a peculiarity of form—would always introduce the one absorbing subject. In the crowd and in solitude it was ever present with him. I well remember when one evening we were wending our way amidst the mountains in the neighbourhood of Loch Katrine, not so much frequented then as it has been since the "Lady of the Lake" appeared: it was near the going down of the sun, when, amidst the wildest scenery, we saw a Highlander on a distant crag, standing out clear and distinct, and seemingly magnified to a large size, and his huge shadow stretching out towards us. The effect for my friend was magical: fatigue was felt no longer, and he at once resumed all his powers of mind and body, and poured out a most splendid dissertation on the history of the Celtic nations—the dark, fearful, gloomy, and savage rites of the Druids—and conjured up the horrors we should have endured, if in those earlier times we had been lonely wanderers in that remote district, and beguiled the weariness of the way till we reached our place of rest at night.[17]

When not on romantic excursions into the Celtic past or absorbed in his medical studies, Prichard was tackling the unorthodox anthropological theories developed by two highly respected Edinburgh men. Lord Kames, a judge and central figure of the Scottish Enlightenment, had claimed in his recent, popular edition of *Sketches of the History of Man* that the environment, climate, or state of society could not account for physical differences among humankind; the human *races* must have descended from separately created co-Adamic, as opposed to non-Adamic, stocks. James Burnett, Lord Monboddo, controversial advocate of the affinity between apes and humans, had asserted in his *Origin and Progress of Language* (1773–92) that humans had progressed from simple tool-makers, through forming social structures, to developing language. The changing environment and progressively developing social structures had allowed language to evolve. But Monboddo's proto-social-evolutionary environmentalism contradicted the biblical account of the instantaneous creation of human beings and their languages. These were the unsubstantiated polygenetic, environmental, evolutionary speculations that Prichard found so vague and conjectural, not to mention unorthodox.[18] Monboddo was like those many writers who "have preferred the more specious and expeditious modes of reasoning which are drawn from probabilities, and founded on arguments a priori, to the tedious process of analytical discussion."[19]

As well as considering Kames's and Monboddo's theories about humankind unacceptable, Prichard was dissatisfied with his otherwise much-admired professor Dugald Stewart's lectures on the subject: "I was induced to investigate the subject the more attentively, as I found that some of my own opinions concerning it did not altogether agree with those of my illustrious Preceptor. This inquiry furnished me with the argument of an inaugural essay."[20] Stewart held the prevailing view that external factors could cause heritable change through some unknown physiological process. Prichard's fellow student's lecture notes quote Stewart: "In what I have hitherto said, I have gone on the supposition that the complexion alters with the climate. And I believe this holds so generally as to establish the fact." Anything that "held generally" did not necessarily hold water, to Prichard's mind. Stewart could not *prove* changes caused by the environment were heritable. He needed to tackle heredity.[21]

Prichard's other teacher, Professor of Natural History Robert Jameson, also lectured on the human species. He followed Blumenbach's classification of five human varieties, explaining how they might have come to be: "It is supposed that there existed in the first pair [Adam and Eve] germs of the after varieties of the human race, which climate &c called into existence. The different races do not pass into each other by the influence of climate. . . . It is supposed that the Caucasian was the original stock whence all the varieties have sprung."[22] So Adam and Eve had ingrained potential for variation that was merely stimulated rather than caused by climate? "Supposing" would not do.

The "First Drafts" of *Physical History*: Prichard's Royal Medical Society and MD Dissertations

Inspired to tackle his professors' unsubstantiated theories, Prichard chose human variation as the topic of his mandatory Royal Medical Society dissertation. It rejects straight environmentalism; an organism's life experiences cannot somehow cause heritable change, as, for instance, this would soon reduce all life to a miserable degenerated state by the accumulation of hardships, acquired mutilations, and diseases. The trigger for variation must therefore reside *within* an organism. Something in the "animal economy" (physiology) causes accidental variation, but never so great as to bring forth a new species. Nearly a century later, the term "genetic mutation" was coined.

Prichard stepped up his consumption of travelogues and histories. He started borrowing books from the university library on October 17, 1805, even before he had attended his first medical lecture. Of course, he started by diligently plowing through standard medical tomes like those of Hippocrates, Galen, and Friedrich Hoffman, but he also explored the classical historians who later made their appearance in his dissertations and books. Soon the balance of his borrowing shifted away from medicine. He read John Pinkerton's *An Enquiry into the History of Scotland* (1789) near the time of his expedition with Joseph Arnould, making this the likely inspiration of his Celtic effusion.[23] The library held several dissertations on the human species question; between 1799 and 1806 three Edinburgh MD dissertations had been written on human specific unity and a steady stream followed thereafter. As for the Royal Medical Society's own collection of members' dissertations, between 1775 and 1835 no fewer than fifteen were written on human unity, variety, or environmental causes of variety. He would have been relieved to find that the great majority were monogenetic.[24] Prichard's early interest in the biological and cultural "history of man" was piqued by his professors' unacceptable theories and nourished by Edinburgh's intellectual climate and the university's resources.

Prichard's "Of the Varieties of the Human Race" is inordinately long. It marshals ancient and contemporary resources to tackle the underlying question of the plurality of the human species. The very next dissertation presented at the RMS, "Is There Any Original Difference of Intellectual Ability amongst Mankind?" was just the sort of topic that Prichard decried as allowing most respectable members of the scientific world to fling about theories tainted with "heterodoxy and impious audacity" on the one side and "ignorance and puerile credulity" on the other. (He was frequently given to fits of grandiloquence.) He admitted both polygenism and monogenism were plausible theories, but they had been so vaguely and inconclusively argued a priori as to render them more like wishful thinking.[25] The study of humankind came within the scope of metaphysicians, physiologists, and political theorists, and he was willing to take it on.

Prichard referred to the famous anatomist John Hunter and to Professor Stewart's lectures, extensively employed Blumenbach's analogical argumentation and applied natural historians' generally agreed definition of what constitutes an animal species. He started with a discussion of skin color because its striking diversity had been the source of polygenists' speculations. Observing that all species tend to vary under domestication, as humans are the most domesticated, they are likely to exhibit the most variation in color and form. However, all species contain individuals of vastly differing hues. The subject of color concludes with his claim that the original form of the human species was not white, but light-skinned with dark eyes and hair, a view he would adjust six years later.[26]

The notion of the environment as a driver of diversity needed to be carefully considered. Prichard suggested that there are cases in which external conditions *might play a role*, but the exact mechanism "must remain a secret until the physiology of the generative process shall be better understood." Rather, it seemed climate more indirectly excites some natural disposition to "connate variety," and these permanent changes in offspring occur suddenly, not gradually as some anatomists claimed. In opposing the theory of species transmutation and the inheritance of acquired characteristics and in qualifying possible environmental causes, he nailed his colors to the mast.[27]

Prichard then considered the structure of skin and hair and variations in features and stature. Concerning the latter, while people of higher social status have superior grace and expression of countenance, these are not inherited. Like skin color, there are great variations in form among any population.[28] In the next section, concerning the effects of climate on skin color, Prichard noted that any darkening is transient. In dismissing Samuel Stanhope Smith's observation that American "house slaves" became whiter than "field slaves," he bitingly claimed it obvious, as the former were not subjected to "the relentless lash of those sons of liberty." As well as bringing to bear on the subject pages of evidence demonstrating proximity to the equator irrelevant, Prichard dismissed as nonsensical the claim that Black skin is caused by trapped black bile.[29] He concluded by setting out his position: as all differences in human appearances are attributable to natural variation *within* the species, there are no grounds to presume the existence of more than one current or original human species; the effects of climate are not transmitted to offspring; and variation is driven by engrained, environmentally stimulated potential. He cited thirty-six authors in eighty-eight footnotes, the three most frequent being Blumenbach, Buffon, and J. R. Forster.

Having read and defended his dissertation at an RMS public meeting, Prichard set to work broadening his research for his MD dissertation. The deadline for submission loomed. He extended the manuscript by nearly a third and translated it into the required Latin as *Disputatio inauguralis de generis humani varietate* (1808), another Prichardian doorstop of a dissertation.[30] This time he contemptuously dubbed loosely reasoned, empty hypotheses "visionary" musings. He also demonstrated his taste for accumulating more and more ethnographic and physiological data, as he would continue to do for the rest of his life. From data obtained inductively or abductively, scientific truths can ultimately be derived—a mantra of the age.

The first 113 pages of *De generis* closely follow the RMS manuscript, but with added citations and extracts from travelogues and classical and natural histories. He described many more ethnic groups and reinforced his views on variation in skin color. After exploring human temperament and physiognomy, he speculated on aspects of primeval humanity and outlined patterns of world migration that indicate humankind's origin in or near biblical lands. He was a committed migrationist.

Significantly, Prichard stressed the new practice of comparative philology for its potential to elucidate prehistory. The notion of language as a reliable historical tool goes back to the seventeenth-century philosopher and historian Gottfried Wilhelm Leibniz, and Prichard cited the contributions of Sir William Jones and subsequent students of language.[31] The belief that language provides key evidence of monogenism would be central to his subsequent anthropology. Most of the more than eighty books cited in *De generis*, ranging from the ancient historians to works published in 1807, can still be found in the University of Edinburgh Library. Seventeen references to Peter Simon Pallas's various works and long extracts from Lucretius's *De rerum natura* and other classical authors are examples of the fuller treatment Prichard gave his subject. He had added to his core biological argument the weight of history and language, two cornerstones of his future anthropology. *De generis* marks his understanding that his future research needed to be as much cultural-historical and linguistic as biological.

Prichard dedicated his MD thesis first to his nonmedical professor Alexander Christison, whose erudition and dedication to scholarship he so admired, and to his wealthy and learned relative John Walker, another paragon of scholarly and scientific endeavor. After taking his degree, studying for a period at Cambridge and Oxford, and then settling into medical practice in Bristol, he carried on his research to build an even more convincing demonstration of the unity of the human species. His would be a lifetime spent mining the publications of linguists, historians, natural historians, and travelers, ancient and modern.

Researches into the Physical History of Man (1813)

Once Prichard had settled in Bristol, he returned to his anthropology in earnest, borrowing more than seventy relevant volumes from the Bristol Library, adding to his own library, and regularly sharing new books with his father. Some unacceptable views had recently come out; for example, Frenchman Jean Baptiste Lamarck's 1809 *Philosophie zoologique* peddled the transformist notion that species continually and progressively develop, adapting to the environment. This was nothing short of a claim that all creatures could take it upon themselves to change without God's guiding hand, and it implied the whole universe comprised nothing but matter—no spirit, soul, or God. Lamarck further posited that individuals that had undergone some alteration during life could pass it on to their offspring by a mechanism termed "the inheritance of acquired characteristics." Lamarckism would both inspire and dog biological thought for decades.[32]

With few patients to distract him during his first two years in medical practice, Prichard amassed material for *Researches into the Physical History of Man*, publishing it in 1813. It brought a greatly developed version of his MD thesis to a wider audience of educated readers, placed him in the ranks of the natural historians of the period, and made him a punching bag for polygenists. From its name, *Physical History* might be considered a biological survey of humankind through time. Far more than that, it innovatively presents both biological and some historical-cultural material. Prichard divided his book into two clear sections. The biological first part lays out physiological proofs of the single human species, describes the variations within it, and suggests some causes of these variations. The mostly linguistic but also historical, geographical, and cultural second part surveys different nations and explores connections between them. This division is roughly ancestral to modern biological and cultural anthropology.

Prichard concluded *Physical History* with what would become his mantra: "We very easily conclude that all men are of one and the same species."[33] In this early comprehensive attempt to demonstrate the unity and single origin of humankind, Prichard organized the world's human groups into a taxonomical system based on both biological and cultural characteristics. He gathered and analyzed anatomical and physiological observations, concluding that the varieties of humankind comprise a single species. As in his dissertations, Prichard attempted to disprove polygenesis without resorting to elaborate speculations or to Scripture except as a source of historical material. *Physical History* forms an early anthropological paradigm—one of establishing the unity and single origin of the human species.

The book cites more than two hundred works of five main types.[34] About one-third are the classical authors, historian-geographers such as Herodotus, Diodorus Siculus, and Strabo. The ethnographic chapters make some attempt to trace the origin of the human species to the Near East, for which the classical histories were invaluable. Prichard also relied on more recent histories such as William Camden's *Britannia* (1586) to describe the European nations. The second source comprises explorers and travelers' accounts, James Cook's *Voyages around the World* being most often cited. A third type of resource consists of a variety of publications of a broadly biological sort, such as general comparative anatomies useful for citation of plant and animal analogies. Prichard found some books of comparative anatomy of *internal* structures particularly useful. Buffon, Cuvier, and Blumenbach were invaluable, while he criticized Camper, White's compilation of data, and von Sömmerring's comparative anatomical dissections of Europeans and Africans.

A fourth source of material is of quite a different nature. Prichard stressed: "The direct authority of history furnishes but a very imperfect insight into the origins of nations. We must therefore often depend on the reflected light which is obtained by the comparison of languages, by the analysis of civil and religious institutions and mythological fables, or by tracing clearly marked affinities in the manners and customs of different tribes. The most important of these aids is the comparison of languages."[35] Language and culture.

As of 1813 Prichard considered his science of humankind to ideally include biological, linguistic, and cultural components. The high proportion of biological and linguistic to cultural data in *Physical History* reflects the proportion of such material then available: physical descriptions of colonized and Indigenous peoples and samples of their languages were gathered for their commercial and administrative value, whereas knowledge of their customs was considered less consequential. Further, not only was access to such evidence limited, but Prichard did not entirely trust it as indicative of affinities (his prime interest), one reason being that a particular custom might be a universal phenomenon.[36] His long chapters on Egypt and India, however, abound in descriptions and comparisons of these cultures for which Prichard had resources to draw on.

Traditionally, biblical scholars relied on an etymological approach to researching the origin of language until German philologists developed Sir William "Oriental" Jones's insights into the relationship between Sanskrit and the European languages. From compiling word histories, philology shifted to the comparative study of grammatical structure and language families—an analytical approach to the study of language. A very early British adopter of this, Prichard believed that traces within the basic elements of a language provide evidence of its descent from a primitive common stock, while apparent language dissimilarity could not be used to prove separate origin. He also valued Jones's suggestion of the relationship between the Indo-European languages and Sanskrit. He hoped that orientalists would soon be able to use their discoveries to shed light on the origin of the European nations.[37] Prichard would continue to employ comparative historical linguistics in his *Eastern Origin of the Celtic Nations* (1831).

Prichard's fifth, arcane resource for *Physical History* was fast becoming obsolete. There had been a long tradition of basing histories on the chronologies and genealogies of nations descended from Noah's son Japheth after the Flood. Attempts to reconcile secular and biblical history were problematic, however, as the chronologies of the ancient civilizations were much longer than those of the Old Testament. The paganism of classical and European nations posed a further challenge: In which order had religion developed? Had pure monotheism degenerated into debased forms such as paganism, or was polytheism the universal original religion that had been gradually distilled into monotheism? Prichard was biased in favor of primeval monotheism, viewing polytheistic and primitive religions as corruptions, a position that led him on a quest for the supposed monotheism at the core of Hindu and Egyptian beliefs. As for the cause of religious degeneration, he could only speculate that while culture could progress, religion did not because it was not the product of the human mind but God's direct revelation. Clearly influenced by Scottish Enlightenment views on social evolution, Prichard claimed humans had originally been primitive in social organization, only subsequently progressing to a civilized state. In sum, and paradoxically, cultures progressed while religions could degenerate. Despite trying to avoid "resorting to elaborate speculations or to Scripture," he did so.

Prichard claimed he was "far from wishing to interest any religious predilections in favour of my conclusions." While drawing information from many sources, he avoided "the writings of Moses, except with relation to events concerning which the authority of those most ancient records may be received as common historical testimony, being aware that one class of persons would refuse to admit any such appeal, and that others would rather wish to see the points in dispute established on distinct and independent grounds."[38] He was also concerned to avoid teleological argumentation. He understood the importance of arriving at useful theories through the accumulation and analysis of evidence, while he once again derided unsupported theorizing. By adopting Baconian scientific method, he would be able to fathom the true history and nature of humankind.[39] These were his clear ideals, if not his reality.

Prichard appreciated Enlightenment science and classicism but avoided the theories of the French Enlightenment *philosophes*, those peddlers of materialism and infidelity. As for the German comparative linguists, they were available to him only in translation, as he had not yet mastered their language. His eleven citations of German sources such as Gottfried Wilhelm Leibniz, Carsten Niebuhr, and Peter Simon Pallas are either secondary or through French, English, or Latin translations.[40]

Physical History's Biological Anthropology

In the first part of *Physical History* Prichard brought several biological arguments to bear on his subject. Notably, he valued physiological over anatomical observations; all humans share the same physiology, such as the period of uterogestation and susceptibility to disease, although more research was needed on the second point. Human interfertility met one of Buffon's criteria of species. Prichard drew on Blumenbach's analogical reasoning throughout the biological section of *Physical History*. He noted that there is even less anatomical variation among humans than among animals of a single species, indicating human specific unity. Similarly, superficial variations within a population are no different than what may be found among human siblings. To drive home these two points, he provided scores of examples of "variation in which Nature chiefly delights." Here Prichard tended to stress the generic characteristics of human beings instead of contrasting them, and he kept his sights on tracing the origin of humankind in an apparently reverse diffusionist approach.[41]

Biological theorists debated whether the environment drove change. As he had in his MD thesis, Prichard countered environmentalists' speculations about the causes of human variation such as the action of the sun. Europeans long resident in hot climates do not pass on their acquired brown skin to offspring, nor do skin color and climate correlate, some Africans being light-skinned and Laplanders dark, for instance. Prichard noted that other animals also retain their original color, even under extreme conditions. Concerning a quite different speculation, the idea that Black skin was the result of the diffusion of black bile, Prichard repeated his ridicule from his dissertation; the notion implied all Africans suffer from some sort of hereditary jaundice.[42]

In considering the mechanisms of biological variation, Prichard importantly contrasted the *temporary* effects of the environment with the *permanent* effects of congenital change in offspring. While he could find no evidence that bodily change caused by the environment can be inherited, it was well known that offspring born with some spontaneous peculiarity pass it on to future generations. He cited two classic examples of this hereditary transmission among humans: the phenomenon of polydactylism and the famous case of a "porcupine"-skinned person, born of normal parents, some of whose children shared their father's peculiar type of skin.

Prichard called his mechanism of biological change the spontaneous "hereditary transmission of congenital characters of body" in a theory he set against Lamarckian "inheritance of acquired characteristics." He believed biological alterations just "happen to arise" or "casually spring up" in the course of procreation. Employing analogy, Prichard noted that animal and plant breeders exploit this phenomenon assiduously in propagating spontaneously occurring desirable qualities while preventing propagation of undesirable ones, thereby achieving new varieties within a species. Searching for a breeding experiment among humans, he cited some despotic Prussian kings' program to increase the stature of their citizens.

Crucially, Prichard thought that congenital heritable alterations do not result in a species changing beyond its bounds, so when he used the word "evolution," he meant evolution of varieties within a species, not the creation of new species. He could illustrate the impermeability of species boundaries by pointing to the almost universal sterility of animal hybrids' offspring, which prevents a chaos of intermediate species. He based his opinion that new species cannot arise not on fear of career-destroying accusations of infidelity such as Charles Darwin would later suffer, but on his unassailable belief in the immutability of species.[43]

Prichard felt that craniometry alone would neither prove nor disprove the specific unity of the human species. He pointed out that Petrus Camper's facial angle formula for gauging intellectual capacity completely ignores brain volume. Similarly, Cuvier's face-to-brain ratio implying Europeans' greater intellectual capacity was a mere conjecture unsupported by any evidence of Europeans' actual intellectual superiority. He respected

Blumenbach's craniological schema of three general forms of human skull: European round head, Mongol square head; and Negro narrow head. But not all individuals of a particular group conformed to one of Blumenbach's types, a case in point being the prevalence of round skulls among extra-Europeans; across human populations there is considerable overlap in form. Just as the shape of the cranium can differ greatly among the members of other animal species, so can the human cranium—another animal analogy. Prichard's consideration of crania, moreover, is not classificatory but descriptive.[44]

Prichard rounded on polygenists' baseless theories. He deemed Charles White's hypothesis that Africans represented a separately created species intermediate between apes and Europeans "absurd" and "fanciful." He also objected to African hair being referred to as wool, noting that across Africa hair form varied greatly from crisp and curly to perfectly straight. His thorough research into hair variation among several animal species demonstrated by analogy that other species have a range of form from wool to hair, sometimes both occurring in the same individual. That trounced any polygenetic argument based on hair.[45] All in all, he argued, obvious and continuous variation is a natural occurrence within a species, and any one characteristic is not exclusively possessed by a particular population. Prichard claimed this true of both human beings and other species.

Bringing in Erasmus Darwin's theory, a variation of which Darwin's grandson would name "sexual selection" in 1871, Prichard described a social means by which human variation is perpetuated—the behavior of selecting mates on the grounds of beauty, a sign of "health and perfect organization." He noted cases of the higher ranks of society's greater power to select the best spouses, a practice leading to diversity of form based on class apparent all around the world. Conversely, instinctive repugnance to defective spouses prevents deformity from proliferating. In a glimmer of what would be called cultural relativism, he agreed with Blumenbach and Camper that what constitutes beauty is not universal; Prichard felt that differing opinions on beauty are partly the cause and partly the effect of differences in criteria. Biological theorist William Lawrence repeated Prichard's view of male choice of mates effecting biological change, while Darwin would read their books and eventually shift it from male to female choice.[46]

"But by far the most powerful cause of the evolution of varieties in the animal kingdom is domestication": here is another example of human behavior instigating biological variation. Prichard drew upon the analogy of domestication's luxury, abundance, and protection of plants and animals as a metaphor for civilization's role in producing human variation. To demonstrate civilization's refining effects, he cited societies in which higher social status correlates with lighter complexion, such as among the elite of the Society Islands and the Brahmins of India. Then he found himself suggesting that certain environmental factors might play a role: "when the disposition to variation is excited by civilization, it is probable that it may proceed rapidly in producing its effects in some climates more than in others" such that "local situation and moderate temperature, promote the tendency to the production of light varieties." In other words, civilization aided by climate lays the foundation for change, stimulating it somehow to produce permanent biological alterations in offspring. Although he included this speculation about the environment, by and large, Prichard leaned more toward spontaneous congenital change perpetuated by human behavior as the mechanism of variation.[47]

Prichard brought the future sciences of biogeography, paleontology, and geology to bear on the subject of global distribution of species. He had to counter polygenists' incredulity of global human migration, especially to isolated islands. He cited biogeographers' demonstrations of genera having particular original abodes from which they had spread. Prichard extrapolated that this must also be true of the human species, whose populations vary greatly because they are spread so widely around the world, are exposed to extreme conditions, and exist at different levels of culture. He predicted "when Geology shall have assumed the character of a science," it will continue to provide evidence elucidating the history of species. It was already understood that continental movement had cut off land routes along which species had previously migrated great distances, and as isolated islands were universally found to have been populated by small animals that are similar to those of the nearest mainland, natural migration even to islands was entirely possible. If other animals had done so, why not humans?[48]

The biological part of *Physical History* concludes with a startling, but not completely novel, claim that "the process of Nature in the human species is the transmutation of the characters of the Negro into those of the European, or the evolution of white varieties in black races of men." As there is no evidence that white organisms become black, "this leads us to the inference that the primitive stock of men were Negroes, which has every appearance of truth." Applying his ubiquitous analogical reasoning, Prichard adapted John Hunter's view that animal varieties get progressively lighter, although exceptionally a white variety called albino springs up among black, but not vice versa. He argued that there was also evidence that Black people, who could better bear the rigors of extreme conditions, lived primitive lives, white people lived civilized ones, and those of intermediate hue possessed an intermediate degree of civilization. As civilization is attended by this whitening effect, he reiterated: "On the whole there are many reasons which lead us to adopt the conclusion that the primitive stock of men were probably Negroes, and I know of no argument to be set on the other side."[49]

Prichard's startling hypothesis of primeval Blackness contradicted the view expressed in his dissertation, as well as Blumenbach's and the generally accepted opinion that Black skin is a degenerated form of original lightness, a view nicely safeguarding God, Adam, and Eve's white credentials. It gave credence, on the other hand, to the already mooted idea that the cultures of contemporary Black-skinned peoples might be that of early humankind. There was undoubtedly some discomfort in reconciling original Black skin with the site of human creation in the Near East. Prichard felt his argument for original human skin being Black was nevertheless sound and would be corroborated through the study of individual nations. He therefore confidently concluded with his refrain: "On the whole it appears that we may with a high degree of probability draw the inference, that all the different races into which the human species is divided, originated from one family."[50] Prichard linked the environment and behavior to human physical variation, posed some limited evolutionary theories, and invested heavily in his migrationist/diffusionist model.

Physical History's Ethnology of Origin

The second half of *Physical History* attempts to be nothing short of a global ethnology. At the time it was ambitious in the astounding amount of data amassed. The balance of the material, mostly descriptions of peoples' physical features and languages, is a reflection of the information available to Prichard at the time. He believed that the analysis of religious practices and civil institutions could provide indications of connections between nations. Of scarcely less importance is the understanding of "habits and peculiar customs," although there are some pitfalls when evaluating such data. A shared custom or behavior might be a universal response to natural circumstances rather than evidence of common ancestry. Prichard more readily trusted language over other cultural artifacts, and he had access to a lot of linguistic data.[51] When he had a wider range of material available, however, he saw the benefits of comparing cultures. This is apparent in his extensive comparison of ancient Egyptian and Indian culture, an approach "invented" decades later and called cross-cultural studies, attributed to E. B. Tylor.

Prichard could describe little more than the language affinities among some of the peoples of the South Pacific and Malaysia, as this was the type of material available at that time, while the African interior and some other areas of the globe were yet to be explored.[52] Even with these drawbacks, he devised a coherent framework for synthesizing and analyzing data: first he ascertained his informant's credibility as an observer; next he classified and cross-checked the data with information provided by others; and finally he analyzed the material and drew conclusions.[53] Prichard often brought in biological points made in the first part of *Physical History* as they pertained to individual cultures.

By contrast to his sketchy descriptions of many parts of the world, Prichard had the resources to compare extensively the Egyptians and Hindus, physically, culturally, and historically, especially to show similarities in their civil institutions and complex mythologies. He played down their physical differences, instead noting that both classical and their own texts, monuments, and art point to their shared ancestry and African origin. He attributed these two peoples' gradual loss of African physiognomy to the whitening effect of civilization. He referred to Manetho's *Aegyptiaca*, a chronology created circa the second century BCE, while he found Indian chronology rather extravagant in its claims of great antiquity, though it correlated with ancient Greek writings that seemed to confirm 2200 BCE as the approximate date of the foundation of its empire by "a very learned people." There are many mentions of affinities (a favorite term) between these two civilizations as indicative of common origins but less discussion of actual causes or processes. Concerning Indian political institutions, for instance, he wrote that "we have at present no concern with the causes that gave rise to these establishments. Our design is to compare together the institutions of Egypt and India, in order to determine whether they are of separate derivation and growth, or manifest congruities so clear and extensive as to leave no doubt of their common origin."[54]

All the nations from Libya to the Tigris are of common descent, Prichard concluded. Following the views of philologist Sir William Jones and referring to articles in the *Asiatick Researches*, Prichard determined that the ancient language of Persia was derived from Sanskrit, making the Persians and Indians of kindred stock, while their similar political institutions and religious beliefs indicate that they are branches of the same ancient culture. Both "stocks" are descended from an African stock, whose peoples had wandered to the four corners of the world, where they remained in their primitive state while the parent stock advanced culturally and diversified. Prichard was attempting to build a genealogy of human culture.[55]

Having demonstrated the characteristically African physiognomy of the ancient nations of the Middle East, Near East, and South Asia, Prichard set about providing historical evidence in support of his ancestral "Negro stock" theory. Calling on the classical historians and adding his own linguistic analyses, he found similarities among the European tribes, indicating they had a common origin in some ancient Eastern stock. He then turned to the inhabitants of Europe displaced by incoming tribes.[56] Their original migration into Europe had been in times too remote for the classical historians to cover, but they shared traits with the aforementioned tribes of Asian origin, including affinities with Indian culture. The Celts must have originally occupied the continent but were driven to its fringes by incoming German tribes.

Anything touching on the Welsh was close to Prichard's heart, so much so that he would devote an entire volume to the Celts. But at this point his task was to link them to other peoples in any way he could. He described the Druids' and Brahmans' shared polytheism and other cultural traits.[57] Prichard's considering Celtic complexion and facial structure to approach that of the "Mongole" type was his cue to turn to further tracings to Indians, not to mention the Finns and Laplanders; the occupants of the remotest parts of Europe thereby hailed from western Asia. Moving on, he even managed to link the Indians with other Asian nations. Peoples inhabiting the most inauspicious locations deviated more from the European type, whereas more civilized peoples, he reiterated, tended to be larger, lighter, and therefore more European in appearance.[58]

Indigenous Americans are briefly described for lack of reliable data. All American tribes are of common origin in eastern Asia, as indicated by their general physical similarity to each other and to the "Mongole" type, as well as some linguistic and cultural affinities. Prichard cited the respected observers Blumenbach and explorer and naturalist Alexander von Humboldt, who had testified to the similarities between the Mongoles, Americans, Mandshurs, and Malays. The Aztecs themselves thought their forebears came from the far North, and the American tribes believe that their ancestors migrated from the direction of Asia.[59]

Prichard's ethnology contains as much evidence as he could muster of similarities in languages, beliefs and customs, and possible historical relationships. So with the biological section of *Physical History* demonstrating the specific unity of humankind and his ethnological section its single origin, he could conclude by summarizing the "probable history of mankind." Its original territory (the biblical lands), bounded by the Caspian Sea, the Nile, the Ganges, and the Indian Ocean, is also the cradle of civilization. Before early humans could hunt, they fished along those shores and gathered vegetation, activities fostering migration that scattered them to the far corners of the earth where they remained in their primitive state. Twentieth-century paleontologists would produce arrow-filled maps illustrating a similar human flow.

Prichard noted that languages cannot be traced to their most ancestral form because early humankind had left their territory of origin before the development of language or culture. This was also before religious degeneration into idolatry. In the primeval seat of humankind, meanwhile, culture advanced somewhat as hunting and pastoralism developed, and migrations northward to Scandinavia and eastward to far Asia and America spread these new skills and their developing worship of the heavenly bodies, Sabaism. With the advent of agriculture in the original home of humankind came the division of labor, allowing a priesthood to elaborate on original Sabaism, and class and political institutions to form. The Celts migrated westward into Europe, carrying their developing polytheism, language, and philosophy of the East with them, but these people were eventually displaced by later tribal migrations.[60] Prichard's successive waves of migration by hunter-gatherers, pastoralists, and then agriculturalists outlined social development in line with Scottish Enlightenment thought.

Prichard hoped *Physical History* would see off claims that the environment and the inheritance of acquired characteristics bring about new varieties and even species. He suggested ways in which superficial biological differences among the single human species had arisen: certain conditions lead to the whitening of animals, and civilization has a refining effect on humans, but the actual mechanism of variation is congenital spontaneous biological change in a process as yet unexplained. He could imply the Blackness of Adam, Eve, and God because he understood that the original couple had existed in a state of perfection they were deprived of by the Fall. All his evidence told against facile polygenism. *Physical History* combined biological and cultural research into a form of early anthropology, establishing Prichard's scientific reputation and helping to lay the foundations of British anthropology.

Physical History's Reception

Physical History was jointly published in London by the Quaker firm John and Arthur Arch and in Bristol by B. and H. Barry.[61] Long summarizing reviews appeared in periodicals, and a few typically non-evaluative notices and abstracts found their way into Continental journals such as the *Journal général la littérature étrangère*. The respectable London *Monthly Review; or Literary Journal* praised Prichard's learning and ingenuity in making a plausible case for monogenism, albeit conjectural and sometimes resting on rather slender foundations. His friend John Bostock noted in the *Critical Review* how he had carefully set aside Mosaic records in his "assiduous research for historical facts," to form "a most valuable and edifying publication." He added that Prichard's hypotheses still lacked proof, however, while his notion that the primeval stock of humans had been Black was particularly shocking. Conflating "original stock" with the dramatis personae of Genesis, the reviewer complained: "Many of the most beautiful poetical images will lose the force of their allusion, if the lovely charms of the first born, Eve, should prove to be a negress." Although Dr. Bostock could not accept that "the most beautiful complexions" (white) were not those of Nature's original design, he still endorsed *Physical History* as "one of the best essays of natural philosophy extant."[62]

Another reviewer wondered rather crossly why Prichard had attempted to prove monogenesis without the aid of the Bible, unless it was to kowtow to his sly, idle, speculating, infidel, sciolist former Edinburgh professors. This Christian *British Critic* reviewer did approve of Prichard's ingenious support of the veracity of the sacred records. Reviews in scientific journals were generally positive; the one in the well-respected *Annals of Philosophy* began by praising Prichard's remarkable achievement in having been the first to succeed in bringing to bear a wide range of discoveries using analogical reasoning on the challenging issue of human origin. This was distinct progress over previous speculative philosophers' piecemeal pronouncements and the myriad of crude and unsubstantiated conjectures by the likes of Lord Kames. Such was the reviewer's regard for *Physical History*, there was no condemnation of the "startling" Black-to-white hypothesis but only the hope that the young author would continue researching the history of humankind. A Scottish journal was impressed by Prichard's methodology.[63]

The era's interest in "deep history" encouraged speculation, even by Prichard. Reviewers pointed out instances of his indulging in it despite claiming otherwise. There was, however, little appetite for establishing links among European nations, never mind extra-European cultures, during this period of political, economic, and social instability, growing Christian fervor, European hostilities, and nationalistic mythologizing. Geological evidence of the great age of the earth suggested a prehuman state that undermined Scripture, and natural historians hesitated to integrate humans into a framework of speculative evolutionary biology, fearful of bringing the condemnation of the religious establishment down on their heads. Prichard had made a start on devising a science of humankind at a time when ethnographical and linguistic material was only just becoming available. In this inauspicious political and social climate, his friend Dr. William Lawrence closely read *Physical History* and began lecturing rather boldly on the science of life and of humankind.

Lawrence and the Lawrence Affair

Six years after *Physical History* came out, a famous scandal involving Prichard's friend William Lawrence illustrates the risks involved in treating humankind as a natural historical object. Prichard was orthodox in being a "mind-body dualist"; mental phenomena are nonphysical, a view compatible with belief in the immaterial soul. Not so Lawrence. He rashly expressed materialist leanings in his *Lectures on Physiology, Zoology, and the Natural History of Man: Delivered at the Royal College of Surgeons* (1819), in which he claimed thought to be the product of the brain. Not only did he point out that scientific proof of the existence of the soul was lacking, but he seemed not to have clearly separated humankind from consideration of the lower animals.[64] This handsome, charismatic, and sometimes titillating lecturer landed himself in hot water for these Continental ideas, fondness for rationalistic arguments, and lack of deference to his British scientific forebears and especially to natural theologians. His attitude bordered on disdain for Scripture itself. Lawrence's neglecting scriptural evidence and treating the human species as a common animal deeply offended and alarmed the Establishment.

Nonmedical commentators were infuriated by Lawrence's apparent doubt of the immortality of the soul, a corrosive view that would surely lead to a breakdown in national moral and social order. The conservative press so relentlessly reviled this flirtation with atheism that, threatened with prosecution for blasphemy and the ruin of his career, he was forced to suppress his book. That helped it to become wildly popular; pirated editions sold on the black market at inflated prices, while its author brazenly distributed privately printed copies. His daughter later wrote, "My father withdrew his 'Lectures' entirely in deference to the strongly urged wishes of his father & his family." Lawrence and Prichard's fathers thought alike. And perhaps the word "entirely" should be stressed, considering Lawrence's involvement with radicalism early in his career. In private he regretted his lack of courage in agreeing to recant, while publicly he admitted his book had been improper. He vowed to one of his employers never to publish on the topic again.

More concise and readable than Prichard, *Lectures* became a resource for freethinkers, agitating radicals, and successive generations of scientists, Darwin included. The bulk of it was actually not all that original, much being derived from Blumenbach and Prichard. Methodologically, Lawrence's concentration on zoological, anatomical, and physiological, rather than linguistic, evidence distinguishes him from Prichard. Notably, he adopted the position of "qualified monogenist," that is, that there is a unity of the human species but insufficient evidence of its unity of origin. It stands to reason that he rejected the role of the environment in creating varieties; instead, he brought French biology (the first to use that word in English) to bear on the new science of humankind. Lawrence's materialist position disturbed Prichard's sincere Christian view of the natural world, and his calling for scientific proof of monogenism hit home. Prichard had failed to accomplish this.

Lawrence dealt with the threat of censure for unorthodoxy by dropping the science of humankind and developing his talents elsewhere. Prichard was sufficiently confident to give *Lectures* a qualified public endorsement in 1826, praising it as the most comprehensive survey of facts demonstrating the unity of the human species. Without mentioning its debt to *Physical History*, he lauded it as a contribution to anthropology and scientific method. The Lawrence debacle provided a stern reminder of the perils of entertaining Continental scientific theories; Prichard avoided criticism and quietly devoted himself to finding the proof of monogenesis Lawrence demanded.[65]

New Data and *Researches into the Physical History of Mankind* (1826)

The respectability Lawrence risked and Prichard valued was typically advertised by a string of postnominals indicating a university degree and some memberships in high-status learned societies. Any gentleman naturalist, Prichard included, would have been pleased to have FLS (Fellow of the

Linnean Society) after his name on the title page of a book. The Linnean Society's resources and its members' expertise would be useful to Prichard in further researching his biological arguments for a revised edition of *Physical History* as well. His relative John Walker, friend Charles Mackenzie, Edinburgh professor Robert Jameson, and young zoologist William Elford Leach supported his application; he was elected fellow of the Linnean Society on May 4, 1813.[66]

Amid the notoriety that the publication of *Physical History* brought him, Prichard was fully occupied in Bristol by his medical practice, charity health care, publishing on other subjects like geology, Egyptian mythology, and fevers, campaigning, and getting involved in establishing a scientific society. He also started spending a few predawn hours every day filling manuscript volumes with notes for an enlarged edition of *Physical History*. He found it beneficial to try out some of his material at the new Bristol Phil & Lit Society by lecturing on topics like the Gauls and on the distribution of plants and animals in 1824, and newly "discovered" African peoples and the Native tribes of America in 1826.[67] Prichard had published a book on neurology and insanity in 1822, and by the summer of 1824 his father had good grounds for being seriously worried about his son's health.

It took twelve years for Prichard to prepare the two-volume, 1,199-page second edition of *Physical History of Mankind*. Published by the same London firm, it was a costly item at 40 shillings, even in basic board binding.[68] No longer of *Man*, but a more scientific *Mankind*, it contains several vocabulary lists, a section of notes, and ten engraved plates, mostly of skulls illustrating the characteristics of human "varieties," reflecting its author's continuing qualified interest in craniology. The frontispiece is a striking colored portrait of the learned Ethiopian Abbas Gregorius. Ethiopians figured in Prichard's opinion of the original skin color of the ancient Egyptians; Gregorius's very dark skin but prominent forehead and vertical facial angle nicely contradicted those old facial angle stereotypes. The book is dedicated "to the venerable and justly celebrated Professor Johann Friedrich Blumenbach, of the University of Goettingen; by whose eminently successful labours, the physical history of mankind has been chiefly illustrated. This work is, with his permission, respectfully dedicated by the author." Its introduction acknowledges the work of the German professor as well as Lawrence's *Lectures*, although he carefully pointed out his disagreement with some of the latter's views.[69]

Frustrated by his inability to provide conclusive biological proof of monogenesis, Prichard turned to gathering more and more linguistic and other ethnographic evidence. The 1826 edition contains a threefold increase in ethnographical material, substantial modifications to his argument concerning the processes of human physical variation, and a much greater focus on historical linguistics. He no longer stressed civilization as stimulative to human biological progress from "rude" to "refined," dark to light. While still opposed to the direct action of the environment, he was starting to think favorable conditions and climate might somehow facilitate change. His ultimate goal was still to prove the unity of the human species and its single origin.

Previously Prichard had claimed that change in what he termed the connate (innate, congenital) structure of organisms happens suddenly and spontaneously in the generation of offspring, not gradually and cumulatively, as transmutationists believed happened in the creation of new species. In 1826 he still felt that variation through spontaneous connate change was a valid theory but that external circumstances might play some role in encouraging changes in offspring to adapt to their situation. While all living things contain a certain set of "germs" that provide all the information that determines its form, there is some scope for external circumstances affecting offspring, a view he adopted from Kant via Blumenbach. He cited many examples of variation that seem related to geographical location, claiming that some varieties are better adapted to extreme climates than others; a case in point is that Black-skinned people thrive in tropical zones while white-skinned ones die out.[70] He was toying with the notion of biological adaptation. A later Darwinian might criticize Prichard for adding the triggering action of the environment to his view of what is essentially random mutation, since through a strict Darwinian lens the most suitable succeed and the least die out. Yet a twenty-first-century observer might note Prichard's formulation of the basis of what is now called gene switching, or gene expression activated by signals from the environment.

Prichard's qualified admission of the environment being an instrument of change reinforced his argument against polygenism's fixity of the human species. Importantly, he held firmly to his view that bodily modifications acquired during life cannot be passed on to offspring. He now minimized his hypotheses on sexual selection and original human Blackness, converting the latter point to an original "melanous," or dark, hue. New evidence suggested to Prichard that dark, "primitive" stocks are more prone to variation, eventually producing lighter descendants in a natural process. This implied a greater susceptibility of "savages" to environmental influence.

Prichard did not explain why he had decided to obscure his 1813 argument concerning the original Blackness of humankind. Public reaction had not been noticeably hostile; fellow scientists like William Lawrence generally ignored it. In this pre-Darwinian, pre-scientific racialism era, implying Europeans' African instead of Middle Eastern homeland may have been considered merely provocative speculation. Probably, while he seemed to still believe humans had developed from Black to white, the theory was proving difficult to substantiate, so he dropped it.[71]

In elaborating his theories of the production of varieties, Prichard incorporated some prevalent attitudes concerning male and female roles in reproduction. Although he thought tales of external influences affecting the fetus in late gestation were absurd, he could no longer entirely dismiss another explanation: the father provides the defining characteristics of the species, while impressions on the mother from external circumstances at or soon after conception may affect her offspring. So the environmental influences on variation operate within the mother, but the exact mechanism, Prichard mused, "we shall perhaps never be able to ascertain." Again, either sudden or gradual congenital changes in an individual are liable to be reproduced in offspring, but outright, externally caused changes are never heritable.[72]

Prichard doubted whether it would ever be possible to explain the exact mechanisms of heredity and environmental stimulation. In replacing civilization with the environment as stimulative of development of varieties, he was asking his readers to accept a vague, limited, and unsubstantiated theory that he hoped would hold transmutationists at bay and shore up his monogenist position.[73]

Prichard retained the first edition's extensive material on the diffusion of plants and animals, its content expanded by a generous supply of new systematically collected biogeographical material linking biological structure and climate. New resources demonstrating relationships between form, physiology, and habitat were highlighted. He particularly valued the contributions of Alexander von Humboldt, Augustin Pyramus de Candolle, and Robert Brown, the last describing the geographical origins of particular plant genera. Some eighteenth-century writers had proposed that there had been multiple centers of creation to account for the obvious relationships between the physical characteristics of animals and their habitats. Prichard feared that extending this notion to the human species would play into the hands of polygenists, however. Instead, his compromise was to suggest that while there had been several centers of creation, each species had only a single locus of creation.[74]

The 1826 edition of *Physical History* draws on many more German resources, as Prichard had learned to read German. Now he cited Julius Klaproth and Franz Bopp for linguistics and Carl Ritter for geography, but he continued to ignore German metaphysical philosophy, French materialism, and any anathematic Continental transmutationist hypotheses that cast doubt on the fixity of species. Instead, overt reference to Scripture did more than just creep in: he appended nine pages of notes comparing his views on the diffusion of plants and animals and the history of humankind with the account of the Deluge in Genesis, including proofs, examples, and inferences. His hypothesis as to why there are different genera of plants and animals in different locations was that once the Flood had subsided, different regions were "supplied with organized inhabitants, suited to the soil and climate of each district." Geology shows that there had been successive perishings and creations, with different forms inhabiting the earth at different times. These catastrophes were associated with floods, each preparing the earth for new and different groups; the earliest ones had decimated species, but some genera had survived. This brought his account down to the most recent deluge, the only one recorded in history. The elevated regions of central Asia where humankind was "created on the banks of the Euphrates and ... survived on the mountains of Armenia" appeared to have been the human species' original place of abode before and after the Flood.[75] This Neptunist, postdiluvian, partial creation had not figured in Scripture because an account of the whole world had been unnecessary and irrelevant: "And it was of no importance for men to be informed at what era New Holland began to contain kanguroos, or the woods of Paraguay ant-eaters and armadilloes." There had been several sites of creation around the world, and as each species had only one place of origin, this must also be true of human beings. His hypothesis thus accorded nature with the Mosaic account that satisfied the vast majority of his readers and himself.[76]

Prichard devoted a special subsection to a clear statement of his position on "race," lest his readers mistakenly conclude that his division of peoples into groups or nations implied separate races or species. Following Blumenbach, he set out the five human varieties: Caucasian, Mongolian, Aethiopian, American, and Malayan/South Sea Islander. He now devised three not very catchy terms for skin color—xanthous, melanic, and albino—and he distinguished the skull forms stenobregmate, mesobregmate, and platybregmate. Prichard dismissed attempts to classify human populations according to skull form: "Hence the hypothesis of a limited number of particular races or principal nations, including all those tribes who have a certain conformation, must be given up; and, if we divide the whole family of mankind into several departments, with reference to the shape of their skulls, or any other particular trait of organization, it must be only with a view to facilitate comparisons, and must be done independently of any design to ascribe a common origin, or a near relation of kindred to the tribes included in each class."[77] All humans are of the same species, which cannot be divided into races because of a lack of exclusively held distinguishing characteristics and the great variations of form within a given population. To Prichard's disappointment, the mechanisms by which variations had arisen had not been conclusively established.[78]

The many descriptions of newly explored parts of the world published since 1813 allowed Prichard to fill 827 pages with ethnography, with the world now divided into the "departments" of Africa, the great Southern Ocean, the Indo-European nations, and so on.[79] The American material swells to nearly two hundred pages, and more than one hundred on Africa benefit from recent, more individual, and systematic descriptions. This mass of material turned out frustrating, however: the obvious complexity of world populations made it exceedingly challenging to establish a grand genealogy of humankind with its origin traceable to the biblical Middle East. Prichard's unwieldy ethnographic material is necessarily more descriptive and classificatory than historical or analytical.

"A Catalogue of Nations, or Index of the different Races and Tribes of Men, as distinguished by their Languages" is the title of Prichard's list of ethnic groups, indicating his increasing reliance on linguistics.[80] Convinced that skin color, skull form, and other characteristics are merely descriptive rather than defining of human varieties, he put greater stress on historical linguistic evidence, which might more reliably and successfully be brought to bear on the question of the origin and unity of the human species. His list of African languages is remarkably accurate, and noteworthy is his exploration of the relationships among African languages, for which he produced comparative vocabulary lists. He convincingly described the Bantu family of languages from their analogous vocabularies and grammar structures. By and large, however, Prichard ended up with more delineations of language groups than proof of their relationships or origins.

Linguistics dominate the ethnographic portion of *Physical History*. As there is an "infinite variety of jargons" among the tribes of New Holland and Papua, Prichard used the German comparative linguistics of Klaproth, whose *Asia Polyglotta* (1823) helped him to tease out relationships between languages based on vocabulary and grammatical forms, offer explanations of the causes of change, and relate language to culture.[81] After equating the simplicity of language with the simplicity of culture, he concluded that early dispersals of peoples and their degradation into a state of barbarity had led to the development of different languages. He then compared Indo-European languages, citing Franz Bopp's analysis of tenses and his geologist friend William Daniel Conybeare's work on nouns, adjectives, and pronouns.

In preparation for his future *Eastern Origin of the Celtic Languages*, Prichard was keen to contradict those authors who had excluded the Celtic languages from the Indo-European family.[82] His stress on language is obvious, but his research was not limited to it. Travelers described physical and linguistic features of Indigenous people more fully than cultural, so wherever there was an absence of "history" or "customs and manners," Prichard turned to language. While he might have thought the evidence of language more measurable than that of culture, he did value nonlinguistic aspects of culture.

The second edition of *Physical History* was not extensively reviewed. The February 1827 issue of the *London Medical Repository* printed a long abstract of it that thoroughly approved of medical men studying human diversity and praised Prichard's devotion to proving the unity of humankind. The *British Critic* considered it "the most complete magazine of general knowledge on [the natural history of humankind] that is to be found in the English language," particularly praiseworthy for its exclusion of fanciful theories and materialist stances and for the author's exposition on the diversity of language. There was fulsome praise of Prichard's orthodoxy, industry, twenty years of indefatigable labor, and eloquence of expression.[83]

There were some foreign reviews of the second edition of *Physical History*. A German reviewer considered it to stand out from anything previously published on the subject and was especially appreciative of Prichard's geographically organized ethnographic material's avoidance of hypothetical racial classification.[84] The reaction of some of the U.S. press was alarmingly negative, by contrast. Americans were taking up race studies, apparently to counter the anti–slave trade movement's shift of focus to antislavery itself. Race theory was useful in justifying rampant Indigenous American genocide as well. For the Kentucky physician Charles Caldwell, *Physical History* was infuriating. He had developed an interest in phrenology for its biological determinism and was so keen to refute Prichard's monogenism that he expanded his long critique of it into a sizable book, *Thoughts on the Original Unity of the Human Race* (1830). Caldwell not unreasonably accused Prichard of bias in his commitment to monogenism: "He never forgets his covenant with himself, that, right or wrong, the affirmative side of the question must triumph." He attacked Prichard's feeble reliance on mere analogy, his implied absolute belief in every sentiment expressed in the Old and New Testaments, his dwelling on the diffusion of plants and animals, and his suggestion of spontaneous biological change in offspring. An example of Caldwell's ridicule of this last notion was that a Caucasian couple, for example, would have had to suddenly produce Black-skinned babies, becoming the parents of the "Negro type." He claimed Caucasians' intellectual superiority, whereas Native Americans' predilections for uncontrolled bloodthirstiness and disinclination to acquire property clearly demonstrated that race's incapability of being civilized. Caldwell's views were summarized approvingly in a Philadelphia medical journal. His was just the first of a tide of American polygenetic publications over the next four decades.[85]

Prichard and Proto-Darwinian Theory

Alfred Russel Wallace, Darwin's fellow developer of the theory of evolution through natural selection, wrote in 1897:

> I was *delighted* with your account of Prichard's wonderful anticipation of Galton & Weismann['s Germ-Plasm theory of heredity]! It is so perfect and complete.... It is most remarkable that such a complete statement of the theory and such a thorough appreciation of its effects and bearing, should have been so long overlooked. I read Prichard when I was very young, & have never seen the book since. His facts and arguments are really useful now, and I should think Weismann must be delighted to have such a supporter come from the grave. His view as to supposed transmission of disease is quite that of Archdall Reid's recent book. He was equally clear as to Selection, & had he been a zoologist and traveller he might have anticipated the work of both Darwin & Weismann! To bring out such a book as his "Researches" when only 27, and a practising Physician, shows what a remarkable man he was.[86]

Prichard has been cited as coming so close to explaining the process of organic evolution in 1826 that it is a challenge to understand how he avoided it. Elements of it had been suggested by others, but his synthesis seems before its time. Prichard recognized the sudden generation of heritable new forms (mutations); that the undesirable do not reproduce (natural selection); that the choice of mates effects change (sexual selection); that varieties of humans are produced in a way analogous to that of plants and animals by way of a "set of germs" (genes and particulate inheritance); and that species somehow physically adapt to their geographical location (adaptive evolution). Rather than suggesting the so-called survival of the fittest, he observed the converse in that "individuals and families, and even whole colonies, perish and disappear in climates for which they are, by peculiarity of constitution, not adapted."[87]

The year Prichard published the second edition of *Physical History*, a teenage Charles Darwin was being inspired by his family's involvement in the antislavery cause. As they had been for Prichard, the iniquity of slavery and the allied search for human unity motivated Darwin, and like Prichard, the younger scientist would combat the institution of slavery not with antislavery pamphlets and medallions but through his quietly pursued effort to prove the common ancestry of all humans. After a voyage spent immersed in the study of the natural world, Darwin returned to London and began secretly filling notebooks with his ideas about how species vary without the guiding hand of God. Unlike Prichard, crucially, he began to consider varieties of a particular species incipient future species.

Darwin was influenced by Prichard's early editions of *Physical History*, either directly or through Lawrence's summary of the 1813 edition. His notebooks contain many examples of analogical reasoning—Prichard's mainstay—and, as had Prichard, he noted the relativity of beauty. As for the skin color of original humans, Darwin was free to suggest that the cradle of humankind had been Africa. While the first written evidence of Darwin's studying Prichard dates from the 1850s, he repeatedly took extensive notes on and annotated the third edition of *Physical History* and noted "the old edition" as he was preparing *Origin*. But after decades of secretly considering biological development, Darwin decided not to include humankind in his magnum opus of 1859, so great was social pressure against such an idea. A dozen years later the climate was ripe to tackle it.[88]

Prichard gave evolutionary theory its fullest expression but confined it to explaining the production of varieties within a species, not the mutability of species themselves. Although he eventually wrote of imagining all life developing from an ancestral form, he turned more toward considering adaptation as the driver of change. So while Prichard remains one of Darwin's sources of evolutionary argument, he is not included in the ranks of the many pre-Darwinian evolutionists, disqualified by his unshakable Christian adherence to the fixity of species.

Was Prichard satisfied that the second edition of *Physical History* had succeeded? His book contains some convoluted arguments in support of monogenism, as he could not demonstrate human biological unity solely on genealogy. Rather, he resorted to the unclassifiability of physical traits and mired himself in historical comparative linguistics.

Prichard became active in societies for the preservation of extra-Europeans and the study of their cultures. He went on to develop, promote, and defend his science in a five-volume, third edition of *Physical History* (1836–47) and several popularizing editions of *Natural History of Man*, adjusting his arguments in response to polygenetic and materialist incursions into his Christian monogenetic science and the increasing volume of ethnographical and scientific material available. His volumes had an international reach and can claim to be among the earliest textbooks of the broader discipline of anthropology. He made humanitarian speeches like the "Extinction of Human Races" and drew attention to the values of Indigenous cultures and the detriments of civilization. In his writing on anthropology and psychology, Prichard would suggest a theory of the universal mind that unified the human species. His high reputation among the learned elite ensured the science of humankind was as he defined it, while rival polygenetic theorizing was held in check, at least in Britain.[89]

7 · Epidemics, History, and Mythology

Building a Reputation in Bristol, 1817–22

> It had long been an impression on my mind, that thy health
> has not suffered so much by the duties of thy profession
> as by midnight studies too assiduously pursued.
>
> —James Cowles Prichard, "Memoir of Thomas Prichard, Part 2"

Death in the form of typhus swept Bristol in 1817, and it struck again the following two years. Prichard was in the thick of it, employing his heroic treatments on the suffering paupers packed together like sardines in ancient St. Peter's Hospital and entering the many fatalities in his casebooks. At home there were a few occasions for joy, but more for anxiety and sorrow. The Prichards' daughter Mary was born on December 6, 1816, while little Francis died suddenly of fever the following February 3.[1] Then there was the physician's occupational hazard; Prichard was seriously ill much of the summer of 1817 with typhus. In these trying times, could he be persuaded to abandon Anglicanism for Unitarianism, an about-turn as sensational as Dr. Stock's disavowal of Unitarianism?

Having a Unitarian divine of renown for a father-in-law could be trying at times. Dr. Estlin might have exercised reserve when chatting with Thomas Prichard, but young churchman Prichard was fair game. Estlin applied some Unitarian pressure, according to a family friend:

> Dr Pritchard too, is by no means to be brought over to the true faith, as preached at Lewins Mead, but continues his provoking orthodoxy, in spite of a most eloquent letter written to him by his Father-in-law, in which he compares his mind to a fine building, with airy and spacious apartments, capable of containing everything that is commodious and beautiful, but unfortunately all the rooms are let out to Prejudice. Whether this inconvenient personage will ever be dislodged from her premises by the arguments of our good friend, or whether Dr Pritchard will die in his belief, is a point which is very doubtful, altho' Dr Estlin told us that upon the whole he was very sanguine upon the subject.[2]

Dr. Estlin had no further opportunity to proselytize. Anna received devastating news from the family's summer home in Wales—he had died from a massive hemorrhage of the stomach. Tributes flooded in; Bristol's Unitarian community deeply felt the loss of their valued educator and influential minister.[3] Efforts to make a Unitarian out of Prichard stalled.

Even during the postwar economic doldrums and epidemics, there was a bit of excitement to be had in Bristol. One intriguing local drama highlights the fascination that the outside world held at this time. While Bristolians were quite familiar with products from beyond Europe, contact with extra-Europeans was rare, aside from glimpses of sailors on the docks or the occasional novelty of the aristocracy and super rich's African servants. The curiosity about "the Other" that had fostered interest in Prichard's *Physical History* got a live specimen to feast on when a bereft foreign princess turned up in April 1817. This destitute young woman, who spoke not a word of English, set Bristolians agog.

The graceful, mysterious beturbaned foreigner was given shelter by the wealthy Worrall family of Knowle Park and instantly became a visitor attraction. The lady of the house and her friends became quite devoted to her as they invited experts to ponder her complex language, orthography, manners, religious rituals, and fastidious personal habits. A regular procession of the carriages of the great and good could be seen drawing up to Knowle Park, eager to be granted an audience by and to proffer suitable regal gifts to the "exotic" Princess Caraboo of Javasu. Her ship had been captured by pirates, but she had managed to jump overboard into the Bristol Channel and swim ashore. Over the next ten weeks there were regular newspaper updates about Princess Caraboo. One linguist concluded she was Circassian, and another expert thought she might be a Muslim, were it not for her weekly sun-worshipping. When Prichard's friend artist Edward Bird had the privilege of painting her full-length portrait, it proved her undoing; a local landlady saw a print of it in the newspaper and identified the princess as Mary Willcocks, a Devonshire vagrant. The game was up. Prichard had luckily kept his distance. Having fascinated Bristol and beyond, Princess Caraboo's erstwhile patrons put her on a ship for America.[4]

Thomas Prichard was now making full use of his son's medical expertise, summoning Prichard to himself at Mary Moline's in Godalming to treat his gouty stomach pains. He had more than just health worries: Tom, then working as an agent for a transatlantic freight and passenger ship, was about to start his new life in America, attracted by a surefire business opportunity. Of course, his father would have to stand as Tom's guarantor.[5]

Epidemics

The epidemic that had broken out earlier in the year in other English cities was then ravaging Ireland. Prichard's university friend Patrick Mackenzie's London Fever Hospital admitted 321 typhus patients in six months. Reminded of his young friend John Pole's death fifteen years earlier, Prichard would fight the epidemic in every way he could, even though the Bristol Corporation balked at spending a farthing on public health measures.

Prichard felt it his duty to warn local government to prepare for an epidemic. The increasingly confident physician to St. Peter's Hospital published a letter in the newspaper addressed to the mayor pointing out that Bristol's most indigent vagrants and beggars were wandering the streets, spreading typhus among their kind. Property owners were having to hire watchmen to root out the miserable wretches from the corners of stables and outbuildings where they had dragged themselves to die. Others huddling in crowded living conditions through the bitter winter were spreading the disease rapidly. Nor were the opulent safe when the diseased were free to roam at large. Prichard attempted to win over his readers by appealing both to their humane impulse and their dread of contagion. He must have hit home with his account of several perishing souls recently found laid at the gates of St. Peter's Hospital, already grossly overcrowded and without facilities for segregating fever patients. Neither could the Infirmary cope with all the typhus cases turning up. He concluded by calling for the establishment of a fever hospital along the lines of the successful ones in London, Liverpool, Manchester, and other large towns. He counted on Bristolians not wanting to be seen as lagging behind rival cities.[6]

Prichard's imputation of civic neglect was met with angry rebuttal; his demands were branded premature and unnecessary.[7] Responding with an update from St. Peter's, he countered with some impressive statistics and positive news. Of its 134 cases of typhus that year, 26 had been fatal, an increase in mortality over previous years that he attributed to the policy of admitting infectious patients. Fortunately, the recent establishment of a temporary charity House of Recovery had resulted in the eradication of fever at St. Peter's. He added statistics on fever cases at the Infirmary and the North and South Bristol Dispensaries to demonstrate the need for a permanent fever hospital in the city. In defending himself and asserting his dignity, Prichard concluded irritably: "I have been informed, that censure has been cast upon me for exciting unnecessary alarm, by the letter inserted in your Journal a fortnight ago. This is ridiculous enough, as I only stated facts, which, if in their nature alarming, ought to be known—If not, there could be no reason for concealing them. I certainly shall not be deterred by the childish clamours of a few imbecile persons from making known to the public facts which are interesting to the whole community, and which I know it to be my duty to lay before them."[8]

In the same issue of the newspaper, Prichard's former Clifton Dispensary colleague Dr. Chisholm chipped in with his own statistics and his own axe to grind. While not criticizing Prichard, he pointed out his priority in having published in the *Edinburgh Medical and Surgical Journal* fever statistics from all the Bristol medical institutions. He added that typhus was not caused solely by infection because typhus patients in the Infirmary did not spread their disease to other patients. Indeed, as the cause of fevers was not merely contact but living conditions, Chisholm concluded that ameliorating the filthy, confined, deprived, and malnourished conditions of the poor was the way to tackle the epidemic.[9] He thus undermined Prichard's call for a permanent fever hospital.

Britain was not as hard hit by the epidemic as Ireland, where the famine of the previous few years had contributed to the virulence of the disease, claiming about one hundred thousand victims. In Bristol, the calamity of this epidemic, Prichard's warning of its spread from the impoverished to the affluent, and his firm belief in isolating fever cases had spurred him to take a public stand that effectively enhanced his reputation as a medical authority. Like Chisholm, he set great store by the belief that knowledge could be derived from medical statistics. With the help of the apothecaries of the Bristol medical charities, he gathered more case histories and data and presented his findings in the prestigious *Edinburgh Medical and Surgical Journal*. It was a bit over the top.

Prichard's "Cases of Typhus" article focuses on treatment, highly praising his bloodletting hero Dr. John Armstrong while berating some medical practitioners' disgraceful, "vulgar prejudice against bleeding." They "deserve to be hanged up, and gibbetted without mercy, as little better than licensed murderers. I have detected many other instances, in which this kind of ruse has been exercised by crafty persons." Aside from extravagantly championing bloodletting for continued fever, he called upon all physicians to record cases and publish their findings. The greater the amount of statistical evidence, the sooner there would be universal acceptance of antiphlogistic therapeutics. As for the etiology of typhus, Prichard rather arrogantly found "repugnant to probability" respected authorities' view that fever arose from a "general derangement of the whole constitution occurring independently and primarily." In his own theory of the visceral seat of fever he had an ally in Dr. Thomas Mills of Dublin: typhus had its seat in some diseased part of the body, rather than being a disease in itself. In the early stage of fever topical bleeding from its originating site was invariably more effective than general bloodletting. In support of his views, he appended many successful case histories, including St. Peter's apothecary Mr. Morgan's staving-off typhus by promptly letting two pounds of blood from his own arm.[10]

Prichard got a bit of a shock; his rather arrogant tone attracted criticism in the rival London medical press. One editor-reviewer claimed he would have rejected the article for its self-indulgence, lack of government, loose terminology, and failure to cite any but a few recent authorities. Someone of Dr. Prichard's respectability and scientific standing should have been more circumspect.[11] This did not make for enjoyable reading.

Typhus kept Bristol in its grasp over the next two years. Prichard traded statistics and fever case histories at the Bristol Dispensaries and St. Peter's with Dr. James Percival, who had similar concerns based on his extensive experience in a Dublin fever hospital. Perhaps Dr. Percival's new book on typhus inspired Prichard's next publication.[12] First, however, he had a Bristol ally in his fight against epidemics. In early 1819 a necessarily anonymous Bristolian attempted to rally the troops. "One Not of the Faculty" was reformer Susanna Morgan. She published *An Appeal to the Good Sense and Humanity of the Inhabitants of Bristol & Clifton, on the Expediency of Forming an Institution for the Cure and Prevention of Contagious Fever*, a thirty-nine-page pamphlet outlining the causes of fever and describing the many fever hospitals established in the principal cities and towns around the country. Like Prichard, she implied Bristol was dragging its feet. After summarizing the opinions of the most eminent medical writers on the subject, she provided local fever statistics and letters from fourteen Bristol physicians urging the establishment of a fever hospital. One of the two dissenting letters considered the Infirmary the proper provider of fever care, but Miss Morgan countered that its staff was fully occupied with their existing obligations and, at any rate, should not have the monopoly of doing good, a veiled reminder that the Infirmary was a Tory institution. The pamphleteer concluded by soliciting subscriptions for a fever institution.

Prichard's letter in Miss Morgan's pamphlet demonstrates his humane concern. He felt assured that a fever hospital would be established, especially as the disease's progress was inevitable and the "luxurious classes" were not exempt from its ravages. Still smarting from being attacked and then ignored in 1817, he pointed out that anyone who took the pains to look into the condition of the poor in their miserable abodes would endorse removing fever patients to well-ventilated hospitals in order to decrease mortality and contagion.[13]

A History of the Epidemic Fever (1820)

Prichard had little success as an epidemiologist—not that this term or specialism had arrived in Britain yet. He continued his medical statistical work, nevertheless, and was one of the founders of the Bristol Medico-Chirurgical Society in 1818, further illustrating his belief in sharing scientific ideas in this pre-microbe era. In 1820 Bristolians were not surprised to see a newspaper advertisement for "Just Published, price 5s / A History of the Epidemic Fever, which prevailed in Bristol, during the years 1817, 1818, and 1819, founded on reports of St. Peter's Hospital and the Bristol Infirmary."[14] His was not the first book to point out the contagious nature of some diseases and identify their correlation with overcrowded, unsanitary conditions; he wished to share his findings more widely and thus add to the evidence on the subject. He stressed the necessity of isolating sufferers, employing "heroic" therapeutics, and using statistics as a tool of science. Of course, he started *Epidemic Fever* by laying into callous Bristolians and praising that lady pamphleteer.[15]

Prichard compared St. Peter's and Bristol Infirmary's fever statistics between June 1817 and the end of 1819. He again attributed the former's higher mortality rate to patients' being admitted nearly expiring or after having been forced from parish to parish and then closely confined with other fever patients. He noted that more than one-third of fever patients had had previous contact with other fever patients.[16] As to the different situation at the Infirmary, its rule banning the admission of fever patients had long been managed or ignored by its humane medical officers. The short interval of time between admission and death there indicated that patients had also been admitted only in the final stages of disease.[17]

Epidemic Fever then outlines the symptoms, etiology, and treatment of fever. It is of an essentially inflammatory nature and is linked to particular diseased organs: "That derangement of the system of functions which constitutes fever, is very nearly allied in its nature to the disease which accompanies the inflammation of particular organs, is an opinion which is gaining ground every day among medical practitioners."[18] As inflammation and fever are somehow related, anti-inflammatory treatments are called for as "fever is only dangerous when it gives rise to, or displays the symptoms of visceral inflammation." The milder, noninflammatory "simple" fevers risk degeneration into the more severe "cephalic" type, which upon dissection unequivocally shows inflammation of the brain, lungs, liver, stomach, or bowels.[19]

Prichard's fever treatment regime is precise. The wretched, filthy vagrants admitted to St. Peter's were stripped, had their heads shaved, and then were bathed, vigorously rubbed dry, and given a warm drink. Only the most exhausted were administered stimulative wine—cases that usually ended fatally. The primary treatment of cathartic vomiting bringing on the "hot stage" served to "break through the chain of morbid actions."[20] Next, venesection from the arm was prescribed; an average of ten to fourteen ounces was considered a moderate first bleeding. Although the more exhausted patients were prone to fainting, this was sometimes necessary before the required relief was obtained; especially effective was bringing on a near faint and vomiting simultaneously. The abstracted blood was analyzed for symptoms like "buffy coat" (white blood cells and platelets). After ten or twelve hours, bleeding might be repeated up to four times. While for simple fevers a single bleeding could suffice, cephalic fevers required sustained bleedings. Only the very weak and the young were leeched instead.[21] Other measures were taken to "reduce arterial action": the head was covered with cold cloths, the body sponged with cold water, and blisters might be applied to the nape of the neck. Children and patients suffering from simple fever might undergo a "cold affusion" (shower). Purgation with regular doses of calomel (mercury chloride), jalap, senna, and yet more medication completed the regime.[22]

The type and severity of fevers varied with the seasons, as did their treatment, with due regard for the patient's constitution. Simple fever cases left unbled for three or four weeks risked degeneration, first into cephalic fever and then one displaying typhoid symptoms or actual "typhus gravior." Patients experiencing delirium and rash were dosed with calomel until the gums were sore and blue, and they were bled, purged, and bathed.[23] A well-established precaution was a "low diet," that is, thin gruel, barley water, and sometimes beef broth, but abstention from meat until convalescent. Fresh air and ventilation were highly efficacious; patients could make substantial progress after just one night in a well-ventilated ward. Prichard admitted having visited patients in foul "confined hovels" who thereby perished.[24]

Prichard did not pretend to understand the true cause of fever; rather he predicted it would eventually be discovered by the "laborious collation of recorded facts and authorities." He was on a quest for knowledge as opposed to some "polemical mania or a zeal for defending paradoxical opinions."

In other words, he was pointing a finger at those who disputed the theory of contagion just to make a name for themselves as an expert in the field. Such doubters could only be suffering from prejudice, as the contagious nature of fever was a matter of observed fact. He provided several examples of this, such as his demonstration that all seventy cases at St. Peter's were attributable to contagion by contact or communication. Further, the admission of a succession of infected vagrants had resulted in a pattern of fever among members of staff, including himself, and a patient who carried the body of a fever victim soon succumbed. Meanwhile, inmates in other wards had remained unscathed. Elsewhere in Bristol, one particular lodging house furnished several victims. If the alternative traditional theory of marsh miasma were valid, the high, dry, and airy elevated Redcliff-Hill district would have been free from contagion, but the opposite was true; a servant there had been seized with fever after having slept in a bed previously occupied by fever sufferer. Once the bedding had been boiled, no further illness occurred. He went on to give several more examples of contagion among his affluent patients to underscore his views.[25]

Prichard felt there was some distinction between contagion (person to person) and infection (some phenomenon to person); he marshaled evidence for this from the incidence of fever at Bristol Infirmary. At St. Peter's Hospital the disease spread from person to person in the cramped, ill-ventilated wards, unlike in the light, lofty, and airy wards of the Infirmary. In the most opulent and well-ventilated homes of Prichard's private patients' fever spread among its occupants, but stopped when measures were taken to segregate the sick from the well.[26] Whether fever *originated* in matter or from lifestyle was debatable. Other diseases such as erysipelas and hospital gangrene had been proven to spread from one individual to another, but just a few diseases spreading this way did not prove that all did so. On the other side of the argument, there were many cases where exposure to extreme weather or fatigue had resulted in fever. Although some deemed these merely auxiliary or contributing factors, until there was actual traceable physical matter to show otherwise as in the case of gangrene, Prichard could not accept that fever had a *strictly* physical cause. He called for further research into it, but until then, the jury was out: "I am persuaded that we must conclude fever to be a disease frequently excited by [conditions], but perhaps requiring other conditions not yet ascertained, and generating in the body affected some peculiar matter capable of exciting a similar distemper in a healthy person."[27] Prichard the contagionist also felt that there might be a predisposition to disease. While it should be possible eventually to ascertain the "peculiar matter" that caused fever, until that time, environmental conditions, the "miasma" of ancient medical theory, provided some evidence, along with the geographical distribution and seasonal variations in fevers. Perhaps it was a combination of environmental conditions and physical matter.[28] Prichard hedged his bets. It would be nearly half a century before the germ theory of disease was confirmed.

Having outlined the fever situation in Bristol, Prichard attempted to convince the authorities of the necessity of epidemic prevention. In a barbed Adam Smithian warning, he predicted Bristol would be greatly relieved of the burden of its aged, infirm, pauper, lunatic, and orphan population if public health measures were not taken. But, assuming there was a will to preserve the lives of all human beings, he allowed that the Infirmary might be reorganized to accommodate Bristol's poor fever patients. He also demanded that a board of health be instituted as a medical police force empowered to remove the sick to isolation wards and ensure the purification of infected dwellings.[29] At the outbreak of cholera at St. Peter's over a decade later, the Bristol Board of Health was formed, with Prichard one of its members.[30]

A History of the Epidemic Fever established Prichard's reputation as an experienced physician, an authority on fever treatment, a campaigner for public health, and an advocate of medical progress through the application of scientific methods of research. His was just one of many books, articles, and dissertations published during this period of epidemics. He must have been gratified by its reviews in the medical press, even if they were not entirely laudatory. The *London Medical Repository* reviewer was skeptical of Prichard's inflammatory theory of fever and the notion that fever could be caused by some "intangible, invisible something around and about us." The *Medical Intelligencer* pointed to some inconsistencies in Prichard's doctrine and considered it a confirmation of Armstrong's theory and practice, while the *London Medical and Physical Journal*'s critical analysis valued the book's contribution to a growing body of clear and precise evidence, though Prichard's view of contagion was merely Thomas Sydenham's "pestilential constitution of the atmosphere." Another reviewer called Prichard learned, judicious, and a talented observer, though some of his theories and facts did not bear scrutiny and his views were derivative of Henry Clutterbuck.[31] This would not be the last time he faced an epidemic.

The Age of Improvement in Bristol

Prichard was frustrated by provincial Bristolians' failure to "improve" in ways he thought needed, the issue of public health being a case in point.

Life in the city nevertheless had its merits, and there were glimmers of progress. Post–Napoleonic War economic dysfunction continued to make life difficult for its poorest citizens, but there were some compensating distractions. When not gripped by election fever, the "lower orders" of Bristol enjoyed entertainments, such as the procession of a decorated bull through the streets on the way to bull-baiting on the Downs. In 1816 there was wider civic ecstasy in the brief appearance of the heroic Duke of Wellington at the head of a lavish procession through a triumphal arch erected over Park Street.[32] There were substantial improvements in transport, too, when John Loudon McAdam was put in charge of the Bristol turnpike roads; his new system of roadbuilding dubbed "macadamization" hugely improved transport efficiency and safety. By 1821 the *Regulator* stagecoach could accomplish the journey from Bristol to London in only sixteen hours. Maritime transport was also making strides; a steam packet service to Cork started in 1821 and to Dublin and Newport the following year.[33]

The June 1818 general election unsettled Bristolians. Reformers were in a difficult position; even though the prosperous and influential Dissenters among them wanted reform granting full civil rights to themselves, they tended to side with conservative Bristolians and the two incumbent MPs in their generally rabid anti-Catholic emancipation stance. After just five days of the usual ribbons, favors, threats, and assaults, the sheriffs cleverly closed the polls prematurely, depriving many country voters from plumping and ensuring victory for Bristol's two anti-reformist MPs.[34]

The hardships and reformist unrest among the city's poor and artisans was tackled by an Act of Parliament intended to bolster their spiritual well-being. Public funds were allocated to the construction of churches in populous districts, but Bristol chose a site conveniently near fashionable Clifton on which to erect neoclassical St. George's. The blessings of the Established Church continued limited in Bristol's slums, where local justices and the Guardians of the Poor ordered whipping for loitering, flogging for being rogues and vagabonds, and the stocks for drunkenness.[35]

When the Bristol elite was not busy managing the parliamentary elections to their satisfaction or vigorously punishing the poor for vagabondage, they could enjoy more personal nest-feathering activities. A prime example involves Samuel "Devil" Worrall, the town clerk and harshest of magistrates, who was forced to resign in July 1819 upon being made bankrupt. He had been a partner in the Tolzey Bank, which had too lavishly printed its own bank notes, precipitating a run on the city's eleven private banks and a period of financial uncertainty. For this contribution to Bristol's economy,

Worrall's Corporation friends rewarded him with an annual pension of a very handsome £400.[36] Meanwhile, there were stirrings of social and political reform in Bristol as in the rest of the nation, accompanied by some beneficial technological innovations sweeping the country, promising a better world. The Prichards were living in an Age of Improvement.

An Universal History, in Twenty-Four Books (1818)

When not treating his typhus patients, gathering contagion statistics and campaigning for a fever hospital, Prichard was tackling a gap in his knowledge. Without access to innovations in linguistic methodology being developed in Germany, he could hardly make a serious start on studying the Celtic languages. He owned a German grammar and dictionary, and his German lessons had been helpful, but he needed a goal. Swiss historian Johannes von Müller's multivolume world history had been recently commended in the *Edinburgh Review*. Prichard set himself the challenge of translating Müller, aided by his study-mate William Tothill. *An Universal History, in Twenty-Four Books* was published in three volumes in 1818 on a profit-sharing basis, eventually earning Prichard £50, 1 shilling, and 9 pence. It went on to have a long life as a popular history book in America, pirated in Boston in several editions between 1831 and 1847, but as there was no international copyright agreement at that time, he did not benefit.[37]

Prichard's *Universal History* went beyond mere translation. He added an extensive preface and peppered its more than 1,300 pages with many explanatory notes and comments. While he praised Müller's impartial handling of the history of religion and comprehension of nations and historical eras, he naturally criticized the German's failure to endorse divine revelation unequivocally, attributing this laxness to a love of being novel. Prichard's translation was positively and widely reviewed in Britain, gaining gratifying comments such as "the translation is executed in a masterly style"; otherwise, it was a "not strictly close, but very good" translation.[38] Throughout the nineteenth century the English-speaking world appreciated *An Universal History*; purveyors of German thinking such as Thomas Carlyle particularly admired it. With his new facility in German, Prichard could now exploit a broader range of authors in his research on anthropology, linguistics and psychology. Yet in 1847 he offered to correspond with a scientist in French or Latin because "although I read German continually, I cannot easily write in that language."[39]

Prichard was becoming one of Bristol's undoubted assets, a popular consulting physician, scientist, public figure, and scholar. An American

Quaker educator visiting Bristol in July 1818 found the city's glory days past, but he valued meeting Prichard:

> This city contains a polished and truly respectable society, in which are several persons of considerable eminence in science and learning. Dr. Pritchard, respecting whose talents and research I had formed a favourable opinion from the perusal of his work on the "Physical History of Man," did not by any means lessen in my estimation from personal acquaintance. His mind is at once excursive and discriminating, and if his genius and industry shall be aided by time and health, he bids fair to become, not only an ornament to the medical profession, but to the literary ranks of his country.[40]

Three hundred gentlemen attended the funeral and interment at Bristol Cathedral of another celebrity Bristolian, Royal Academician Edward Bird, on November 9, 1819. This friend and supporter of Prichard in his bid for the Infirmary post was a genre and then history painter, one of the founders of the Bristol School, whose work had recently gained favor in London and among the Royal Family. Prichard and his friend John King, apparently his medical attendants during Bird's long illness, rode in the principle mourning coach.[41]

Faith and *An Analysis of the Egyptian Mythology* (1819)

Religion continued to inform Prichard's personal and professional life. Between 1814 and 1820 he borrowed scores of religious commentaries from the Bristol Library. As his scientific opinions evolved, his 1818 notes on Müller offer a glimpse of his attitude toward the important issue of religious orthodoxy. He was discomforted to the point of annoyance at the historian's "deviation" from unreservedly endorsing divine revelation. Müller

> admits that the Hebrew Scriptures contain the history of a people destined by Providence to preserve and transmit to posterity the true religion or the revealed declaration of his will, and shows that the course of human events was so controlled and guided by a peculiar ordination, as to promote this end by concurring circumstances through a long succession of ages. The events which completed this chain of singular dispensations are allowed by the author to have been altogether out of the usual course. It seems, therefore, strange to find him so anxious to represent the circumstances which led to this miraculous consummation as natural occurrences described under

a veil of allegory; to regard the prophecies which point in every age at the predestined conclusion as so many efforts of human intellect; or to call in the aid of some mysterious and unheard-of powers of the spiritual world, rather than coincide with an explanation which demands no other cause than what has been already conceded to exist. In order to preclude every attempt of this kind, we need only remark, that the sacred writers refer to miracles as the evidences that they were invested with supernatural powers. Either these persons therefore were impostors, or the facts they recorded were out of the usual course of nature, or in other words miraculous.[42]

Prichard could not countenance religion being the product of the human mind, nor just some allegorical account of natural phenomena. Miracles, phenomena "out of the usual course of nature," occurred. His father warned him that "the Bible is a book of principles which are not to be disputed, they are to be received as the voice of Revelation & the man who refuses so to receive them has nothing in common with me." He took the leaders of Prichard's cherished Established Church to task, for instance, in his anonymous article in the *Christian Observer* critical of the bishop of St. David's. Thomas Prichard pulled no punches, accusing the bishop and more than half the established clergy of being swallowed up by the corruption of secularity as they fixed their eyes "upon the golden fleece instead of the souls of their flock, they pant after promotion, treading down in the pursuit all the graces of the New testament Christianity." When not discussing illnesses, Prichard and his father were carefully combing through their faith in revealed religion.[43]

Amid his reading on epidemics, history, philology, and theology, Prichard had time to study many travelogues and the classical historians' descriptions of Egypt, the Middle East, and India. Having previously put forward his view on the affinity of the Egyptians and Indians, he returned to this topic in October 1816 upon reading the linguist Alexander Murray's edition of Sir James Bruce's *Travels to Discover the Source of the Nile* (3rd ed., 1813). Murray's appendix claimed "that the Egyptian religion is the produce of the country, peculiar to itself, and without any marks of foreign improvement or innovation." This not only flatly contradicted Bruce but implied the uniqueness of Egyptian people and their culture, thus calling into question the notion of the single origin and species of humankind and "the Sacred Records, the earliest memorials of mankind." Asserting the uniqueness of the Egyptians was also "at variance with the general observations that result from a survey of the organized world, and the distribution of species over the globe."[44] Prichard's analogically based, diffusionist argument about the spread of plants and other animals extrapolated to that of early humans was under attack. Nations could not be unique; he would continue his research into links between the Egyptians and Indians that would refute Murray and defend Holy Scripture.

Egyptian civilization and its undeciphered script had huge romantic appeal. The mysterious Egyptian treasures looted during the Napoleonic Wars had sparked the European imagination. Young Prichard's aforementioned study of the Zodiac of Dendera is a case in point. While Britons indulged in general Egyptomania, Prichard set his sights on the thorny issue of Egyptian culture being evidently older than what the Bible allowed for human history. How could this be reconciled? In *Physical History* he had expended considerable effort on proving the common origin of the Indians and Egyptians, comparing their governments, mythologies, theologies, and physical characteristics. Now his *An Analysis of the Egyptian Mythology: To Which Is Subjoined, a Critical Examination of the Remains of Egyptian Chronology* (November 1819) addressed these points in more depth. With five black-and-white plates and one in color, it sold for a costly £1 and 7 shillings in boards, royal octavo. He apparently wrote the ten-page promotional abstract of it in the *Classical Journal*. *Egyptian Mythology*'s comparative material from beyond India and Egypt signaled Prichard's intention to continue his anthropological research.

The 445-page tome is no page-turner; the American educator John Griscom predicted correctly: "Dr. Pritchard's book has gratified me very much. Like his other productions it evinces elaborate research, penetration and discrimination, and will do more for his reputation the more it becomes known. It is questionable, however, whether, in this novel-reading age, his merits will be appreciated in any proportion to their extent. While Scott and Byron are 'lords of the ascendant,' such recondite works as those of Dr. P. must be confined to the choice few who seek for instruction as well as amusement."[45]

Prichard hoped *Egyptian Mythology* would further his monogenetic agenda, reveal the monotheistic foundation of Egyptian religion and bring biblical and Egyptian chronologies into line. It begins with a careful summary and review of Paul Ernst Jablonski's *Pantheon Aegyptiorum* (1750).[46] This otherwise praiseworthy author had "been led into some errors, the result of his fondness for refined and erudite explanations, and for eliciting from every popular superstition a dignified and philosophical meaning." Vague, fanciful theorizing was unacceptable to Prichard whether the subject was fever or Egyptian mythology. The holy records and classical literature were factual, while the tittle-tattle of superstitious people was untrustworthy. And to underline his orthodoxy lest readers misconstrue his interest in "heathen superstitions," he avowed that while his goal was to establish historical facts, he wished to show the world how fortunate it was that "Divine Providence has been pleased to deliver us from the atrocious barbarism and unmitigated depravity, in which our pagan ancestors were involved." *Egyptian Mythology*'s ethnological content explores the influences upon and the relationship between India and Egypt and attempts to find kernels of Christian doctrine in their beliefs. This book may be considered a pioneering form of what is now called cross-cultural research.[47]

Prichard adopted the structure and some of the resources of his illustrious predecessor Jablonski. Drawing on the classical authors, he compared Hindu and other mythologies with that of Egypt, and he considered German scholars' theory that myths were attempts to explain natural phenomena. After a section on Egyptian fables, he went on to explore their cosmogony, notions respecting the soul, morality, and some of their colorful religious customs. He compared Egyptian rites with the ordinances of Moses and extrapolated that all primitive peoples had originally shared a pure but primitive form of monotheistic revealed religion that had subsequently become debased. This important point he would return to in future editions of *Physical History* to further his ultimate goal: proof of the unity of the human species based on the universality of religious and moral doctrines. First, leaving no stone unturned, Prichard thoroughly explored the civil institutions of Egypt, India, and the Israelites.[48]

Egyptian Mythology's section on Egyptian chronology, a crucial issue in Prichard's opinion, appears something of a digression. He thought he had discovered the source of the discordance between the biblical account of the creation of the earth, calculated to be 4004 BCE, and Egyptian chronology's indication that human life had existed at an earlier time. This project appealed to his desire to create order, and correlating the biblical and Egyptian chronologies would shore up the integrity of the former. His analysis of fragmentary Egyptian records led him to conclude that scholars had double-counted the length of some of the Egyptian reigns; the records of the Memphite and Diopolitan kings had been misconstrued as referring to two separate and successive reigns. Once that discrepancy was corrected, the Old Testament and Egyptian chronology were in accord.[49]

The reviews of Prichard's book were mixed, to put it politely. The strident *Antijacobin Review, and Protestant Advocate* (its name tells it all) decisively dismissed all but classical and Christian European culture. It cuttingly proclaimed Prichard to be "a man of patient discrimination and sound judgement" in making abstruse inquiries into what was hardly worth knowing; the book was "a waste of the talents Dr. Prichard so evidently possessed." Mythography was going out of fashion in Britain, anyway; myths were increasingly seen as merely the unhistorical product of the imagination. The influential *British Critic* agreed that the learned author had thrown away his time on an unprofitable subject. Worse still, there was a suspicion that men who engaged in arranging the mystical nonsense of all religions into a single origin had surreptitious materialist motives. But far from finding Prichard guilty of religious skepticism, he was judged perfectly orthodox in his Christian professions. His adjustment of Egyptian chronology was particularly successful and indicative of indefatigable industry. The *Monthly Review* considered Prichard's inquiries abstruse, seemingly uninviting, "occasionally too verbose for the intelligible enunciation and simple development of its propositions" and too conjectural, although it did delve deeply into the important task of authenticating the biblical account of the single origin and distribution of the human species. The reviewer was pleased Prichard had been mindful of his duty to prove the truth of Scripture and the universality of belief in a single deity and a future state.[50]

Not everyone questioned the relevance of *Egyptian Mythology*. Prichard's loyal friend Conybeare thought it "a model of judicious, sober, and philosophical criticism, applied to subjects where we are accustomed to meet only with extravagant conjectures, and still more extravagant etymologies."[51] But if Prichard had expected *Egyptian Mythology* to be appreciated abroad, he must have been disappointed. German scholar of Greek mythology Karl Otfried Müller deemed Prichard somewhat overconfident in basing his views on weak sources, and he lacked understanding in his attempt to find analogies between Greek and Egyptian gods. He thought Prichard's book was based on confused principles, contained blunders and lacked objectivity. To top it off, Prichard had allowed his religious views to compromise his methodology. His only saving grace seems to have been his appreciation of German biblical scholarship. Another reviewer claimed Prichard had wandered from one authority to another without sufficient reason. At least the *North American Review* considered Prichard ingenious in devising a corrected Egyptian chronology.[52]

Egyptian Mythology was unfortunate in predating the watershed in Egyptology brought about by Jean-François Champollion and rival Thomas Young's decipherment of hieroglyphics. German scholars' disdain did not dampen the young Danish linguist Rasmus Rask's interest in Prichard's work on Egyptian chronology; his *Den gamle Ægyptiske tidsregning* (Ancient Egyptian Chronology, 1827) attempts to correct Prichard's errors and inconsistencies. The 1837 German translation of Prichard's book, with a preface by the illustrious August Wilhelm von Schlegel, praises the intelligence and learned industry of the author who had to write in a pre-hieroglyphic era; he kindly omits noting that this had rendered the book somewhat obsolete. With curious modesty, Prichard wrote to thank Schlegel for sending him a copy of this German edition. Perhaps in competition with German scholarship, another English edition came out the following year, now with Schlegel's preface translated into English.[53]

Prichard hoped *Egyptian Mythology* would support his argument for the unity of humankind and universal primeval, pure theism, defend biblical chronology, and shed light on an era closer to Creation. But it was most remembered, cited, quoted, and praised by authors throughout the century for its innovative methodology and contribution to the development of Egyptology, earning Prichard citations in dictionaries and histories of the field.[54]

Bristol Life and Private Life in the Early Twenties

Following national mourning upon the death of George III in January 1820, there were lavish celebrations of George IV's accession. The Corporation processed around Bristol in splendor, distributing wine and porter to its loyal citizens. Later that year the lower orders of Bristol ecstatically celebrated the failure of the unpopular new king's attempt to divorce Queen Caroline, while their betters kept their homes in darkness in sympathy with the frustrated monarch. In the ensuing general election Tory Davis, having undergone heavy losses as a result of scandalous speculation, nevertheless agreed to stand against the Whig Henry Bright of the Bristol banking family and Radical J. E. Baillie. The Radicals found Davis an easy target in his support of the repressive "Gagging Acts" of 1817 and 1819, which empowered the government to do just that to newspapers and public meetings. Baillie withdrew early from the poll. Bright astutely and noncommittally declared himself friendly to parliamentary reform, while in a bid for Bristolian votes both candidates declared themselves opposed to Catholic emancipation. Victorious Bright had the most opulent "chairing" that Bristol had ever witnessed.

The following summer, the members of the Corporation had their own procession, a banquet with thirty-five toasts, some glees, and a ball, the last said to have cost the ratepayers nearly £700.[55] Throughout the 1820s Bristol politicians continued impervious to criticism. In keeping their snouts firmly in the trough, they were hardly exceptional, although perhaps less subtle than elsewhere in Britain in their nepotism, lavish salaries, self-aggrandizing ceremonies, and reluctance to invest in public works. The "Old Corruption" endemic throughout the upper levels of eighteenth-century British society lingered on.[56]

Another privileged profession was the clergy. Preferment, the appointment to a position in the Established Church, appeared unconnected with either merit or a sense of vocation. These often highly lucrative benefices "in the gift of" individual landowners and organizations such as the Bristol Corporation and Oxbridge colleges were more often bestowed for social reasons. The second sons of the aristocracy and the sons of the rich, professional, or socially skilled could accumulate multiple "livings" in a practice called pluralism. The young Rev. F. W. Blomberg, a royal ward and the spitting image of the Royal Family, held ten such lucrative livings simultaneously, one of which was prebendary of Bristol Cathedral. His successor, Lord Somerset, possessor of four livings in the gift of his noble family, managed to deliver a total of two sermons in twenty-three years. The majority of churches in the nearby county of Somersetshire had "nonresident" clergy. Apathy and slothfulness did not diminish among self-serving clergymen promoted to a bishopric; several bishops of Bristol resided comfortably elsewhere.[57] In this Age of Improvement, however, discontent over squandered taxes and nonresident, neglectful Establishment clergy grew, spurring on both evangelicalism and reformism. While Prichard attributed his ancestors' dissent from Anglicanism to its former lamentable corruption, his father continued to remind him that the evils of Anglican secularism were unabated.

Those who did not benefit from the system began criticizing it more openly. Criticisms by the articulate trickled down to the poor, who in their poverty and distress expressed their discontent by turning to radicalism. Young apprentices and laborers, the traditional volunteers of Tory and Whig violent election gangs, were in the vanguard. Even the "middling sort's" evangelicalism and reformism spiced with the boldness of radicalism kept Bristol in the 1820s in turmoil. The next decade would bring the Bristol riots, national legislation for local government reform, and other reforms like the Pluralities Act of 1838, which limited clergymen from holding multiple livings.

Births and deaths in the Prichard family were frequent; their son Augustin was born on July 16, 1818, and Constantine on April 5, 1820, while brother

Edward's family seemed doomed. News was received of relative Samuel Prichard meeting his death while struggling on the prairies of Illinois, and in the spring of 1820 Prichard became the executor and beneficiary of eccentric cousin Joseph Cowles, who had died in the lap of Bath luxury.[58]

After naming their first three children after themselves and Prichard's sister and mother, Prichard and Anna chose significant names for their remaining offspring. Augustin acknowledged their respect for the first archbishop of Canterbury and Christianizer of England, while the first Christian Roman emperor Constantine the Great was a respected reformer and builder of churches. Prichard read William of Malmesbury's history of the first Anglo-Saxon king's half sister Edith of Wilton, a Wiltshire nun famous for her sacrifices, learning, beauty, and saintliness. Francis might have been named after the early seventeenth-century statesman and philosopher Francis Bacon, the father of the empirical approach to science and advocate of inductive reasoning, the avoidance of misleading oneself, and the careful observation to comprehend the truths of nature, tenets Prichard and his contemporaries held dear. Admittedly, they may have had the baby's rich great-uncle Francis Fisher in mind. Arminius, or Hermann, the defender of the Germanic tribes against the Romans in the Teutoburg Forest and a popular symbol of German nationalist, anti-Napoleon sentiment, provided a heroic middle name for baby Albert Hermann. The seventh-century scholarly archbishop of Canterbury Theodore of Tarsus was remembered as a great church reformer and political peacemaker. Finally, Illtudus Thomas combined Prichard's father and grandfather's name with a sixth-century hero of Welsh history. Saint Illtud was a defender against enemies and founder of monasteries and what is thought to be the first center of learning in Britain. He was also connected with a village near the Estlin summer home. The Prichards invested their offspring with the qualities they greatly admired.

While the Prichard children were generally thriving, eight of the eleven Bristol adolescents and adults sentenced to death at the April 1820 Bristol Assizes had been found guilty of theft. Some were reprieved, but there were still some executions for Bristolians to relish.[59] The city was transfixed by the 1821 trial, hanging, and dissection of the hapless teenager John Horwood. Prichard's colorful Bristol Infirmary colleague Dick Smith combined his passion for publicity and the macabre to serve as ringmaster of these events.

It was not Smith's first encounter with the country lad's case. On January 26, having been spurned by Eliza Balsum, Horwood petulantly threw a stone at her from a great distance. Unfortunately, it struck her on the head, creating a wound that her family's bread and ointment dressing would not heal. After some days in the Infirmary without improvement, Smith trepanned her skull to reveal an abscess under the sawn-out disk of bone; the wound soon proved fatal. Smith even managed to testify at Horwood's trial, but little reference was made to the surgery as contributing to the death. His reward was a rather festive pre-execution breakfast with the sheriff, after which the condemned lad was exhibited to an exclusive gathering of pious citizens who prayed and shed fervent tears for his soul. At the new jail's scaffold, so great was the volume of spectators that special measures had to be taken to prevent them from falling into the river in their excitement. Even the executioner bolted and had to be fetched back to his duty, while Dick Smith suddenly decided not to watch. After Horwood prayed a bit more, he dropped his handkerchief, the signal for launching him into eternity. The onlookers skirmished to take advantage of the curative powers of touching the dead man's hands. Although the Kingswood colliers waited for an opportunity to rescue Horwood's body from the surgeons' scalpel, the following day Smith had it stashed in a coach and driven to the Infirmary, receipt attached.[60] According to statute, executed murderers were fit for dissection.

Smith was in his element, conducting dissections of Horwood on four successive days to audiences of about eighty lucky citizens. After thus demonstrating the infinite wisdom of the Almighty, he suspended Horwood's skeleton, complete with cap and hanging rope, in the Infirmary Museum, accompanied by a cast of his head and memorabilia. An avid collector of documents and ephemera, Smith had Horwood's skin tanned to form the gold-tooled cover of a large scrapbook, which until the 1970s was cheerfully displayed in the Infirmary's Board Room. The Horwood case had been a boon to Bristol culture, stimulating the production of newspaper articles, broadsheets, doggerels, and sermons. Throughout the spring of 1821, Smith was in his element, his fellow Bristolians were variously entertained or outraged, and young Horwood was not in his grave.[61]

The Prichards deserted College Green that same year to the quieter, more elegant residence of 12 Berkeley Square. They were grateful for the safe delivery of Theodore Joseph on June 27, 1821, but death and serious illness marked 1822. Thomas Prichard described Edward's son's death on March 23: "His decease has been occasioned by a complaint very similar to that of your little Francis—extensive inflammation of the viscera, high fever & determination to the head. The dilation of the pupil of the eye was very great. The progress of the disease was however much more rapid."[62]

After Prichard himself suffered a near-fatal illness in 1822, he convalesced in the bracing air of St. David's and provided his father with the opportunity to advise: "It has long been an impression on my mind, that thy health has not suffered so much by the duties of thy profession as by midnight studies too assiduously pursued. If these were relaxed, for a while even totally given up, I am persuaded that the exertions that thou art called upon to use in the daily routine of business would rather help than injure thy strength." Once restored to health, Prichard had the strength to counter his father's strictures on the Established Church and its ordained clergy. And whatever was Prichard suggesting about the dreaded Church of Rome? Thomas Prichard claimed the last word: "I do not think we shall gain any valuable point by fighting battles in the field of theology. We differ and must agree to differ.—Were thy argument respecting Apostolic Ordination admitted, we must consider the Reformation as an act of rebellion against the ordinances of God, and if we allow two true churches of Christ, we may as well allow two hundred."[63]

Of course, Prichard bore his father's observations respectfully, but begged to differ and got on with his career. In his medical charity work he was thought dedicated and diligent, and in publishing *Physical History* he was considered learned, but as for enhancing his standing as an innovative physician, his descriptive *History of the Epidemic Fever* had made no breakthroughs—fever was a tough nut to crack. An advertisement bound in this 1820 volume indicates that he had already struck out on a new path; Prichard would establish his credentials as an expert on neuropsychiatric conditions based on much more challenging research and his professional experience. He had had early encounters with the insane, and the captive lunatics and epileptics at St. Peter's had furnished him with almost a decade of case histories. Prichard's new medical textbook was advertised on November 16, 1822, as lately published, *A Treatise on Diseases of the Nervous System*, octavo, 12 shillings.[64] Its subtitle, *Part the First: Comprising Convulsive and Maniacal Affections*, signaled his intention to publish a second volume on chorea, hysteria and comatose conditions. He soon abandoned volume 2, turning from the as-yet-unnamed discipline of neurology to the as-yet-unnamed one of psychiatry. Those "midnight studies too assiduously pursued" were also devoted to researching the unity of the human species; he was working on a second edition of *Physical History*.

As Prichard studied, however, he longed for opportunities to engage in discussion with like-minded men. Although he might have considered philistinism his city's predominant quality, Bristol was not without literary and scientific figures; the *Bristol Memorialist*, a little periodical published between 1816 and 1823, produced bibliographies of "living authors, natives of Bristol, or residing in that city and its vicinity." There was James Rawlins Johnson's succinct *Treatise on the Medicinal Leech*, Prichard's father-in-law's many pamphlets in defense of Unitarianism, and Prichard's own impressive list.[65] No wonder he was described as always reading.

Not all work, no play, Prichard was a keen but sober host and a person worth inviting to dine, serve on committees, and chair meetings. Dining with friends at home or in public was a favorite middle-class pastime. There were clubs just for dining and drinking, or there might be a token activity such as discussion, debate, or meeting to get out of the way before the eating, drinking, and singing of glees commenced. Charities, societies, and associations advertised their supporters' status and beliefs while providing opportunities to socialize; they all had annual dinners. These usually started out moderately enough, but later in the evening, after the more sedate participants had retired, the banter and singing would start, accompanied by many sacrifices to Bacchus. The Infirmary's annual divine service and special sermon at St. James Church was swiftly followed by a long session at The Nag's Head; even the Library Society had an annual dinner. Making toasts was a must; the 1839 Dolphin dinner boasted seventeen formal and nine informal toasts, each preceded by a speech and followed by a glee. At the meeting of the Provincial Medical and Surgical Association in 1840, after Dr. Prichard had "left the Chair," Dick Smith led the carousing until midnight. Prichard did not join his medical colleagues at the frequent public breakfasts that ended with champagne and dancing or at the various dances and balls, such as the Annual Clifton Fancy Dress Ball, which went on merrily until dawn.[66] The prodigious quantity of alcohol consumed was proudly recorded in the press.

Prichard and some of his more sedate medical colleagues found the regular meetings of the discussion clubs and reading societies more congenial. One was the not very soberly entitled, long-established Bear's Cub Club. Prichard's fellow "bears" were the Clifton surgeon John King, the Rev. John Eden, and some schoolmasters, educated tradesmen, and businessmen. In the eighteenth century its discussion topics had been lighthearted, such as Dr. Wallis's "Which are the most grateful to the human mind, the pleasures of hope or the pleasures of memory?" The club gradually sobered both its name and the tone of its discussions; by 1824 it had become the Bears' Debating Club, where the topics for discussion were seriously scientific and literary. It continued to exist into the 1830s, apparently becoming a foster parent of the Philosophical and Literary Society of the Bristol Institution, an almost private society of about a dozen men.[67]

Bristol's thriving glee clubs, drinking clubs, a True Blue and a Jacobite club were not as attractive to Prichard as the city's medical societies and the medical and religious charities. He enjoyed dining at friends' homes or inviting guests to dine at his. Far from being alcohol-fueled, an evening at the Prichards was remembered as intellectually stimulating. Invitations, usually for 5:00 or 5:30, were to a meal of several courses lasting for hours. If there was no lecture to go to afterward, there might be music or the display of some "curiosities." Later, tea would be taken in the drawing room, and supper followed at about nine o'clock. At other times, he would send a written invitation to just tea at 8:00. When the Prichards moved to the Red Lodge, entertaining took place on a more lavish scale. A sought-after host and guest, by the end of the 1820s Prichard had become a "lion," as such men were called, albeit a rather tame one.

Looking back on the twenties, Prichard could reflect that he had consolidated his position as a leading Bristolian, produced medical publications such as *Epidemic Fever*, and campaigned for public health. He perfected his German by translating *An Universal History*, and in his *Egyptian Mythology* he redoubled his efforts to fathom the history of humankind in preparation for an expanded edition of *Physical History*. Volunteering at medical charities allowed him to conduct research for *A Treatise on Diseases of the Nervous System*. Dr. Prichard could be more often seen riding in his carriage around Bristol or on his way to distant patients. The Prichards welcomed new babies into the world and buried some of them.

Over the following few years Prichard's homelife and his professional and intellectual goals would continue to evolve. He could remember the evenings at Edinburgh's Royal Medical Society and dream of a scholar's life in quiet Oxford libraries or at London's learned societies. But if he could not be there, he would recreate Bristol versions of them. He would devote his indefatigable energy to shaping Bristol to his liking, helping to establish several institutions and associations designed to promote education, science, medicine, and charity—contributions to the Age of Improvement.

8 · Nervous Diseases

Neurology and Psychiatry, 1822–47

> [I am] not without suspicion that there is something in the state of civilization which tends to promote the existence of that congenital state of bodily structure on which predisposition to mental disease depends.
> —James Cowles Prichard, *Treatise on Insanity*

Back in the late summer of 1811, Prichard bought some notebooks and was keen to start filling them. The appointment to the post of physician to St. Peter's Hospital was just what he needed. His voluntary work at Bristol's workhouse and pauper lunatic asylum would help him build a public profile, gain clinical experience, and fulfill his father's desire that he should benefit society. It would also be a valuable opportunity to collect his captive patients' case histories, not only on their communicable diseases such as typhus but on neuropsychiatric conditions and mental states. The scientific approach to studying medicine lay before him.

Long before starting at St. Peter's Prichard had witnessed the challenges of insanity, including the misery of depression among his friends and close family, his mother included. As a medical student he had seen for himself the effective and humane treatment of the insane when he visited the Quaker asylum in York. The Scottish Enlightenment "science of man" and Prichard's own commitment to Christian doctrine informed his understanding of the human mind. At university, his professor of moral philosophy Dugald Stewart described forms of insanity, and his medical training furnished him with a system of therapeutics he could use to treat its abnormal states, but clinical experience had not been provided.[1] Through his service to St. Peter's and other charity medical institutions and his later private practice, government appointments, and publications, he contributed to the development of the fields of neurology and psychiatry.

Knowledge of the nervous system was considered foundational to comprehending the body and mind. In an era before much medical specialization, Prichard studied French, English, and eventually German textbooks and periodicals covering the subject where he found nosologies (classifications and descriptions) of neurological and neuropsychiatric conditions and disorders of the mind. These resources also offered some advice on care and treatment. The British lagged behind their European counterparts in psychiatric theorizing; they tended to publish more practical books on therapeutics and asylum management. The most respected British writer on the etiology and therapeutics of insanity and the humane management of its suffers was Dr. Thomas Arnold, a Leicestershire public asylum physician. Closer to home, Bristolian Dr. Beddoes's *Hygeia* included a section on psychology and nervous diseases.[2] As for Dr. Prichard's immediate concerns, overcrowded St. Peter's warehoused insane and disabled inmates hardly got care, never mind cure.

The liberal-minded citizens who considered it their duty to push for reforms in this Age of Improvement, whether it be the extension of civil rights, prison reform, the antislavery cause, or the welfare of the poor, had their attention drawn to the plight of the insane by a cause célèbre. An 1815–16 House of Commons Select Committee Report revealed shocking cases of neglect and abuse in workhouses and the few public and private asylums. Who should be responsible for mad people? The state reluctantly assumed the duty of establishing institutions to house the increasing number of people with psychological and neuropsychiatric disorders who were either too dangerous or unable to be at large or whose families could not care for them. The planning, administration, and inspection of these asylums fostered the development of the psychiatric profession.

At the top of the social scale during the opening decades of the nineteenth century, the British monarch George III's final period of derangement gave impetus to the study of insanity. As for the other strata of society, the aristocracy and the wealthy might find themselves the subject of an ancient legal procedure called a commission in lunacy, at which a family member would petition for a finding of insanity in order to gain control over the person's finances and care. These sensational de lunatico inquirendo cases relied on the testimony of family and other witnesses, but also that of some new experts dubbed "mad-doctors." Members of the middle classes, like the Prichards' friends the Crosses, might care for their insane at home, calling on the services of a medical practitioner known for his ability in such cases. Otherwise, the well-off insane could be lodged discreetly at the country home of a medical man. As for the poor, if they could not be left to roam at large, then it was the workhouse or prison for them.

It was a growing industry. Concentrating solely on insanity, some mad-doctors established private asylums that might lucratively house the fee-paying insane as well as local authority-funded patients. These medical gentlemen were fit to associate with wealthy private patients, local government officials, and the legal profession. Bristol's Edward Long Fox and son are cases in point. Mad-doctors also found their way into a not very receptive justice system to testify in cases involving criminal responsibility. One of these was Prichard's friend Dr. Alexander Morison, who apparently was the first to give a course of lectures on insanity in 1823, another contribution to the professionalization of psychiatry. The care of the insane thus gradually passed from clergymen and the family to a new branch of the medical profession, aided by societal factors, the founding of institutions, and the development of psychiatric theory. It was a respectable profession for a physician like Prichard.[3]

Psychiatry's Foundations

In Western medicine the notion of insanity as a derangement of the nervous system can be traced to the Hippocratic medical literature of the fourth century BCE, when the idea that insanity originated in the brain established medicine's hegemony over it. Galen's first-century psychiatric therapeutics were still recognizable in Prichard's day. In the early Christian era, the writing of Saint Augustine showed psychological introspection. During the Middle Ages, when insanity was generally thought the result of diabolical possession, the prevalence of the occult and the witchcraft craze afforded opportunities for clerical and civic engagement in psychological and psychic phenomena. The seventeenth-century philosopher Descartes postulated the distinction between body and mind; the theologically compatible nonphysical mind is invested with consciousness, rationality, and immortality. This notion of dualism, or the interaction of the physical body and immaterial mind, and the quasi-psychological topic of hypochondriasis were explored by Prichard. Eighteenth-century rationalists defined insanity as the experience of delusions leading to erroneous reasoning. Importantly, it became viewed as an illness that might be managed and cured.

The study of the mind and soul known as psychology developed in relation to anthropology, a subject that had been of philosophical concern on the Continent for more than two centuries. In France, where there was early medical specialization, there was a school of thought with a well-developed psychophysiological element confusingly denominated *anthropologie* that would inform future French psychiatric theory.[4] Psychotherapy was a university subject in Germany by 1811. French and German doctors with experience of asylum management also began developing theories and nosologies of insanity, gaining adherents to their varying approaches and reinforcing the notion that insanity was an illness requiring medical expertise. The medical model of insanity did retain one component redolent of the past: the pastoral care and consolation of the insane traditionally provided by the Church became the purview of a system of psychiatric care called moral treatment.[5]

The first mental hospital was established in Damascus in 800, while Britain's Bedlam dates from about 1403. The government of Florence legislated on insanity in 1774, and in the 1790s French physician Philippe Pinel worked in public custodial institutions to reform the care of the insane. Spurred by general reformist zeal, the British government's attempts to address the ills of a growing and increasingly restless population coincided with the professionalizing efforts of alienists. The 1828 County Asylums Act aimed to strengthen earlier legislation and establish and better regulate county asylums. This would eventually lead to the construction of large, imposing, and segregating asylums. A further benefit to the nascent psychiatric profession was the law's requirement that asylums employ medical officers to care for and keep records on their patients. But their official reports to central government were incomplete and haphazard, as there was no recognized list of conditions and symptoms for asylum medical officers to use.[6] Prichard set to work on this lacuna.

Mad-Doctoring: Theory and Culture

With the insane paupers of St. Peter's Hospital at his disposal and the benefit of recent European research on the nervous system and its diseases, Prichard planned a two-volume textbook on the etiology, symptoms, and treatment of conditions of the nervous system and mind. Soon after the publication of the first volume in 1822, he obtained the county government post of visiting physician to Gloucestershire private madhouses, cementing his professional commitment to mental health. He embarked on a career in a new medical subdiscipline and would contribute to its nosology, theory, and professionalization.

Always wary of theorizing, Prichard made much of applying Baconian observationism: theories should be derived from evidence. He never tired of criticizing those who he thought neglected this essential approach to science proper, and he attempted to apply it to every scientific subject he tackled. But instead of taking the physicalist approach of conducting research into the human mind through dissection of the brain, Prichard engaged in what might now be considered meta-analysis. He analyzed others' work on cerebral morbid anatomy, for instance, and solicited asylum statistics widely. To these he added the weight of his own large collection of case histories. Prichard was among a generation of researchers, the harbingers of evidence-based medicine, but not free from the prevailing views of his era.

Prichard appreciated German and French alienists' theories, with some exceptions. In Germany, where the asylum medical profession was already well developed, there were some fascinating and conflicting views on the mind and its ailments. He found unappealing the claims of the German atheist and materialist neuroanatomist Franz Gall, founder of the science of phrenology, who held that mental phenomena were localizable in the brain. Also suspect were the ideas of Franz Anton Mesmer, proponent of wonderous "animal magnetism," later called mesmerism, ancestral to hypnotism.[7]

Mesmerism and phrenology, that new science of the mind, lacked scientific rigor, in Prichard's opinion. Phrenological theory also implied a materialistic conception of the mind, a seismic notion in early nineteenth-century Christian culture. Could all life, including the mind itself, be reduced to a physical entity? The question had wider social and political implications, at the core of which was materialism's denial of a God-granted "immaterial" or spiritual element of the mind and soul. This assault on scriptural authority threatened to lead to the breakdown of civil society as the selfishness of the masses would prevail and revolution ensue. The British Establishment duly cracked down on anyone daring to express materialist beliefs, considering them revolutionary notions in themselves. Materialists were the enemies of "Church, King and Country," as Prichard's friend William Lawrence discovered in 1819. Being known as a materialist risked social and professional condemnation for one and one's family. Prichard had no reason to pay lip service to religion; his belief in the immaterial nature of the mind and soul made him a thorough dualist. His study of the mind unified his psychological and anthropological research.

Prichard grappled with some hotly debated issues of the era concerning where the mind/soul is located, how it functions, its relationship with the physical brain, and, more specifically, the locus of insanity. In opposition to a materialist conception of the mind, dualism, the belief in the existence of a physical body invested with a separate immaterial (nonphysical) mind, accommodated religious tenet, and was thus acceptable to the Establishment. Prichard prevaricated, revising his opinions over time. He was acutely aware of the brain's role in madness somehow but wary of those who claimed this at the expense of involvement of an immaterial element he believed was a reality in itself. He countered claims that insanity arises solely in the brain and attempted to keep the condition, if not out of the mind, as least out of the immaterial soul by maintaining the traditional view that some forms of it originate in the viscera. As to why insanity seemed to be on the rise and much more prevalent in civilized societies, he suspected the ills of civilization. Society might be advancing technologically, but selfishness and deterioration in piety and social order were taking their toll on the human mind. And as for psychiatric therapeutics, there was an array of medical, social, and psychological approaches to explore.

Prichard lighted on the medical subdiscipline of mental health where he could carve out a reputation in a fiercely competitive profession. It offered greater scope for him to collect and analyze data, derive theories, and devise classifications than his work on fevers, where progress had stalled. Prichard began to focus on understanding the human mind, its diseases, and their origins, and he experimented with various methods of treatment. He joined new professional organizations and published his research, acquiring both international recognition and considerable opposition to some of his views. Prichard's contributions to what would become neurology and psychiatry can be traced through his several medico-neuropsychiatric, psychiatric, and medical jurisprudential books and articles and their reception and impact. His work was at the core of nineteenth-century British psychiatry and, with Benjamin Rush's textbook of 1812,[8] dominated American psychiatry. It stimulated generations of psychiatrists, influenced government policy and even found its way into Victorian literature. As his father had hoped, Prichard benefited society in identifying and naming certain neuropsychiatric and psychiatric conditions; introducing Continental theories of medical psychology into Britain; refining and expanding psychiatric nosology; establishing some consideration of the insane under law; and being involved in asylum regulation, reform, and inspection.

A Treatise on Diseases of the Nervous System (1822)

Prichard's *A Treatise on Diseases of the Nervous System* tackles the relationship between the nervous system and the mind and begins to formulate a nosology of insanity and various neuropsychiatric conditions such as epilepsy and dementia. Most notable for introducing to the English-speaking world the French medical psychology of Pinel, Jean-Étienne Esquirol, and the French nosographers, it systematically describes the etiology and symptoms of neuropsychiatric and psychological disorders and suggests effective treatments, supported by detailed case histories.[9]

Importantly, the book maintains that madness is not a primary disease but symptomatic of other latent disease, particularly of the vital organs. By adopting the novel mode of classifying the various types of insanity according to their primary or causal site, such as the brain or abdominal viscera, their etiology and therapeutics become apparent. This naturally led Prichard to suggest that treatment should be aimed at the primary disease rather than its manifestations. To this arrangement he added observations on the effects of noxious agents on the brain.[10] Prichard also noted that physicians' failure to discover remedies for convulsive and maniacal diseases had led them to consider them incurable; rather, he more optimistically asserted that cases in which symptoms spontaneously disappear provide clues to their cure. Tracing the course of these spontaneous cures and ascertaining any constitutional changes in the patient would lead to the successful choice of therapy.

Rather incongruously, *Diseases of the Nervous System* starts with a disquisition on some of the deeper interests that would permeate Prichard's later psychological, physiological, and anthropological work. In exploring the nature of the brain and nervous system, he distinguished the natural and vital functions (physical), from all the animal (mental) functions that arise from the existence of a nervous system. He recognized that the nervous system is the organ of the mind, as mental processes and affect cannot occur when the brain is incapacitated. He provided a physiological survey of what was known of the functions of the nervous system and its connection to intellectual faculties such as memory, sensation, imagination, reasoning, passions (emotions), and volition. The location of these qualities in any specific part of the brain was yet to be discovered, contrary to phrenologists' claims.

Prichard held to previous generations' philosophy of physiology that suggested the existence of two general "faculties" of the brain. While some mental functions, such as perception, memory, and dreaming, necessarily arise from events in the real world, emotions and moral and rational judgment, by contrast, do not have physical causes. This latter group, aspects of the soul or mind, cannot reside physically in parts of the brain because this denies the immateriality of the soul, an unacceptable, religiously unorthodox view. Prichard's version of what is known as faculty psychology is that the mind is divided into separate functions, but without any specific physical locations in the brain.[11] Unlike the brain and body, the "soul, spirit, mind" is immaterial. "According to this, all the phaenomena of which we are conscious, such as sensation, thought, volition, passion, appetite, &c. are to be termed affections, not of the nervous system, but of the soul, which is acted upon through the instrumentality of that system; the possession of which principle must, therefore, according to the notions of the Platonic school, be regarded as co-extensive with the endowment of animal life, and not limited, as Christian philosophers have generally thought it incumbent upon them to limit it, to the human species."[12]

Human beings cannot be reduced to mere physical bodies. As the mind is not *physically* in the brain, there must be an as-yet-undiscovered link between the physical nervous system and the nonphysical mind: "every series of [mental] operations begins with the body, and ends with the body, though the more remote links are withdrawn from this intimate connexion with the organized instruments." The mind accounts for all properties accessible through consciousness, but because there is entire ignorance of the essential properties of the mind itself, "there must ever continue to be a wide chasm in the chain of our observations respecting the theory of the mental operations."[13] Prichard thought that the body somehow aids and cooperates with the mind/soul to create trains of mental actions, a view that opened the door to the idea that mental disorder arises in the temperament, which has its humoralist seat in other parts of the body. His model of the constitutional and somatic origin of mental disorders diverted attention from the idea of a diseased immaterial mind. Insanity is a natural phenomenon.

Diseases of the Nervous System digresses into claiming the universality of the human mind, a topic that he would develop in his anthropology in support of human specific unity. Drawing on his view of the essence of religious beliefs explored in *Egyptian Mythology* (1819), he suggested that superstition is not mere fancy but the manifestation of conscience. The propensity to consider the future with gloom and fear is natural to the human mind because of a universal feeling of "demerit" or "delinquency." People naturally hold themselves accountable to "certain unseen powers, before whose tribunal they may, and probably will, be arraigned." Prichard pointed out that Christian doctrine is able to "tranquilize the evil forebodings of the mind."[14] This discussion of universal religious belief prefaces his observations on the causes and treatment of religious mania. He pointed out the greater incidence of insanity among the congregations of "fire and brimstone" preachers than among those who receive the reassuring absolution provided by the "Romish" Church. Notwithstanding this implying a social cause of insanity, sufferers' symptoms must be traced to their bodily origin in order to ascertain the correct course of treatment.[15]

Prichard introduced yet another related topic. An extended note outlines physiological processes and concludes they are reducible to chemical and mechanical actions, making it unnecessary to claim any kind of peculiar agency otherwise termed the "vital principle," a theory about which he would later publish. That a process has not yet been explained was no excuse for speculating that some special mechanism for it had to exist. In a second long note he underlined his concept of the soul, calling on what he had learned from Dugald Stewart and dismissing the materialist conjectures of Joseph Priestly. Prichard concluded that the nervous system provides the instrumentality through which a separate sentient principal comes into relationship with the body. As higher animals also have a nervous system and feelings, he stated what he acknowledged might seem a quaint and singular notion: "If all animals feel, all animals have souls."[16]

Prichard noted some affinities among diseases such as apoplexy, palsy, and epilepsy in that they can transition into each other. Some were traceable to a source in another part of the body, though the comprehension of this process was still in its infancy, while other nervous diseases were idiopathic, arising from no ascertainable lesion but from strong emotions such as terror or grief. Yet others were inflammatory in nature. Before moving on to his survey of diseases of the nervous system, Prichard stressed that further progress on this topic would be made by dissecting the dead, closely observing the living, and studying accurate case histories.[17]

Prichard called upon both ancient and contemporary authorities in forming his definition and description of epilepsy. His chapter on it lists the stages of an epileptic attack, beginning with an acute observation of the initial "aura" stage, then peripheral convulsive tremors progressing toward the head, and then general paroxysms and their variations.[18]

The next portion of *Diseases of the Nervous System* established Prichard's reputation as an expert in psychological medicine, if initially only as its nosologist. He explained that madness cannot be defined variously as having erroneous judgment or reasoning, derangement of emotions, impairment of sensation or perception, being a matter of degree of eccentricity, or even the philosopher John Locke's idea of correct reasoning from false premises. Instead, there are two states of the mind: active realistic thinking and imaginative reverie; a person's inability to distinguish between these two states characterizes insanity. Reflection and imagination occur in the brain, but a morbid state of that organ accounts for any confusion between those two aspects of thinking. Some organic fault could cause miscommunication between the physical brain and the immaterial mind as well. He admitted this hypothesis would have to await the scientific discovery of the physical operations of the brain.[19]

The business of classifying the types of insanity was as complex as defining it. Prichard first and importantly dealt with Philippe Pinel's *manie sans délire*, "mania without delirium." The French alienist believed this form of insanity was characterized by the propensity to paroxysms of violent rage in people who otherwise display no evidence of intellectual impairment. Prichard, however, rejected Pinel's claim that such people can actually be in full possession of their intellectual faculties; rather, in his experience, some insane people adeptly hid their delusions, especially under repeated questioning. It was likely that people who ordinarily behaved perfectly sanely might fall into a hallucination only at the precipitation of their insane act, though it might have been nothing more than a vague and undefined impression of grievance. Some latent "morbid bias of the understanding, some hallucination, more or less strongly marked" that accounts for the insane behavior might always be discovered.[20] Prichard would reformulate his view of *manie sans délire*, publishing his influential concept of "moral insanity" in 1833.

Was insanity necessarily a cerebral condition? Dissection of the brains of the insane had not revealed any distinctive evidence of morbidity other than the vascular fullness which is commonly found in those who have succumbed to apoplexy, epilepsy, nervous fevers, or convulsions.[21] This was a satisfactory state of affairs in Prichard's opinion. Had it been shown to be merely a brain disease, the mind/soul would have been reduced to a physical function of the brain—that dangerously materialist view again. Rather, madness resides in the nervous system and is caused by some disease of the body or even of the brain itself, but not directly by the brain. Essentially, there is a malfunction in communication between the brain and the mind. The soul/mind operates through the intermediary of the brain; only the brain can be diseased, not the immaterial mind. Understanding exactly how the brain interacts with the nonphysical mind was beyond the scope of scientific inquiry, Prichard concluded.

A major cause of insanity is "determination of blood." Prichard's several examples include disorders in "uterine function"; menstruation, pregnancy, childbirth and breastfeeding all offered opportunities for physiological derangement leading to psychiatric symptoms. His chapter 5 finishes with fifteen case histories of "uterine epilepsy" and its treatment. In the absence of the curative properties of marriage, he advised depletive medical treatment.[22] Prichard then turned to the "translation of morbid action from other structures to the brain"—metastasis. The disordered state of the intestinal canal can lead to epilepsy and mania, and diseases of every organ through the mechanism of "sympathy" seemed to be able to affect the nervous system adversely in some unknown way.[23] Other causes of these two conditions are brain trauma or disease, alcohol abuse, and some medicines such as mercury, as well as the better-known causes, namely mental overexertion, sudden fright, emotions, and pessimism. Should a condition prove chronic, Prichard recommended his usual "heroic" physical intervention, such as the insertion of setons, issues, and drains, painfully invasive procedures designed to set up counterirritating suppuration.[24]

The final chapters tackle local convulsions, "partial epilepsy," convulsive tremor, and somnambulism or "ecstasis." For instance, partial epilepsy, somehow linked to epilepsy, is a condition involving sudden dimness of sight and stupor, later termed *petit mal* by Esquirol. Prichard described somnambulism, again stressing the importance of tracing symptoms to their sources. Having planned a second volume of *Diseases of the Nervous System*, he provided no concluding remarks.[25]

Case histories and treatment regimens are plentiful in *Diseases of the Nervous System*, as is a lot of theorizing. But there is one recently devised treatment Prichard particularly stressed; "moral treatment," the behavioral training of asylum inmates had replaced the barbarities of the past. "The cruel methods which have been adopted in some establishments, to the disgrace of our nation, must have owed their origin to carelessness and indifference, rather than to any mistaken ideas; since it is impossible that any medical practitioner could be so stupid as to suppose that any beneficial effect could result from inflicting corporal severities in the cure of a disease of the brain. At least, if such things have been, the time for their existence has passed."[26]

One of the earliest and unfortunately reprinted reviews of *Diseases of the Nervous System* appeared in the January 1822 number of the *Quarterly Journal of Foreign and British Medicine and Surgery*. The author began by taking Prichard to task for muddling his interest in the history of man and Egyptian mythology and his flights of philosophical fancy with what busy practitioners wanted and needed—practical facts. Worse still, the book contained too much useless lumber, being illustrated with mere commonplaces, larded with deceptive jargon, and bristling with errors. Nevertheless, once the practical portion of the work was untangled, one could find detailed, accurate, and valuable case histories and sound practice. Further uncomfortable reading came from the pen of Andrew Combe, then building his reputation as a physician and champion of phrenology, whose thoroughly condemnatory review piled on the negative adjectives. Countering Prichard's assertion that there is no *proof* of the reasoning faculties being an organic process, Combe claimed that the Phrenological Society's writings, casts of heads, and all living heads were "undeniable proofs" in themselves; his science even provided the key to crime prevention.[27] The phrenological community would keep Prichard firmly in their sights.

Other reviews were more positive. The *London Medical Repository* thought it "an excellent work. It evinces an accurate observation of the phenomena of the diseases which it embraces, and a sound pathology, giving rise to an active and judicious method of cure." The reviewer most appreciated what the previous one had dismissed; he regretted the lamentable progress hitherto made in understanding "the mysterious union of mind with matter." He approved of Prichard's organ-of-origin nosology of insanity, predicting it would enhance understanding and lead to more rational therapeutics, and he valued Prichard's definition of madness as the inability to distinguish imagination from attentive reflection. The *London Medical and Physical Journal* was impressed by Prichard's novel nosology of nervous diseases, while the *Medico-Chirurgical Review* considered his fine reputation based on his two previous publications a guarantee that *Diseases of the Nervous System* would command the attention of all thinking medical men for being both practical and full of "ingenious physiological and even metaphysical reasoning and enquiry." Prichard's antimaterialist, antiphrenological stance was praised, and although it presented hardly anything new, the book was the best in the English language by a writer of accurate observation, unwearied attention, and profound thought. Long extracts, summaries, and reviews in American and German medical journals indicate a similarly positive reception of Prichard's ideas.[28] So it was not all bad press.

Diseases of the Nervous System was frequently cited and extensively paraphrased in subsequent textbooks. For instance, George Gregory's standard *Elements and Theory of the Practice of Physic*, published in five editions between 1825 and 1846 in Britain and America, contained chapters on epilepsy, mania, chorea, palsy and apoplexy, for which he acknowledged Prichard "from whose valuable work I have derived great assistance." He was also referred to in John Mason Good's *The Study of Medicine* (1825) and in a textbook by Thomas J. Graham. Robert Hooper's popular general medical reference book of the time, *Lexicon Medicum* (1839), contains extensive material from all three of Prichard's books on the subject; Hooper acknowledged its section "Insanity" as a summary of Prichard. German author Moritz Romberg considered him "a most careful observer," while he was cited as a "high authority" in Edward Henry Sieveking's *On Epilepsy* (1858) and in several publications in the 1860s.[29]

A Treatise on Diseases of the Nervous System is considered an early and comprehensive British nosology of neuropsychiatric conditions. It provided the first in-depth descriptions of the premonitory indications of epileptic seizure, improving on the mere "aura" of classical medicine. It also contains the first mention of the post-epileptic muscle condition now called Todd's paresis and the dangerous, rapid succession of fits known as status epilepticus. Prichard acutely described what he termed "epileptic delirium" as possibly occurring without fits and "epileptic somnambulism," a kind of ecstatic state later termed "psychic equivalences." He established "partial epilepsy" in the literature, devoting a whole chapter to these localized convulsions later called petit mal.[30]

Diseases of the Nervous System marked a transitional point in Prichard's career. By 1822 he had gained clinical experience, gathered and carefully analyzed data, outlined and arranged what was already known on the subject, and formulated some views in preparation for making a greater impact on the understanding and treatment of sufferers from mental conditions. He would go on to concentrate on psychological medicine, continue at St. Peter's, make medical inspections of Gloucestershire private asylums, and refine his concept of moral insanity.

Toward Psychology and Psychiatry, 1824–33

The January 1824 issue of the *London Medical Repository* contains Prichard's "Remarks on the Treatment of Paralysis, and Some Other Diseases, by Issues and Blisters," a description of his two-stage method of treating paralysis. After vigorous antiphlogistic (anti-inflammatory) measures were taken to the utmost limits of safety, "as much as [the patient] could bear," "issues" were applied (wounds were made) to establish long-running suppurating "drains" (continually emitting pus) along the spinal column. In cases of severe paralysis, nothing was as effective as internal stimulation with generous doses of oil of turpentine. His advocacy of heroic treatment and attention to pathology attracted wide attention, with abstracts appearing in British and foreign periodicals.[31]

Bristol Infirmary's House Apothecary William Swayne's assiduous dissection of fatal cases of chorea (St. Vitus' dance/Huntington's disease) inspired Prichard to repeat his call for the systematic practice of "morbid anatomy."

This important shift from dissecting for the purpose of understanding anatomy to dissecting to determine the cause of death was a watershed in scientific medicine: the transition from the traditional, more holistic conception of the causes of disease to an approach that traced disease to tissue level. Prichard could only look forward to it, but in the meantime, there was little choice but to continue with the antiphlogistic therapeutics as described in his next publication.

Events spurred Prichard to continue publishing on insanity. Around 1829 some notorious court cases about the illegal confinement of the insane destroyed the reputation of Britain's preeminent mad-doctor George Man Burrows and by association impugned the respectability of the young psychiatric profession in general. In this period of intense political reformism, campaigners voiced concern for the civil liberties of the insane. The following year a chapter in a book by iconic mad-doctor John Conolly laid out the criteria for diagnosing insanity that evidently disturbed Prichard. Liberal Dr. Conolly was on the side of patients, assuming that they needed to be protected from wrongful diagnosis. He also felt that doctors should prioritize the liberty of patients over family interests, so diagnosis should be based on examination of the patient without reference to the opinions of family members, whom he instinctively distrusted. This did not endear Conolly to many mad-doctors, whose fees depended on their satisfying lunatics' families. Conservative Dr. Prichard had the welfare of both the patient and family at heart; a patient's deviation from family values was enough to tip indications of eccentricity into symptoms of what he would term moral insanity. He was concerned for the preservation of family wealth from a member's profligacy, a central motive of those commissions in lunacy, at which he was a profession-enhancing expert witness. In July 1833 he testified at one of these de lunatico inquirendos on the earl of Kingston, quoting five German experts on the gradations of imbecility.[32] As for unfair deprivation of liberty (and life), Prichard was clearly on the side of defendants at risk of execution for crimes for which they were not responsible on the grounds of insanity.

In an era of encyclopedias, Prichard was recruited by his friend Dr. Tweedie, who with Sir John Forbes and John Conolly was bringing out the *Cyclopaedia of Practical Medicine*. Prichard's six articles, "Delirium," "Hypochondriasis," "Insanity," "Soundness and Unsoundness of Mind," "Somnambulism and Mesmerism," and "Temperament," appeared in volumes published during the early 1830s. The *Cyclopaedia* was reprinted under a new title in 1840 and in revised and several reprinted American editions from 1845 onward.[33] Prichard's articles in it reinforced his reputation as an authority on psychological medicine around the English-speaking world.

Prichard's *Cyclopaedia* articles outline the general topic, make new observations, suggest treatments, recount case histories, and cite relevant experts. As it turned out, they generated enough related material for him to recycle into a full-length textbook on insanity. He confined his first article "Delirium" to the causes, symptoms, stages, and treatment of a fever-induced state in which the sufferer cannot function, is temporarily unaware, and yet recovers when the cause is removed. While sympathetic delirium, Prichard wrote, was caused by a lesion elsewhere than in the brain and should not be treated with antiphlogistics, idiopathic delirium indicated disease of the brain or its meninges and should be tackled with measures such as topical bleeding, blistering, counterirritation, and cold applications. The article is enriched with anecdotal accounts of cases such as one in which the delirious patient speaks a long-forgotten language or undergoes a permanent change in ability.[34]

"Temperament" explores the ancient humoral doctrine of the four basic constitutions or personalities: sanguine, choleric, melancholic, and phlegmatic. One's constitution and personality were considered determined by a corresponding superabundance of one of the humors: blood, yellow bile, black bile, or phlegm. For example, a constitution dominated by blood results in a sanguine temperament, characterized by red or fair hair and complexion and thin skin. At the same time Prichard deemed this theory fanciful, he suggested there might be some correlation between temperament and medico-psychological conditions; for instance, the views that a choleric person is prone to being disputatious while melancholics are timid he considered to have some merit. Whole nations had characteristic temperaments. Prichard concluded that temperament is an attractive but vague and speculative concept. That did not inhibit John Conolly from citing the temperaments as predisposing factors in his lectures on insanity published in *The Lancet* in 1846.

"Temperament" also allowed Prichard to reconsider evidence of the structure and function of the brain and its relationship to the mind. He accepted Samuel Thomas von Sömmerring's demonstration that the seat of reasoning and perception is in the brain, where the moral (emotional/affective) and active (physical) powers originate. He also discussed the fascinating phenomenon of instinctive behavior and its unknown location in the body. The topic of brain anatomy brought him on to Franz Joseph Gall's praiseworthy scientific research on every aspect of *intellect* originating in a different part of the brain. Gall, however, in the course of researching the material nature of the operations of the mind had devised organology, or phrenology. This was Prichard's cue to renew his attack on that science: locating aspects of *personality and behavior* in different areas of the brain is alarmingly biologically deterministic and a denial of free will; its materialist subtext was dangerous and some of its advocates unworthy of respect. As for phrenology's lamentable lack of scientific rigor, he referred to his personal examination of Esquirol's extensive collection of crania of the insane and that eminent alienist's confirmation that there is no correlation between skull shape and mental endowment.[35] Phrenology haunted Prichard's psychiatry as it did his anthropology. He never stopped attacking it.

In seventeen dense pages "Soundness and Unsoundness of Mind" explores the nature of madness and the issue of the insane in society. Prichard summarized several German and French alienists' views on the three basic types of insanity. He admitted that unsoundness of mind could arise from disorders or defects in the structure or function of the brain, making the scientific study of insanity imperative. Prichard introduced the term "irresistible impulse" for actions without motive or delusion, the principal component of what would become his concept "moral insanity." And here, in his obvious concern for the insane in wider society, are the seeds of his 1842 book on jurisprudence.[36]

Like phrenology, animal magnetism was a popular topic of the time. This late eighteenth-century creation of German physician Anton Mesmer was initially a medical therapy, but over time, Mesmer and his licensed practitioners broadened it into a complex ceremony involving magnets in which patients were "magnetized," with results varying from convulsions to artificial somnambulism. It was an early form of hypnotism. "Somnambulism and Animal Magnetism" admits that these related phenomena were not yet understood. The state of ecstasis or cataleptic somnambulism consisted of selective perception and rapid changes in the state of the mind, but with perception achieved in the usual manner. Sleepwalking was a modified type of dreaming symptomatic of disease.

"The supporters of animal magnetism carry back its history, as do the historians of free-masonry, to a period of high antiquity," Prichard jibed. Nor was he the only detractor of this new form of therapeutics: Mesmer had merely revived the "visionary" (Prichard's favorite term for unsubstantiated) ancients' claims that some subtle, imperceptible fluid pervades all life. Prichard linked the topics of animal magnetism and sleepwalking because mesmerists had been claiming to be able to produce a range of effects from strange feelings to profound sleep. They could conduct "vital fluid" in the brain around the body via the nerves to sites of healing, a "bold speculation" (again, for "bold," read unsubstantiated), in Prichard's opinion, as he reprised his recent book on vitalism. He concluded it was unnecessary to resort to the unfounded theory of magnetic fluid when the effects of magnetism could easily be attributed to the imagination. Prichard had tried the services of a mesmerist on one of his epileptic patients, to no effect. Rather than dismiss it, however, he thought it should be further investigated, given evidence that magnetism was an imagination-induced anesthetic. What he thought was left of animal magnetism after discounting its tendency to charlatanism approaches the later practice of hypnotism. The *Cyclopaedia* article outraged mesmerists. Eventually, like phrenology, itinerant mesmerizers and entertainers eroded mesmerism's reputation, and when its principal proponents died out, so did its popularity as medical therapy.[37]

When Prichard sent a copy of his article "Hypochondriasis" to his father, back came the reply: "I was amused by some parts of thy paper on hypochondriasis, & I could not help fancying that I found in it something like a sketch of myself."[38] This was not exactly Thomas Prichard admitting his illnesses were imaginary. Hypochondriasis, long considered a real disease with a recognized array of symptoms, was then in the process of migration into the realm of medical psychology. Its supposed locus gave it its name: *hypo* meaning "under"; *chondros* meaning "cartilage"; together the unpleasant feeling at the top of the abdomen under the rib cage. In an age when the boundary between bodily and mental illness was blurred, hypochondriasis was thought not merely psychological in nature but a serious condition causing spiritual and physical pain of physical or psychological origin. The condition was also known as the English malady. Eighteenth-century physicians had found that the higher up the social scale the patient, the greater its prevalence; in effect, having it was something of a status symbol.[39] Hypochondriasis was further elaborated into hysteria, the feminine version of the disease. Belief in its "nervous" origin gradually gained ground in popularity, spawning a plethora of new terms until later in the nineteenth-century "neurasthenia" replaced "hypochondriasis," completing its transformation into a nervous condition and eventually to purely psychological "neurosis."[40]

Prichard defined hypochondriasis and described its causes, symptoms and location in the nervous system and then suggested some treatments. He thought hypochondriacs suffered from perverted or unnatural feelings or affections that they dwelled on, discussing them at length until they were at risk of becoming depressed and suicidal. Diagnosis was particularly challenging as patients typically presented with a multiplicity of confusing symptoms. They tended to have a lifestyle requiring little bodily but great mental exertion, anxieties and disappointments; this *morbus literatorum* was a disease of literary men. The brain could be instrumental in the disease without being its original site; causes could act upon the mind and nervous system without affecting the brain. In other words, hypochondriasis originated in the brain and nervous system. After citing the case history of a gentleman (his father, perhaps), Prichard moved on to treatment. The first impediment to management was that the patient was likely to have already read every medical treatise on the subject and tried every suggested remedy to no avail (his father, again). The best treatment was therefore nutritional and lifestyle management rather than medication. If, however, the digestive system seemed affected, an antiphlogistic approach was necessary.[41] By basing hypochondriasis in the mind through the brain and nervous system, Prichard fostered its eventual transition from a somatic to psychological condition.

One of Prichard's earlier articles for the *Cyclopaedia* would significantly affect his career and reputation. "Insanity" was published in volume 2 in 1833. A reviewer wrote that "it proves the author to be a humane, learned and judicious physician."[42] Most importantly, Prichard revised his previous doubt of the existence of insanity without delirium by clearly defining moral insanity as a condition characterized by a perversion of the natural feelings, affections, "without any notable lesion of the intellect." He claimed that no single English, French, or German publication had brought together up-to-date views on insanity and that there was confusion and inadequate consideration of it in respect to the law.[43] The whole subject would fill a book, so drawing on his *Cyclopaedia* articles, especially "Insanity," he started writing what would become one of the nineteenth century's most important textbooks on psychopathology.

A Treatise on Insanity and Other Disorders Affecting the Mind (1835) and Moral Insanity

A medical man could reach the height of his profession by claiming expertise in one aspect of medicine or surgery and publishing a textbook on it. Prichard set about doing this. He researched his chosen topic extensively, gaining advice and encouragement from Alexander Tweedie. He also visited Philippe Pinel's Asylum de Bicêtre in Paris and received Esquirol's "personal kindness" at Ivry. Both French alienists influenced him. Pinel stressed the use of observational statistics and considered the "passions" (emotions) instrumental in insanity; he pioneered "moral treatment" in asylums, where he treated patients as morally (behaviorally) managed individuals. Concerning the physical origin of insanity, Pinel believed mental derangement begins in the stomach and affects the head, whereas Prichard maintained that aside from emotional and social causes, mania is the result of inflammatory disease. Dr. Esquirol is considered the first complete psychiatrist based on his contributions to psychiatric theory, asylum management, and psychiatric education. He combined sociopsychological observations with a theory of the organic origin of insanity and published a classic textbook noted for its clarity and use of statistics. Prichard followed Esquirol in his nosology of medical psychology.[44] The most influential British author on insanity well into the second half of the nineteenth century, Prichard was one of the last great alienists to publish before the biomedical revolution. He was interested in late eighteenth-century consideration of cerebral pathology, and he followed Thomas Arnold in reporting cases of dissections. Prichard welcomed the prospect of physiological and structural research shedding the light of science on medical psychology.[45]

In 1834 Prichard asked Samuel Tuke of The Retreat, York, for descriptions of any patients with intact understanding but with a "perverted state of feelings, temper, inclinations, habits, and conduct. Such individuals are sometimes unusually excited and boisterous; at others dejected (without any hallucinations), sometimes misanthropic or morose."[46] He was gathering case histories of patients suffering from emotional disturbances and mood swings to support his theory of moral insanity. He trebled the length of his *Cyclopaedia* material on insanity, adding a good deal of asylum statistics, many case histories, material from his article "Somnambulism and Mesmerism," new chapters on jurisprudence and mental impairment, plus his usual attack on phrenology. His textbook on insanity and its treatment was published in 1835.

Prichard hoped that *A Treatise on Insanity* would lead to improvement in the treatment of the insane. It presented his theory of a nonphysical mind and called for the early diagnosis, medical treatment, minimal confinement, and better management of the insane; their protection from unjust punishment under the law; and the abolition of capital punishment. This compact, well-documented, and closely argued volume relies heavily on French nosology and theory and entertains the latest German ideas on the subject. It especially explores whether insanity originates in the brain or the mind, and concludes that civilization somehow causes insanity. In favoring Pinel's "sympathetic" concept, which traces mental disturbance to visceral disorder requiring antiphlogistic response, he could insist that insanity requires medical treatment.[47]

Prichard described insanity as a chronic disease manifested by deviations from the healthy and natural state of the mind, such deviations consisting either of intellectual insanity or moral insanity. He first outlined monomania, "partial insanity," in which the patient is unable to think correctly about a particular issue, whether in optimistic or pessimistic terms, and is otherwise intellectually unimpaired. Mania, or raving madness, consists of derangement of understanding unlimited in its scope and duration. The patient constantly raves most vehemently, sometimes focusing on a particular general subject such as religion, and at other times expressing a hurried jumble of ideas. Mania has various manifestations and stages, ending in mental decay. In fact, monomania, mania, and mental decay can blend into each other.[48]

Prichard thought one condition deserved special attention. He reconsidered Pinel's *manie sans délire* with its limited application, further researched the work of French and German psychiatrists, and was inspired by his friend Thomas Hancock's recent book on instinct. These led him to enlarge and refine his concept of moral insanity, dropping the symptom of mood swings he had previously asked Tuke about. Prichard believed everyone possessed a basic God-given sense of correct behavior from birth, but it could be affected by adverse circumstances, feelings such as the hopes and apprehensions for the future, and aspects of civilization itself. His concept of moral insanity became central to his reputation in the field.

Prichard's definition of moral insanity, quoted by generations of psychiatrists and historians, is "a morbid perversion of the natural feelings, affections, inclinations, temper, habits, moral dispositions, and natural impulses, without any remarkable disorder or defect of the intellect or knowing and reasoning faculties, and particularly without any insane illusion or hallucination." This type of insanity arises in a person's habits or feelings rather than in the intellect; "behavioral," "affective," or "emotional" are more modern synonyms for Prichard's "moral," while "moral causes" indicates "social factors." Prichard suggested "pathomania" might better define the condition. While not entirely free from implied moral judgment, he did try to confine moral insanity to emotional abnormality, choosing illustrative case studies of patients possessing socially "wrong" feelings and behavior rather than immorality. He pointed out that the morally insane demonstrated a decay in "social affections" that could only be diagnosed by those who know the patient well. This type of insanity could vary in severity from mild eccentricity to behavior requiring confinement for the protection of society. Crucially, it was not necessarily manifested in violent fits of anger as Pinel had maintained. Sufferers were unable to resist the power of an emotion either because they failed to understand right from wrong or they were overwhelmed by the passion itself. The morally insane might exhibit alternating excitement and melancholy and dejection (depression); they might have a passion for drunkenness and debauchery or a propensity to create mischief, steal, and engage in habits such as "erotomania." In fact, "morally insane" seemed a bit of a catchall term. There was generally little hope of recovery. In modern jargon, moral insanity comprises both affective and volitional insanities that accommodate states such as bipolarism with no psychotic features.[49]

Prichard's goals in gaining acceptance of this subtle type of insanity were to secure appropriate treatment of the morally insane, protect families and society from harm, and prevent miscarriages of justice. He was against capital punishment, and particularly keen to prevent executions of the morally insane. The courts, however, did not accept a class of insanity among defendants who manifested no delusions or disturbance of the intellect and who could reason and justify their actions. Prichard kept up his efforts to convince jurists, eventually publishing a separate volume on the jurisprudence of insanity and mental capability. In formulating the concept of moral insanity, Prichard effectively shifted the notion of madness from cognition to the moral faculties. The term became a commonly used and often disputed diagnosis, especially on the Continent, where French and German alienists otherwise thought their British counterparts had contributed little to the science of mental illness beyond the practice of "non-restraint."

Prichard then described two deteriorating mental states, incoherence or dementia and the general paralysis of the insane. The first is characterized by rapid, unconnected, and evanescent emotions, ideas, extravagances, forgetfulness, lack of judgment, unawareness, and perpetual activity. The mind is incapable of continued attention and reflection and at length loses the faculty of distinct perception or apprehension. He admitted that dementia's status as a type of insanity was a matter of dispute, but as it is generally caused by disease, it was madness irrespective of cause.

Prichard produced a table of causes of dementia divided into physical and moral, and he outlined its four stages from forgetfulness to loss of instinct and volition. In his description of its fourth stage, it is clear that he found the task of examining such patients emotionally draining. Concerning this condition in the elderly, he coined the term "senile dementia" and is credited with being the first to have thoroughly described it.[50] His second degenerative and distressing condition is the "general paralysis of the insane," whose course differed in duration and was remarkably more prevalent among males. It would be decades before this condition would be understood as the final stage of syphilis. It too was greatly distressing to observe, and dissection reveals alterations in the brain of its sufferers.[51]

Prichard wrote: "Insanity is not to be reckoned among the diseases which are very dangerous to life." He noted that while the insane often suffer from diseases and disordered bodily functions, these were not necessarily the cause of their condition. It seemed more accurate to qualify recovery as being from the manifestations of insanity rather than insanity itself. If the brain was diseased, and especially if complicated by epilepsy or general paralysis, the prognosis was poor. Once incurable paralytics, epileptics, and "idiots" (not yet a pejorative term) were removed from the equation, it was clear that mania was more curable than incoherence. The sooner a "maniac" came under medical supervision, the greater the chance of recovery, according to asylum superintendents' testimonies and statistics. Prichard analyzed data from many British, French, and German asylums to demonstrate how the rate of cure diminished with age and how women were more likely to be cured, but he could not account for different rates of recovery among the asylums.[52]

Prichard admitted that "there are many questions connected with the theory of mental disorders, which are yet and will perhaps always remain involved in obscurity," but there were some predisposing conditions and necroscopic evidence. There were clearly more moral (sociopsychological, emotional) than physical causes of insanity, as the French alienist Étienne-Jean Georget indicated. Prichard pondered one particular social cause: he was "not without a suspicion that there is something in the state of civilization which tends to promote the existence of that congenital state of bodily structure on which predisposition to mental disease depends." He noted the greater incidence of insanity among the refined and its relative rarity among the uncivilized even though such peoples possess unrestrained passions of all kinds, just the sort of behavior that was believed to cause madness. Perhaps poor and "rude" nations did not have the social restraints, diverse interests, arduous pursuits, anxieties, disappointments, and taxing intellectual exertions that some considered causal factors.[53] He cited statistical evidence of social psychological causes of insanity such as anxiety, passions and emotions, apprehensions of the future, and religious anxiety—about this last he produced a lot of examples. As in Prichard's anthropological views, there is a sense of despondency concerning the detriments of civilized life.

Chapter 5 concerns "necroscopical researches" into the physical causes of insanity; in it he reviewed English, Italian, and several French researchers' findings on the physical causes of insanity. These include head injuries, the effects of heat, metastases from other diseases, use of alcohol and drugs, sensuality, intestinal or uterine conditions, and childbirth. Evidence of sensuality as a cause was the prevalence of female prostitutes in French asylums suffering from the late-stage general paralysis of the insane.[54]

Prichard's discussion of therapeutics is divided into behavioral and medical. Inclined to the latter, he would have been fascinated by modern psychopharmacology and psychosurgery. First, any diseased condition of the brain must be treated with an antiphlogistic regime and cooling of the head. The condition of the bowels was paramount, but good diet, fresh air, and exercise were also required. Importantly, therefore, the most senior officer of an asylum should be a physician.[55] Prichard then outlined the "moral treatment" of the insane and the asylum conditions appropriate for it, based on the work of Samuel Tuke of The Retreat. The Quaker asylum keeper's book about moral treatment and asylum management was widely circulated, and his presentation to a Parliamentary Select Committee in 1815 had helped shape views on insanity and guide asylum reform. Prichard stressed that asylums must segregate patients according to their conditions and sex and provide comfort, cleanliness, access to pleasant exercise, trained staff, and vigilant supervision. The four elements of moral treatment are seclusion from society, distraction from negative associations, development of self-control, and self-awareness of illusions.[56]

By the time Prichard published *A Treatise on Insanity*, moral treatment carried out in an asylum was becoming generally considered superior to medical treatment. But it was too labor-intensive to be used on pauper lunatics crammed into workhouses and the new county asylums, nor did it deal with the causes of insanity. Its regimen was, in fact, a reflection of successful family life, in which a child internalizes the rules of acceptable behavior. Some reformers started viewing this treatment as abusive psychological restraint.

Having discussed the causes, symptoms, and suggested treatments of different types of insanity and mental impairment, Prichard explored certain topics in greater depth and returned to sociocultural factors. He described puerperal madness, idiotism, and mental deficiency, drawing together data from around Britain as to the prevalence and class basis of insanity. Concerning the popularly held apprehension about the number of the insane increasing rapidly, he noted that the preponderance of asylum patients were "pauper idiots." He suggested that this problem might be addressed by taking measures such as confining them in order to prevent procreation, and prohibiting marriage between close relatives. He returned to the issue that concerned him so deeply—Esquirol's observation that insanity is a disease of civilization. Prichard thought that just as civilization had given rise to expanded brains and awakened intellects, it had also led to the development of diseases. During this process structural variation of the brain had occurred through the "efforts of nature," some imperfections had resulted, such as the forms of insanity he had outlined.[57] Prichard's psychological, biological and anthropological interests were again brought together.

After devoting a chapter to a global statistical survey of the prevalence of insanity, Prichard introduced two related topics.[58] The first, the medical jurisprudence of insanity, he had included in his 1822 book, and he would develop it further in his 1842 publication on the subject. He stressed that madness is a much more subtle condition than the merely raving state recognized by the law at that time. He called for a clearer relationship between the legal and medical professions in which physicians have the prerogative of setting the standards on which soundness or unsoundness of mind is judged, while lawyers formulate and apply the law. Prichard hoped jurists would be convinced of the existence of moral insanity and recognize the medical profession's exclusive expertise in the matter of mental health.

Legal cases hinging on the question of a defendant's insanity attracted wide publicity. In John Bellingham's hasty trial for the assassination of the prime minister in 1812, the question of his mental competence had been decided by magistrates without the aid of medical opinion. Another quite different type of legal case was a commission in lunacy, the process to determine a person's insanity or sanity. These posed the risk of wrongful deprivation of liberty and property by grasping relatives, as well as the threat to the financial and social position of the families involved. Where people were clearly delusional or mentally deficient, there was little basis for legal challenge or suspicion as to their incompetence to face trial or control their own affairs, but when they appeared rational, confusion could arise. Moreover, medical men who became involved in such cases by either signing committal certificates or testifying at commissions in lunacy risked accusations of collusion with families or avaricious asylum owners, or charges of incompetence. Although Prichard admitted it was challenging to diagnose moral insanity with demonstrably scientific accuracy while grappling with its fuzzy border with eccentricity, he felt a diagnosis of moral insanity could often be useful both in preserving a family's wealth and respectability through control of disruptive family members and in determining exemption from criminal responsibility. The wealth and respectability of affluent families should be preserved and wrongful executions prevented.[59]

Prichard hoped to set a standard by which physicians could soundly and convincingly testify to a defendant's mental state. He organized his chapter on psychiatric jurisprudence on the plan of German professor of philosophy Johann Christoph Hoffbauer. The stages of mental incapacity ranged from lack of judgment and comprehension to fatuity, with relative positions under the law. For example, imbeciles of the third degree should not be left to administer their own property.[60] Of the next pair of mental afflictions, mania was undisputed between medical and legal experts, but in cases of monomania or partial insanity, the law should not attach criminality to actions that are the result of particular delusions, nor should monomaniacs be deprived of their rights. In conclusion, although English law clearly absolved lunatics from criminal responsibility and deprived them of civil rights, it did not actually define lunacy, leaving it, for instance, to the chancellor to receive information about a person, issue a writ of de lunatico inquirendo, and obtain a jury verdict.[61]

Prichard's goal in getting moral insanity recognized in law was to extend the criteria for determining a defendant's insanity beyond manifested delusion, illusion, or hallucination. Particularly sensitive was his qualification of moral insanity as the "irresistible impulse" to commit a particular crime or destroy things but without manifesting delusions.[62] Prichard admitted that it would always be a challenge for the courts to distinguish criminal from insane acts, but this task would be rendered less critical

> when the good sense of the community shall have produced the effect of abolishing all capital punishments. That this will sooner or later happen I entertain no doubt. Many persons have begun already to hesitate as to the moral rectitude of putting men to death. . . . A single private individual would scarcely think himself justified in taking upon himself the office of the Almighty, and inflicting mortal punishment on a person whom he knew to have perpetrated a crime. If such an

act would be, not meritorious, but culpable, when executed by one individual, it does not seem clear how it becomes more righteous when that person has any given number of accomplices, ... say twelve men.[63]

Prichard considered the issue of suicide as indicative of insanity. Those who took their own lives were often judged insane out of compassionate avoidance of the barbaric laws pertaining to suicide. The suicidal, Prichard wrote, often had an impulse to homicide, showed symptomatic behavior, or most often had a precipitating disease. Although a hereditary propensity and more prevalent in different seasons, suicide was not generally an example of insanity as delusion was not involved; rather the act was a perversion of the instinct of self-preservation.[64]

A Treatise on Insanity concludes with further development of Prichard's *Cyclopaedia* articles on somnambulism and animal magnetism, which he now classed "ecstatic affections." In renewing his attack on phrenology, he started by exploring the innate talents and propensities in animals analogous to those of humans. For this approach he apparently coined the term "comparative psychology." He accused phrenologists of selecting a few coincidences, ignoring contrary evidence, and conjuring up excuses in order to baffle opponents with their organology. He was simply fed up with pretentious phrenologists and their "converts," "proselytes," and so on. He predicted that "the time is not far distant when the whole theory will be abandoned. This persuasion is founded on the prospect of more substantial and secure discoveries in the real physiology of the brain and nervous system." He contrasted the hollow claims of phrenologists with Continental scientific anatomists' remarkable research into brain physiology; well-devised experiments were being conducted to establish localization of brain function by, for instance, vivisection of animals and the study of brain-injured humans. One impressive discovery was the apparently discrete functions of two organs within the skull of vertebrates: one controls sensation, conscious perception, and the psychical phenomena related to intelligence, while the other is the seat of voluntary motion.[65] He was clearly enthusiastic about such examples of scientific medicine.

Prichard's research for *Treatise on Insanity* included delving into the rich variety of Continental literature on insanity and the nature of the mind to explore the rival theories of French and particularly two German schools of thought. German psychiatric theories were founded on the intellectual movement called German Romanticism, whose "psychicists" or "mentalists" tended to take a somewhat metaphysical approach, supported by clinical observation. Key proponent J. C. A. Heinroth maintained that the seat of insanity was in the mind/soul, with some exceptions such as in the case of epilepsy.[66] Prichard disagreed with Heinroth's implied sinful origin of insanity. For instance, when Prichard cited alcohol abuse as a cause of insanity, he meant a physical cause rather than a moral one. An undercurrent of the notion that sin and depravity caused insanity would haunt psychiatry much later in the century.

In opposition to the psychicists were the German somatists such as C. F. Nasse and K. W. M. Jacobi. This group of Romantic philosophers opposed French Enlightenment rationality and phrenology's physicalist location of madness in the brain. Somatists helped Prichard understand that mental faculties themselves could be diseased and that there was a complex interaction between the mind/immaterial soul, body, and experience. In 1824 their journal published an excerpt from Prichard's earlier work, and *Treatise on Insanity* cites Jacobi's articles in that same journal. Jacobi believed insanity the result of underlying physical disorder, and it could be precipitated by conditions such as alcohol abuse and parturition. His research, disdain of speculation, and views of asylum design also impressed Prichard.

The Nasse school of somatists attributed most cases of insanity to deranged emotions caused by bodily disease, especially of the visceral organs. According to Jacobi, the emotions, unlike the intellect, were governed by a person's temperament, a notion based on traditional humoral understanding of the body's constitution. Prichard found this framework of a holistic interaction of body and mind/soul attractive. It also justified the continued use of the humoral medical therapeutics he had always relied on. He was pleased to understand that passions and emotions could be diseased and that insanity arose not just in the brain but from the general constitution of the sufferer. In these cases, pathological brain lesions might be the effect and not the cause of insanity, which might be located in the brain or elsewhere. So in 1835 he could confidently maintain that while the brain was the seat of some mental illnesses, they should also be considered in relation to conditions in the rest of the body, particularly the viscera.[67] Aside from the Germans, Pinel, and Esquirol, Prichard drew on Belgian Joseph Guislain and Frenchman Pierre Laromiguière on delusions, Georget and others on insanity without delusions, and François-Emmanuel Fodéré and Georget on mental deficiency.[68]

A Treatise on Insanity was widely reviewed, ranging from a long positive one in the *Medico-Chirurgical Review* (April 1835), to its being described as a competent compilation in *Göttingische gelehrte Anzeigen* (1838). Thomas

Wakeley's medical reformist *Lancet* deemed it "an essential index to the literature of the disease," and a long abstract in the *Medical Quarterly Review* ended: "Though inferior to the works of Haslam in depth of thought and felicity of style, it is nevertheless the most elaborate, comprehensive, and useful treatise on insanity that has yet appeared in this country." Prichard was, of course, looking forward to Esquirol's opinion: that respected alienist was more appreciative of Prichard's attempt to formulate a definition of moral insanity than he was convinced of its accuracy, as he seemed to consider it a type of monomania. He nonetheless praised Prichard as a learned man whose book "is the most complete work we now possess on mental diseases."[69]

The detractors of Prichard's concept of moral insanity were legion. One medical writer claimed it a false and dangerous doctrine that blurred the boundary between depravity and insanity. The *American Journal of Insanity* published dozens of articles refuting it, helpfully including a translation of an Italian anti-moral insanity article that provided a bibliography of many other similar condemnations of Prichard's theory. Xenophobic British authors bemoaned his overreliance on German and French sources as well. Many extracts, abstracts, reviews, and references appeared in German medical journals, and German textbooks referred to and quoted Prichard at length.[70] Carl Berthold Heinrich reviewed Prichard's concept of moral insanity in 1848, beginning by acknowledging that Prichard's name was synonymous with that of moral insanity, but then he complained that such was his authority British writers dared not contradict the "infallible oracle." He objected to the extreme elasticity and inadequacy of Prichard's definition, both as to the psychological and, to a far higher degree, to the somatic nature of moral insanity. Heinrich concluded that Prichard's lasting contribution would not be the concept of moral insanity, but the improvement of the educated public's attitude toward their unfortunate, suffering fellow creatures:

> And, indeed, Prichard and psychiatry may claim to have played rather an important part in the great process of intellectual agitation which we live with right now, but is still hidden to the majority. When [Prichard's] doctrine was developed, its founder will scarcely have been aware of the implications, as its consistent application in real life will be a nail in the coffin of the English High Church. Evaluating Prichard's merits as a practising psychiatrist, however, we can ascribe only minor importance to them. Although we have to approve of the

fact that Prichard added a new collective term, which is based on psychic symptoms, to the established forms of insanity at the expense of these, mainly of that of madness, we miss the clear statement of a condition which is absolutely necessary if he does not want this term to become a mere formality in the eyes of a pathologist: we miss the clear statement that all kinds of moral insanity are conditioned by certain pathological processes and a somatic foundation.[71]

As for Prichard's immediate influence on his fellow alienists and the medical psychology of the period, John Minson Galt's 1846 *The Treatment of Insanity* contains seven pages of material on therapeutics abstracted from Prichard, and the celebrity mad-doctor John Conolly in *Familiar Views of Lunacy and Lunatic Life* quoted Prichard approvingly, agreeing with him on moral insanity. Antiphrenologists often cited Prichard as well.[72] Abroad, Karl Schaeffer considered him to have successfully introduced German psychiatric knowledge into England. Harald Selmer, the "father of Danish psychiatry," translated *A Treatise on Insanity* into Danish in 1842.[73]

Americans modeled their asylums on The Retreat and adopted many of Prichard's and other British psychiatric views. There, however, the developing humane treatment of the insane was coupled with the most extreme of humoral-based heroic medical therapies. The two American editions of Prichard's *A Treatise on Insanity* (1837) received positive reviews. The country's leading forensic psychiatrist, Isaac Ray, in his *Treatise on the Medical Jurisprudence of Insanity* (1838), agreed with Prichard's idea of moral insanity. Other leaders in the field such as Pliny Earle, preeminent psychiatrist and proponent of progressive asylum management, and Amariah Brigham also accepted it, though Earle dubbed it the great *quaestio vexata* of psychological medicine. Some American psychiatrists eventually used the term "moral insanity" as a convenient catchall for any condition where there was unimpaired or usually unimpaired intellect.[74]

Prichard's was the standard textbook on the subject for decades. Toward the end of the century, the later editions of John Bucknill and Daniel Hack Tuke's *A Manual of Psychological Medicine* acknowledged: "Dr. Prichard's excellent 'Treatise on Insanity' has undoubtedly been the one which hitherto has most nearly afforded the desired information; but it was written a quarter of a century ago, at a time when the Treatment of Insanity bore an aspect entirely different to its present one; and, moreover, it is now out of print." Its authors then cited Prichard thirty times, indicating how similar their views were to Prichard's, as they agreed on the ultimate organic basis of insanity; a simple intellectual/emotional classification; a stress on pathological mechanisms although some evidence of duality of the mind is acceptable; and avoidance of theories of the mind (metaphysics/psychology). In 1871 another psychiatry textbook reviewed the contemporary definition of insanity as comprising elements that are intellectual (ideational) and emotional (affective), with the latter subdivided into moral alienation (insanity of the moral sentiments) and insanity of the propensities (impulsive insanity). The author summarized: "Here we come to the *moral insanity*, concerning which so much contention has arisen, and which is so often said to have been invented by doctors as an excuse for crime. The great teacher of the doctrine of moral insanity was Dr Prichard, who, in his well-known Treatise on Insanity, published in 1835, insists strongly on this division." The author then extensively paraphrased *A Treatise on Insanity*, ending, "Dr Prichard's work, however, is to be found in most medical libraries, and I must refer you to it."[75]

During the early decades of the nineteenth century, when Prichard was among the few Britons publishing on insanity, *A Treatise on Insanity* brought him international eminence in this new subdiscipline of medicine. His gathering of hospital statistics from around the world marks an early contribution to this approach to understanding disease. Concerning the organic causes of insanity, he described some of the exciting new discoveries made in laboratories. Prichard's nagging question as to whether insanity originates in the brain or mind led him to ponder, for instance, whether brain lesions recently identified by morbid anatomists were the cause or effect of insanity, especially as brain function and mental processes were so little understood. From weighing conflicting Continental theories to drawing on British asylum statistics and his long personal and professional experience, Prichard helped lay the foundation on which the comprehensive study of the mind and its illnesses would be built.

Prichard vs. the Materialist Science of the Mind

Prichard's work on psychology and psychiatry addressed some burning scientific questions of his era. Is there a universal quality of mind despite humankind's superficial dissimilarity? Are thought, emotion, memory, and understanding the products of the immaterial mind or soul, or merely manifestations of the brain's conglomeration of chemicals and cells? If the latter, might personality and mental capacity be fixed in the physical fabric of the brain? These had serious implications for science, religion, and society.

In an era when scientists could not challenge Scripture with impunity, phrenologists started rocking the boat. They offered an attractively straightforward scientific approach to human psychology: the shape of the skull reflects cerebral organization beneath, revealing a patient's personality, abilities, and potential. Phrenologists claimed to be uniquely qualified to diagnose psychological defects in individuals and in society generally. Their practical science spread rapidly and widely. It fostered international scientific cooperation and aspired to make major contributions to human welfare during the Age of Improvement. Prichard despised phrenologists and their alleged science.

Phrenology's roots lie in Franz Joseph Gall's late eighteenth-century cerebral anatomical research. His materialistic "organology" mapped the brain's twenty-seven "faculties," or departments of the mind, a system based on traditional faculty psychology. Gall "anatomized" these metaphysical views of the mind to create a psychological map of the brain. In Britain Johann Spurzheim renamed organology *phrenology*, an impressively Greek construction meaning "mind science." Phrenology also drew inspiration from Swiss theologian and mystic Johann Caspar Lavater's highly influential popularization of the ancient art of physiognomy, the analysis of character based on facial features, in which facial "perfection" indicates moral worth. Unsurprisingly, the European visage occupied the summit of Lavater's hierarchy, while whole nations were condemned—the "Negro" and the "Lapp" coming in for particular excoriation.

Phrenologists' fellow citizens were not immune to scrutiny. Combined with the facial-angle-based aesthetic as used in polygenetic theory, phrenological analysis of the heads of prisoners and lunatics reinforced prejudices.[76] Armed with measuring instruments, skull diagrams and those ubiquitous ceramic "phrenological busts," phrenologists were soon generating satisfying, quantifiable data that would aid the ordering of society at home and in the colonies. A better and safer society was on the horizon. To Prichard, however, this popularist, biologically deterministic, unorthodoxically materialistic, and obviously unscientific science threatened the hegemony of his psychological medicine and anthropology.

Phrenology's British home was in scientifically liberal Edinburgh, where iconic phrenologist lawyer George Combe became one of the founders of the Edinburgh Phrenological Society in 1820 and its *Phrenological Journal* in 1823. Soon the society could boast a large reference collection of skulls. For more than twenty years George Combe was at the hub of the flourishing discipline. He and his associates promoted their science, created jargon, founded societies, gave lectures at the new mechanics' institutions and philosophical societies, devised apparatus, and published books, periodicals, manuals, charts, and affordable pamphlets. Combe corresponded extensively with friends and with opponents such as Sir William Hamilton and Prichard. He wrote to the archbishop of Dublin and to Queen Victoria's physician about Prince Albert's interest in employing phrenology to educate and shape the character of the difficult young Prince of Wales.[77] His textbook *Essay on the Constitution of Man, and Its Relations to External Objects* was one of the international best sellers of the century, estimated to have sold 350,000 copies in nine editions between 1827 and 1860. It contains respectful references to Prichard, with quotations from his *Physical History* about the transmission of hereditary qualities among humans and lower animals.

Although the leading British phrenologists occupied "respectable" professions, they did not shun the less elite, such as younger, ambitious, marginalized medical men. They were generally non-Anglicans, even avowed atheists like Gall himself, materialists, reformers, and sometimes downright Radicals, all socially unacceptable to the likes of Anglican Tory Prichard. Phrenology was ridiculed for its popularity among the less-educated and women, neither having legitimate business dabbling in science. It had a too easily mastered methodology; medical training was unnecessary, much to the deprecation of the status-minded medical world, of course. Recognizing British class bias at work, Combe grumbled privately: "I am actually shunned & disliked by all those influential classes; and my admirers belong to a different sphere, highly intelligent, respectable, & excellent, but not possessed of a public character sufficiently powerful to overbalance my opponents." While phrenology aimed to tackle the ills of individuals and of society and the weakness of whole "races," such a utilitarian science was unappealing to Christian elite Oxbridge cultivators of experimental, pure science for the sake of uplifting knowledge.[78]

Despite phrenology's somewhat déclassé reputation, it continued to thrive, paraphernalia sales boomed, and phrenology lectures and head-reading sessions drew large audiences. Phrenological societies sprang up in several countries. Phrenology's provision of a comprehensible guide of character and aptitude suggested the benefits of nurture as well as the facts of nature, couched in an optimistic and progressive social philosophy devoid of the Church's depressing doctrine of the corruption of original sin. Its adherents believed it was a respectable and promising science demonstrating divine intelligence, along with a panacea for personal and societal ills—salvation here and now. Like Prichard, others doubted its religious orthodoxy, scientific validity, and philosophy. Two of the earliest key criticisms of phrenology came from Prichard's university friend John Gordon, writing in the influential *Edinburgh Review*, while the *Encyclopaedia Britannica* article on phrenology was from the pen of the socially acceptable antiphrenologist Dr. Peter Mark Roget.[79] Establishment periodicals and the medical profession, for the most part, closed ranks against the new science.

The idea that the brain was the repository of the mind did attract several prominent alienists to take an interest in phrenology, however, Dr. John Conolly among them. Phrenologically inclined Amariah Brigham, foremost advocate of American asylum reform, was perplexed: "I am in correspondence with Dr. Prichard of Bristol—this arises from my having reviewed his work on Insanity in the North American Review two years since—Dr P. I find is not a Phrenologist—but is I judge from some cause or other somewhat sore & sour upon the subject."[80] Prichard had no intention of falling in with phrenology's view of the material nature of the brain's operations. Instead, his modified version of faculty psychology, with the mind divided into separate functions but without particular locations in the brain, obviated recourse to materialist and biological determinist notions. He thought he had firm grounds for challenging Gall's theories on the brain development of lower animals. Prichard had studied the effects of domestication of animals on behavior and structure. Finding that behavioral modification is always linked to change in form, he challenged phrenologists to demonstrate localized cerebral changes caused by domestication.

Recognizing the threat such an eminent scientist like Prichard posed, phrenologists plotted to convert or discredit him. He and his theories of the mind were frequently singled out for criticism in the *Phrenological Journal*, the *American Phrenological Journal*, the *Zoist*, and in phrenological textbooks.[81] The nearby Bath Phrenological Society organized Combe's highly successful course of lectures there, and he was invited to speak to his Bristol followers as well. Dr. Edward Barlow of Bath pointed out Prichard's "little lurking unsuppressed sarcasm" of phrenology in his *Cyclopaedia of Practical Medicine* article "Temperament." Winning him over would have been a coup. Barlow thought Prichard's "arguments appear to me weak in the extreme, and it is gratifying to see how little of substantial reason even such a mind as Prichard's can array against us.—They may not merit formal refutation, yet as Prichard stands high as a philosopher, and as he is both a respectful and respectable opponent, it may not be wise to disregard his opposition, which is very likely to carry weight with the unreflecting, and those who, as yet, have no knowledge of Phrenology."[82] Failing to convert Prichard or at least put a stop to his sniping, Combe tried a more personal appeal, sending him copies of his Edinburgh City Council testimonials. Prichard replied diplomatically that he was not phrenology's opponent, and in fact, some (unspecified) phrenologists whose efforts he respected were uncovering interesting facts and opinions that merited respect.[83] Their correspondence at an end, Prichard redoubled his campaign against phrenology.

That phrenology was making inroads into democratizing access to science and playing a part in developing the Victorian culture of self-help literature did nothing to recommend it to Prichard. Nor did he like phrenologists' seeming disregard of the accepted view that science was at one with Scripture. As for its faulty science, he repeatedly pointed out its dearth of proofs, contradictory observations, tendency to make excuses for the many exceptions encountered, citation of case histories that were merely coincidences, and risible analogical reasoning. Their vaunted correlation of skull form and size with intellectual capacity had not a shred of evidence to support it, for instance. Not only was it unscientific; it had both alarmingly reformist and inhumane implications.

Confidently dismissing phrenology's claim to be able to divine personality, national character, and "race" qualities, Prichard lectured against it at the Bristol Phil & Lit and attended a course of lectures on it there in 1837. He predicted phrenology's demise, and he ridiculed phrenologists as "zealous partizans who go about in search of such facts in favour of this doctrine" and "sanguine votaries." Phrenology's "votaries" could only condemn Prichard for retarding the progress of the greatest discovery of the age.

The fortunes of phrenology on the Continent were somewhat different. In 1831 the Société Phrénologique was founded to study the brain intensively, profiting from the Parisian scientific ferment of the time. French phrenology advocated programs for improving society by maximizing individuals' differing potential through tailored education, including the management of children, women, and criminals. But like British phrenology, it drew the hostility of the French scientific elite. The revolution of 1848 left organized phrenology in disarray. But because Gall's neuroanatomy and phrenology stimulated later French scientists' research into brain localization of function, phrenology receives some recognition in the history of neuropsychology and neuroanatomy.[84] Its less positive legacy was its focus on the form of the head, which became a preoccupation of later nineteenth-century anthropology, psychiatry, and criminology.

Prichard had the satisfaction of seeing some decline in British phrenology's popularity as a growing number of showman-like practitioners tarnished its reputation, and the popularity of mesmerism distracted attention from it. It took several decades for phrenology to bloom, flourish internationally, and ultimately fail to live up to its promise.

On the Different Forms of Insanity, in Relation to Jurisprudence (1842)

Prichard's chapter on the jurisprudence of insanity in *A Treatise on Insanity* signaled a new direction he would take in his efforts to improve society: he would work to secure the humane treatment under the law of sufferers from disabling mental conditions and insanity. He had a high profile as premier British mad-doctor, but the legal profession remained unsympathetic to his notion of insanity without symptomatic delusions. He published *On the Different Forms of Insanity, in Relation to Jurisprudence, Designed for the Use of Persons Concerned in Legal Questions Regarding Unsoundness of Mind* in August 1842 (reprinted as a second edition in 1847). Its dedication to the then–high chancellor Lord Lyndhurst was an obeisance to the head of British justice, an affirmation of Prichard's Tory disdain of political reformism, an expression of gratitude for his recent appointment as a metropolitan commissioner in lunacy, or likely all three.

Prichard's previous publications on moral insanity and jurisprudence had done little to lessen prejudices among professionals and the public. He complained to a barrister: "I observe your remark on Lunacy. It is quite well founded as far as it relates to the Incompetency of most barristers in questions relating to Lunacy. But I am sorry to say that physicians are not often much better informed. Dr. Conolly is an exception."[85] By minimizing the medical details and omitting therapeutics, Prichard produced a compressed and easier-to-read outline of the different types of mental health conditions and insanity, especially moral insanity. Far from making strident demands about the protection of the insane from undeserved punishment or the preservation of society from the dangerous insane, he appeared merely to promote jurists' awareness of an array of psychological and neuropsychiatric conditions.

The law dealt with the insane case by case, referring to famous legal precedents, including Lord Matthew Hale's introduction of the concept of "partial insanity." Although the philosophical definition of madness was mistaking false impressions as truths and then acting upon them logically while the general powers of the mind are intact, some medical writers had insisted that the insane have a deluded imagination, a definition adopted by jurists Thomas Erskine, Hale, and John Singleton, Baron Lyndhurst. This was a valid definition of partial insanity, but it neglected an entire category in which the sufferer's values, emotions, and propensities are diseased without outward manifestation of delusion. Prichard wanted to convince the legal profession to adopt moral insanity as a category in law.[86]

The section on moral insanity defines it and lays out Prichard's views in great detail, providing several case histories. There are sections on monomania or partial insanity, chronic melancholia, and the difficult-to-grasp condition "instinctive insanity," in which atrocious acts are carried out on irresistible impulse. He provided a set of five points to apply to the diagnosis of "homicidal propensity" or "insane homicide" and described propensities to suicide, pyromania, and cleptomania.[87] Prichard then tackled the degrees of irresponsibility for crime and for undertaking civil acts, praising French and German law and criticizing English rulings that required obvious defective understanding, mania, or senselessness. He next outlined what the legal response to the various types of insanity ought to be, noting as key issues the suspension of civil rights and protection of society from danger. In the case of actions performed during lucid intervals, Prichard was concerned with both criminal responsibility and the validity of wills, for instance.[88]

The book ends with a description of other types and degrees of deteriorative and congenital mental conditions, grading them according to a person's right to perform civil acts. He did admit that a jury must determine a person's mental capacity on an ad hoc basis, accepting Lord Hale's guidance that behavior similar to that of a fourteen-year-old should be considered a standard of civil and criminal responsibility. Also, irreversible dementia, both senile and arising from organic disease, should absolve sufferers from legal responsibility.[89]

Different Forms of Insanity underscores the existence of a subtle type of insanity, moral insanity, whose recognition could prevent unjust sentences and unacceptable suffering. Well aware that the legal profession and the public generally believed the insanity plea was nothing more than an excuse for murderers to get off scot-free, Prichard expected criticism. There were reviews in several British general, medical, and legal periodicals, as well as in the foreign press. The *Athenaeum*'s was prompt and positive, stressing the importance of determining each defendant's *degree* of insanity. The *British and Foreign Medical Review* contrasted a book by Forbes Winslow with that of Prichard, the former being a mass of "inaccuracies and fallacies." The *London Medical Gazette* was entirely positive, noting that a certain flexibility in determining insanity does not invalidate moral insanity as a valid category. The *British and Foreign Review*, on the other hand, doubted Prichard's claim that the morally insane might evince no observable trace of their condition, nor were his arguments about partial insanity and motiveless crime convincing, the latter tantamount to giving the defendant the benefit of the doubt.[90]

Among the several French, German, and American reviews, the *Legal Observer, or Journal of Jurisprudence* recognized Prichard's threat to the legal profession and charged him with neglecting to distinguish between having an uncontrollable desire to commit crime and failing to control it. The reviewer deplored the presence of medical witnesses in criminal trials; doctors, with the air of Delphic oracles, erroneously claimed complete knowledge of the defendant and the case, thus interfering in the proper domain of the jury, who could better weigh up all evidence without being confounded by medical witnesses. Besides, monomaniacs' escaping punishment would encourage others to do the same, hoodwinking the public and creating a climate of insecurity. Alienists were just meddling in the law. Later authors cited Prichard's manual of jurisprudence and its subtle classifications. In the United States decades later, the author of a standard work on psychological law vehemently condemned Prichard's concept of moral insanity, while the influential editor of the American *Journal of Insanity* was strident in its condemnation at the 1881–82 trial of President James Garfield's assassin.[91]

Prichard had hoped that a diagnosis of moral insanity might be used to protect the insane under the law, but events were against him. In Victorian Britain, assassination attempts on the queen and political figures by the mentally disturbed occurred alarmingly regularly. The year after Prichard's book on jurisprudence was published, Daniel M'Naghten was tried for the assassination of a public figure. After the testimony of medical experts on the defendant's insanity, M'Naghten was found not guilty on the grounds of insanity *inspired* by a delusion. It sparked a debate leading to the formulation of the M'Naghten Rules, which established that in order to be considered not guilty on the grounds of insanity, a defendant must manifest delusional notions and be unable to distinguish right from wrong at the time of the act. These rules were a setback as far as Prichard's concept of moral insanity was concerned, especially since he viewed the condition as a disease of the emotions that caused people to do wrong even though they understood it to be wrong. Strenuous resistance to the insanity plea did not slacken. Hostility to the idea of moral insanity continued, and the

M'Naghten rules prevailed. In sum, the effect of the moral insanity plea on legal decisions was limited and sporadic.[92]

Insanity and Pessimism

In *A Treatise on Insanity*, Prichard traced many cases of insanity directly to affections of the brain that could be revealed upon dissection but noted that many other cases originate rather obscurely in the viscera and then affect the brain. Several years later he published an article more fully endorsing the generally visceral and constitutional origins of insanity. Prichard thought some French alienists' claiming the brain the locus of morbid incitement both somewhat excessive and with dangerous implications. German research favoring the idea of insanity originating in visceral conditions suited Prichard; he started praising K. W. M. Jacobi more fully. An example of this is the case of a patient considered insane for refusing to eat. It was discovered postmortem that she had had intestinal ulcers, which Prichard concluded were the cause of her insanity rather than the cause of her refusal to eat.

This 1844 article in the *Provincial Medical and Surgical Journal* marks Prichard's final stand against phrenology and affirms that insanity originates principally in the viscera, a view consistent with humoral medicine. He claimed insanity was not at all, or only in a minor way, linked to the brain, a qualified position that avoided materialism. While still believing in the somehow holistic interaction between body and mind/soul, he carefully noted that the points made by the psychicists also had to be mentioned. This article was widely noticed.[93]

No longer in his prime, Prichard was tired of being a Bristol physician, dogged by petty rivalries, worn out by constant travel. He was depressed, with good reason: tuberculosis was taking his children, one after another; his academically driven son Theodore's socially unacceptable behavior was being remarked on; his countrymen appeared unconcerned for the plight of their fellow humans in bondage and those being driven to extinction by colonial rapacity; polygenism and racism were on the rise; and there was social unrest and the clear threat of revolution on the Continent spreading to Britain. Like Jacobi, he lamented the moral deterioration of society as typified by the disgraceful French, whose lack of self-control and disregard of religion were faults manifested in their predilection for lower passions and vices. Even Esquirol agreed that religious decline in France had led to increased superstitious mania, egotism, and selfishness.[94] The old values of social order that religion had kept firm were deteriorating as society advanced, and not just in France.

Prichard's idea of the universality of proto-religious thought characterized by feelings of gloom and apprehension of the future tied his natural history of humankind to his natural history of the human mind. He observed that the morally insane are prototypically gloomy and that this form of insanity was more prevalent in "civilized" societies. In fact, the more "refined" people become, the more susceptible they were to feelings that might precipitate mental disturbance. And as eccentricity could tip over into insanity, perhaps sanity existed on a continuum, potentially manifesting itself in everyone—a pessimistic view in itself. Insanity was thus an inescapable part of the human condition, inbred in the species and exacerbated by modern life. A faulty mind was but the symptom of a faulty society. Further, if primarily social and psychological factors were at the root of insanity, the utility of Prichard's physical causes and medical treatments came under doubt.

A Legacy?

Even as the issue of insanity began to emerge from the shadows of previous centuries, the very idea of it continued to shame, horrify, and fascinate Victorians, stirring imagination, whether through sensational newspaper accounts of criminal trials, asylum scandals, and lunacy commissions on the aristocratic or wealthy, or in spicing up the plots of novels. Charlotte Brontë's *Jane Eyre* (1847) paints Bertha's mania in the most nightmarish terms, while *The Strange Case of Dr. Jekyll and Mr. Hyde* (1886) explores the nature of moral insanity and Victorian values. Captain Ahab's monomania is a clear example of American Herman Melville's insanity plot. Prichard himself neither cared for nor needed to read fiction to experience the horrors and too frequent hopelessness of insanity.[95]

By the mid-1840s Prichard had little to show for all his effort on behalf of the mentally ill. His post as a commissioner in lunacy involving the design, regulation, and inspection of asylums had proven just as problematic as the theories he grappled with. The new asylums were filling up with the barely treated, and the criminal insane were still being sent to the gallows. The language of insanity remained medical, despite medicine's inability to deal with it, and the fabric of his science of the mind was being pulled about by the conflicting interests of the medical and legal professions, government constraints on administration and finance, and the hostility and suspicion of the general public. A case in point is the reformist Alleged Lunatics' Friend Society's claim that moral treatment is nothing but a social and psychological straitjacket used to oppress the insane into conformity.[96]

Amid growing pessimism, a generally confident young psychiatric profession nonetheless prospered, benefiting from legislation, the stimulation of professional associations, journals, and textbooks, and the construction of monumental county asylums. A few generations of psychiatrists acknowledged Prichard's psychiatric nosography as the standard, often noting the concept of moral insanity to have been his most important contribution to the discipline. Toward the end of the century he was cited in major textbooks of psychiatry by Daniel Hack Tuke and Henry Maudsley. Hack Tuke wrote optimistically that "Prichard's sagacity laid, it may be said, the foundation stone of modern criminal anthropology," in which if the facts bear, will deserve respect; in fact, he had written "the best work on insanity in his day." The *Dictionary of Psychological Medicine* (1892) referred to Prichard on the topics "Classification," "Ecstasy," "Insanity, moral," and "Trance." Psychiatrists wanting to stamp their own name on the discipline enthusiastically set to work on moral insanity, variously clarifying, modifying, elaborating, distorting, or dismissing it. Notwithstanding, Prichard's role in the development of psychiatry is still apparent.[97]

While Prichard was optimistic about the coming benefits of scientific medicine, he would have regretted the course psychiatry embarked on not long after his death. Some laboratory-based alienists adopted the trappings of science to measure patients' heads, calibrate physiognomy, and conflate phrenology's biological determinism with somatists' organic basis of insanity. They made generous use of hereditarian doctrine to reinforce their theories of the mind, devising notions based on analogies with recently emerging evidence of heritable physical diseases and mutations. Meanwhile, German scientists came to the fore, dissecting brains and claiming physical explanations for psychiatric conditions. They seemed disinclined to search for cures.

The growing negativism that led to scientific racialism in post-Prichardian anthropology found fertile ground in psychiatry as well. The eighteenth-century notion of degeneration as a cause of human varieties was rehabilitated. Denigration of the Other in this period of colonial expansion and exploitation also spread to denigration of the social Other in one's own society; mental conditions became seen as evidence of degeneration. Drawing on Darwinism, degeneration theory gained acceptance as a natural process: the descendants of "tainted strains," the mentally unfit, progressively degenerate and are doomed to extinction. Only civilization's compassion allows the unfit to survive and procreate. Laboratory alienists took measurements, amassed photographs, and analyzed evidence to evaluate their fellow human beings. They found them wanting. An element of moralistic condemnation of the insane and of people with learning difficulties fostered a degeneration psychiatry that would inspire later movements to advocate the elimination of these so-called degenerates from society.[98]

The notion of degeneration spread further, spawning a new science underpinned by old-fashioned physiognomy. Cesare Lombroso's measurement-based criminology claimed to detect criminal tendencies in society, just as biological anthropologists of the period, using similar methodology, enthusiastically evaluated and ranked the intellects of "races."[99] The later decades of the nineteenth century were an era of making damning measurements of the Other at home and abroad that would have deeply disappointed Prichard.

As to the fate of Prichard's theory of moral insanity, detrimental to its integrity as a class of mental illness was an increasing tendency to associate it with immorality and psychopathy. In the United States, moral insanity, sin, asylum medicine, and the law were conflated in a long-running, unprofitable debate.[100] Diagnosis could lack credibility; as it was often based merely on the patient's family's testimony, misinterpretation or abuse was possible. Jurists tended to prefer intellectual derangement as the clear-cut criterion of insanity, and they shared conservative Christians' hostility to a vague "illness" that allowed the guilty to escape punishment. Remnants of the concept of moral insanity nevertheless survived in psychiatry's ever-changing nosography: It can be traced in Isaac Ray's "moral mania" of 1871, Spitzka's "moral imbecility" of 1887 and Koch's "psychopathic personality" of 1891. Cleckley established "psychopathy" in 1941, and the 1952 *Diagnostic and Statistical Manual* records "psychopathic personality disturbance." Variations on this theme continued until "sociopathy" came into use. As some of Prichard's case histories cite depression of spirits interrupted by bursts of excitement, "manic depression," that outdated term for bipolar disorder, could be thought at least a collateral relative of moral insanity. Some recent encyclopedias of psychiatry deem moral insanity an "affective condition" and compare it to a form of sociopathy currently called antisocial personality disorder.[101] It is no wonder that some frustrated historians of the discipline have simply considered it any behavior that falls midway between normal and psychotic or even any disorder without delusions. The meaning of moral insanity became distorted by later misinterpretations that failed to separate definitively medicine from morals and insanity from wickedness, disputed by jurists and medics alike. Despite its descent into psychiatric terminological chaos, Prichard's formulation of moral insanity as a class of mental illness remains a milestone in the history of the field.[102]

For those who appreciate lists of firsts, Prichard was the foremost nineteenth-century nosologist of insanity writing in English. He introduced French and German psychiatry into Britain and shares the fatherhood of British psychiatry with Thomas Sydenham and Thomas Arnold. He was the first to provide a clinical description of moral insanity, a concept that influenced psychiatric theory throughout the transatlantic world. Prichard established that the prognosis for those suffering from long-established psychiatric conditions was poorer than for those whose insanity had been brought on by transient events. He was the first to identify accurately the stages in an epileptic seizure, and he coined the term "senile dementia." Instrumental in the early days of forensic psychopathology, he helped shape the discipline of psychiatry, driven by his humane desire to improve the lives of sufferers.

9 · "Irksome Things"

Improving Bristol and Medical Practice, 1823–26

> I pay many penalties for being a physician & none more irksome than the almost total alienation from the society which I should most desire.
> —James Cowles Prichard to James Yates, August 10, [1826]

How would he get a chance to read the books weighing down his greatcoat pockets? Prichard was in his carriage and headed for Ross. Creaking along the icy turnpike road, he arrived at the ferry crossing to the Welsh market town of Chepstow. From there the peaceful, undulating route took him along the picturesque River Wye, past the frosted ruin of Tintern Abbey, through bustling Monmouth, by romantic Symonds Yat and imposing Goodrich Castle to Ross. There were no tourists to be seen preparing to embark on the fashionable Wye Tour downstream this January day in 1823. Prichard was returning to his birthplace; his father had summoned him for comfort and advice yet again.

Thomas Prichard laid out his worries. Aunt Newman's state of mind was as poor as ever. Then there was his daughter Mary Moline's situation; he had been pressing her and her husband to settle in Ross, whereas the Moline family wanted them to remain in their hometown of Godalming. A Quaker elder brought in to mediate settled on the latter. Brother Tom and his wife were struggling in a harsh New Jersey winter and strapped for cash so Prichard dispatched them a draft for £50. His April in Somersetshire spent recuperating from another serious illness was cut short when events drew him back to Bristol. While he might have been gratified by the successful publication of *Diseases of the Nervous System* and the prospect of developing a reputation as an alienist, there was no escaping the family crises of 1823.

The theological debates with his father boiled over. Thomas Prichard was dismissive of his son's interest in German Higher Criticism, distrusting newfangled attempts to trace elements of the New Testament to Plato and the like. His faith was simple and straightforward: "all truths on which my salvation depends are written with a sunbeam." Why get mired in abstruse inquiries when one could rely on the Bible and surrender oneself to pure faith in redemption from a polluted world and ultimate regeneration of the evil heart of mankind under the guidance of the Holy Spirit? And to the elder Prichard's mind, theologians deliberately obscured doctrine lest congregations realize that there was no need of a clergy to mediate between their souls and the Redeemer. How he needled his son with Quakerism's handy trope.[1]

Bristol Civic Life and the Idea of Science

Bristol in the 1820s kept up its reputation for not keeping up with the times. The Corporation remained indifferent to calls for reform, and its devotion to self-aggrandizement continued unabated. Its plans for an impressive new Council House were financed with harbor dues so exorbitant, shipowners started deserting the port for cheaper alternatives in the north. The wealthiest Bristolians were complacent; trade and manufacturing need only continue sufficiently to keep them in their lovely suburban residences, or they might even attain their goal of giving up commerce and the professions altogether to ape the aristocracy by acquiring country estates where they could engage in a bit of gentlemanly agriculture and sport. Some middling Bristol businessmen frustrated by local government's inertia and greed formed a lobbying chamber of commerce. The Corporation, having thoroughly alienated reforming religious minorities and even some of the city's bourgeoisie, became the butt of satire and critical contemporary histories.[2] Its reputation would be further tarnished by its bungled handling of the famous 1831 riot, when it treated the rioters as dangerous revolutionaries. Not only did local government and the Bristol elite continue to put pomp, status, and self-interest before the welfare of the poor and minorities, but they evinced little enthusiasm for education, science, or the arts.

Bristol's older charities, often quasi-local government-administered endowments, functioned primarily to foster cultural, moral, and religious values and promote prudence and conformity among the poor. The growing need to "do something about the poor" also reflected a desire both to counter local Methodists' recent efficient and well-developed aid and education programs and to neutralize imagined French revolutionary tendencies among the poor. Bristol charities flourished. Citizen subscribers organized new ones addressing whatever issue inspired them. Membership typically comprised men of commerce, earnest Anglicans and their clergy, Dissenters, a large number of enthusiastic recent converts to Anglicanism, and medical men. A few ladies' names appeared on the subscription lists, but their participation was limited to fundraising activities or serving as inspecting "Visitors" to the domestic or feminine aspects of a charity.

Some of these new charities were local branches of national organizations. They published reports of their regular meetings and annual dinners, listing their officers (almost invariably including some prominent or aristocratic inactive president or patron), members, and the value of their subscriptions and donations for everyone to see. Bristol charities were exclusive, directly or indirectly religious, and nearly always supportive of the conservative values that dominated the city. As Bristol charities established their members' class credentials, maintained conservative social control, and did a bit of good, Prichard supported them enthusiastically.

Bristol offered plenty of opportunities for Prichard to associate with men interested in improving their knowledge of medicine and the medical, spiritual, and general welfare of the poor. But as for making progress through science, his fellow Bristolians were not known to value the active and earnest pursuit of knowledge, even when practical outcomes for industry were involved.[3] Bristol had a tendency to complacent reliance on traditional methods of manufacturing, aversion to risk, and suspicion of and disdain for the novelties of those freethinking, upstarts in the rival northern cities, and anyone involved too ostensibly "in trade." The city was not totally devoid of casual higher learning, however. There had been sporadic meetings of a Bristol scientific and literary society during the early years of the century, and itinerant lecturers and medical men such as Prichard's teacher Dr. Pole had found audiences for their "improving" lectures. Stimulating for a time were Dr. Beddoes's medical charities and his empirical approach to developing the curative properties of gasses as he struggled to revolutionize medicine by establishing it on a foundation of chemistry. Medical men gradually became the mainstay of Bristol's scientific and educational initiatives, experienced as they were in organized learning at local private anatomy schools, medical societies, and the city's medical charities.[4]

Elsewhere in Britain attitudes were different. Scientific discoveries and their technological applications transformed the nation into a powerhouse of science and industry that astonished the world. Northern towns blessed with good ports or navigable rivers overtook Bristol in wealth production and associated science. To foster this progress, provincial and more liberal versions of metropolitan and universities' elite learned societies started springing up, often allowing the membership of less socially acceptable men who earned their livings in industry. Establishing a similar scientific society in Bristol would make quite a change from attending charity dinners.

Laying the Bristol Institution Foundation Stone, February 29, 1820

News of rival cities' new scientific and literary societies reached Bristol. In 1818 Leeds emulated ones founded in Manchester and Newcastle. The Leeds institution's dual objectives were explicit: manufacturing and medicine required understanding of the physical world, and the organization itself advertised Leeds as possessing "polite society." Keen geologists in Cambridge started organizing their Philosophical Society in 1819.[5] Aware of such a tangible mark of cultural attainment, Bristolians planned the Bristol Institution for the Advancement of Science, Literature and the Arts. Merchants, bankers, and professional men promised to purchase £25 shares in it, and an architect was hired.

This demonstration of optimism, altruism, and the desire for improvement needed reification in the form of an edifice, complete with columns. Prichard and his fellow Bristolians gathered to lay the Institution's foundation stone on Leap Day 1820, and two years later the impressive neoclassical building on respectable Park Street was nearing completion. The Tory editor of *Felix Farley's Bristol Journal* must have had men like Prichard, the antiquarian George Cumberland, and the clergyman-geologist William Daniel Conybeare in mind when he rejoiced at the prospect of showcasing the literary and scientific stars of Bristol.

The Bristol Institution's (BI) new temple of knowledge featured a suitably temple-esque portico surmounted by a famous architect's allegorical alto-relievo frieze. The Reading and Committee Rooms on the ground floor were spacious; a grand staircase led to the four first-floor rooms "of noble proportions" accommodating the Museum, Gallery, Library, and other rooms. The Theatre and its adjacent Laboratory were ready for use, and the resident curator, Prussian-born Mr. J. S. Miller, was installed in his own apartment.[6] Every means to quench Bristolians' thirst for knowledge and achieve triumphs in science were now to hand. But where were the scientists and intellectuals to fill it? By the time of its inaugural meeting, it was in debt, a feature of its entire history.[7]

The shareholders ran the BI and selected annual subscribers, ensuring the elite nature of the enterprise. A key figure in it was wealthy Whig banker and fossil collector Richard Bright, father of a Bristol MP and of Prichard's friend the future eminent Dr. Richard Bright. He had the ability to "induce men of all parties to meet together on that neutral ground,—the formation of a scientific society." Another was John Scandrett Harford, Quaker

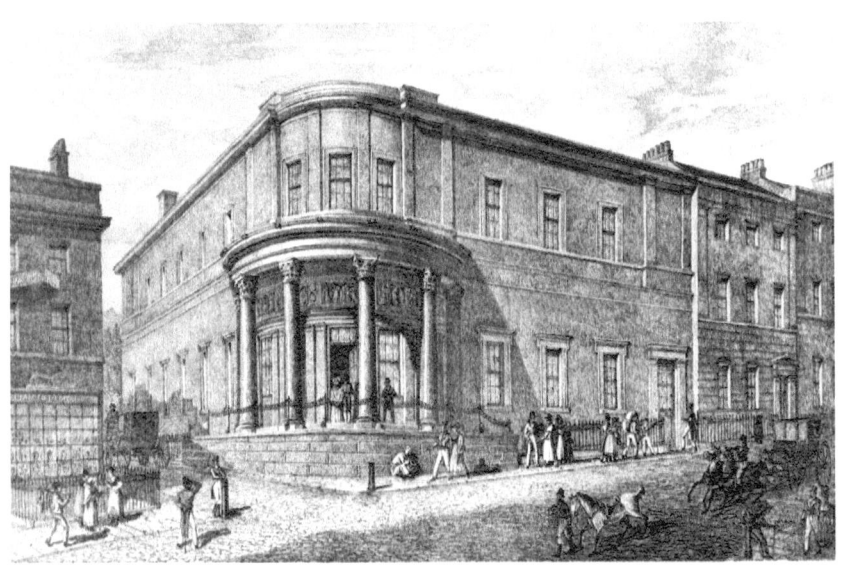

6. Advertising cultural worth. Bristol Institution, Park Street, 1823. Used with permission of Bristol Archives.

convert to evangelical Anglicanism and scourge of radicalism; he was active in national political and intellectual circles and possessed of considerable brass and banking wealth that allowed him to devote his energies to the benefit of the BI.[8] In November 1822 Prichard joined the committee that formulated the rules, drew up a program of lectures and oversaw all necessary arrangements.

Unusually for Bristol, political and religious animosities were suspended at the BI, thanks to the society's rule forbidding direct discussion of religion or politics. Tories, Whigs, and some Dissenters interacted freely. While businessmen managed the BI, generally the city's professional men provided the lectures. It was an elite organization, "designed for and supported by the higher classes" for the acquisition of knowledge and preservation of "the fabric of society." Only once did it memorably and cautiously permit "mechanics" to attend a series of unusually practical lectures.

The BI's lectures on geology, chemistry, biology, natural history, zoology, physiology, literature, history, art history, and philosophy attracted a cultivated and polite audience. Its members and guests were in no danger of being subjected to any assaults on Revelation; for example, Infirmary colleague Dr. Wallis's course on comparative anatomy was carefully described as illustrating the principles of natural theology. In the BI's early years, there were lectures on the Druids and on an "electrometrical" instrument.

Surgeon John Champney Swayne lectured on the properties of blood and blood transfusions, while Prichard's two-part history of pestilences was very popular. Occasional exhibitions of art broadened interest and refined the atmosphere.

Within the elite BI there was an even more elite society, with Prichard at its center. Established in 1823, the Philosophical and Literary Society was the more active and intellectually focused element of the BI, made up of the city's moderate portion of intellectuals, professional men, gentlemen of independent means, and clergymen with antiquarian and scientific interests. It was remembered as very much like a private club of about a dozen men.[9] The Phil & Lit's two pro-directors, Prichard and William Daniel Conybeare, were firmly in control, and with John Estlin and Prichard's Infirmary colleagues Drs. Carrick, Wallis, Riley, and Stock, they provided most of its lectures. The Phil & Lit also welcomed visiting savants to its meetings, and by electing them honorary members, they extended their contacts internationally. Prichard's election as honorary corresponding member of the Academy of Science of Siena on April 29, 1825, was reciprocated a few months later by his proposal of Professor Stanislaus Grottanelli of Siena to honorary membership of the Phil & Lit. Even ladies were allowed to attend suitable lectures.[10]

Prichard's closest Phil & Lit friends were the antiquarian John Eden and the voluble, volatile, and well-connected Anglican clergymen geologist William Daniel Conybeare. A model scientist in Prichard's opinion, Conybeare had just published with William Phillips the religiously orthodox *Outlines of the Geology of England and Wales*, and he continued to do acutely observed, groundbreaking geology throughout the 1820s. His BI lectures carefully pointed out the beneficial relationship between science and industry and the importance of Baconian scientific method, all within the scope of divine truth, of course. His stance against species transmutation satisfied Prichard, and he benefited from the clergyman's wide and influential network of contacts, including in Oxford. Conybeare was a Whig, and of course the two were agreed in their dismissal of Radical ideas, political or scientific. While their personalities and political beliefs were poles apart, they kept up their friendship and cooperated in their efforts to stimulate scientific and educational progress in Bristol, without losing sight of the Almighty's hand in the natural world. Conybeare is remembered for instructing and mentoring the next generation of great geologists.

Geology, that controversial epitome of modern science, was particularly popular. The famous fossil hunter Mary Anning kept the Bristol Institution well supplied with specimens from the fossil coast near Lyme Regis. The BI's growing fossil and mineral collection connected the Institution to a national network of eminent geologists such as Henry De La Beche, Charles Lyell, William Buckland, and Roderick Murchison who visited or corresponded and traded specimens with the BI's members. The first discovery of prehistoric human remains was made in Paviland Cave in nearby South Wales in January 1823. Archaeological and geological discoveries, the BI's interesting lectures, and its expanding collection of specimens stimulated public support of the Institution well into the 1830s.[11] Particularly acceptable to Prichard were Conybeare and Riley's lectures on some Bristol fossils that described changes in form over time as "succession of creation." The earth, meanwhile, was yielding up more and more discoveries that challenged Genesis.

As well as serving on the Institution's library and lecture committees, Prichard was one of the two secretaries of the Phil & Lit. Their printed circulars announced the private business meetings in the Committee Room and public lectures in the Theatre, held two Thursdays per month from October to May. Members were entitled to bring three guests to the lectures, which began at either 7:00 or 7:30 p.m. Prichard regularly attended, chaired meetings, organized, or lectured at the Phil & Lit and the more widely attended Bristol Institution.

Prichard chaired the Phil & Lit's second monthly meeting, at which his friend John Eden read a paper on the druidical monuments of Brittany, while Conybeare excitedly brought news of a perfect specimen of a plesiosaurus recently discovered at Lyme Regis. At their third meeting, February 26, 1824, Prichard's long paper "On the Distribution of Plants and Animals," read by the stronger-voiced Eden, was illustrated with many fine examples of plants. A newspaper sensationally reported that Prichard had demonstrated the single origin of plant species, evidently panicking him into concluding part 2 of his lecture by stressing that his findings accorded with those of recent geology *and Scripture*. This lecture traced the origin of humankind to the southern declivity of the Asiatic mountain chains and the two "Paradisiacal" rivers. Prichard described later postdiluvian creations and suggested that the Sacred Record had omitted descriptions of animals because they were irrelevant to the Bible's business of dealing with human history, a notion that explained recently discovered phenomena.[12] This lecture was based on material destined for the second edition of *Physical History*, then in preparation. He chaired the meeting of July 29, at which he read his "Memoir on the Abraxean Stones," outlining the

Bristol Institution.

THREE LECTURES
ON
EGYPTIAN MUMMIES, EGYPTIAN ANTIQUITIES,
AND THE
ROSETTA STONE,
ARE ABOUT TO BE DELIVERED,

FOR THE BENEFIT OF THE INSTITUTION,

BY

J. C. PRICHARD, M.D., F.R.S., &c.

AND

G. T. CLARK, Esq.

This Course has been undertaken in consequence of the liberal offer of a Gentleman to allow a splendid Egyptian Mummy belonging to him, to be opened for the purposes of scientific information, and for the benefit of the Institution. Other Specimens will be brought from the Museum.

———o———

First Lecture .... MONDAY, March 31st ⎫
Second .... WEDNESDAY, April 2nd ⎬ At Half-past Seven o'clock in the Evening.
Third .... FRIDAY, —— 4th ⎭

Subscription to the Course, 7s. 6d.—Single Ticket, 3s.

Every Member of the Institution, subscribing to the Course, is entitled to a Set of Privilege Tickets, transferable to any one of his Family residing with him, to a Lady, or a Minor.

Subscribers to the Course may have Tickets to admit Minors at 4s.

☞ Tickets to be had at the Institution.

———o———

During the Month of April will be commenced a Course of Ten Lectures on GEOLOGY, by SAMUEL WORSLEY, Esq.; also in aid of the Funds of the Institution.

Printed at the Bristol Mirror Office by John Taylor.

7. Middle-class Bristolians' entertainment. Advertisement for Dr. Prichard and Mr. Clark's lectures on Egypt at the Bristol Institution, 1834. Used with permission of Bristol Archives.

beliefs of an early Christian sect and acknowledging the donation of some gems by one of the Brights.[13]

Unwrapping a Mummy, December 9, 1824

"Dr. Prichard who has (as is well known to all our scientific readers) published a very ingenious work upon Egyptian Antiquities, made many pertinent remarks, explanatory of the subject, very much to the satisfaction of the assembly," the local newspaper reported.[14] With the nation in the grip of Egyptomania and Prichard's qualification for the task, he was put in the spotlight. A real Egyptian mummy had been presented to the BI, which Prichard, a Dr. Gapper, flamboyant surgeon Richard Smith, and the BI's curator were appointed to unwrap before a specially invited audience. It would be a sensation—and add a bit to the Institution's coffers.

Prichard's mummy lecture was such a hit, he was prevailed on to deliver another one at the following month's meeting of the Phil & Lit. Long before the scheduled hour the Theatre was crowded to excess. He started by confessing discouragingly that he had long given up the study of Egyptian antiquities and had nothing novel to report. After describing the religious beliefs of the Egyptians and the place of hieroglyphics in the history of writing, he patriotically defended Dr. Thomas Young's priority over Frenchman Champollion in deciphering hieroglyphics. Prichard concluded by congratulating Bristol for having shed its reputation for indifference to the acquisition of knowledge. He was immensely proud of the Bristol Institution and looked forward to contributing to its future prosperity.[15]

Throughout the twenties, Prichard periodically drew on *Physical History* for his lectures at the Phil & Lit and the Bristol Institution. An appreciative audience attended "Observations on the Races of People who Inhabit the Northern Regions of Africa," the same evening his brother-in-law lectured on "Some Egyptian Curiosities," quoting Prichard's *Egyptian Mythology*.[16] Keen to make a success of the BI, Prichard's next lecture was a highlight of the winter of 1826:

> Dr. Prichard read before a very numerous assembly of the Members and their friends, "An Essay on the Native Races of America, with some general Observations on the varieties of the Human Skull." The Paper was replete with matter of the most interesting kind, and the whole displayed striking proofs of acute penetration and deep research. The concluding observations respecting the varieties of the Human Skull were particularly ingenious, and strikingly calculated to demonstrate

that, notwithstanding the modifications under which the crania of different nations at present appear, the whole human race must have originally sprung but from one parent stock.[17]

This lecture outlined the geography and languages of the two continents, referring to German and American linguists. He explained that the eleven great nations of the Americas had common origin in the far northwest. When comparing American and Asiatic skulls, he fascinated his audience with an array of genuine crania arranged into European, narrow-elongated, and broad-faced types. Craniology was of great interest, especially as phrenology was then gaining in popularity.[18]

The following May Prichard and his friend John Eden's double act at the Phil & Lit reflected their shared pastimes. While Eden's lecture was on how published interlinear literal translations aided the learning of the dead languages, Prichard described Santes Pagnino's 1584 interlinear translation of the Old and New Testament in Hebrew, Greek, and Latin. He displayed a copy of this work, pointing out how some scholars had criticized it. This lecture pleased Prichard's father when it gained national notice in the *Gentleman's Magazine*. Less pleasing was Johann Spurzheim's sell-out BI course of twelve lectures on phrenology in 1827, which Prichard countered a few years later with his own lecture critical of mesmerism and that upstart science. After his 1828 lecture on pestilences, Prichard's next contribution was so successful he was urged to publish a book on the subject; the following year he brought out *Review of the Doctrine of a Vital Principle*.[19]

Deprived of the benefits of London and Oxbridge, Prichard pinned his hopes on the Phil & Lit. With himself clearly in mind, he asked the BI's 1828 annual general meeting whether "it would not advance the cause of science, and increase the respectability of the Institution, to appoint *Professors* as Lecturers in the various departments." He imagined the BI as the foundation of a university, providing facilities, scientific recognition, and dignity. After a great deal of discussion, the society unanimously resolved to consider his proposal—but it was quietly dropped. There would be no "Professor Prichard."[20]

The BI did not flourish. By 1829 its shares were changing hands at a considerable discount, causing the curator to complain that "there are more Shares in the Market than Philosophers in Bristol."[21] Soon, with 169 out of its 600 shares unoccupied, the BI was burdened with a debt of nearly £200. Its tangible assets had been a drag from the start, but its museum, which functioned as a diffuse depository for gentlemen's "collections," its sparse library, basic scientific apparatus, dwindling membership subscriptions, dearth of lecturers, sporadic annual reports, and its short-lived journal also point to its ever-parlous state. Outsiders considered the BI's collection of specimens not as good as boasted.[22]

The intellectual climate of the region did not improve, and Bristol merchants and bankers, distracted by their own economic stresses during the 1830s and 1840s, neglected the Institution. Several members gave their lectures gratis for the benefit of its funds; for example, Prichard and Clark's 1834 lectures raised £71, 6 pence. Upon deserting Bristol for London, Prichard was voted honorary member in 1846. The BI and Phil & Lit events continued sporadically. The Bristol Institution struggled on, missing a later opportunity to gain security by amalgamating with the Bristol Library, and sorely in need of subscribers, it gradually slid downmarket, some shares falling into the hands of mere tradesmen. Another development took its toll on it: instead of science being accommodated under a single umbrella institution like the BI, as the nineteenth century progressed, so did the proliferation of single-issue scientific societies such as the Bristol Microscopical Society, the Statistical Society, and the Archaeological Society. This fragmentation of science diverted support from the generalist BI.[23]

For a time, the Bristol Institution served as a venue for public intellectual activity, a mark of elite Bristol culture and a bastion of natural theology. It provided a social structure around which some other initiatives took shape such as the Bristol College and the 1836 meeting of the British Association for the Advancement of Science. But as its lectures generally lacked practical application to industry and its facilities were limited in scope, the BI remained a pleasant, mostly scientific, elite, harmonious, Christian society. Later in the century it faded from existence.

A Holiday among the Appalling French, September 3, 1823

Back in 1823, when the Bristol Institution was just being launched, Prichard must have surprised even himself by risking a journey through conservative Britons' terra incognita, if not *terra horribilus*—France. He had been poring over several of the Bristol Library's volumes describing the wonders of the Alps and decided to trace their authors' routes, accompanied by his wife, Anna Maria, and a relative, Mr. Grundy. They cheerfully set out, destination Mont Blanc, keen to drink in the wonders of nature—and meet some famous scholars and scientists, of course. The couple took it in turns to describe their progress and impressions in a joint diary of their trip. It candidly documents their thorough dislike and suspicion of anything French as they struggled on their dusty, wearisome journey on an array of execrable vehicles to their awesome destination. Both their route and attitude were typical of English tourists of the period.[24]

On September 3 they jostled their way by stagecoach to Southampton, where amid the noise, smoke, smells and bustle of the busy port they boarded one of the new steamboats bound for Le Havre. This short voyage across the channel afforded Prichard "scarcely any recollection: only a general, undefined impression of misery, greater than usual in a voyage." The holiday went on as it had started. The French were thoroughly "grotesque." The party first lodged in "a vile cabaret in the middle of a stinking street: passed thru a filthy kitchen, up a prodigious number of stairs to a little close apartment, where we opened the casements to admit air, loaded with the fetid exhalations of a street which answered the double purpose of a driving way and a common drain." While poor Prichard headed to bed to sleep off his seasickness, Anna and Mr. Grundy explored Le Havre and attempted to dine "with 7 or 8 french people, whose volubility of tongue, exceeded only by the rapidity with which they devoured dish after dish, quite bewildered me, not yet accustomed to a table d'hote." The next day, they endured what was to be the first of the nearly daily tasks of haggling over transport. So repulsive was the prospect of taking a steamboat up the Seine, they took seats on the "derriere of a Diligence" headed for Rouen, their carriage knocking the apples, pears, and plums from the trees along the narrow lanes.[25]

Occasionally, the suffering diarists grudgingly admitted to having seen a fairly pleasant view, but for the most part, France was condemned as mean, ugly, and filthy, the architecture undistinguished and devoid of gentlemen's residences, the people all seemingly of the "lower orders," the meals and inns utterly disgusting, and the rattling vehicles uncomfortable, exorbitantly priced, and exhausting to be in. Anna Maria attempted a positive sentence: "Caudebec is very romantically situated, and the bustle of the people, the singular costume of the women, who were all dressed in the high white Normandy Cap, short petticoat and wooden shoes, the eagerness of men women and children to dispose of their goods and to cheat the strangers formed an amusing scene." The exterior of Rouen Cathedral was magnificent, and she felt drawn to the site of William the Conqueror's tomb. But the people around her were "by no means remarkable for civility." Anna witnessed with mixed feelings a mass being said at the Abbey of Saint-Ouen and women attending confession.[26]

From Rouen, Prichard recorded the more tolerable views of vineyards, the "pleasant, gay town" of Louviers and a telling encounter with fellow passengers, one of whom was

> going to Paris on business, a great republican who disputed not a little with an old lady who was a warm adherent of the royal and catholic cause. The woman had the best of the argument and declaimed against the demoralization of France with much eloquence. "How many fathers do you think there are now in F. who teach their children religion or morality?" The man acknowledged that this was not the care of the men. The old lady talked about the misfortune of the English, "Qui ont perdu la foi" and I took occasion to tell her that the English never hold markets on a Sunday, and that the men go to church as well as the women.

Prichard damned Paris as "fitter for the ancient Romans than for a congregation of petits maitres, harlequins and men-cooks." Securing their passports, they set out on the overnight mail coach for Dijon.[27] At the best inn in Troyes they were subjected to the indignity of dining in the same room as the guard of the mail and his companions, who "roared, swore and scolded like so many bedlamites, while they devoured a meal sufficient for so many bears which had just issued from their winter dens and swallowed a proportional quantity of wine." Prichard enjoyed recording another example of French character: "the Mercury who conducted us found no little difficulty lighting his candles owing to a violent wind. This so disconcerted him that he exhibited a fine specimen of french petulance and violence—swore, exclaimed, stamped in the most furious manner and at last absolutely cried like a child. I never saw such a want of self government in any other country. I believe from this and other circumstances which have come under my notice or have been related to me, that even the Irish have generally more restraint on the ebullitions of temper than the French."[28]

Beyond Châtillon the countryside became somewhat more picturesque, but they could not stop more than once a day for refreshment. They found the towns and inns as horrible as the inhabitants themselves. Dijon had not a single good street, nor any gentlemen's carriages and dwellings. In an exorbitant hired unsprung charabanc, they bumped to Dole, where Anna described a meal in a kitchen swarming with cockroaches, a hot bedroom "smelling just like a dripping pan," and their haggling for "a Char a Cote, to take us to Geneva for 100 francs." Dusty roads and vineyards eventually gave way to mountain views as they approached Poligny at the foot of the

Jura Mountains. After French vermin-filled beds, bad dinners, and abominable impositions, Prichard found the Swiss civil, "more like English than French, [with] clean and airy apartments and everything that an antigallican, after breathing the dust and wallowing in the filth of France[,] most anxiously wishes for."[29]

Instead of being treated to breathtaking views of the Alps from the shore of Lake Geneva, all was shrouded in mist, so the little party skipped a visit to the local Roman ruins and jogged on to Geneva through the drenching rain. Prichard decided he might just tolerate living in Switzerland.[30] A distinctly pleasurable day in Geneva then unfolded. He was fortunate to have a letter of introduction to Professor Marc-Auguste Pictet. This highly respected elderly Swiss scientist was editor of a periodical that published translations of British and other European scientific literature. He kindly took his visitors to see the curiosities at the great public library, including some illuminated manuscripts and a pile of John Calvin's original correspondence. Prichard enjoyed being introduced to a Homeric scholar, chargé d'affaires of the Holy See at Geneva. But he was "rather scandalized at espying by the side of some original pictures of the Reformers, a bust of Jean Jacques and particularly at observing that these degenerate descendants of the stern Jack were even more proud of the polluted Sophist than of their citizens who were among the foremost champions of religious liberty. But they are now rational enlightened people. However as the pastors complain of the growth of methodism we may hope that a different way of thinking may gain ground & that the bust of Jean Jacques may be burnt for quick lime."[31]

Like so many tourists to Geneva, Prichard, Anna, and Grundy were drawn to an enterprising citizen's must-see scale model of the Alps. With a long pointing stick he directed them on a tour through its passes, describing everything as if they were actually traveling through the mountains. Back to reality, they set off for Chamonix the following day, their fog-shrouded goal ahead of them. This leg of the journey took them out of the (Protestant) Swiss canton and into (Roman Catholic) "dominions of a royal potentate, the miserable extortionate king of Savoy, Sardinia &c. Everything had the appearance of discontent and bad government: the people we had to do with were often the example of their master, knavish & insatiable." En route to Sallanches, they marveled at the cascades of Nant d'Arpenaz dashing and foaming into the beautiful countryside, a scene Prichard sharply contrasted to the squalid, old, wretched, dirty town where he had to pay "an extravagant price for vile accommodations to a cringing sycophant who endeavoured to curry favour while he was cheating us." In another pricey charabanc, they looked forward to seeing the romantic scenery ahead and were not disappointed, despite being harassed by the rustics' petulant begging.[32]

The vale of Chamonix was absolutely stunning, and at the foot of the Mont Blanc Massif,

> the heat of the midday Sun at length dissipated the mist and opened what we might term a way thro the sky: midway between the plane of the horizon and the zenith we discovered first the snowy side of the High Alps on which the sun was shining. Notwithstanding all that we had read and imagined of the height of mountains, we found it difficult at first to believe our own eyes when we saw a vast mass of the earth thus raised among the clouds, and almost above our heads. We descended into the level valley of Chamouny, by a declivity indescribably beautiful: the whole range of the High Alps immediately in our front, with clouds below their summits, and glaciers reflecting the light of the sun with scarcely diminished splendor between the dark masses of the projecting mountains. . . . Thro' the valley we now descended along the side of the avenue to the Priory, where we got an excellent reception at the Union Inn, and getting mules and a guide, the weather being fine immediately set out to visit Montanvert and the Mer de Glace.

After a few miles the mules started climbing like cats up a rough track through the trees. They dismounted at a visitors' tent for some wine, then took up alpenstocks and ventured onto the sea of ice:

> Of the scene we now witnessed no description can convey any idea. A vast river of ice and snow coming down from the sky, with their shining clouds or rather mists flitting over all the higher and more distant parts. As they dispersed momentarily and the sun shone thro them we caught a view of the mountain tops above, shooting their black pyramidal points which are termed aiguilles or needles partly covered with shining snow. . . . The sea of ice itself was of all colours, blue, sea green and red. Immense fissures in it opened beneath our feet passages which appeared to lead into an unfathomable gulph. . . . We descended immediately from Montanvert by the help of long poles, rather jumping than walking down a declivity almost precipitous.[33]

Fifteen days of arduous travel had taken them across the channel, through Paris to Geneva and up breathtaking Mont Blanc. The Prichards' diary ends abruptly on the glacier.

Therapeutics and Theology, Friends, Family, and Foes, 1824 and 1825

After his Continental holiday, Prichard settled back into professional life and private research in Bristol. He kept the Bristol Library porter busy bringing him travel books, natural histories, several biographies of clerics, and Thomas Young's newly published *Account of Recent Discoveries in Hieroglyphical Literature, and Egyptian Antiquities*. He needed that one for his upcoming Bristol Institution lecture. He was also working on a revised edition of *Physical History*, so he sent his brother-in-law Alfred Estlin to a London map dealer to exchange his old engraved maps for some more useful ones, such as d'Anville's atlas of the ancient world.[34]

That autumn Prichard penned a short article on quite another topic, sending "Remarks on the Treatment of Paralysis, and Some Other Diseases, by Issues and Blisters" to the *London Medical Repository* on November 29. This article made quite a splash in Britain and on the Continent, promoted his recent book on nervous diseases, and encouraged him to continue his research on this topic.[35]

In 1824, as Prichard worked to get the Bristol Institution off the ground, he was distracted by his father and Aunt Newman's issues; the latter's depression Prichard attributed to ill health. Prichard delighted his father with John Wesley's *Sermons*. The dispute with his daughter's in-laws behind them, Thomas Prichard looked forward to his yearly sojourn of several summer months with the Molines. There he enjoyed the company of Mary's growing family and his days spent in their cozy library. He even fancied trying the newfangled steam ferry that had recently started plying the Bristol Channel between Chepstow and Bristol.[36]

That year Prichard got involved in some initiatives that were out of character. The idea of gas lighting had got off the ground, and he joined the management committee of a company promising to supply a greatly improved type of gas lighting to Bristol homes.[37] He also got caught up in a distant political struggle stirring the Romantic imagination of Britons; he helped establish the Bristol branch of the London Philhellenic Committee. The plucky Greeks' long struggle for independence from Ottoman control had recently become a cause célèbre for some educated Europeans and Americans, not the least owing to the growing fashion for Hellenism, an engrained respect for classical civilization (and distrust of their non-Christian Turkish oppressors). Lord Byron's poem on the subject and his active and financial support of the Greek freedom fighters effectively promoted their cause. The Whig-backed London Greek Committee's plan to fund a revolution held little appeal to the Tory government. When the committee's agents started proselytizing in the provinces, Prichard's Whig friend Conybeare became actively involved, and to his surprise, so did some Bristol conservative gentlemen such as Prichard. Only the very wealthy of Bristol seemed unmoved by the "Cause of the Greeks."[38]

Prichard chaired the inaugural meeting of the Greek Committee's Bristol branch at the *Felix Farley's Bristol Journal* office on January 24, attended by thirteen men, four of whom were clergymen and most of whom were friends such as Conybeare, Eden, Seyer, Bright, and Elton. They launched a public appeal for donations and produced a rousing manifesto. For the sake of Christianity and the civil liberties of the downtrodden representatives of a glorious ancient civilization, the barbaric, despotic Turks had to be defeated. Bristol patriots were exhorted to add their mite to the cause.[39] But just as interest in the cause of the Greeks started growing in Bristol, it started waning in London. The whole affair was a touchy political subject for the government, finding the freedom fighters as deplorable as their oppressors. It then became apparent that huge donations and loans had been grossly mismanaged and squandered. British panhellenists' enthusiasm fizzled out, and Prichard later considered the organization corrupt.[40]

During the summer of 1824 Prichard was deep into writing about the Celts and the peoples of the Middle East for *Physical History* while Anna and the children were holidaying at the Estlin seaside home in Southerndown. When he finally joined them, barely fit to travel following an illness, his father knew where to pin the blame yet again: "it has been brought on by too close application, which for want of thy monitor [Anna], may have been pursued to excess. . . . I should be glad to see a second and enlarged edition of thy Researches, but I cannot recommend thee to much laborious employment of thy head & thy pen for some time to come." As for James Jr.'s illness, his grandfather diagnosed overstudy too. Like father, like son.[41]

Thomas Prichard closely monitored his son for lapses in spiritual reflection, and he continued to needle him about the corrupting tendencies of Establishment clergy. After reading hardly any religious commentaries for some months, Prichard incensed his father by announcing that "I have no doubt that every thing is predestined in its proper place and time." Predestination smacked of Calvinism. Had he picked up this notion in Geneva the previous year? Prichard dug himself into a hole attempting to explain his position, only strengthening his father's view that the notion of predestination served to "undeify the Deity." But about politics, they were in accord when Thomas Prichard penned: "I am afraid the death of the present Louis of France, will be followed by an exhibition of character which will do the French nation no credit. I cannot help fancying that France & Spain are verging towards the limits of that desolation prepared for Popery & its adherents."[42]

In the autumn father and son resumed working their way through Christian literature, such as the seventeenth-century divine John Lightfoot's weighty *Opera Omnia*. Prichard's enthusiasm for the new Bristol Institution earned him a stern parental warning of the perils of materialist science: how vain are men's attempts to understand and explain natural phenomena independently of Scripture! Some knowledge is beyond human understanding. His father's lecture had been brought on by reading *Essay on Instinct, and Its Physical and Moral Relations*, by Prichard's university friend Thomas Hancock. He reminded his son of his duty to uphold Scripture in the face of any doubts and temptations to skepticism that he might encounter. The Bristol Institution must be a platform for Christian science.

The year 1825 was one of conflict, reflection, loss, and research. Battles at the Bristol Infirmary were sapping Prichard's energy. Ill will among the members of the faculty and with the administration came to a boil, precipitating the mass resignation of its surgeons and physicians. The ensuing drawn-out, publicly aired dispute ended in compromise, the resignations were withdrawn, and the dust settled—for a time.[43]

Amid these hostilities, Prichard took refuge in making translations of Greek and Latin religious verse and sending them to his father. He also wrote an essay on the ancestry of Jesus, which a pleased Thomas Prichard promised to "take care that it has a place in the Christian Observer."[44] This anonymous article exercised Prichard's proclivity to collect, coordinate, and analyze; in six closely argued pages he tidied up the account of the Blessed Virgin's ancestry by untangling ancient genealogies and chronologies. To correct errors and reconcile the gospels of Saints Matthew and Luke, he drew on theologians from the third century to the most recent authors. In the course of this he dismissed Joseph's genealogy as biologically irrelevant and finished by claiming that "our Lord was really of the seed of David" and Mary herself was the daughter of Heli, a descendant of Adam. This fitted nicely with God's promising Adam an "avenger come of woman."[45]

As for Prichard's friendships, John Eden, vicar of St. Nicholas and St. Leonard's Church and minor canon of the Bristol Cathedral, was active in the Bristol Institution and Library Society. He and Prichard particularly enjoyed discussing Christian history and theology and sharing their translations of classical texts and sacred poetry.⁴⁶ It was certainly not Unitarianism that bound Prichard in friendship with James Yates. This independently wealthy, former Unitarian minister was devoted to antiquarianism, the future field of archaeology. During the 1820s and 1830s they corresponded and met at the British Association for the Advancement of Science meetings. Prichard could only dream of Yates's scholarly life of leisure; when told of his friend's plan to study abroad, he replied candidly: "I could envy you the prospect which you have before you of joining the society of such men as you will find in Berlin. I pay many penalties for being a physician & none more irksome than the almost total alienation from the society which I should most desire." At least he got Yates to obtain some books and information while in Berlin.⁴⁷

Undergoing tough times in New Jersey, Tom Prichard might have better appreciated more practical gifts than an engraved portrait of his successful brother. Family and friends had much admired Nathan Cooper Branwhite's portrait of Prichard in oils, so an engraving of it was made for distribution.⁴⁸ In other American news, Thomas Prichard's erstwhile friend pious-Quaker-turned-atheist Morris Birkbeck, had lured relative Samuel Prichard's family to his utopian settlement in the United States. On learning Birkbeck had accidentally drowned on a visit to Robert Owen's utopian New Harmony, Indiana, Thomas Prichard could only regret Birkbeck's delusion as to the natural goodness of human beings. Prichard more harshly considered such socialist leanings a form of mania.

Relative Josiah Merrick nearly drowned, too, in a close shave with new technology. While crossing the Humber the steamboat he was on ran afoul of a brig, the shock of which stove in the timbers, threw down the mast and chimney, and burst the boiler in a hellish scene of devastation. Lucky Josiah lived to tell the tale. Even luckier Uncle Lewis sold his estates and retired from medicine to the life of a gentleman. Prichard and his father discussed their relatives' fortunes, far and wide.⁴⁹

The scourge of tuberculosis was ever-present in Prichard's life, professionally and personally. It took a Bristol colleague and a relative in 1825. Infirmary Apothecary William Swayne was a conscientious medical officer, firm adherent of heroic therapeutics, and an exemplary student of morbid anatomy; he systematically and effectively dissected nearly every Infirmary fatality. After a stay in Barbados failed to alleviate the symptoms of *phthisis pulmonalis*, he returned to Bristol to a slow and painful Christian death. Prichard composed his obituary memoir for the Bristol newspapers, and in it he stressed Swayne's freedom from "the baneful skepticism, often reputed to the medical profession, which darkens and embitters the mind."[50] Prichard's promising young brother-in-law shared Swayne's fate. Infirmary pupil and champion body snatcher Edward Rochemont Estlin had been his brother John's intended medical partner. When just twenty-two and barely able to carry out his duties, he managed to keep a most affecting diary charting his deterioration, futile sojourn in Barbados, and return to Bristol to surrender himself to God's will. His exemplary Victorian "good death" obituary spared no details, including his sudden hemorrhage and cry, "Pray for me—it is all over."[51] Prichard's more pleasant tasks around this time involved providing references for former Infirmary students and MD testimonials for local colleagues.[52]

In the autumn of 1825, while infant Augustin was dangerously ill, Thomas Prichard moaned about his own ill health. This time it had been brought on by social unrest and the national economic crisis, precipitated by a rash of speculative commercial ventures and the policies of the Bank of England. Upward of seventy British banks failed that year. Would there be a run on Ross Bank, on which his wealth and reputation and his son Edward's occupation depended? He was in an "agony of suspense" over this threat and the disgrace his bank's failure would bring. Luckily, its depositors did not lose faith in the Quaker firm, and the bank survived. Thomas Prichard returned to his theology and anxiety over Tom's harsh New Jersey winter ahead, asking Prichard to send his brother some household goods and the usual bank draft.[53] Perhaps the happiest event of the year was the birth of the Prichards' son Illtudus Thomas on December 16.

The Medical Profession in Transition, January 1826

In an era when the medical profession was in the process of being radically reshaped, professional disputes were rife. Prichard's quarrels were typical of the time and not confined to the Infirmary. Ever conscious of his professional dignity, he fell out with a Bristol medical man, MD, and proud member of the Royal College of Physicians, whose transgression, to Prichard's mind, was to practice simultaneously as a physician and surgeon. It started in January, when Dr. David Davies requested that Prichard join him in a consultation on his patient. Having ascertained that Davies had been acting as a physician, Prichard acidly replied in formal English: "Dr. Prichard presents his compliments to Dr Davies, and is very sorry that he is under the necessity of declining to meet Dr. Davies in consultation as a Physician, Dr. Davies being a Surgeon, witness his appointment to St. Peter's Hospital. Dr. P. begs to assure Dr. Davies that nothing disparaging to him or his professional character is intended by Dr. Prichard, who is solely activated by a necessary regard to customary modes of proceeding in thus declining to meet Dr. Davies."[54]

As if breaching medical etiquette wasn't bad enough, Davies was poaching patients who should have been paying physicians' fees to properly practicing MDs. This spat over demarcation went public, of course. Prichard laid out the superior claims of physicians in a series of letters to the editor of *Felix Farley's Bristol Journal* and Davies, like a dog with a bone, topped it with a pamphlet detailing the whole sorry episode, namely the patient's injured feelings; the Act of Parliament allowing Davies to practice in both capacities; precedents for his mode of practice; and Prichard's unlicensed status as a physician outside of London. Davies threatened further action to boot. Faced with these valid points, Prichard uncharacteristically refrained from having the last word, and two months of public quarreling ended with no apparent detriment to either's reputation.[55] This argument over professional etiquette is symptomatic of the general disarray in medical philosophy, education, and regulation during medicine's long period of modernization and reform.

Prichard could well remember his childhood encounters with medicine. When anyone in his circle became ill, a doctor would be summoned and expected to prescribe treatments so dramatic in their effects, they were noticed by the entire household; purging, vomiting, blistering, bleeding, "low diet," and cold water affusions, the armory of heroic therapeutics, were favored by his family. Then, while a student at Dr. Pope's, Prichard briefly encountered the opposing "expectant," supportive form of treatment, involving warmth, food, fortifying drinks, and tonics. At Edinburgh Prichard's fellow medical student Henry Holland had his doubts about both:

> I am often disposed to regret that I cannot increase my faith in the efficacy of Medicine, & in the value of the functions which the physician performs. I confess to you that the more I look into the matter, the more does my confidence diminish; and if it were allowable to apply numbers to express an opinion of this kind, I should say that four fifths of the medical practice which I see going on around me, is either entirely nugatory, or something worse than nugatory. The quantum of quackery in regular practice is really very great. I have been more especially struck with this (& my companions have partaken in the sentiment) in making these preparations for our approaching examination. It is amusing to observe the great diversity of opinion,

not only as to the theory, but also upon the practice proper to every disease; & the equally positive declarations of success from modes of treatment diametrically the reverse of each other. In the statements too with respect to the value of particular medicines, there is often something infinitely ridiculous—what is extolled by one set as next to infallible in particular cases, is censured by others as perfectly inert—and while one physician celebrates the success of a couple of grains, another is giving the very same medicine in doses of fifteen times the amount.[56]

Unlike Dr. Holland, Prichard seemed confident in his choice of heroic medical therapeutics.

There was an element of ceremony in a doctor's visit that comforted and inspired faith as patients saw the doctor take complex measures on their behalf. Physicians possessed profound understanding of the inscrutable interior of the human body based on arcane principles, the application of which necessarily required a prescription and a substantial fee. Extreme effects of treatment showed the doctor was doing something tangible. As late as the 1830s, physicians rarely physically examined patients and were slow to adopt beneficial apparatus such as the stethoscope, speculum, and thermometer. The more successful and fashionable the physician, the more likely he would do little more than look after the general well-being of his patients, a prime example being Sir Henry Holland, who with minimal faith in physic could still become physician to royalty and senior politicians.[57]

Although medicine could stimulate or facilitate the natural actions of the body, it could not alter the natural functions of recovery or decay. So if a patient died, it was not for want of their physicians' palpable efforts; it was the result of uncorrectable disequilibrium. Doctors were protective of their remedies; informative medical periodicals only gradually became popular during Prichard's lifetime. New nosologies boasting impressive Linnaean-styled Latin terms like the ones Carrick and Prichard listed at the Clifton Dispensary led to proliferation of classifications and confusion. Medical men keen on making a name for themselves also propounded extravagant and contentious remedies requiring increasingly bold and extreme treatments.[58] By contrast, there was minimal interest in determining the cause of disease; patients paid to be cured of symptoms rather than educated in the etiology of some abstract condition.

Prichard could hardly have been comfortable with the coexistence of two diametrically opposed approaches to medical therapeutics, nor was he complacent about the state of medicine in general. Where was the science in medicine? Unlike progress in chemistry and geology, for decades medicine had been all but stagnant; an ancient Greek physician would have felt at home with early nineteenth-century medical philosophy. The less prestigious practice of surgery, on the other hand, had been making strides owing to improvements in anatomy education, war casualties providing plenty of practice, and the greater technical quality of surgical instruments that allowed a range of procedures to be completed quickly and efficiently on unanesthetized patients. Operative procedures steadily became bolder and more sophisticated, despite the risk of sepsis. It was not until decades after Prichard's death that modern surgery was revolutionized by the introduction of anesthesia and antisepsis.[59]

Prichard and his fellow medical men published their innovative treatments, but they were at a loss to explain how they worked. One idea was based on the observation that what effectively controlled a symptom in one disease might do so in another. He had faith that medicine would make strides equal to those of surgery; properly conducted science would result in better understanding of the causes of disease. In the meantime, the medical philosophy of the ancients held sway, its cornerstone the notion of the body's humors. Prichard adhered to humoral medical theory and heroic therapeutics for lack of an effective alternative. It had the weight of centuries in its favor.

Whether medical practitioners employed heroic or expectant remedies, their understanding of illness was founded on analysis of the general workings of the human body. When Prichard was being educated, the body was thought to function as a series of input and output events; illness was caused by an imbalance in secretions arising from the body's four humors. There had been little further development of this ancient philosophy of physiology and health other than some recent elaborations such as "excitement" of blood or muscles, "corpuscular flow," "determination," and "debilitation." Humoral medicine premised on equilibrium meant that health is restored by stimulating a physiological reaction while simultaneously managing diet, allowing for the age, situation, and the patient's character. Diagnosis and treatment were therefore systemic because patients are more than the sum of their body parts or any discernible morbidity.

Rebalance of the system is achieved by regulating secretions, echoing natural bodily evacuations of blood, urine, feces, and perspiration. After all, the body itself functions similarly in the course of illness, such as in its excretions of vomiting, sweating, and diarrhea. For example, by the 1830s, second to bloodletting, physicians widely advocated the use of mercury. Because mercury stimulates secretion, notably in its laxative and salivatory effect, it must counteract inflammation, the object of treatment. Medicine confined itself to managing particular diseases and their symptoms.

Even when a condition had an obvious local cause or, as in the case of inoculation, did not fit into the accepted forms of treatment, doctors would elaborate their prescriptions with a regimen of cathartics and diet. It was a matter of personal choice whether they favored expectant treatment or took heroic, drastic measures to rebalance patients' systems. Designed to manipulate the patient's general constitution, humoral medicine was a holistic, comprehensible system in an era before the biological or physical causes of illness and disease were understood.[60]

Expectant therapeutics did not imply doctors' inertia or disbelief in heroic treatment. Its advocates understood that most diseases debilitated and exhausted the vital excitement of the system. The body required support with stimulants such as alcohol, opium, and Peruvian bark (quinine). Lacking the reassuringly dramatic effects on patients that rival heroic treatment offered, during the early part of the century it lost ground. These two modes of treatment might have contrasted greatly, but they were based on a shared philosophy of medicine that gave little incentive to investigate the actual causes of disease.

There Will Be Blood: Prichard's Heroic Armory

Heroic medicine was championed by Edinburgh men in particular.[61] They published a steady stream of influential volumes on bloodletting, and other heroic forms of treatment. Student Prichard ordered James Hamilton on purgative medicine, James Currie on cold water in fever, and William Cullen's *First Lines* from his London bookseller.[62] He attended Dr. James Gregory's Practice of Medicine course, where almost every condition demanded bleeding and purging.[63] Another Edinburgh physician, Benjamin Welsh, wrote about an epidemic of fever in that city in a book titled *A Practical Treatise on the Efficacy of Bloodletting*. Welsh, an acolyte of Prichard's teacher Dr. Hamilton, accused the great physicians William Cullen and John Brown of having held back progress by casting doubt on bleeding for fever. Welsh even provided a history of the bloodletting revival, citing American Benjamin Rush as the preeminent proponent of copious bleeding.[64]

This heroic approach was enthusiastically advocated in 1807 by the eminent London physician Henry Clutterbuck, particularly for fever. His

Lectures on Blood-Letting in the 1820s does not explain why it works but describes it as a sort of countershock to the system. Another physician hazarded: "bleeding to syncope, during the active stage of inflammation, diminishes, in a great degree, the power of the brain and nervous system; and, as a consequence of this, the action of the heart and arteries; so that the blood is carried with less force into their capillary extremities, than it was previously to the bleeding; subduing thereby active inflammation."[65] Tackling inflammation, no matter how subtle, was central to heroic medicine. Prichard's prime bloodletting role model was Dr. John Armstrong, an Edinburgh contemporary who in 1816 claimed success in bleeding away congestion, though he urged caution in the late stage of fever. His excellent reputation arose from his publications on puerperal, typhus, and other fevers, whose inflammatory nature demanded copious bleeding.[66]

Although he was committed to bleeding for fever and other conditions, Prichard's interest in blood did not always involve its extraction. While he was inordinately fond of self-bleeding, he did not experiment on himself when it came to the novelty of transfusing blood. One heroic pronouncement brought him international notice; he claimed "that many lives may be saved by injecting good blood into the veins of exhausted patients."[67] Bleeding had until only recently been carried out as a seasonal prophylactic, and it was often prescribed to achieve "relief"; Prichard's unhappy brother Tom would beg for it. Their father felt he had to ration his own more restrained form of bleeding: "I am endeavouring by the use of blisters occasionally to my head, to diminish the frequency of leechings: it is now more than six weeks I believe, since I used the latter remedy: an extraordinary interval of late: but my head at night begins to remind me that I must not longer defer the use of the leech." Prichard preferred taking the more efficient lancet to himself, and so boldly as to alarm even his father.[68] When reading his son's criticism of hypochondriacs, Thomas Prichard teased: "but as thou art, as well as myself, something of an experimentalist among the varieties of the Pharmacopoeia, I am content to take my share with thee."[69]

Prichard would order various methods of bleeding depending on a patient's condition. General bloodletting was done with a lancet to the arm or temple, while local bloodletting focused on the site of the ailment and required more precise control. "Wet-cupping," done by creating a vacuum with a special heated glass enhanced by a multiple-bladed lancing device, effectively sucked a glass full of blood from the patient, while "dry cupping" merely reddened the unbroken skin. Prichard fearlessly prescribed the lancet and leeches. But as each little leech extracted only about an ounce of blood, they were applied in groups or relays, or at set intervals from one to twenty at a time. Being slow suckers, they were more appropriate for children, weaker patients, and those with certain conditions such as menstrual problems for which Prichard prescribed leeches to the groin.[70] The leech business thrived in Bristol.

Prichard prescribed the most vigorous forms of treatment he could for the poor of the local medical charities and his private patients alike. If, for instance, a postoperative cataract patient was suffering from pain, bleeding to twelve ounces was ordered, as was the judicious placing of leeches. Dr. Symonds described Prichard's approach diplomatically: "He weighed their symptoms anxiously, and was most conscientious in carrying out the appropriate treatment. He was particularly successful with cases that required a decided uncompromising line of action; and his boldness, consistency, and fearlessness met with their best rewards. Of the little matters of detail that must have their share of attention in many cases, he was rather impatient. He liked in practice . . . broad views rather than a fine analysis of symptoms and minutiae of treatment."[71]

These "uncompromising" treatments drove one of Prichard's patients to verse:

> You'll want some news—Well, first poor me
> Have been unlucky, as you'll see.
> For full five times I've leeches had,
> Five blisters too, almost as bad,
> Then medicines of all sorts and kind
> Enough to suit each different mind,
> At last the issue of it all
> Was in my arm an issue small,
> And tho' I am not yet quite well
> Of progress I at least may tell,
> And hope that surely very soon
> Perhaps before the next new moon,
> That Harrison and Prichard's firm
> Will stop their business for a term.
> No time is fix'd for us to go,
> Uncertain like all else below.
> To Doctors of all men alone
> The name of mercy is not known.[72]

As well as bloodletting, Prichard favored using counterirritants. A moxa was made of a corrosive substance fixed to the skin of the affected area to burn it, and the subcutaneous implantation of an irritative seton was even more drastic and long-lasting in its suppurating action. He famously refined and published on the drastic counterirritant dubbed the "tomahawk," or "Prichard issue." His son Augustin rather proudly recalled:

> My father originated the plan of making the long issue in the scalp in Brain diseases; and although a strong remedy, it was sometimes undoubtedly the means of saving life. A cut was rapidly made with a sharp scalpel, through the thickness of the scalp from just above the occipital protuberance to the edge of the hair in front, and filled with a string of peas, which soon set up the needed suppuration as counterirritation to the morbid process going on within the skull. We had, in addition, not unfrequently to insert setons, or make an issue in the arm or elsewhere by incision or caustic.[73]

Counterirritation restored patients' humoral balance. It drew the morbid excitement from elsewhere in the body to itself, where they drained the body of morbid matter. Use of the "tomahawk issue" spread beyond the Bristol Infirmary when Prichard advocated it in articles published in 1824 and 1831. His use of it for hemiplegia was cited in American, French, German, and Italian medical periodicals.[74] He further promoted it in a paper read to the medical section of the British Association for the Advancement of Science meeting in Bristol in 1836, when he claimed its efficacy in adjusting the vascular condition of the brain by lessening the "hypoplethoric" state of the blood vessels; he regretted it was the only intervention that medical knowledge allowed at that time. Doctors wrote approvingly of "the tomahawk practice of Bristol" as a powerful remedy for formidable diseases and superior to setons, blisters, or moxas. Prichard's advocacy of counterirritation attracted international coverage.[75]

Medical Progress

Recurring typhus, gnawing tuberculosis, and the arrival of cholera in the early 1830s spurred some improvements in public health during Prichard's lifetime. The rich started demanding solutions, especially as these diseases spread among themselves as well as the poor. In this era of pre-biological medicine, although it was understood that physical contact could spread disease, doctors still referred to ancient Galenic miasmic theory: putrefying materials caused atmospheric corruption, leading to infection among people with predisposing conditions such as malnutrition. Lingering belief in miasma and lack of systematic investigation hampered progress in understanding contagious disease.

Prichard was tasked with reporting on medical progress in his speech to a meeting of the Provincial Medical and Surgical Association in 1835. Some new ideas were making waves in the medical world, though Prichard's frustration with the lack of tangible progress is apparent. He started by rounding on some outmoded, fanciful theories concocted by the safely deceased Scottish physicians Cullen and Brown, and he reminded his audience of the scientific invalidity of phrenology, his customary jab. He then turned to some recent advances in medicine and medical technology, especially in mental illness and the physiology and pathology of the nervous system, having himself published on these subjects. As for the important issue of contagion, he equivocated, referring his audience to the writings of his friends Drs. Hancock and Symonds. Getting to his main point, he called for a disciplined, scientific approach to medical research. Progress would be made if medical men more systematically studied the history of diseases and applied technology, carried out dissections, experimented, and compiled and analyzed data using statistically sound techniques. Of course, he stressed that the truths of science and religion were compatible and would continue to be revealed.[76]

During the second quarter of the century interest turned more to the prevention of disease, or at least its spread. Infectious disorders comprised a large part of medical practice. While their associated inflammation and fever were the subjects of varying theories and treatment regimes, most medics agreed on the benefits of disease prevention and control, as Prichard did in his call for a fever hospital in Bristol. The deleterious effect of poor ventilation was most often cited. Steps were taken to implement improved hospital ventilation, a hygienic measure the Bristol Infirmary was noted for even while patients suffering from different diseases were put in shared beds.[77]

Medical progress lagged behind that of other forms of science and technology, but not for want of effort. Some doctors did collect case histories, employ empirical methods, and share their observations. Prichard's early publications of typhus and epilepsy case histories and his blood transfusion experiment exemplify his own attempts. Nevertheless, entrenched suspicion of theorizing and disdain of hands-on experimentation continued to inhibit scientific medicine. Rather, the norm remained publishing monographs on single diseases, bristling with meticulous case histories and treatment regimens but with little appetite for etiology.

Heroic and expectant therapeutics continued for lack of practicable alternatives, nor would doctors admit that previous practice had been wrong, as this would lessen confidence in the profession. When the key practice of bloodletting did wane, some agreed with Dr. William Pulteney Alison's "change in type" theory, which held that bloodletting had declined because the nature of inflammations themselves had changed, making the treatment less effective.[78] Patients' constitutions had also changed from robust to feeble: modern conveniences had rendered people too soft to be bled.[79] Some controlled clinical trials revealed bloodletting's low rate of cure. Heroic therapeutics in general also faced growing competition from "alternative" practitioners such as homeopaths, hydropaths, healers, and quacks who provided cheaper and less painful treatments. The mid-nineteenth century turned out to be less an Age of Improvement in therapeutics than an age of therapeutic nihilism.[80]

The Doctor and His Patients

Being a physician was a tiring, time-consuming way for a gentleman to earn a living. Patients could call at Prichard's home, and house calls often took him out of Bristol, either by carriage or post chaise by day and by night. Most of his income came not from his own private patients but from being called into consultation by medical practitioners. He was particularly popular among the well-to-do of more distant Wales.[81] One Welsh patient got a friend's advice:

> Ascertain what day of the month the steamer starts for Bristol at 6 or 7 in the morning; having done this, write immediately to Dr. Prichard—Red Lodge, near Park street to enquire whether he will be at home on that day, as your time is valuable,—if he answers in the affirmative, start by the latest train the evening before, so that you may sleep at Cardiff and thus be in time for the morning voyage. In your letter to the Doctor you should give a most ample description of your symptoms, the duration of your illness, whether you have been under medical treatment and what that was, he will thus be prepared with some knowledge of the course you require, you will give him a sovereign and a shilling he will give you a prescription which on your return to Merthyr after turning out all your pockets you will find you have lost, imprison it therefore in the bottom of your fob—the journey and fee will cost about three pounds.[82]

Having taken the conventional approach to building a successful practice, Prichard was fortunate that it did not exclude his main scientific and scholarly interests—far from it. He noted that his nonmedical *Physical History of Man* (1813) had brought him more private patients, something that perplexed a visiting American physician who assumed that patients disapproved of physicians having avocations:

> Dr. Pritchard is so well known at Bristol, where he resides, and throughout Europe, for his scientific pursuits, and for his valuable publications on the collateral branches, as to induce me to ask, if such studies never interfered with his professional business, by inducing his patients to believe that he did not devote sufficient time to his legitimate and proper concerns; to which he replied, certainly not, for although he every now and then came out with a book, or paper, on natural history, or some similar subject, he next appeared, perhaps, with a work on insanity, or something else so closely connected with his business, as to render it impossible for such an idea ever to enter their heads; and that, at any rate, so far from proving injurious, he believed it would be considered, by most of them, good ground for strengthening their confidence; inasmuch, as the more diversified and extended a man's knowledge was, provided he did not neglect his profession, the more entitled he should be to the character of a good physician.[83]

Patients were typically referred to Prichard by their family doctor. They paid for this consultation by discreetly leaving a guinea on the table. The bishop of Bristol and Gloucester, having the excuse of cataracts, made an embarrassing error in this regard. Augustin related: "One day, after a visit to the Red Lodge, he gave my father the fee wrapped up in paper as usual, but when opened it turned out to be two shillings, the bishop with his dimness of sight having mistaken a shilling for a sovereign; and at the next visit my father told him of the mistake, and told me afterwards that the bishop was so vexed and appeared to take it to heart so much, that if [Prichard] had known that would have been the case, he would never have said anything about it."[84]

A lady who had returned to Lancashire after having been under Prichard's care in Bristol wrote to him that she still felt unwell. He replied: "I was sorry to hear that your health is not reestablished. There is no disorder more disappointing to physicians as well as to patients than a disposition to frequent headaches, depending on the constitution, I have at this very time under my care a young lady from Scotland, whose case much resembled yours. I thought I had cured her by advising her almost to starve herself, leaving off all animal food &c, but the disorder after a long interval has again troubled her."[85]

Reputation and Family Life, 1826

Prichard was as concerned about his social status as his professional status. Exercising his passion for collecting information, he copied references from the Society of Friends registers of births, marriages, and deaths, corresponded about his ancestry with distant relatives, and constructed genealogical charts to compile a respectable pedigree. So prepared, he wanted tangible evidence of his family's status in the form of a coat of arms. He was informed that there were three available Prichard coats of arms already registered. He went for "Gules, A Fess, Or between 3 Escallops"—three rather modest-looking scallop shells.[86]

A long genealogical chart and a coat of arms added to the obvious pride Prichard had in his Welsh and Quaker background; researching these was satisfying in itself. Another satisfaction came in the form of a post-nominal FRS. With the publication of the second edition of *Physical History* in 1826 and supported by his friends Conybeare and Bright, he was nominated fellow of the Royal Society. This was a great honor and mark of his eminence in science, even if the society was at that time less of a progressive force in science than a source of prestige. Twenty-one years after student Prichard had the privilege of attending his first lecture at the Royal Society, he began the election procedure: notice of his candidacy posted at ten meetings between June 1, 1826, and February 1, 1827, led to his election the following week. In later years Prichard invited his friends to lectures at the Royal Society, and a copy of *Physical History* is in its library.[87]

Family concerns weighed on Prichard. His father had a lot to complain about in 1826, aside from his gout. Aunt Newman's mental health continued fragile and not at all helped by her husband's decision to quit Pearhill in Gayton, near Ross, a country home Thomas Prichard let to them cheaply. He soon disposed of this idyllic home, a source of Prichard's fondest childhood memories.[88] Meanwhile, from Bloomfield, New Jersey, came Tom's thanks for Prichard's invaluable recent supplies and bank draft for £30; it had been a bitter winter and spring of privation. He still hoped to establish himself as a surveyor and accountant, sanguine that land speculation sparked by the proposed Morris Canal passing through Bloomfield would profit him.

During the family's autumn visit to Ross, Anna was unwell and could manage only a walk in the garden, while according to Thomas Prichard, their son James sorely needed some fresh country air after his cramming. Even on holiday, the boy was made to grind away at his studies, with only a short break allowed to read his great-aunt Elizabeth's sensational three-decker novel *Waverley*. His grandfather claimed: "We are not idle though we do not fagg. I never was a great fagger, and now fagging is beyond my powers. I have found for James an Eton Grammar, so that you need not send one." His home became something of a schoolroom, as he was also engaged in teaching his son Edward's two children.[89]

Thomas Prichard's missives kept Prichard's nose to the theological grindstone too. They shared books on and corresponded about biblical history and Christian doctrine throughout 1826. George Stanley Faber's *Difficulties of Romanism*, the newly published bishop of Bristol's book on Tertullian's ecclesiastical history, John Wesley's *Travels*, and Ebenezer Henderson's *Biblical Researches and Travels in Russia* topped their reading list. Wesley's writing appealed to Thomas Prichard, especially as he had been slightly acquainted with the great father of Methodism. Politics came in for discussion as well; Prichard was lectured on the sorry state of governments' tendency to warfare and unchristian behavior. Unfortunately, "in a world like this, Christianity cannot prevail. If Christianity were allowed all its influence in changing the nature of Man we should hear of no more wars. This is fully allowed of writers of the Church." For both father and son, the "nature of Man" would remain forever disappointing.[90]

Prichard sent a copy of *Physical History* to his father for approval. The verdict arrived in mid-December:

> I have read thy book through and am much pleased and satisfied with it. There were a great many hard words which sent me to the medical dictionary, & some relating to Botany which I could not quite unravel. Some of thy English readers will complain for want of a translation to many passages in French, & it was very spiteful to bore one with so many German quotations. Thou hast forgotten thy spleen against the poor Dutchmen because their language was not intelligible to thee. Art thou quite right in saying that the Hebrew tenses are never formed by means of the verb substantive? . . . It is however more sparingly used than in other languages. I am astonished at the amazing quantity of matter collected from travellers in all parts of the world. Where didst thou meet with the necessary books for all these purposes?[91]

Obviously proud of his son's achievement, Thomas Prichard nevertheless chided him for showing off his proficiency in German.

As the year drew to a close, Prichard could reflect on recent events with a degree of satisfaction. He looked forward to Bristol's becoming a city of science and literature, fostered by the Bristol Institution and its elite Phil & Lit. The publication of the second edition of *Physical History* and a medical article and his election to the Royal Society assured his reputation as a physician and man of science. There had been some annoying professional squabbles, but there had also been a fascinating Continental holiday, the happy birth of another son, and frequent, intense, but rewarding correspondence with his father. Before starting his third edition of *Physical History*, he planned to do more medical research and make a notable foray into what would become known as biological theory. As for family responsibilities, Prichard found himself with several growing sons in need of an elite but affordable education that would prepare them for the University of Oxford. Another opportunity to improve Bristol came to mind.

10 · The Early Red Lodge Years

Improving Institutions and Publications, 1827–32

> It is only by the hand of man that any race of human beings has been exterminated; and perhaps we may add, that it is only by christian nations that such a work of total extermination has ever been totally accomplished.
> —J[ames] C[owles] P[richard], "Horae Africanae, No. 2"

The Red Lodge, Friends, and Family

"I really do not know what to say to the Red Lodge. Its external is certainly not inviting.—I always looked at it as only one remove from a prison. Yet it is very possible that it may be a good & roomy house. Its situation is sufficiently elevated. I suppose there are gardens to it. I would advise thee not to engage it on a long lease, so as not to be shackled with regard to future movements," wrote a perplexed Thomas Prichard.[1] Why would anyone want to move from upmarket Berkeley Square to a dusty, rambling ancient Tudor pile in a less fashionable part of Bristol? The Prichards took on the tenancy of a large, ancient house in need of redecoration and new life. As it turned out, the move to the Red Lodge in the summer of 1827 ushered in a new phase of family and professional life. The recent publication of the second edition of *Physical History* had furthered his national reputation as a scientist and his local reputation as an extraordinarily learned physician. Committed to using linguistics as a key to human history, Prichard resumed studying the Celtic languages. The Bristol Institution was surviving, if not thriving, so he offered to support it by giving a lecture on a controversial physiological theory. There was just so much that needed improving in Bristol as well. At home, there were sons to educate and their careers to secure; the death of another baby and Anna's protracted convalescence marred the start of the following year.

The Prichards were not strangers to the old mansion. Early in their marriage they had spent pleasant evenings at the historic Red Lodge visiting Anna's relative the Rev. William Jillard Hort, who ran a school there. In about 1589 Sir John Yonge had built it as guest accommodation for his mansion lower down the steep hill. Over the centuries, it passed from owner to owner. Narrowly escaping being rebuilt as the Bristol Infirmary, it was for a time a gentlemen's school and eventually a young ladies' boarding school.

The Red Lodge became something of an intellectual tourist destination as Prichard's fame increased. Its symmetrical facade overlooked the garden on the cityside of the property. Visitors were astonished upon entering the house through an unimposing door on a dusty lane at the top of the hill to find themselves in a richly oak-paneled Elizabethan hall dominated by a grand cantilevered staircase. Just as surprising was the principal room on the ground floor, modernized in the early eighteenth century in fine, light, austere, pastel-painted Georgian style. The strikingly large arched windows of this airy reception room opened onto the gardens via a modest door and exterior stone double staircase.

The Prichard children played in the sheltered garden or ranged around the spookier parts of the Red Lodge. Its deep well and traces of a previous ancient building in the several dark, dank, and fearsome chambered cellars fired the imagination. They might have noticed the small window on the Red Lodge's outside wall that had no corresponding one on the inside. Upon pulling up some floorboards of an upper room, an opening was discovered to a very dusty little room lit by the telltale window. Was it a "priest's hole" for post-Reformation security, or could this have been the Bristol hiding place of Charles II for a brief period just after the Battle of Worcester? The Red Lodge intrigued the Prichards and their visitors.[2]

On the first-floor the large Oak Room provided the main drama of the Red Lodge, plunging the visitor back into Tudor times. Except for its "modern" windows, it was then as it had been in 1590. Ornately carved exuberant decorations vied with each other in covering its rare, oak-paneled interior porch, high-relief marble fireplace, and darkened oaken walls. Pattern book classical motifs inspired the richly carved classical columns, pilasters, pediments, arcaded dados, strapwork spandrels, coats of arms, cartouches, allegorical figures, and pairs of atlantes and caryatids, and the whole was topped with a highly ornamented plaster ceiling.[3] A steady stream of guests was entertained in the Oak Room; Prichard held meetings of the Bristol College Committee and private medical societies there. One of the smaller adjoining chambers became the Doctor's library, while several more rooms, outbuildings, and a covered play area in the walled garden completed the Prichards' family home.

The fame of the Red Lodge and its occupants grew. Future economist and social theorist Walter Bagehot, son of Anna's sister-in-law by a second

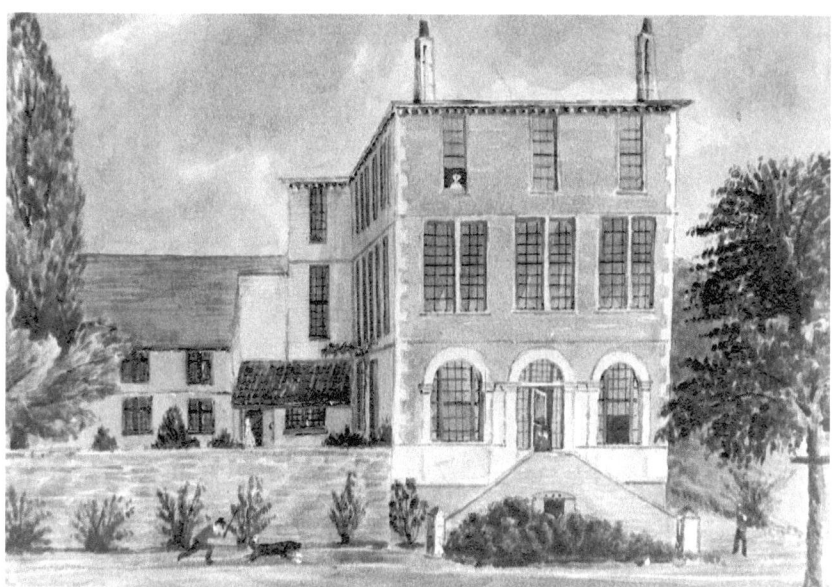

8. Unimposing red sandstone exterior. The Red Lodge's facade and garden. Watercolor. Property of the Orton family.

marriage, was a pupil at nearby Bristol College. He sometimes boarded at the Red Lodge, where he was fascinated by the discussions at the soirees, meetings, and family dinners. Prichard could be relied on to bring up fascinating subjects such as Niebuhr's philosophy, the existence of Agamemnon, and the origin of the Etruscans. The schoolboy reported enthusiastically: "I dined at the Prichards a day or two ago. The Doctor had two friends there talking about the Arrow-headed character and the monuments of Peutapolis, and the way of manufacturing cloth in the South Seas." Banker Thomas Watson Bagehot recognized the benefits to his fourteen-year-old son, replying that he was "glad to hear of your intellectual employment at the Red Lodge, and hope you will avail yourself of every opportunity of acquiring the habits and tastes that pervade the house."[4] Soon Walter was borrowing skulls from Prichard's collection to help him distinguish the principal forms of crania outlined in his host's essay on craniology.[5]

Like the Prichard children, Bagehot was a bit of a swot, desperate to please his father. Young Mary Prichard kindly kept him supplied with interesting books. Less enjoyable was the Doctor's physic: "Being rather an invalid, means that I was rather giddy all day yesterday and towards the evening became worse so that Dr Pritchard observed that I ought to have some medicine and accordingly wrote a mysterious looking prescription;

which being hastily translated into drugs became nothing more or less than a 'calomel pill and black draught.' This was of course taken, and made me very poorly all the morning."[6] Dosing with mercury and a hefty laxative would take its toll on any sick child. Bagehot's relationship with the Prichard family did not end when he left Bristol College for the equally liberal University College London. He visited the family at their later London home and remained close to Prichard's son Constantine. In his *Physics and Politics*, Bagehot's theory of civilization as a process was inspired by reading Prichard.[7]

As well as the Bristol College boys, young Bristol Medical School students came to dine and enjoy conversing with Prichard and his distinguished and often quite remarkable visitors, as documented in the family's albums. One January, young Mary Prichard was drawn to a famous guest sitting with their father and examining some Egyptian seals. The poet Robert Southey had called by to ask some background questions about Quakerism, as he was writing a biography of the Quaker George Fox. He had some erroneous impressions of the sect. Prichard seemed to appreciate his relationship with the then-conservative Southey; they continued to correspond on several subjects. The poet laureate delighted Mary by inscribing a quote from Ovid in her album.[8] Life in the Red Lodge was not all learned discussions. There were family fun and games for young and old. The year 1827 marked the start of a comfortable and productive period for the entire family.

Prichard's Anglicanism never led him to be proscriptive in his friendships. While his in-laws' Unitarianism continued to disgust him, he valued his relationships with several Unitarian intellectuals, serious thinkers worthy of his time. Dr. Estlin's successor in the Bristol ministry was Dr. Lant Carpenter, whose children William Benjamin (physiologist) and Mary (educationalist) came into the Prichards' orbit. Dr. Carpenter's former pupil James Martineau, brother of the famous Harriet, became a teacher at Lant Carpenter's school in 1827. Keen on botany and later a well-known Unitarian theologian, he was part of an intimate circle based at the Phil & Lit including Prichard, Estlin, Conybeare, chemist William Herapath, and Baptist ministers and theologians John Foster and Robert Hall. Their politics and religious affiliations were varied, but they found common ground discussing "the newest questions of the time, and the greatest questions of all time."[9]

Family duty occupied Prichard in January 1828. Reports of Aunt Newman were now dire; her life had been dominated by nervous complaints, an unsatisfactory homelife, and preoccupation with a sense of spiritual unworthiness. In a lingering decline, she was frequently longing for death. Prichard hoped his aunt's passing would put an end to their relationship with impulsive, tiresome Uncle Newman. Instead, he and his father were all too soon commiserating over the widower's scandalous marriage with his deceased wife's nurse-companion. Thomas Prichard knew it was useless to remonstrate with his brother-in-law over this "repugnant" turn of events. He could only hope that as Newman would naturally no longer be able to socialize on the same terms as previously, he might temper his inordinate fondness "for what the world calls Dash." The Prichards agreed that un-Quakerly Newman and his nurse-bride were unequal only in the weight of their purse; the best policy would be to avoid their erstwhile relative and keep silent on the matter of his inappropriate marriage.[10]

Prichard was not known for any fondness for art, popular novels, or poetry other than sacred or classical verse. His family's albums, in contrast, contain poetry, sketches, dramatic scripts and riddles. Even his father was taken with an epic poem, hot off the press, sweeping British middle-class drawing rooms:

> Have you read the *Course of Time* by Pollock? A poem sent to the press by an author who died soon after? Byron, Scott, Wordsworth! hide your diminished heads. Surely nothing ever written equals the Course of Time! I know not how to turn over its pages, particularly in the fifth book, where I get into an ecstasy at every line. Do get it. It has passed with unexampled rapidity through three editions, and I am told that during the dearth of the book between the second and third, a guinea was offered in London for the mere perusal of it. I could weep for the loss of such a man. If we compare him with any other writer, it must be with Dante. But how does the Italian kick the beam! The one I could never read; the other I could read for ever.

Thomas Prichard's copy of Pollok's 394-page poem was one of a phenomenal seventy-eight thousand in twenty-five editions sold in Britain and America. His son was not at all enthusiastic about the blank verse religious effusion, detecting in it signs of Arminianism.[11]

Thomas Prichard's contemplation of sacred poetry was interrupted by worldly matters: "It is not improbable that Dr Stock's departure from Bristol will throw more practice into thy hands, & I would advise thee to rise earlier & begin the business of the day at an earlier hour. Fashion would, I suppose, forbid thy rising with the lark & beginning business with the Bee, for nobody would be ready for the Doctor at so early an hour: but there is a Via Media in all things."¹² He followed his son's and grandsons' achievements avidly; he looked forward to reading the latest *British Critic* review of *Physical History*. Jem's literal prose translation of a Greek sacred poem was even better than expected; he could not, however, refrain from observing that the boy's indisposition might be addressed by giving him a short holiday from his books. His views were not without contradictions: he believed "a christian is the same Being all the world over," and followed the comment with an anti-Catholic jab. Swallowing a prejudice in endorsing Dr. Hancock's latest publication, Thomas Prichard penned over-optimistically:

> I have ordered Dr Hancock's new work for our Reading Society, as well as a copy for my own use.—This was a little work recommending the Peace Society or its objects—I was for a long time discouraged from joining the Peace Society, observing so large a proportion of Unitarians crying up the cause in a way that excited much disgust in my mind, but I have since thought it necessary to put away this objection & give my subscription. I am surprised to see so many of the clergy advocating this case. A time will come, I have no doubt, when war will be as strange a thing in Christian countries, as the worship of Jupiter & Juno.¹³

Over the winter of 1828–29 Prichard continued working on languages, supplementing his own reading of theology and the classical historians with books on Sanskrit and Celtic borrowed from the Bristol Library. He read Dugald Stewart's *Philosophy of the Active and Moral Powers of Man* and De Candolle's *Elements of the Philosophy of Plants* as he was preparing a Phil & Lit lecture on physiological theory. A dutiful Christmas visit to Ross was followed by family illnesses as spring arrived.¹⁴

The Vital Principle

In his Edinburgh student days Prichard had enjoyed Dr. John Allen's chemistry course, in which "the vital principle," or the "immaterial" force that controls the function of living things, was explored in the context of "animal economy," that is, physiology. At first glance, Prichard's tackling this topic appears tangential to his commitment to improving society. But for him the concept of the vital principle was central to his exploration of the brain and mind relative to mental illness, a topic on which he was planning another textbook. It also bore on his views of heredity and on the psychic unity of humankind, so central to his anthropological program. The ancient theory of vitalism had been hotly debated during the second half of the eighteenth century, especially among French academics, and it was still contentious but already losing its credibility when Prichard started researching it. The issue was that a demonstrably sound alternative to it was nowhere to be found.

Sniffing out unscientific theorizing, Prichard was motivated to counter the vague and erroneous views held on vitalism. In attempting to fathom the laws governing the generation and development of life, he hoped to establish a revised biological theory that would also see off religiously unorthodox materialist notions. His November 1828 lecture on the vital principle at the Bristol Phil & Lit so impressed some members of his audience, they encouraged him to publish it. He dedicated his book to the founders and patrons of the Bristol Philosophical Institution, and in particular to Richard Bright and John Scandrett Harford, two of its staunchest supporters.[15]

Since ancient times the idea of an immaterial force controlling the function of living things had been a subject of debate; no matter the name given to the idea of a cause, a principle, power, or faculty, its ultimate nature was unknown. A Montpellier academic specializing in philosophical medicine, Paul Joseph Barthez, produced a highly influential revised edition of his synthesis of vitalist ideas in 1806, in which he argued that as the exact nature of the vital principle is completely unknown, it is pointless to consider whether it is a substance; rather it is a necessary "abstraction" used to describe phenomena. Barthez carefully couched his views in Christian orthodoxy.[16] An alternative materialist explanation of the nature of life started gaining ground, disturbingly. Both vitalist and materialist theories lacked the scientific credibility Prichard cherished; he wanted vitalism proven, disproven, or replaced by another more useful explanation. His book managed to dismiss vitalist theory without taking a reprehensible materialist stance. Rather, Prichard steered a middle path that retained the presence of divine inspiration in living matter, thus creating a textbook that was culturally acceptable and appropriate to the mores of contemporary science.

The aim of *A Review of the Doctrine of a Vital Principle, as Maintained by Some Writers on Physiology* (1829) was to dismiss unsupported theorizing and inspire a scientific approach to the long-held idea. The French Enlightenment desire to explain all phenomena through chemistry was at odds with orthodox Christian belief. Closer to home, materialist Joseph Priestly had maintained that chemistry was the basis of science through which all properties of life and even the mind could be reduced to matter. Prichard hated this. More to his view was John Hunter's idea that a vital principle or power distinguished the living from the dead. The chemist Humphry Davy contributed to this opinion when, affected by Romanticism, he became an antimaterialist and a believer in the distinctness of living and dead matter: the blood had "ethereal parts," and the connection between the mind and the organs of the body was unfathomable, for instance.[17] Prichard dismissed these views as speculative.

There were some basic scientific tenets to begin with. Physiologists had made substantial progress in demonstrating that matter was not inert: some was self-propelled, some self-regulating, and some thinking. Modern chemistry helped to distinguish organic and inorganic matter: oxygen in the atmosphere caused inorganic matter to change, whereas it did not affect living matter. However, upon death, organic matter became subject to the atmosphere and changed. What had departed from organic matter to allow this? As chemical reactions occurred in living matter, a chemical explanation was necessary. Physiologists could neither prove living things to be mere explicable mechanisms, nor could they prove them to be invested with a mysterious property that governed them. If there were a vital principle, an active power superadded to matter which was independent both of mind and of material substances, what was it?[18]

Some scientists accepted the inexplicability of the vital principle, just as they understood that gravity existed, though it was unexplained. They were both facts. This attitude allowed the vital principle to function as a catchall for unknown causes, however. When the physician John Abernethy opined it a "subtle, mobile, invisible substance" superadded to matter and working as magnetism and electricity do, controversy came to a boil. Some scientists, including Prichard, rejected Abernethy's view that his hypothesis was sound because there was none better.[19]

Prichard's argument against the existence of a vital principle required him to tread carefully. The experience of his friend William Lawrence served as a warning to all who sought to challenge the existence of a divine or independent element in living things. Lawrence's lectures at the Royal College of Surgeons clearly rejected the concept of a vital force, likening the idea to the propensity of men to account for what they do not understand by claiming the effects of mysterious and imaginary higher beings. His lectures published in 1819 had landed Lawrence in seriously hot water for daring to extend his antivitalist stance to the human mind; he claimed that mental functions were the products of the brain rather than of any immortal, immaterial soul. This earned him wide censure, forcing him to withdraw his book. It was enough to make anyone think twice before uttering a view that might be construed antireligious.[20] A decade later, Prichard approached his task with no intention of falling into the theological and cultural pit that had nearly swallowed Lawrence. Instead, he proposed that there is no mysterious force that controls the physical functions in plants and animals: all that an organism needs to exist is physically present in it. A harmony of mechanical structure with chemical composition has no need of something tantamount to an immaterial soul within it to ensure its function. So far, so materialist. He then reminded his readers of the fact that plant and animal life had been created and is controlled *overall* by God; there is thus no need of His presence *within* structures. Rather than speculating about some essential, intangible organizing substance, Prichard called for scientists to buckle down to more disciplined physiological research on, for instance, the nervous system.

Prichard followed his physiological theory with an exposition on what constitutes sound scientific methodology, including Sir Isaac Newton's demand that causes of phenomena must be limited to the fewest that are both true and sufficient for the task. Sometimes the only evidence of a cause was its effect, in which case two issues must be considered: the degree to which a supposed cause provided a solution to the question, and whether a factual or probable cause was actually independent of its effect. Just being a possible cause should be considered the weakest form of evidence.[21] Prichard believed that scientists would eventually be able to explain all phenomena of life without invoking the existence of some internal mysterious agent like the vital principle. His closely argued and persuasive book then turns to describing the phenomena of digestion, secretion, animal heat, the prevention of putrescence, muscular contractility, latent life (the seed), and embryonic differentiation, laying out and discounting vitalist arguments as he went along. About one issue, he was sorely challenged, however. Either the seed contained all the information required for the future organism, or, lacking proof of that inbuilt program, development could be "accounted for by ascribing it to the universal energy and wisdom of the Creator." In other words, while ascribing the phenomena of life to natural materialism, aspects of developmental differentiation were so complex as to require divine guidance.[22] In conceding what is called First Cause in this instance, Prichard established an intermediate ground in the debate between natural materialism or reductionism (that biology could be reduced to the action of chemistry and physics) and transcendental superintendence. He viewed the seed materialistically but tentatively allowed Creation to drive development. This effectively preserved him from criticism by both materialist and orthodox partisans.

Prichard then moved on to issues relevant to the research on insanity that was then occupying him. First, there were some observations on the instrumentality of the brain and nervous system in the operation of the mind, in which he defined the brain as the "instrument or the medium through which the mind becomes affected by external agents, and by which it reacts in giving rise to voluntary motion;—in other words, the connexion between the soul and the body." He considered it a "subject involved in the deepest mystery," unlikely ever to be understood. He then reviewed some evidence and conjectures pertaining to sensation, its locations in the nervous system, and whether sensations and ideas had traceable physical effects on the nervous system. Do all mental processes take place in the brain, or do some occur without the assistance of material organs? He distinguished volition from emotions, speculating that the "higher powers" of the mind might not have a connection with the structure of the brain; they reside in the realm of the immaterial mind, though they require the brain in order to produce results. Prichard thus asserted the brain to be a sort of intermediary between the immaterial mind and the material body.[23]

Prichard went on to welcome the disciplined approach of some modern physiologists, particularly the French, thoroughly discussing Blumenbach's theory of *nisus formativus*, the doctrine of creative power, and other evolutionary theories like that of Étienne Geoffroy Saint-Hilaire. But he warned that the notion that external agencies could transmute an organism into another species was nothing more than the imaginative extravagance of men of genius. As in *Physical History*, he repeated his anti-transmutation position: gradual changes in an organism are confined within the bounds of its immutable species in conformity with Christian doctrine.[24]

Prichard's perceptive critique of this ancient theory explored the reasons for invoking it and the untenability of most of the arguments in its favor while still managing to be a successful reconciliation of theology and naturalism.[25] He sent a copy of it to his father, who kept watch for the reviews, proudly writing, "It is gratifying that J. J. Gurney was pleased with Dr P.'s book on the Vital Principle—The eclectic Review spoke of it with very high encomium lately."[26] The reviews were positive and respectful. A medical periodical focused on Prichard's discussion of the immaterial soul, while the *Eclectic Review* expressed interest in his views on the power of generation and formation and on the properties of the mind. They thought *Vital Principle* "remarkably luminous and dispassionate, and exhibit[ing] a happy combination of extensive reading and sound judgement." Two other reviewers pointed out the difference in British and Continental science culture. The Anglican *British Critic* found Prichard had written "with much good sense, as well as with a complete knowledge of all the hypotheses which have been advanced from the days of Aristotle to those of Dr Darwin." He was praised for contrasting the ingenuity of the French school of physiology with the religious principles of British physiologists.

A long review in *Göttingische gelehrte Anzeigen* took a different view: *Vital Principle* contained nothing unknown to even an elementary German physiology student, but it was an impartial, intelligent, and well-organized survey of the main issues, even though Prichard sadly suffered from typically British religious inhibition when dealing with the issue of materialism. As this reviewer would have predicted, Prichard's friend Dr. Symonds's anonymous review in the *Bath and Bristol Magazine* lauded him for disposing of Dr. Priestly's materialist argument, even if the outcome remained inconclusive.[27] Prichard's *Vital Principle* elegantly succeeded in replacing both materialism and vitalism with compromising, superintending, *external* divine guidance.

In *Lehrbuch der vergleichenden anatomie* of 1834–35, Rudolph Wagner (*Physical History*'s later translator) declared that while both humans and animals possessed bodies and souls, only humans had minds. Not only was there no evidence to *disprove* the existence of a soul, but the moral order of society required the assumption of humankind's possession of one. Belief in a soul or mind independent from the body and disbelief in transmutation and materialism went hand-in-hand. Prichard's approach was certainly novel and an example of his desire to accommodate scientific thought with cherished religious doctrine.[28]

Prichard managed to divorce vitalism from metaphysical consideration of the existence of the soul or mind. He argued carefully, precisely, and comprehensively as he led the reader through to a rejection of untenable vitalism by applying an array of empirical facts gathered from decades of science. *A Review of the Doctrine of a Vital Principle* was for some years a valued and standard text on a subject that had been intensely debated since 1780. Reference to it began to fade, especially when his friend John Bostock's widely read *Elements of General Physiology* (1836) followed his analysis.[29] The vital principle's validity was ultimately maintained only from the point of view of strict religious orthodoxy. Decades later, when Gregor Mendel's pioneering genetic research was recognized, the idea was consigned to history altogether, as was Prichard's role in its demise.

Family Matters

Tom and his wife's hardships in New Jersey cast a shadow over 1829. He had been ruined in commercial speculations probably concerning that local canal construction project and was attempting to eke out a living as an accountant and surveyor. Prichard and his father continued their consignments of provisions and money, but Tom was miserable and never satisfied; he felt he lived an exile's life in America, needy for what support his brother and father provided. Their attempt to find him employment in Canada came to nothing, nor was there relief from Tom's in-laws, those "scurrilous bankrupts," the Lawrences.

Prichard's idea of a winter holiday for his son Jem was to send him to his grandfather's for yet another round of swotting, reducing his grandfather to plead for mercy: Jem "reads Greek & German to me, but he has almost abandoned in despair his version of Milton, finding it too hard. Canst thou give him some other task? say Gray's Elegy. They had fine sport last night in company with their Uncle Edward, with a clap-net and took about three dozen unfortunate sparrows, upon a part of which they are going to dine to day."[30] Uncle Edward knew how to have some fun.

Edith was born in July, while Prichard's sister Mary Moline was already the mother of ten. In the autumn he set out for the Continent again, accompanied this time by Jem and a Professor Tulloch of Aberdeen. They visited several of the German universities and met with some of their most distinguished professors. They took in the town of Koblenz, but the highlight of their tour was a visit to Göttingen to meet Professor Blumenbach, the inspiring naturalist to whom Prichard had dedicated the second edition of *Physical History*. Blumenbach gave him a signed copy of his own book, which occupied pride of place in Prichard's library. The sight of the German scientist's magnificent craniological collection was inspirational. On returning to Bristol, Prichard got embroiled in local controversy, and he had to travel to South Wales to treat his friend Conybeare after his near-fatal carriage accident.[31]

Bristol College

Access to liberal education was just one of the issues occupying some middle-class British reformers, but this did not apply to charitable and strictly Christian education for the working classes, toward which attitudes were less than liberal. The four oldest Prichard boys needed preparing for university and respectable careers in the Church. Bristol's private teachers did not, however, provide the necessary prestige and focused instruction found at the elite ancient so-called public schools such as Eton or Harrow. With these boarding schools out of Prichard's price range, how could his boys be educated most effectively and economically?

Bristol happened to be the home of a famous Baptist seminary later called Bristol Baptist College. Prichard and his father read, appreciated, and had great respect for the Baptist ministers and their evangelical commitment. Two of them, the Revs. John Ryland and Robert Hall, came under Prichard's medical care, while others were fellow members of the Phil & Lit.[32] When he was invited to be one of the College's annual classical examiners in June 1829, his report was full of praise for the scholars' performance in Greek, Latin, Chaldee, and Syriac, and he noticed that the young seminarians were also receiving a liberal education in modern languages, mathematics, and logic, as well as theology. Every June until he left Bristol in 1845, Prichard spent a day carrying out these examinations, and he donated copies of his books to their excellent library.[33] Could he obtain a similar education for his boys?

Prichard's positive experience at the Baptist College convinced him that the piecemeal education provided by tutors, himself, and his father was insufficient for his sons' needs. He resolved to enter public life as the driving force among a group of Bristolians who would establish a private college. Instead of this initiative being welcomed as advertising Bristol's progressive attitude and an asset to the city, the scheme caused a sustained barrage of hostility from the local Anglican clergy. Prichard and his colleagues expected some opposition to the liberal principles of their proposed college but were nearly overwhelmed by the Establishment's intolerance of any school that was not *exclusively* Church of England in its worship, faculty, and pupils. It turned into a struggle for Anglican hegemony in education.

Sectarian hostility in Bristol was as virulent as ever. Any Protestant dissent, like political radicalism, was suspect in the eyes of the Establishment. Both lacked patriotism. Roman Catholics and Jews were beyond the pale; Wesleyan Methodists joined Anglicans in vociferous condemnation of Roman Catholics for their potentially subversive support of the pope's supposed quest for political domination. Invective against Catholics was a cornerstone of Protestant Bristol culture that also expressed itself in the denigration of the city's impoverished Irish immigrant population. The devastating 1798 Irish Rebellion was only yesterday in Bristolian minds. Some civil rights won by Protestant Dissenters in 1828 were viewed by Tories as a slippery slope leading to dreaded Catholic emancipation. The following year had been rife with newspaper wars, handbills, speeches, and rallies, while the lower orders of Bristol contributed to the debate with an anti-Catholic riot. One huge rally in Queen Square evidently supported by extremist elements of the Anglican clergy whipped up the antipapist fervor of some twenty thousand Bristolians. A thirty-five-thousand-signature petition was got up, and the city's window-breakers set to work on Irish Catholic properties. After the Catholic Emancipation Act was finally passed in 1829, hostility toward Catholics increased. Societies founded to proselytize Catholics and Jews flourished, while Anglican Tory loathing of scheming, ambitious papists possibly outweighed their disgust of Jews; at root both groups were foreign and therefore threatening.[34] Dissenters, Catholics, and Jews could not possibly be allowed to mix with nice Anglican schoolboys. Prichard and his friends' plan to provide broad, nondenominational education outside of Church of England control threatened Anglican supremacy during this volatile sectarian period. The battle over Bristol College was acrimonious, but while the school existed, it afforded Prichard and his family new and broader enriching relationships, lasting friendships, and an excellent education for young Jem, Con, Gus, and The.

The organizing committee of Bristol College treaded carefully. Prichard and several other prominent Bristolians, including his friends Drs. Carrick and Symonds, William Tothill, and surgeons John Champeny Swayne and Estlin, intended their school to prepare pupils for Oxbridge. Minister Lant Carpenter had to be discouraged from joining the Bristol scheme, as Unitarian involvement would have put ammunition in its adversaries' hands. Impressed by how the new liberal London University was organized, Estlin inquired for details of its curriculum to serve as a model for the level and breadth of what Bristol College would offer, particularly in science. Any similarity between the proposed Bristol College and nonsectarian and dangerously Godless, Whig- and Scottish-influenced London University would be grounds for condemnation in the eyes of the Bristol Tory Establishment.[35]

Bristol College's initial planning meeting attempted to assuage furious opposition with a compromise: while pupils would be admitted without religious discrimination, independently funded Church of England worship would be provided.[36] The Establishment was less than impressed and deluged the Bristol press with criticism. The *Prospectus* informed the public that applications for shares could be obtained from several gentlemen, Prichard's name heading the list.[37] Estlin privately acknowledged the financial and social challenges facing the nascent college:

> We have had a meeting of shareholders to the new College[—]more than half the required sum has been subscribed—the ultra orthodox tory churchmen still think us a dangerous D. of Wellington sort of set, and denounce us: but the evangelical party in the Church are less

opposed: many have joined[.] A concession to the church has been found expedient;—permission to have a theologl. tutor, but not as a college appointment—to be paid for by those who attend him, and not from the [general] funds.—I see no harm in starting in this way: a violent opposition would otherwise [have] been started.[38]

Far from pacifying their opponents, the theological lecture proposal fanned the flames of intolerance. A circular on the subject by the bishop of Bristol, Robert Gray, was obligingly reprinted in the local newspapers. He initially insisted that the College provide an integral chapel, properly employ Church of England instructors, and provide divine service. When this was ignored, he instructed his clergy to boycott the scheme on the grounds it did not meet the law requiring places of education to teach the precepts of the Established Church. The Bristol College committee was attempting to "set up a scheme of vague and precarious tuition, enforced by no prescribed rules and responsibility, and subject to every change." The bishop dismissed their offer to provide extrinsic religious instruction.[39] Censure from such high quarters plunged the school's prospects into doubt.

Public attack notwithstanding, a few days later Prichard chaired a well-attended meeting of subscribers at the Bristol Institution to elect a provisional committee and demonstrate that the College would not be Godless. They elected a twenty-seven-strong council and set up a theological lecture fund. Prichard donated a generous £5 to the fund and subscribed a guinea annually. The list of subscribers included men of business and the professions, Dissenters and Anglicans, Whigs and Tories alike. The seventh regulation put this fund under the control of a special committee of members of the Church of England.[40] Their enemies not in the least bit pacified, the newspaper battle raged on.

Thomas Prichard received a blow-by-blow account. He could understand Establishment domination of seminaries, but the consciences of Dissenters should not be burdened in schools.[41] John Estlin sought advice from Thomas Coates, who had had a good deal of experience struggling to establish nonsectarian London University in 1826:

> I hope you have seen in the Bristol papers the first Manifesto of the new Council? It was rather strong, but I think not more than the virulence of the attacks on us demanded on first starting, to show that we had spirit as well as perseverance in our undertaking. Dr. Prichard wrote it: he has always been a "true-blue" Tory & churchman, but is rather ashamed of the Cloth on this occasion.

Three sub Committees have been appointed from the Council-Educational—for Laws and Regulations,—for Building & Finance and we shall soon be ready with a sketch of the general plan of Instruction for the public, as something of this kind more definite that the original prospectus is necessary—

My object in writing to you is to ask if there may not be within your knowledge some persons of distinction & influence who if applied to, particularly under the circumstances of the episcopal & clerical opposition we have met with, would be willing to countenance the Institn by taking a share? a few names of this kind would be useful to us in many ways. Would there be any impropriety in such an application? What persons occur to you as proper ones to be written to? Any advice of this kind your knowledge of persons connected with the L. Univy will enable you to give would be valuable to us. Hitherto no applications hardly have been made <u>out</u> of Bristol, except to a few officially connected with the City as the D. of Beaufort, and our Members. All have declined even Mr Bright, our <u>whig</u> member. <u>He</u> thinks a college <u>useless</u>!!!

Perhaps we may be able to get the Marquess of Lansdown when the time comes, to lay the first stone! Mr E. Protheroe Jr M.P. has written for a share, I believe without any solicitation, merely on hearing of the college, & has offered us his services.[42]

A rumor circulated that some Anglican clergymen initially supporting the scheme were now refusing to pay for the shares they had ordered. This was hardly surprising, given the bishop's decree and the three anonymous threatening letters in *Felix Farley's Bristol Journal* directed at any Anglican clergymen who supported the plan. "A Member of the Royal College of Surgeons" enterprisingly charged a shilling for his eleven-page printed diatribe against the College, embroidered with Latin quotations and references to the sacrifice of the Redeemer.[43] Bristol College Council responded in kind, inserting an official riposte in the newspapers calling the opposition self-righteous fanatics, designing men, malign accusers, inciters of feverish excitement, votaries (one of Prichard's favorite words) of prejudice and bigotry, and so on. It also clearly stated that a chapel would be of no use to Bristol College because as a day school, its boys would be taken by their fathers to their own places of worship on the Sabbath, leaving the college chapel deserted.[44] This letter had Prichard's fingerprints all over it.

More printer's ink was lavished on the subject. The Rev. James Shackleton's invective on the evils that would befall the students of Bristol College so angered Prichard, he applied the prestige of his signature to a long *Felix Farley's Bristol Journal* riposte. Dealing with the clergyman's criticisms one by one, he asserted that there were financial resources in Bristol adequate to maintain the College and insinuated its citizens lacked only the desire to foster higher education. As to the claim that a multiplicity of educational establishments was unnecessary, especially if it exposed *all* classes to mental cultivation, he contrasted Scotland's positive attitude toward education and resulting international reputation for excellence in many fields with the lesser achievements of England. Prichard also noted while English universities exclusively educated clergymen and sons of the more affluent, the several Scottish universities encouraged all respectable young men to expand their minds. Who would want English education and attainment to lag behind Scottish? The otherwise conservative and conventional Anglican Tory Prichard was actually advocating broader access to education. He had more to say; he ridiculed those who feared the more democratic diffusion of knowledge would jeopardize the supremacy of the Established Church, a sentiment more appropriate "from the mouth of a poor ignorant Spanish friar." This jibe at "popery" would surely hit home. In Prichard's opinion, the Established Church could bear any scrutiny; minds should be expanded by learning and judgment strengthened using the sound principles of critical investigation.

Turning to the merits of Bristol College, Prichard assured his readers its curriculum had been carefully modeled on those of the universities. He promised that it would be zealously and assiduously conducted on sound financial and educational principles and would therefore obtain the support of "sensible" Bristolians. There was no question of its competing with existing gentlemen's private schools, which educated younger boys only. In fact, the single stumbling block in the whole project was the local clergy's hostility, a situation every man of sense and candor would realize was the result of present social conditions. Prichard predicted acidly that the success of the Bristol College would be a triumph of wisdom over folly.[45] The letter was an appeal to Bristolians' pride and a defiance of the Establishment that risked losing him patients. His patience was already gone.

In the face of this unrelenting opposition, Bristol College needed to enlist an Anglican clergyman unafraid of a scrap. Prichard had just the man. There could hardly be a more respectable one than his friend and Bristol Institution stalwart Conybeare, whose incumbency was safely in another diocese. He had an international reputation as a geologist and could command the attention of the public. Conybeare agreed to give a course of theological lectures at the College and become its Visitor. Prichard published his letter of total support. At last, they had the approval of a respected Anglican clergyman.[46]

The proprietors of the College made halting progress. Understanding that building a noble, purpose-built edifice would delay the College's opening, they opted for rented temporary accommodation in a house just opposite the Red Lodge, hired tutors, and prepared to admit upward of a hundred boys.[47] More trouble loomed. An impressive candidate for the well-paid principal's post suddenly demanded an Anglican chapel in the College and a new rule requiring all future principals to be Church of England clergymen. The bishop was at work again. By May 1830, still with no principal, Estlin concluded that the Established Church had a stranglehold on education. Confidence in Bristol College was waning.[48]

Still in the eye of the storm, Prichard took his friend the eminently Establishment Reverend Eden to beard the lion in his den. Bishop Gray admitted his opposition had been the result of "misrepresentations;" he was not actually opposed to the College. Reverend Biddulph, so-called unofficial bishop of Bristol, had obviously been the culprit. A *Felix Farley's Bristol Journal* report of a special meeting of the shareholders summarized Prichard's long speech explaining the satisfactory resolution with the bishop.[49]

With the active opposition of the Establishment seemingly in check, better progress was made. Joseph Henry Jerrard, a Cambridge graduate not in holy orders, was appointed principal, and the committee circulated *Outline of the Plan of Education to Be Pursued in the Bristol College*, candidly reporting their meetings and detailing the school's liberal syllabus. The "Infidel College" officially opened with thirty-four pupils on January 17, 1831. This low figure was not unexpected considering the era's general political and economic turmoil and Anglican hostility. That evening they celebrated their victory with an inaugural dinner. In reply to a toast expressing the school council's indebtedness to Prichard, his central role in the venture was outlined:

> Dr. Prichard was well entitled to the compliment now paid him. Dr. P. might not say it himself, but Mr. E. saw no reason why he should not say it, that Dr. P.'s position at the commencement of the affairs of the College, was one of great delicacy and difficulty. Dr. P.'s high attainments, the respectability of his character, and the part which he took

in forwarding the scheme, rendered him a kind of mediator between contending parties; and so numerous were the fears, the forebodings, almost the threatenings he had to combat with, that had he been disheartened and had he deserted the cause, it would not have been a matter of wonder: but thanks to him, he did not leave the helm; and though the circumstances alluded to might have made him less sanguine than others of ultimate success, now that we have proceeded so far on our voyage, (though, perhaps not exactly by the track which Dr. P. thought the only one), we had not merely his best wishes (which had never deceived us), but his full confidence in our triumphant success.[50]

Bristol College attracted teachers and pupils from beyond Bristol who became family friends, guests at the Red Lodge and later at the Prichards' London home. Francis William Newman, brother of the future cardinal John Henry Newman, was its classics teacher for six years and highly successful in preparing his students for Oxford. Newman and Prichard became friends.[51] Physiologist William Benjamin Carpenter and economist Walter Bagehot had fond memories of their time at Bristol College and the Red Lodge. The Prichard boys' names were in the college register and in the reports of the school's annual examinations and prizes.

Amid Prichard's efforts to promote Bristol College as more than a cut above a boys' private academy, he took some pride in his son Jem's joint editorship of its short-lived school magazine, the *Collegian*, to which Prichard contributed an article on demonology. He was also thoroughly cramming Jem in preparation for a Sanskrit scholarship exam at Oxford. Prichard had been corresponding with his friend Dr. Symons, master of Wadham College, about this scholarship and the possibility of having his forthcoming *Eastern Origin of the Celtic Nations* published at the university's prestigious Clarendon Press. Symons's gratifying reply encouraged Prichard to apply for the vacant professorship of Sanskrit. He had also successfully brought his son's scholarly pedigree to his Oxford friend's attention.[52]

In the Bristol College examination report of 1835, Prichard attributed his son's recent success at Oxford to his excellent preparatory education. Dr. Jerrard's evidence before the 1836 House of Commons Education Committee was similarly laudatory.[53] Bristol College provided a sound foundation for its pupils' future studies and careers. Prichard was proud of it. A medical man reminisced:

[Dr. Prichard's] erudition impressed me at my first interview with him, when I was about 15 years of age. [One day while he was driving me in his carriage, he] asked me what Latin and Greek we were doing at the College. I mentioned amongst others *The Clouds* of Aristophanes, and referred to the very long words it contained. He asked me to quote one, and I gave [a twenty-two-letter word]. He made me give him all the derivations of this compound word, and when I came to grief over one he corrected me, and quoted not only many other of the long words, but also several passages from the comedy. In fact, he seemed to know the whole play by heart.[54]

The descriptions of Bristol College printed in the annual *Matthews's Bristol Directory* trace its development throughout the 1830s. Unlike other English schools, Rugby excepted, its curriculum remained remarkably broad and liberal. There was a junior and senior school, and the variety of subjects taught included several modern languages and even drawing. Bristol College proudly printed accounts of its examinations and progress, and Conybeare's theological lectures were made much of, published with an exceedingly long title advertising their orthodoxy: *Inaugural Address on the Application of Classical and Scientific Education to Theology; and on the Evidences of Natural and Revealed Religion. Delivered as Introductory to a Course of Theological Lectures for the Use of the Pupils of Bristol College, Being Members of the Established Church*. In 1832 the principal suggested affiliation with London University, a step on the ladder to Bristol College granting BA degrees. Wakefield College had recently been founded on the same lines as Bristol, having benefited from Prichard's advice. In 1834 amalgamation with the Bristol Medical School was narrowly voted down and the construction of a proper school building urged.[55] That year's *Proceedings of the Fourth Annual Meeting* recorded its educational and financial progress. The College had to be constantly on the defensive, though Prichard was doing all he could to attract positive publicity. He sent copies of the new edition of Conybeare's theological lectures to the periodicals hoping for reviews, and for good measure, he enlisted a friend's help:

> Will you write a puff, saying how great an advantage it is (notwithstanding that Xnity is plain to the unlearned but sincere) in these days when false learning & vain Philosophy have poisoned the minds of the higher orders, to find the Ch. Religion treated in its elements by one of the most distinguished scholars & philosophers of the age, & so set forth as to be recommended acceptable to the most cultivated minds, & that this is a contingent result of the establishment of y Bristol College? If you will do this, I will get it inserted in some of the Newspapers.[56]

In 1837, 111 boys were receiving a fine education, but decline set in. Bristol College launched an appeal in 1841. The literary man and temporary Clifton resident John Sterling gave a rousing speech in support of it and higher education in general, and John Estlin outlined the school's recent troubles, first noting the seven clergymen and the bishop who had tried to sabotage the school. He further admitted that some supporters' departure from Bristol and others no longer having sons of school age were lessening commitment to the cause. And regrettably, some of its former teachers had set up private schools in competition with the College, while the Anglican clergy had hatched another plot: they were founding rival Bishop's College. The patronage and name of the bishop and its promise of strict Anglican conformity intentionally set it in direct competition with Bristol College. Estlin predicted that some pupils would transfer to the new rival, and he was right.[57] Bristol College could not be threatened out of existence, but local events had affected it and the foundation of a rival crushed Bristol College within a year.

Science and Humanitarianism

Amid his Bristol College and Bristol Institution commitments, Prichard found time to publish a short article that enhanced his national standing as a physician: "On Hemiplegia, and Particularly on an Important Remedy in Some Diseases of the Brain" appeared in the *London Medical Gazette* in 1830. He kept up his efforts on behalf of the Bristol Institution, chairing its annual general meeting that year. He continued his pro-directorial duties at the Phil & Lit, and in the autumn gave a lecture on Palestinian geography as illustrating sacred history.[58] In the spring of 1832, his increasing use of linguistics to demonstrate the unity of humankind is evident in the title of his Phil & Lit lecture: "Remarks on the Application of Philological Researches to the History of Mankind, with Some Observations on Baron Cuvier's Division of Nations into Three Distinct Races."

Bristol's new institutions of learning and health care acquired a zealous supporter and new physician. John Addington Symonds, MD, Edin, a sixth-generation Oxfordshire physician, arrived to make his fortune in Bristol—and he did just that, soon gaining a lucrative practice as a consulting physician of great skill. He was often to be found at the Red Lodge, having much in common with Prichard. A serious, sedate, intellectual, dignified, thoroughly honorable, courteous, and kind man, he inspired confidence in his patients. Symonds expertise in medical, psychological, and literary topics, and his dedication and diligence brought him the wherewithal to acquire a magnificent Clifton mansion, where he wrote, remained involved with learned associations, and brought up a family that included the Victorian poet and literary critic of the same name. With filial piety, this son collected his father's prose and poetry, publishing them as *Miscellanies*. It includes an obituary memoir of his friend Prichard.

Symonds divided his efforts between doctoring, literature, and science. He published on cholera and on psychology, and he explored apparitions, somnambulism, sleep and dreams (his son was a sleepwalker), emotions, perception, and criminal responsibility in insanity. He supported Prichard's theory of moral insanity, supplying *A Treatise on Insanity* with an excellent case history. Like Prichard, he wrote for the *Cyclopaedia of Practical Medicine* and was involved in the Provincial Medical and Surgical Association. Unlike him, politically liberal Symonds was a willing and suave public speaker, served the General Hospital, taught at the Bristol Medical School, and was, in essence, an aesthete. He later wrote to fellow biographer of Prichard, Daniel Hack Tuke: "But I am prosing on poetry. Forgive me; and above all do not betray me. Nine-tenths of the world would not let me prescribe for them if they thought I cared two straws for poetry."[59]

Prichard's considerable institutional involvement during the late twenties had not distracted him from his central goal, one that *Physical History* (1826) had not conclusively accomplished. His Bristol Library borrowings of mostly explorers and travelers' accounts show he was continuing his anthropological research, and he commissioned an American friend to acquire some pictures of a variety of Native Americans.[60] Exploration and colonial expansion was bringing not only new ethnographic material for Prichard to mine but alarming reports of the barbaric treatment of colonized Indigenous populations. Frustrated, he was moved to an uncharacteristic action; he chose a sympathetic periodical in which to come out in a humanitarian stance.

Thomas Prichard had not hesitated to set his son to work writing for the *Friends' Monthly Magazine*. In one article Prichard described three basic types of poetry, ascribing the highest form to Hebrew literature. To this he added his translation of the Song of Deborah (Judges 5:2–31).[61] Members of the Society of Friends were highly active in humanitarian causes, not only in holding their "Meetings for Sufferings" but in their dedication to the anti–slave trade and antislavery causes. The Quaker magazine was therefore ideal for another of his articles calling for the humane treatment of humankind.

Obviously Prichard regretted the decimation of Indigenous peoples for the resulting loss of ethnographic and linguistic material, but this is not at all obvious in his 1830 article on the Guanches, the inhabitants of the Canary Islands thought to have been driven to extinction. He was forthright in declaring: "The institutions of nature, or rather of Providence, tend to the preserving and multiplying of tribes, and to their renovation when partially decayed. But the destroying daemon is the selfishness of men. It is only by the hand of man that any race of human beings has been exterminated; and perhaps we may add, that it is only by christian nations that such a work of total extermination has ever been totally accomplished." Prichard continued indignantly that mummies of Guanches were displayed as curiosities in European private collections and museums. His article is necessarily historical and particularly notes Spanish rapacity and Roman Catholic proselytism, but there is also criticism of colonial policy, albeit of non-British nations. It airs his despondency about civilization not only for its destructive propensity but as evidence of the general moral degeneration of modern society. In sharp contrast, he clearly admired the moral qualities the Guanches were said to have possessed, such as their "simple" and peaceful lifestyle. Importantly, their religion had been monotheistic; they believed in a single supreme being and the devil. For Prichard they embodied the original, uncorrupted state of divinely created human beings.[62]

In another article for the *Friends' Monthly Magazine* Prichard considered African cultural attainments and found much to appreciate. European knowledge of Africa was still severely limited, but he could enumerate many great discoveries made by its peoples: "Africa has contributed her full share towards the advancement of mankind in arts and civilisation. If indeed, her claims were fairly estimated, it may well be doubted whether they would not exceed those presented by any other quarter of the world." Among the many distinguished men of science, philosophy, and Christian theology, particularly from Egypt, Ethiopia, and Carthage, Prichard cited Abbas Gregorius, the learned Ethiopian and historian of his country. This was the first of his series of articles praising African achievement.[63]

Bristol Life and Reform

Government repression obvious in the Peterloo Massacre of 1819 had served to further radicalize an element of vocal working people already stirred by hardship and injustice. The following year brought an event that long remained fresh in the memories of the fearful middle classes and ruling elite: the Cato Street Conspiracy, a workingmen's plot to assassinate the prime minister and his cabinet. The plan was foiled, and the discontent of

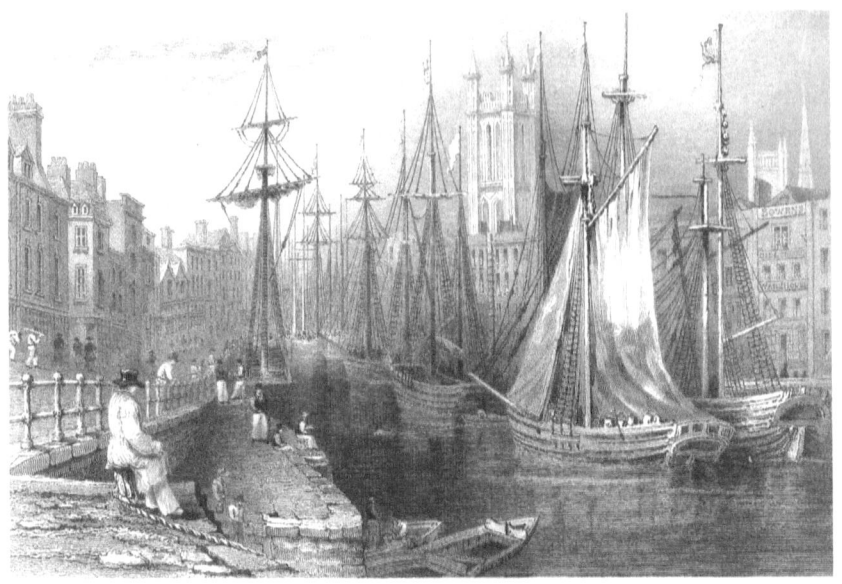

9. A window to the world. The quay, with the tower of St. Stephen's, Bristol, 1830. Engraved by C. Mottram. Courtesy of Bristol Libraries.

the disenfranchised and the sufferings of the poor went on as before. Britain's social and political unrest in the twenties looked like it would turn into revolution in the thirties. Several Continental revolutions and rebellions set the tone for 1830, spreading fear among the British ruling elite. One solution to the problem of the very poor was to export them. Tom wrote to his father that shiploads of shiftless and destitute English families were arriving in America. In the autumn of 1830 Prichard's other brother Edward was making rather un-Quakerly preparations against a possible attack on the family's bank in Ross. Rumors of arson swirled around nearby Hereford, instigated by the "absurd popular movement," Thomas Prichard moaned.[64] There were some rather ineffective attempts at parliamentary reform. The Tory prime minister, the heroic Duke of Wellington, fell from power.

Reformist John Estlin looked forward to political change. He was frustrated by Bristol Tory intransigence when he described the wind of change to Whig grandee Lord Brougham in April 1831: "That influence upon the working classes which the high party have for the last 40 years so powerfully exerted, is for the present at least, paralysed. They refuse upon the question of reform to be guided by their masters. Meetings of different Trades are held every night, and resolutions of independent voting passed."[65] Bristol's local party bosses must have been alarmed to discover that the small proportion of artisans who had voting rights were actually declaring that they would no longer be bribed with brawls, food, and drink, that time-honored electoral tradition.

As the working classes found their voice, they organized political protests rather than just rioting or being led by middle-class Radicals as in the past. An undercurrent of dissatisfaction bubbled among more "middling" folk, too; they called for local as well as national political reform. Increasingly dissatisfied citizens such as unenfranchised men and members of religious minorities dared to put their heads above the parapet. Strident reformist pamphlets and newspapers proliferated.[66] Society was at a crossroads.

The three Prichard brothers' preoccupations in 1830 typified them. The eldest was preparing his book on the Celtic languages; bright, restless, disaster-prone Tom was losing his shirt speculating, complaining, and suffering in New Jersey; and the youngest, Edward, was defending his father's bank from the rabble. Prichard and his father seldom discussed Edward, the brother who had obligingly taken up the career his elder brother had shunned and then spent his life managing the bank and living conveniently at hand. He married three times, had and buried several children, and then died.

Edward Prichard's first wife was Quaker Rebecca Merrick. His second marriage to his first cousin Elizabeth Wilkins in 1822 sparked a family crisis. The Society of Friends disowned them for breaking the rule against first-cousin marriage. This prohibition put constant strain on Quaker membership. During the nineteenth century, among middle-class Britons, Quaker or not, the family reigned supreme; relationships tended to be exclusive, intense, and permanent. First-cousin marriages were common, as the opportunities to find spouses outside the family circle were limited. And after all, those who one grew up with were a known quantity, and marriage with them cemented family bonds.[67] Cousin Elizabeth was part of the family and would be a mother to Edward's surviving children. Alienated from the Society of Friends, Edward and his family were baptized at Ross parish church on March 9, 1836, to his father's grief and Prichard's relief.

In 1842 respectable widower Edward challenged British law. He and his first wife's younger sister, Sarah Merrick (another safe family member) were wed in Germany, as marriage with a deceased wife's sister was illegal in Britain. He published pamphlets on currency fluctuation, the Poor Law, and *Marriage with a Deceased Wife's Sister* (1849). His only surviving child, Maria, married Thomas Gee and died on the island of Madeira, aged twenty-six; Edward died on January 22, 1859, and his widow ten years later.[68]

While Prichard was greatly occupied with the birth of Bristol College, on February 3, 1831, Anna was similarly occupied with Albert Hermann, their last child. And as the bitter winter lingered and Prichard was deep into Indigenous American languages, his father's study of biblical history seemed to reawaken a fondness for reconciling the pagan histories with biblical chronology, an outmoded form of historical study called "connection."[69] Scottish Episcopalian minister Michael Russell set out to right the wrongs of previous chronologists in a hefty three-decker work. Prichard and his father read the second volume hot off the press and discussed it thoroughly, but it was not until April 1832 that Prichard's anonymous review of *Connection of Sacred and Profane History* appeared in the *Westminster Review*. He used Russell's book more as a vehicle for expatiating on historiography and exercising his own passion for "connection." Prichard applied his wide knowledge of sacred and ancient histories to the challenging issues of dating, referring especially to the works of contemporary German biblical historians. At this point he switched his Bristol Library borrowing from theological treatises back to histories and accounts of travel.[70] Work on the mammoth third edition of *Physical History* was getting under way.

Celtic Linguistics and the Unity Question

Ever since *Physical History*'s first edition of 1813, Prichard had been gathering material on the Celtic languages, benefiting from access to contemporary German comparative linguistics like Jacob Grimm's groundbreaking historical grammar *Deutsche grammatik* (1819). Prichard's *Eastern Origin of the Celtic Nations*, conceived as a supplement to *Physical History*, demonstrates his increasing appreciation of language as a key to human history. In seeking the ancestry of Celtic deep in the Indo-European linguistic past, he hoped to make some progress in revealing relationships between nations and from thence shed light on the unique original language consistent with Scripture—the Holy Grail of traditional philology. For Prichard the migration of language was the migration of nations; he aimed to trace Celtic migration from its origin in southwest Asia. This book was another battle in his campaign to demonstrate the specific unity and single origin of humankind.

Prichard's more personal axe to grind spurred him to demonstrate Celtic as a member of the Indo-European language family. Entrenched in English culture was a dismissive, denigratory attitude toward anything Celtic. He hoped his research would bolster the status of Welsh, the language he loved and culture with which he identified. He was of Welsh ancestry and called the Welsh "my countrymen" and "true-born Britons." At eighteen he had subscribed to Edward Davies's *Celtic Researches*, and he always enjoyed traveling, geologizing, and holidaying in Wales.[71] Prichard learned Welsh, thought it beautiful, and was proud of the language, offering to translate for Welsh-speaking Infirmary patients. An Englishman deigning to speak Welsh was a rarity. His anthropological interests were stimulated in part by this cultural tension.

The English commonly considered Welsh a strange, uncouth language; only a few antiquarians recognized the antiquity and richness of Welsh literature. A sort of Anglo-Saxon superiority myth was rooted in the English church's break with Rome during the sixteenth century and consequent propagandistic interest in older, purer Christianity and basic freedoms, aspects of Anglo-Saxon and German tribes rather than of subjugated Indigenous Britons. Subsequent writers glorified the sturdy incomers; eighteenth-century interest in the ancient inhabitants and languages of Europe provided opportunities to contrast cultures and claim superiority over its earliest inhabitants, the Celts. Because incoming tribes were thought to have displaced them, a belief in Celtic inferiority took hold. An example of this attitude can be found in the famous, virulently anti-Celtic author John Pinkerton, who wrote in 1787 that the Celts "have been savages since the world began, and will be for ever savages." Nineteenth-century phrenologists proclaiming the superior form of the Anglo-Saxon skull reinforced this delusion of superiority.[72]

Negative attitudes toward the Welsh and its language hardened during the nineteenth century, following the rise of racialist views in general. The marginalized Welsh were discouraged or prevented from using their language and learning about their history and culture. A Victorian government report attributed Welsh indolence to adherence to their language and dissenting religion. Perhaps there was some concern that the submissive Welsh might become as unbiddable as their fellow Celts, the Irish and those unruly Scots of not very distant yore. The author of *Celtic Gleanings* (1857) pointed out that Britain had university professorships in the Romanesque and Teutonic languages but not in Celtic, a language spoken by four million inhabitants of the British Isles. Later in the century, a Bristol biological anthropologist helpfully contributed an "Index of Nigrescence" that found Celts to be darker than the English population, clearly implying inferiority.[73] Twentieth-century Welsh speakers could still expect ridicule.

Amid and despite denigration, something of a revival of Welsh language and culture flourished among a segment of the early nineteenth-century

British cultural elite, a manifestation of the Romantic ideals of late Georgian Britain that allowed some English-born and Welsh "respectable" members of society such as Prichard to feel confident enough to express an interest in Welsh. Once his *Eastern Origin* qualified him as an expert in and supporter of the ancient pedigree of the language, he was called upon to be an adjudicator of prize essays submitted to new festivals celebrating Welsh culture, history, and language.

Prichard's long title, *The Eastern Origin of the Celtic Nations Proved by a Comparison of Their Dialects with the Sanskrit, Greek, Latin, and Teutonic Languages. Forming a Supplement to Researches into the Physical History of Mankind*, indicates his methodology—comparison. Latin and Greek, symbolic of the great civilizations of the past, were considered an essential part of an English gentleman's education, closely followed by Sanskrit. "Sanskritmania" infected particularly studious gentlemen and clergymen, hence his recent Oxford correspondence on the subject. His use of "Teutonic" instead of "Germanic" in the title conjures Romantic nationalistic notions developing during this period and some historians' opinion that the Teutons were a Celtic tribe. Prichard's title thus links Celtic with the highly valued Sanskrit, Greek, Latin, and Teutonic languages.

Taking a cue from the newly developing sciences, philology was being repurposed as a science. From its traditional focus on classical studies and the history of words, it evolved into the systematic description of individual languages and the affinities among them. The comparative Indo-European linguistics developed by Jacob Grimm, to whom *Eastern Origin* is dedicated, and much-cited Franz Bopp provided Prichard with the method he needed: he compared Celtic to other Indo-European languages to counter the prejudice that Celtic was unrelated to any other language or merely the vestige of some "barbaric" Indigenous tongue.[74] He found that the Celtic dialects were, in fact, of the same original stock as the European and ancient Sanskrit and Persian languages. He compared vocabulary, choosing universal expressions, phonemes and their pronunciation, verb roots, grammatical structure, and conjugations. Of great importance was word transformation according to grammatical function among the several Indo-European languages he compared to Celtic. Finally, he rather sketchily provided examples of Celtic in the above categories, such as in the formation of plural nouns by the addition of suffixes or the alteration of interior vowels.

As well as raising the status of Celtic for personal reasons, Prichard's anthropological agenda is apparent. Affinities among languages imply cultural affinities. If languages on the western fringes of Europe are traceable to a distant eastern location, it is reasonable to conclude that their speakers had migrated from there. And if Celtic migration from the distant southwest of Asia can be inferred, the argument for the region being the original home of humankind is strengthened. While this last point was not ostensibly the subject of *Eastern Origin*, it served one of his two basic monogenetic arguments. Celtic's membership of the Indo-European family was as far as he could go with any certainty, though he did indulge in some speculation about links with the Hebrew language. Prichard had revealed a branch of humankind's genealogical tree; the Welsh are not anomalous outsiders. He concluded:

> the Celtic people themselves are therefore of eastern origin, a kindred tribe with the nations who settled on the banks of the Indus, and on the shores of the Mediterranean and of the Baltic. It is probable that several tribes emigrated from their original seat in different stages of advancement in respect to civilization and language, and we accordingly find their idioms in very different degrees of refinement; but an accurate examination and analysis of the intimate structure and component materials of these languages, is still capable of affording ample proofs of a common origin.[75]

In demonstrating the validity of British philologist Sir William Jones's hypothesis of Celtic's membership of the Indo-European family of languages, Prichard was taking on some respected scholars who suggested otherwise and daring to enter the philological arena dominated by German scholarship. He must have awaited the reviews with trepidation. The *Eclectic Review* considered Prichard to have creditably summarized the subject, exposed the erroneous theories of Pinkerton and Vans Kennedy, and demonstrated that when history is inadequate, linguistics can come to its aid. The *Quarterly* reviewer, philologist Richard Garnett, began with praise, describing Prichard as having undertaken the task with considerable success, but he could have explored the subject more and was guilty of oversights, errors, and unwarranted conclusions. Nevertheless, "he has, to a certain extent, proved his point, and is entitled to the merit of being the first who has investigated the origin of the Celtic tongues in a rational and scientific manner. If we are not mistaken, one part of his researches throws a new and most important light on the formation of language."[76] The Rev. Thomas Arnold, headmaster of Rugby and later Regius Professor of Modern History at Oxford, was also impressed: "You know Dr. Prichard's book, I take it for granted, the only sensible book on the subject which I ever saw written in English. This and Bopp's Vergleichende Grammatik, should be constantly used, I think, to enable a man to understand the real connexion of languages, and to escape the extravagances into which our so-called Celtic scholars have generally fallen."[77] Less gratifying was one of the two long reviews eventually appearing in the more academic *Asiatic Review*, pointing out Prichard's imprecise terminology and unfortunate attempt to link Indo-European to Semitic languages.[78]

Prichard faced considerable rivalry from Continental linguists, as authoritative anthropologist E. B. Tylor noted in 1891: "I have wondered that Prichard's merit as the philologist who first proved the position of the Keltic languages as a branch of the Indo European, is so often left unnoticed. Adolphe Pictet made his reputation by a treatise on the same point, which was received with applause, no one seeming to know that Prichard had done it before."[79] Among his contemporaries, his German friend the scholar and diplomat Bunsen said there was nothing like *Eastern Origin* in Germany, while the eminent professor Grimm, not noted for praising English scholars, admitted the "author doubtless has given further evidence to this thesis and established it more firmly."

Some German linguists credited Prichard's contribution to knowledge even as they pointed out his errors. August Friedrich Pott noted that Prichard had not dealt with the "eastern origin" claimed in the title, while Franz Bopp rather desperately claimed to have preceded Prichard in *suggesting* that Celtic was an Indo-European language, admitting only that the Englishman's proofs were irrefutable, though he had not properly investigated the uniqueness of the language nor accounted for the presence of Sanskrit content possibly being the result of cultural contact. A. W. von Schlegel did not venture to deny the veracity of Prichard's conclusions, but he had his reservations: more exact, extensive, and thorough research was needed. A few years after *Eastern Origin* was published, Bopp claimed Pictet's 1837 proof had been firmer than Prichard's. The Englishman's book irritated German linguists, aside from Grimm, who had to consider the debt of Prichard's dedication. There was certainly national rivalry on Prichard's part too; he privately lamented the relative inferiority of British philology compared to its thriving Continental counterpart.[80] But all in all he felt he had taken up the Celtic question posed by Jones decades earlier and had come up with the goods.

Eastern Origin inspired the wave of German Celtic scholarship that followed, but some views expressed in it marred the book's reputation.

Prichard's extensive command of philological treatises unfortunately included some outdated resources, and his indulging in speculations such as that Celtic was possibly a language transitional between the Semitic and Sanskrit left him exposed to criticism and dismissal by some contemporary Continental scholars.[81] In this field crowded with scholars and university professors, the interference of an English physician was not appreciated. Later elaborations on or independent demonstrations of the place of Celtic in the Indo-European language family are therefore better remembered.

In Britain *Eastern Origin* was highly regarded: some general textbooks and the *Encyclopaedia Britannica* article on Celtic were based largely on it. Modern historians of linguistics credit him with introducing the Continental science of linguistics into Britain, creating the tone for later British research, as well as having been the first to establish Celtic as an Indo-European language. He is generally considered one of the three founders of Celtic linguistics. Prichard had adopted a theory and wrote a thorough, well-documented, and inspiring treatise on it using sound methodology.[82]

Prichard's international reputation, *Eastern Origin*'s contribution to Celtic linguistics, and his known pride in his Welsh background made him an excellent choice as honored guest and prize essay adjudicator at the Abergavenny Eisteddfod. Previous Eisteddfodau had been rather literary and entertaining festivals disdained by Prichard. He preferred to foster serious Welsh scholarship; he urged Welsh antiquarian and politician John Montgomery Traherne to found a more scholarly society with elected officers who would engage in worthy activities such as publishing Welsh literature.[83] Traherne obliged. The moving forces in another development, the Abergavenny Cymreigyddion, were Sir Benjamin (as in Big Ben) Hall, Whig MP, soon to become Baron Llanover, and Lady Llanover, a relative of Prichard's friend Baron von Bunsen. Hall was then successfully campaigning to require the Established Church to permit religious services in Welsh. Prichard was involved in some of the ten Abergavenny Eisteddfodau the Halls helped organize. Emotionally invested, he wrote to a philologist friend:

> I had lately the gratification of hearing some gentlemen from Britanny deputed by King Louis Philippe, sing some Breton songs composed by themselves in their native Armorican, before a Welsh assembly termed Cymredgyddion, & of observing that the Welsh understood them & evinced the most enthusiastic pleasure in recognizing their common nationality. It is a most curious circumstance that this branch

of our old British language should be still preserved to such a degree of purity as to be intelligible after a period of 15 centuries of separation, for it is so long since the Britanni of Gregory of Tours migrated across the channel.[84]

With Prichard in the audience that autumn day in 1838 were the Bunsens, Sir Benjamin Hall, philologist Dr. K. R. Lepsius, and the interesting Breton scholar Vicomte Hersart de la Villemarqué. Afterward, the party made their way to the Red Lodge, and the following day Prichard guided them on visit to Bath and Stonehenge. Villemarqué described Prichard as "a scientist whose work honors England, . . . one of the most learned men in England [and] one of the most excellent scholars I have seen in my life."

Baron von Bunsen was well connected, having friends in Rome, Prussia, and the Court of St James's. Along with his busy diplomatic career and a wide, elite social circle, he was a diligent scholar, particularly in biblical history and philology, and shared Prichard's interests in the Welsh language and Egyptology. Bunsen wrote expressing his appreciation of his time at the Red Lodge: "Your excellent work, I hope will be continued with the same alacrity as it was begun with. You know we have nothing like it in Germany, and thus you are sure of grateful readers in that part of the world. But it must not be done at the expense of your health, with wishes for the continuation of which & of all other blessings for you & yours I conclude these lines of farewell."[85]

As well as being an adjudicator for the Abergavenny Eisteddfod, Prichard was a corresponding member of the Society for the Publication of Ancient Welsh Manuscripts, founded in Abergavenny in 1837, donated £5 to it, and subscribed to the publication of the *Liber Landavensis* (1840). He reprinted his description of the Celts in *Physical History* as a 152-page bound pamphlet, *Ethnography of the Celtic Race*, which he gave to Hodgkin, American linguist Peter Stephen Du Ponceau, and others. Prichard continued his commitment to Welsh scholarship, agreeing to judge the prize essays for 1842 and 1845.[86]

Prichard got into a panic over the 1842 competition, owing to a dearth of Welsh or any other submissions. With just two months to go, the only two were "both so extremely bad that either would be a disgrace." One author had read nothing published within the last twenty years on the subject and blotted his copybook by citing the execrable Pinkerton as an authority. The other was a blatant polygenist, had the temerity to correct Moses's error as to the number of distinct human races, and espoused phrenology to boot.

"Now what is to be done?" Prichard moaned, soliciting von Bunsen's and Lepsius's confirmation of his condemnation. The situation was delicate, especially as these two blind submissions were likely from the pens of Welshmen. When a "more hopeful" third one materialized and von Bunsen came to Prichard's rescue with another one that seemed to have been by Dr. Lepsius himself, the situation became even more problematic. Prichard applied his usual pejorative adjectives to the fourth composition, complaining it contained some "startling, visionary, speculative" assertions about a language called Caucasian being the ancestor of both Indo-European and Semitic languages. He feared that the members of the Cymreigyddion would rush to conclude that Celtic was directly related to the primeval mother tongue. Were it not for his belief that his friend Lepsius was the author, he would have considered it nonsense destined to attract the disgust of Continental linguists who already considered the British absurdly ignorant "adventurers in philology." What was he to do with the claim that Egyptian was a Semitic language? Embarrassingly, Bunsen replied that he had been working on this very same theory. Prichard then had to admit that his friend Francis Newman had found evidence of Semitic in the Berber language and that linguist Edwin Norris had proposed a similar theory. His adjudication report would have to skate over the author's more extreme claims. And so it was that Prichard awarded the prize not to Lepsius, whom he had mistakenly believed was the author, but to its actual author Dr. Karl Meyer.[87]

The Cymreigyddion y Fenni met on October 12 and 13, 1842, in a specially erected pavilion accommodating a "fashionable assemblage" of two thousand spectators, including three members of the aristocracy. Meyer's essay "on the place which the Welsh language occupies among the members of the Celtic family, together with the other branches of the same among the languages of the Indo-European race" was outstanding for its author's scholarship and ability, according to diplomatic Prichard. Privately to Bunsen, he continued to lament the absurdities of all the essays, but he admitted some of the Welsh scholars displayed learning. He was "afraid the Welsh people will get tired of subscribing for prizes which are to be gained regularly by foreigners, and I do not think any of my countrymen, the true-born Britons, will for some time have much chance in competition either with Germans or Englishmen." In public his characteristically lengthy speech at the Cymreigyddion praised the remarkable progress Welsh had made in public estimation; noted that the best of the British and German naysayers had come to accept Welsh as an Indo-European language; and stressed that philological research was "capable of throwing light on the original development of human language, and of illustrating the history of the human mind in the very infancy of nations." He ended with a little Prichardian quip to the effect that although the winner was a German, at least his language and Welsh were members of the same family.[88]

The adjudication of the 1842 Abergavenny Cymreigyddion temporarily distracted Prichard from three books he had in the works: his third edition of *Physical History*, *Natural History*, and *On the Different Forms of Insanity*. He was pleased that more and more scholars working exclusively on Indo-European were effectively turning philology into a new science. The time was ripe to give it a satisfying scientific name. He was frustrated with Bunsen's neologism "linguistic science," complaining, "This word does not quite suit English ears. What do you think of Lexiological or Lexiolytical as a substitute?" He later tried out "glottological science." "Linguistics" soon caught on.[89]

Prichard awarded the 1845 prize on ancient Welsh literature to "Carnhuanawc," his friend Thomas Price, treating his audience to a "most elaborate, critical and learned" adjudication, extracts of which were read to the Abergavenny Eisteddfod. A grand dinner followed; among the many toasts there was one to Prichard, but he skipped the Grand Fancy Ball.[90] Even while fully occupied and often traveling as a commissioner in lunacy, he still had time for his Welsh friends and their studies. With some pride he reported:

> Dr Meyer, a learned German, a friend of the Chevalier Bunsen, has now in the press a work on Welsh literature which he expects to produce a considerable sensation in Germany, and that it will induce many Germans to visit Wales. He forms a very high estimate of the ancient poetical literature in the Welsh language. I hope the work will be translated into English. It seems that the Germans are already aware that a new source of curious information will be opened to them by the study of the Welsh language.
>
> The Welsh booksellers here say that a great demand exists for Welsh books in Germany & that they send abroad many grammars & dictionaries.[91]

Prichard's *Eastern Origin* was in demand for a few decades, at least in Britain. In 1857 his Ethnological Society of London friend Robert Gordon Latham came out with a new edition. Reviewers were perplexed if not annoyed by it, as by that time it had been superseded by the likes of Johann Kaspar Zeuss's *Grammatica Celtica*. Instead of correcting Prichard's blunders of omission and commission and incorporating new research, Latham had simply added a great quantity of his own, in the opinion of the *Saturday Review*. A German reviewer felt Latham had thrown linguistics into disrepute. Prichard would not have found the publisher's fee paid to his heirs worth the embarrassment.[92]

In *Eastern Origin*, Prichard fulfilled his early promise to develop his views on Celtic, and the book gave him an opportunity to improve the status of the Welsh language and celebrate his Welsh background. His selection to be a Cymreigyddion judge undoubtedly gratified him. But considering his admiration for German scholarship, German linguists' variously grudging, lukewarm, or sometimes hostile opinion of his work must have been disappointing, even if he might claim he had spurred them to further efforts. His compatriots, especially those who were not linguists, held his work in high esteem. Not only had Prichard succeeded in establishing Celtic as an Indo-European language, but by adopting the new method of comparative historical philology, he contributed to the development of the modern discipline.[93]

Tom and Change

Around the time Prichard's *Eastern Origin of the Celtic Nations* was published and the parliamentary election of June 1, 1831, resulted in a landslide victory for the reformist Whigs, Thomas Prichard was distracted by the plight of Tom in America. Their latest bank draft and some supplies were reciprocated with tales of woe from New Jersey. Jane was ill and their home so cold they had to chop their frozen bread and meat with an axe. Early the following year Tom returned to Bristol briefly, mired in a lawsuit into which his father was dragged. The Prichard children were simply fascinated by their exotic uncle. Con remembered:

> My uncle Tom was a remarkably handsome man, with a very animated intellectual face, . . . his conversation was interesting, and his manner kind & warm hearted. We were too young to be told of the circumstances which had brought him to England, which were harassing pecuniary difficulties, but only knew of his having suffered a good deal of distress, and were interested in hearing of his travels. He was a man, as I have often heard my father say, of unusual talents, especially for mathematics, and also of much taste; but he never seems to have succeeded in business. He returned to America in the autumn.[94]

The eldest Prichard boy, Jem, worried the family too. After breaking his arm jumping over a chain on the Bristol docks, he got a serious earache, "swallowed" a lot of Sanskrit for his looming Oxford scholarship examination, and was looking not at all robust. His siblings had it easier, holidaying in Ross with their grandfather and cousins Roger and Maria and in lodgings near Chepstow.[95] When Jem set out for Oxford that autumn, his grandfather reflected on how a Quaker such as himself could have a grandson in the heart of Establishment Oxford, destined for the Anglican priesthood. On this momentous occasion, his message containing his usual criticism was for the benefit of both son and grandson:

> I told [Jem] when here last, that if ever he became a Bishop, I hoped he would be a liberal one, and not consign all Dissenters to the uncovenanted mercies of the Deity, but before he reaches the Bench, many changes will take place in ecclesiastical affairs, and I hope they will be effected without confusion, & when effected tend to the purification and firmer establishment of the Church—for I am certainly not one of those unrelenting Dissenters who would rejoice in pulling down the Church; but it will never flourish until its clergy consist of religious men.[96]

To warnings against intolerance, bigotry, and worldliness, Thomas Prichard added complacency. Unlike Anglicans, Dissenters had to be diligent to succeed, ever consciously considering their religion, and sometimes extreme in their religious views out of defensiveness. So allowances should be made when reading their religious works. Prichard and Jem were in danger of becoming thoughtlessly self-satisfied members of the Establishment.[97]

The British Association for the Advancement of Science, 1831

After the great strides made in British science and technology during the height of the Industrial Revolution, progress seemed to stall; Britain was lagging behind its Continental rivals. Government was hardly supportive, and the all-important status of those engaged in science was not high. As the third decade of the century opened, some lamentations were published on the state of British science, an expression of that ubiquitous desire for improvement and reform. What was needed was a national organization dedicated to promoting science. The English term "scientist" had just come into use; it was high time to professionalize science, just as doctors and geologists had been doing. The elite but ineffective and insular Royal Society was distracted by internal quarrels; science was all but absent from universities; the government was uninvolved; and British periodicals tended to ignore innovative foreign science. Meanwhile, a rival influential, peripatetic, German scientific association was holding ostentatious meetings, glorying in the Prussian monarchy's support. French science could also look to government aid.[98] The proposed British Association for the Advancement of Science (BAAS) would enhance the status of British science and its Christian gentlemen members.

Well-connected Rev. William Vernon Harcourt's Yorkshire Philosophical Society was chosen as the ideal location for the inaugural meeting of the BAAS. The Yorkshire society itself was born of scientific gentlemen's aspirations. York was neutral territory, aligned with neither the learned factions of London and Edinburgh nor of Oxford and Cambridge that would have immediately sparked stultifying hostilities. Prichard set out for York, meeting old friends in Liverpool and visiting three asylums en route. About 350 men from around Britain attended this inaugural meeting on September 27, 1831. There Prichard made useful contacts with like-minded provincial British scientists.[99] Although impressed with his son's invitation to the archbishop of York's palace, Thomas Prichard hoped that his "mind will escape the leprosy of Bigotry—he has seen some of the monster's dark side in his negotiations about the Bristol College." The "monsters" in question referred to those Oxbridge reverend professors who did get involved and needed placating. Thomas Prichard was glad that his son had returned from York safe and sound, if not completely satisfied with the new association:

> I was not a little curious to hear something respecting the meeting at York of so many learned men-yet perhaps the result has rather disappointed thee; however the journey and the gratification of seeing thy old friends Drs Hancock and Gilby must have been highly gratifying. I hope one expedition on the new rail will satisfy thee, for I have just put out of my hands a newspaper, which narrates another fatal accident which has occurred there; it is almost impossible that machinery effecting such rapid movement, can be altogether free from danger.[100]

These new "flying machines," as Thomas Prichard called them, might have been a danger to life and limb, but the railway made it possible for Prichard to join this national scientific community. Conybeare had encouraged his involvement, enthusiastically writing to Harcourt on his behalf. Prichard agreed to serve on the Zoology and Botany Subcommittee, having been unable to set one up for the science of humankind. While he thoroughly approved of the Baconian approach to science that underpinned the BAAS, the association attracted some unsettling criticism from those who feared orthodox religious views would be undermined by skeptical, atheistic elements (read: Continental-influenced Edinburgh and London men). The participation of Unitarians and other religious deviants boded ill. The BAAS's exclusion of religion from its proceedings actually implied religious promiscuity, if not irreligion. Tractarians, the stalwart defenders of the Established Church's essential governing core of the universities, were on the alert; there was a fear that Dissenters would somehow infiltrate the universities. Prichard wanted to be labeled neither a religious skeptic nor a liberal, but the BAAS offered an opportunity to promote his science of humankind and benefit science in general, so he gave it his support. The predicted evils did not materialize, and the BAAS established itself as a religiously orthodox organization built on sound natural theology. It dropped its initial promise to seek government support for science and developed an evangelical British individualism and voluntarist style.[101]

Some drawbacks of the BAAS were much more mundane. As Bristol treasurer, Prichard felt himself above the task of collecting subscriptions, especially as the procedures were unclear. He also deplored the fact that applicants' scientific bona fides were not vetted; he was receiving membership inquiries from men "but indifferently qualified to be very creditable associates." The BAAS risked degenerating into more of a social than professional scientific association, a not-unfounded concern.[102]

Not only was the BAAS too inclusive to Prichard's mind, but because each annual meeting was held in a different city, an unfortunate tendency to one-upmanship soon developed. Each year the host city rolled out lavish events, trivial activities, excursions, and luxuries that inevitably drew criticism for clubbery and ostentation. More and more middle-class, amateur attendees and their ladies flocked to the annual meeting intent on diversion. The lampooning press had a field day.[103] Prichard was not pleased. On top of that, his subjects of humankind and medicine were obviously poor sisters to the dominant physical sciences. He continued to attend, support, and lecture at the thriving BAAS, nevertheless.

Discontent and Epidemic, 1831–32

Discontent among the increasingly politically active working classes nationally was felt in Bristol, where just one of the issues was poor access to health care. Dissenters, Quakers mostly, were frustrated by the Bristol Infirmary's notorious overcrowding, as well as their own lack of influence and virtual exclusion from election to its faculty. It seemed as if the Infirmary accepted little from Dissenters and Whigs except their cash. The time was ripe to establish another hospital. The General Hospital opened in makeshift accommodation on November 1, 1832, during a cholera epidemic.

This new hospital by the docks on Guinea Street did not stem discontent among Bristol's working classes. Disrespect for local government deepened generally; the Corporation became the butt of satires, poems, and contemporary histories.[104] It did at least cooperate in one progressive activity at this time. A group of local businessmen, Prichard's friend William Tothill prominent among them, revived a scheme first mooted in 1828. To foster the commercial regeneration of Bristol they would build a railway. With a competitive eye on Liverpool and Manchester's new railways, they planned the future Great Western Railway.[105]

Suffering disproportionately from disease and economic hardship, the working classes were also frustrated by the failure of the House of Lords to pass the Electoral Reform Bill. Amid these raw feelings, the arrival in Bristol of the antireform judge Charles Wetherell sparked protests and then rioting resulting in the destruction of many valuable properties during three terrifying autumn nights of conflagration. Conybeare's was a typically liberal reaction:

> All my friends at Bristol were happily beyond the actual dominion of mob law & suffered only from thinking it unsafe on the Sunday night to retire to bed—having the flames rising from many points of the city beneath their eyes with the momentary expectation of their extension to their own neighbourhood for many houses in Clifton were known to be marked for destruction but were saved by the People finding so much to plunder & drink in Queen square that they could not leave that quarter—Whig as I have always been I must now confess a strong reaction in my own mind—it is high time I think for all honest men to lay aside all factious spirit of Party & to rally strongly around <u>real conservative</u> principles—of course I dont use that term in the sense of the Tories whose ignorant obstinacy I fully believe to have been the main cause of this alarming crisis—but I trust all honest men will now unite in a <u>safe & moderate</u> plan for reform which certainly I cannot consider the last to have been—on the one hand we must frankly sacrifice old borough mongering abuses so inconsistent with the spirit of the age & admit to a just share of political influence the real middle classes (the great bulk of the moral & intellectual force of the country) thus interesting them in the preservation of institutions against which the Tory system has fearfully prejudiced their minds.[106]

Cholera had entered Britain in the autumn of 1831, making matters even worse, and it was only a question of time before it would scourge Bristol. The impending epidemic precipitated a reluctant Prichard into his next public role as a member of the Board of Health. The disease, not yet understood to be a bacterial infection of the gut caused by drinking contaminated water, had been gradually spreading around the world since 1817, like a slower version of COVID-19. The health of the poor could no longer be neglected or left to voluntary schemes. Cholera threatened everyone.

As if an epidemic were not enough, there was the issue of "Burking," or body snatching, as in the infamous case of Burke and Hare's Edinburgh crimes. The developing scientific approach to medicine demanded more and more corpses for dissection. Between 1829, when Prichard was one of the signatories of a national petition calling for reform of the rules of dissection, and July 1832, when the Anatomy Act was finally passed, the topic of dreaded "anatomizing" plagued public imagination. This was not unreasonable, given the documented cases of wholesale dealing in corpses. The Infirmary had its own generous supply.[107] When the new law extended the source of cadavers from executed criminals to any unclaimed bodies (mostly the pauper inhabitants of workhouses), the poor understood the implications and were furious. Medical men could not be trusted.

Faced with a national cholera epidemic, the usually laissez-faire central government was stirred to create a central board of health and provide troops to isolate infected communities. Aside from squabbling, little was actually done. The mayor of Bristol asked the city's most senior physician, Andrew Carrick, to plan and form a local board of health comprising the medical men of the principal institutions. Then there was some local squabbling over extending the membership; the Corporation of the Poor's participation was refused. The Bristol board complained of its powerlessness to the Central Board of Health. After a compromise was forced, some more Bristol board meetings were held, but the task was daunting in a riot-damaged, cash-strapped city, rich only in the number of its miserably and densely housed poor.[108]

Parochial committees started a home-cleaning program, and the board called for four isolation hospitals to be set up. When the Corporation refused to have the fetid docks cleaned, Prichard and four colleagues conducted an inspection and published a graphic condemnation of the stagnant, filthy, dead-animal-polluted waterway running through the center of the city. On November 19, 1831, the *Bristol Mirror* published the board's public announcement that as the disease was understood to spread among squalid, unventilated, and intemperate conditions, cleanliness and improved sustenance were required, and the sick would have to be isolated. Prichard subscribed the remarkably generous sum of £10 to a fund for the relief of the poor and the prevention of cholera.[109]

As the winter dragged on and cholera failed to make an appearance in Bristol, complacency set in. A voluntary program to aid the poor lost momentum. The Board of Health and St. Peter's Guardians started worrying about the money squandered on disease prevention. On May 15, 1832, a call for isolation hospitals was rejected. Meanwhile, when the Reform Bill was finally passed, the artisans of Bristol celebrated with a grand march through the streets on June 18, while the antireform Anglican clergy refused to ring their church bells on the occasion. A few months later, Prichard made his own antireform stance clear when he attended a meeting at the White Lion for the purpose of adopting Richard Rawlinson Vyvyan as the Tory candidate for Parliament.[110] As for the Reform Act's moderate achievements, there was the abolition of some Parliament-packing corrupt "rotten boroughs" and the extension of the franchise to about two-thirds of Britain's men. Would this be enough to stave off revolution?

On a sultry July day in 1832, when the first three cases of cholera in Bristol were reported, its citizens had to get their heads out of the sand. Prichard attended daily meetings of the Board of Health and helped organize home inspections and burials.[111] The disease hit Bristol harder than elsewhere, and nowhere harder than the slums, jail, and workhouse. Ancient, overcrowded St. Peter's Hospital held six hundred at this critical juncture, with its eighty boy inmates sharing sixteen beds in a single room. St. Peter's death toll was seventy-one in the first month, compared to the rest of the city's twenty-nine, and Prichard was one of its physicians. A rumor spread among the poor that its medical men were killing its inmates for anatomizing. And a visitor reported ominously: "The most remarkable circumstance I hear of at Bristol is that the people hate the doctors who are laboring for them, and believe that the sick are poisoned and buried alive."[112] Prichard and his colleagues were insulted and threatened in the streets. Disturbances broke out so that the dead had to be taken from the workhouse in the middle of the night to keep them from being seized by the furious population.

Bristol's betters were alarmed at the prospect of further social unrest, considering the track record of the lower orders for violence. The affluent fled Clifton, and the poor continued to die. One observer wrote in August: "Bristol dreadful. They are burning tar brands in the streets constantly, 60 were buried from the hospital yesterday. . . . 14 dead this morning in

Temple Street."[113] A national politician's letter from Clifton revealed that Bristol's disease and mortality rate was being underreported for the sake of the city, followed by being further underreported nationally for the sake of the country.[114] The hell of St. Peter's was Prichard's last straw.

"On the Cholera encreasing, at its return, Dr Prichard resigned his post at St Peter's Hospital, and Dr Fox retired, on being censured for 3 yrs Non attendance.... These two Men were considered as wealthy, and in full practice for many years," a disgruntled local gentleman observed on August 7.[115] The Corporation failed to respond to the urgent demands of the Board of Health; its plans for temporary fever hospitals were more discussed than acted on. Some Quakers finally set one up. The voluntary anti-cholera association recommended distributing blankets and feeding the poor, while the Corporation's contribution was to ban part of the annual St. James Fair, one of the few entertainments for the city's lower classes. The Tory newspaper *Felix Farley's Bristol Journal* eloquently blamed the infidelity of liberalism for the epidemic and proclaimed that the outcome was in the hands of the Lord. A greatly relieved Thomas Prichard reassured his daughter: "Dr P and his family have taken a house at Almondsbury Hill about eight miles from Bristol on the road to Gloucester where they will probably remain until the Cholera has left Bristol. I am glad he is out of town, as I know he was very anxious about his family. We hear of no increase of the malady in the city, but it is most probable that it will linger there some time."[116]

In the family's Almondsbury refuge, Prichard worked on his *Cyclopaedia of Practical Medicine* articles and his landmark definition of anthropology for his upcoming lecture at the BAAS. His father started expressing more socially liberal views, influenced by his young companion, "republican" grandson Tom Moline. He criticized Prichard for lumping Whigs and Radicals together; the former were capable of being respectable, cool-judging characters.[117]

Two months after the cholera outbreak, the worst was over, allowing its official end in Bristol to be declared on September 26. In its eighteen weeks, 1,612 cases and 626 deaths were recorded. All in all, the disease was tackled with more philanthropy and Christian rhetoric than public funds. The well-off became more aware of the extent of poverty in the city, Bristol Corporation's interest in public health soon waned, the population continued to grow, and cholera struck again in 1849.[118]

In five years Prichard's life had changed: he had moved house, become a more prominent citizen, helped to found Bristol College, broadened his scientific influence through the BAAS, published articles on a wide variety of topics and books on physiological theory and Celtic linguistics, made lasting friendships with Francis Newman and Dr. Symonds, continued his close relationship with his father, sent his eldest son to university, supported his wayward brother, served on the Board of Health, resigned from St. Peter's Hospital, weathered local political turmoil, and survived an epidemic. It was time for a new direction.

11 · Life and Reputation at the Red Lodge

Family, Friends, and Science, 1833–39

> [We Prichard boys administered laughing gas] occasionally to the members of the family and friends as a kind of entertainment, the ladies and younger persons being always secured behind a barricade of chairs and tables, on account of the irrepressible and boisterous character of the proceedings.
> —Augustin Prichard, *Some Incidents in General Practice*

Eight Prichard children ranging from toddler to young adult, parents, visitors, and servants kept the Red Lodge buzzing. On one evening there might be a serious discussion among the members of the Medical Reading Society, on another, a family party enlivened by a drama written by and starring the irrepressible Prichard boys. It was hard to keep up with the constant comings and goings to school and university; visits by friends, relatives, patients, and famous men of letters; teas, dinners, soirees, and *converzationes* for socializing and hearing about the latest theories on a myriad of subjects. There were meetings for planning and plotting; patients to examine and prescribe for; local and national events to reflect on; and illnesses to worry about. Then there were Prichard's books and articles to prepare, honors to receive, and achievements to celebrate.

The Bristol Institution was attracting the attention of a somewhat wider circle of scientists, and Bristol College was bringing the Prichards new relationships among local and regional families, dissenting and Anglican. Prichard became involved in new national scientific and medical organizations that aimed to understand and improve the world. As for Bristol and the nation, the thirst for reform was unabated.

Humanitarian Causes and Reform

John and Mary Anne Estlin's activism helped put Bristol on the antislavery map. It started in the autumn of 1832, when Prichard advised his brother-in-law to winter in the West Indies for his health. During a visit to a Saint Vincent estate, its scheme gradually to "civilize," Christianize, train, and liberate its slaves impressed him. Estlin returned to Bristol in better health, determined to dedicate himself to the antislavery cause. Prichard's apparent acquiescence in Estlin's somewhat qualified observations on Caribbean slavery earned Thomas Prichard's rebuke. He sent his son a book exposing its intolerable reality:

> That thy Brother-in-law has given a correct account of all he <u>was permitted</u> to see, I entertain no doubt whatever—but the Colonists take the most watchful care that visitors from England shall see nothing of the horrors of slavery—& hence arises the contradictory accounts we receive. They well know that if they can hide from the observation of their visitors the horrors of field labour, they obtain so many advocates to their cause. This has been exemplified in a hundred instances—The present state of the question as it stands in the view of the British government, will not allow us to believe that the representations of the abolitionists are only a parcel of lies. But my own opinion is, that Jamaica is about to be given up to judicial destruction—the measure of her iniquities is full, & the Day of the Divine vengeance is at hand. The Planters could have done nothing more effectually to hasten this crisis than by adopting the wicked religious persecution that is every where practised on that island.

This reminded Thomas Prichard of slavery closer to home as he again turned his opprobrium on the powerful who put profit before human dignity:

> Hast thou read the Examination of several medical men before Parliament relative to the oppressive labour of factory children? The prevarication evidently the effect of Bribery in these cases consigns the names of these Doctors & surgeons to eternal infamy. I could not have supposed that men of Education could have thus disgraced themselves. This affords another instance of the difficulty of getting at the truth, when the interests of powerful men are enlisted against its discovery. I hope the time is at hand when these two deep stains on the moral purity of the British nation may be removed.[1]

For months there had been heartrending press coverage of the plight of child laborers in British cotton mills; previous legislation to ameliorate conditions had been generally ignored. Although a government commission investigating the situation failed to cooperate with a reformist organization called the Ten Hour Movement that urged tougher legislation, it seemed quite cooperative with the owners of the factories under inspection. One commissioner observed complacently that factory children had it easier than child miners. A reformist MP campaigning for the Factories Act at this time was Lord Anthony Ashley-Cooper, under whom Prichard later served in the Lunacy Commission, another "improving" body.

Child exploitation in the nation's thriving factories was just one symptom of Britain's dysfunctional social structure teetering on the brink of chaos in the 1830s. The 1832 Reform Act's extension of civil rights to a minority of skilled workingmen had excluded the vast population of the unskilled. Working people up and down the country continued meeting, publishing pamphlets, and communicating with like-minded groups to start their own reform campaigns. By mid-decade their charter demanding six main political reforms had struck fear into the hearts of the Establishment. Britain hovered on the brink of revolution throughout the 1830s and 1840s while the government concentrated on suppressing so-called Chartism. Meanwhile, the socially liberal addressed this threat by pressing for various ameliorative social, economic, and political reforms such as in welfare, prison, education, religious discrimination, and economic protectionism. For all of Thomas Prichard's agonizing over child labor and slavery, he and his son remained aloof from active reformism and reformists.

The year 1833 found Prichard preoccupied in researching and publishing articles on insanity; he served as secretary of the Medical Reading Society, steered Bristol College through stormy waters, and saw to his father's welfare. Now that "republican" grandson Tom Moline had emigrated to Gratz, Thomas Prichard was lonely. A companion was engaged, and family members took it in turn to visit him throughout the year.

Prichard, Anna, Jem, and Mary set out in the phaeton for Paris on the morning of August 21. Near midnight they had the pleasure of passing by Stonehenge, romantically lit by moonlight. "We could almost sense our ancestors," Mary enthused. After visiting an ancient fortification near Amesbury the next day, they traveled to the coast, calling in on Thomas Prichard and cousin Mary Wilkins, who were convalescing on the Isle of Wight and in Southampton. Arriving by steam packet in Le Havre, they found it necessary to slip some money into the palm of the "searcher" to avoid being searched "impolitely."

Mary was much more positive about France than her parents had been a few years earlier. Their first stop was Rouen, where Prichard had arranged to meet M. Achille-Louis Foville and see around his madhouse. In Paris they stayed at an excellent hotel overlooking the Jardin des Tuileries and became thoroughgoing tourists. On the Avenue des Champs-Élysées were plenty of shops and diverting entertainments, including one in which electricity was demonstrated by shocking members of the audience—literally. Less exciting was their visit to an exhibition of real "Indians," the morose and idle-looking last members of a decimated tribe, Mary recorded. Prichard did not feel the same way about these South American Charrúas whom he remembered ruefully in his speech on the "Extinction of Human Races" and whose images later appeared in his *Natural History* (fig. 13). After a tour of the ancient Hôpital de la Salpêtrière, where the famous Dr. Esquirol was in charge of the asylum, the ladies were not allowed to accompany Papa to the Institut de France, nor did they dine at Esquirol's a few days later. Prichard's idea of a holiday was to absent himself from the party to visit various contacts; he even managed to attend a demonstration of animal magnetism. On the way back home via Dover, Mary longed to see the sights of London, but fearing the cholera there, Papa vetoed it. Prichard returned to Bristol with some new material for his *Cyclopaedia* articles and the book he was writing.[2]

Busy as he was, Prichard also spent a lot of time reading pious tomes, reinforcing his Christian faith. John Sheppard had recently presented him with his *Essays Designed to Afford Christian Encouragement and Consolation*, a book Prichard highly recommended to his father. In return, Thomas Prichard thought Alexander Keith's tenth edition of *Evidences of the Truth of the Christian Religion Derived from the Literal Fulfilment of Prophecy* a foolproof aid to returning skeptics and even infidels to the true path. There was simply no excuse for apostasy. The Prichard children's literature was of a lighter nature—slightly. The *Listener*'s moral stories were thought highly appropriate, unlike the deluge of tales causing irreparable mischief to young people's tender minds. Undoubtedly, tale-reading led to distaste for the Bible. Thomas Prichard thought children's neglect of active research into the evidences of Christianity was nothing short of criminal.[3]

Medical Education, the Profession, and Yet More Charities

Prichard was more overt a reformer when it came to the regulation and professionalization of medicine and medical education. His own early experience of medical lecturing, the growing disregard for traditional medical apprenticeships, recent legislation on medical practice and qualifications, his strong sense of social status, and the recurring local squabbles over the Infirmary's pupils led him to support the formation of a medical school in Bristol. He hoped it would help establish medicine as a subject of English higher education and redound to the reputation of Bristol and its medical men, himself included. The Bristol Medical School, amalgamating Dr. Wallis's School of Anatomy and Medicine and Dr. Henry Clark's Bristol Medical and Surgical School, opened its doors to twenty-three students in October 1833. Prichard's Infirmary colleague Dr. Carrick gave the opening address, noting it would be desirable for Bristol College to have a school of medicine. This proposal to form a proto-university that would bolster the status of Bristol College came to nothing. The Society of Apothecaries and the College of Surgeons soon recognized the Bristol Medical School.[4]

Around the time the Medical School was getting off the ground, the new Bristol Medical Library Society acquired premises in a former Huguenot Chapel on Orchard Street at the bottom of Park Street. For an annual subscription of 2 guineas, members could meet for discussion once a month from October to April. By 1837 it had fifty-six members and a library of two thousand books. That year Prichard was elected its third president and remained so for several years.

The Bristol Medical School, Bristol Medical Library, and the several smaller medical societies enhanced the status of Bristol medical education and medical practitioners, and promoted professional standards and solidarity. Elsewhere, provincial medical men with similar goals formed a national association to promote and share medical knowledge beyond the dominant metropolis. In the reformist ferment of 1832, more than two hundred doctors gathered at the Worcester Infirmary to found the Provincial Medical and Surgical Association (PMSA), the forerunner of today's British Medical Association. Although Prichard could not attend its inaugural meeting, he immediately subscribed and was elected a member of council, a post he declined.[5]

Bristol medical men were pleased that the PMSA's first anniversary meeting was held in Bristol on July 19, 1833, with senior physician Dr. Carrick as president and Prichard appointed one of the four members of the Bristol council. After a tour of the Infirmary's wards, lecture theaters, library, museum, and new outpatient room, Dr. Carrick gave a rather optimistic address in which he predicted the association would lessen professional antagonisms among medical bodies. The equally optimistic business meeting noted the doubling of the PMSA's membership and plans to publicize foreign medical news. Members then repaired to a dinner admired in the press for the quality of its wine and turtle.[6]

Bristol medical men attended the PMSA's annual meetings and contributed papers to its *Transactions*. In 1840 Prichard chaired the inaugural meeting of its Bristol branch.[7] His presidential address stated that the threefold aims of the association were to promote friendly feeling, preserve the rights and status of medical men and further science. Concerning the first, the association should help to smooth the occasional ill will medical men were sometimes prone to harboring toward each other. (Perhaps Prichard had his feud with David Davies in mind.) Had he been a Radical artisan on a soapbox, he might have been accused of advocating a "combination" or trade union in the way he went on to advocate solidarity and strength in numbers. He stressed the need to uphold the dignity of the profession and protect its rights and interests, using as an example the government's offering impossibly ill-remunerated Poor Law contracts to medical men to the detriment of the service. He regretted the replacement of traditional Christian care of the needy with "the sordid penury of . . . a so-called utilitarian age."

The highlight of Prichard's "interesting and entertaining" speech to the Bristol PMSA was his rousing call for a university or medical university in Bristol. He proclaimed the superiority of Bristol to any of its rival northern cities, and it already possessed the intellectual capacity to staff such an institution. His speech was enthusiastically received. The meeting ended with Prichard's chairing a sumptuous dinner for more than forty members at the Royal Western Hotel, where "the hours winged their flight during a delightful flow of conversation."[8]

The next year the Bristol and Bath branches of the PMSA merged, increasing the their influence.[9] Their quarterly meetings were followed by *conversaziones*. Once Prichard had begun his duties as a metropolitan commissioner in lunacy, he attended less often, but he did speak about medical reform at its fourth annual meeting on June 27, 1845. Tory Prichard was pleased that the Medical Reform Bill had been withdrawn, as he saw no need of such legislative interference in the profession. Medical education had never been so good, and if medical men could not make themselves valued and respected, no law would do it for them.[10]

Liberalization of medical regulations and the establishment of medical organizations raised the status of the profession and Prichard's satisfaction with it. He looked forward to seeing progress in medicine through the exchange of ideas on a national, less London-centric scale and through new medical periodicals. With local organizations like the Medical Library, Medical School, Bristol PMSA, Bristol College, and the Bristol Institution, the city seemed destined to become a seat of higher learning.

Another Bristol organization deserved Prichard's support. John Estlin's Eye Dispensary put him in constant contact with Bristol's poor, making him aware of their hardships and vices. In this era of reform, alcohol abuse became identified as the lower classes' social evil. There was considerable consternation about the huge increase in public drunkenness, crime, and disorder thought exacerbated by the 1830 liberalization of alcohol licensing law. To stamp out the disgrace of alcohol abuse among the poor, the better off founded temperance societies. Estlin got involved in the Bristol Auxiliary Temperance Society, the Bristol branch of the British and Foreign Temperance Society later renamed the National Temperance League. It targeted "ardent spirits" and published pamphlets with catchy titles like *Drink No Distilled Spirits* and *To the Working Classes*. As Prichard and fellow alienists cited drunkenness as a physical cause of insanity, his involvement in the charity was inevitable. He served on the committee from 1832 to 1836 when the more potent force of a rival teetotal temperance society overtook it.[11]

The Raja Ram Mohan Roy Controversy

Amid Bristol's decade of institutional developments, occasional conflicts distracted Prichard. In the autumn of 1833, the famous Raja Ram Mohan Roy's visit to Bristol started with all the excitement that the presence of a handsome, noble foreigner naturally mustered, but it ended in tragedy. This highly educated reformist Bengali Brahmin and master of ten ancient and modern languages had swept into Britain the previous year as a newly created raja and ambassador to the king. He came with an established reputation for Indian political liberalism that had alienated him from his elite, conservative background. In Christian Britain, by contrast, his Hindu social and religious reformism brought him fame; for example, he sought the abolition of sati (the immolation of widows) and stressed that Hindus should discontinue the practice of idolatry and return to what he considered the original monotheism of their religion—all music to Prichard's ears.[12] For Europeans keen on "Europeanizing" India, Ram Mohan Roy was an asset, as he was to those passionate about reform at home or in the colonies. His linguistic virtuosity and commitment to monotheism secured Prichard's respect.

For his own part, the raja was conducting a bit of reverse anthropological fieldwork in Britain: he needed to comprehend his country's rulers. He professed admiration of British culture, positive aspects of which he wanted India to adopt, but he also boldly sought India's political representation in British government. Ram Mohan Roy found himself constantly on the defensive, lest anything he said or did sullied his own status as a Brahmin and representative of his government. In London he attended a relentless round of soirees, religious services, and balls, where the ladies were quite taken with him; his interest in women's rights was certainly novel. At one event a colonial officer wondered loudly what "that black fellow" was doing in the presence of ladies. All the while his conversation was of the most serious and perplexingly erudite nature. In Liverpool, as elsewhere, adherents of various religious sects vied to enlist the raja's support for their particular beliefs. In Manchester the common folk hot on reformism got wind of the visit of the reformist "King of India" and mobbed him enthusiastically until he had to be rescued by the police. After a visit to the Continent, he arrived in Bristol, exhausted and suffering from a cough.[13]

Ram Mohan Roy was comfortably accommodated at the elegant Stapleton home of a Miss Hare and her brothers, whom he had previously met in London and India. There his arduous regime continued. In early September, John Estlin started visiting him almost daily, recording the serious conversations between the raja and his rounds of guests. Eager visitors included Drs. Symonds and Carpenter, the principal of Bristol College, and some prominent Baptists. On September 15 the raja and Estlin attended Sunday service at Lewin's Mead Unitarian Chapel and Estlin lent him Prichard's *Physical History*. A few days later a fever set in, which Estlin treated until Dr. Prichard was called in for consultation. The patient was impressed with Prichard's countenance, which he thought indicated talent, and he expressed himself satisfied with his treatment. Prichard attended daily until it was thought expedient to call in Dr. Carrick, as the raja's prominence required the inclusion of Bristol's senior physician. They decided the seat of the fever was his brain and accordingly had leeches applied to his head. After four more days of assiduous care, there was nothing more to be done, and Ram Mohan Roy died. A postmortem revealed prurient inflammation of the brain—possibly meningitis. As a Brahmin he was interred in unconsecrated ground.[14]

Then came the aftermath. Tiresome Infirmary colleague surgeon Henry Daniel seized this opportunity to score a point against a rival. Just as bold a bleeder as Prichard, Daniel could hardly criticize Prichard's antiphlogistic therapeutics. Perhaps he had felt a bit left out of the limelight since the notoriety he had gained during the recent Bristol riots. Dr. Daniel indiscreetly gossiped about how the raja had been "sacrificed by his friends" in being put under Prichard's care. When confronted by offended Prichard, he at first assured him that observations he had made in a letter to John Hare had been misconstrued. Little did Daniel know that Prichard had actually seen the damning letter that took Hare to task for 1) not bringing in more physicians for their opinions; 2) not calling in senior physician Dr. Carrick first; 3) not calling on the aid of Daniel himself; and 4) not calling in Dr. Wallis, the Hare family physician. It had been a mistake to engage Prichard at all.[15] Daniel had also rashly boasted that his exposé would soon appear in print. Unfortunately, he had been prolific in his written communications on the subject, one of which, when correlated with an anonymous letter in the local newspaper, made his intention clear: Prichard's public discredit. It was a variation on the Davies controversy of the previous decade. Prichard responded emphatically: "Under these extraordinary circumstances of conduct in which the maxims conventionally governing the medical profession are so completely broken through, I believe that even yourself, and certain I am that the professions & the public, will hold me justified in declining for the future all professional, as well as personal intercourse with you."[16] He kept to his resolution.

Accounts of Ram Mohan Roy's beliefs, life, and death were widely published. Prichard had lost an illustrious patient, a man he admired, and had his competence impugned by a colleague. He honored the raja's memory by using his image as the frontispiece in a later edition of *Physical History*.

When not distracted by the Ram Mohan Roy fallout, Prichard was drawing together what he had learned about insanity and neglecting his anthropological research. As national transport was improving, he could travel more widely to meet fellow scientists, visit libraries and other institutions, attend conferences, and further widen his circle of patients. Two of his articles in the *Cyclopaedia of Practical Medicine* had been recently published, and he was continuing to volunteer at the Bristol Infirmary. He visited his father in Ross two or three times a year and spent at least part of the summer holidays with his family at the seaside. His father complained: "Dr Pichard has promised me a visit, but if one degree of uncertainty hangs over mankind in general, 10 degrees hang over his movements." This was soon amply illustrated in May 1834, when he had to make several trips to Cirencester to attend his aunt Wilkins in her final illness and care for his father as he was deeply affected by his elder sister's death. As if to prove his father's point about always being on the go, a fortnight later he and his friend John Eden attended Sir Charles Bell's famous lecture on the brain at the Royal Society of London.

The following summer Prichard was prevented from joining his family at Ross, being kept busy on a round of professional visits among his many patients in the neighborhood of Cardiff. His cousin Mary Wilkins was also his patient. Her depression was now getting beyond the ability of her family, but attempts to secure her consent to being committed to the Quaker asylum, The Retreat, had been futile. Thomas Prichard marked the fortieth anniversary of his wife's death in Bristol with a visit there. Worryingly, nothing had been heard from Tom for months. The year ended with the familiar negotiation over which grandparent would have the pleasure of hosting the Prichard children for Christmas. Thomas Prichard was particularly anxious to spend some time with Jem, hoping to stem the growth of Oxford bigotry in him.[17]

The Bristol Institution, Its *West of England Journal*, and Bristol College

The struggling Bristol Institution badly needed a boost. So with Egyptomania as strong as ever, the offer of a second "splendid" Egyptian mummy for unwrapping provided an ideal fundraising reprise of Prichard's 1824 performance. He asked young local surgeon and keen geologist George Thomas Clark to help him prepare and assist at the event. Their three lectures planned for the week of March 31, 1834, were on Egyptian mummies, Egyptian antiquities, and the Rosetta Stone. Middle-class Bristolians keen to improve their minds snapped up tickets at a costly 7 shillings, 6 pence; ladies and minors were allowed to attend. A fine leaflet produced such good results, there was a shortage of standing room (fig. 7).[18]

The audience of three hundred filling the stuffy lecture theater was transfixed. The two mummies laid out on a table were surrounded by statuettes of gods, illustrations of hieroglyphics, a large-scale copy of the Rosetta Stone, and some illustrative drawings. Prichard's two-hour lecture, "remarkable for historical research," ended with a cliffhanger: one of the mummies would be unwrapped during the following lecture. A newspaper criticized: "The theatre was crowded to excess. The Doctor sat behind a small candle screen, which had the effect of deadening his voice, and prevented his audience from hearing him distinctly." And when he begged the indulgence of his audience for the imperfect state of his lectures, he won a round of applause.[19] Wednesday's lecture began with a history of Egyptian literature in which Prichard patriotically championed Dr. Thomas Young's attainments in deciphering hieroglyphics over those of the rival Frenchman Champollion, of course. His audience patiently waited for the main attraction. The painted sarcophagus lid was lifted, revealing the precious mummy. Carefully, it was unrolled, and the method of applying the 330 yards of bandages was minutely described, as were the enclosed wax figures and preserving materials.

After pouring more scorn on Champollion in his Friday lecture, Prichard read a translation of the Rosetta Stone and described the various Egyptian artifacts on display. He ended by praising Egyptian theology for its seeming belief in a form of resurrection and expressing gratitude that Christians are not subject to moral debasement and superstitious dogmas like those of the ancient Egyptians. This brought down the house.[20] Public appetite thus whetted, a fortnight later his assistant Clark further expiated on Dr. Young's achievements, contrasted with the "inflated and supercilious style of the French archaeologist," carefully citing Prichard as an authority on Egyptian chronology.[21]

These lectures were praised at the Bristol Institution's subsequent annual general meeting for their interest and pecuniary benefit. The BI's finances remained precarious, nonetheless; they could not even afford display cases for the museum's artifacts.[22] Further schemes to bolster the reputation of the Bristol Institution were entertained, starting with the Lecture Committee's encouraging Prichard and Clark to publish their highly successful lectures. But where? In the summer of 1834, they discussed starting a periodical to stake a claim for the BI as a national body of scientific and cultural excellence, just like the national societies that published transactions and journals. It would be "honourable to this Institution." Prichard recruited Conybeare, and the planning meetings began.[23]

As the proposed *West of England Journal of Science and Literature* took shape, it transmuted from a literary and scientific magazine as outlined in Dr. Symonds's original *Prospectus* to an overwhelmingly scientific journal with some literary content. At a meeting at the Red Lodge, Clark reluctantly agreed to be joint editor, provided it would not be a mere magazine and he would have complete control over its content. That was the promise. Subscriptions of £5 financed the project, and from among its twenty-four participants a committee of five would referee authors' submissions. Despite claiming to represent the West of England, there were no subscribers from Bath; indeed, the editor of the ailing *Bath and Bristol Magazine* felt aggrieved at the competition. The meetings dragged on. In early December 1834, Clark's revised *Prospectus* was printed.[24]

Conybeare could not resist interfering, starting with insisting Clark include Prichard's article on Slavonian gods in the inaugural issue because "we must have his name." Prichard tried to persuade Clark to omit it, but Conybeare prevailed. Rather optimistically Clark's introduction in the first number of the *West of England Journal* lauded Bristolians' growing taste for science and literature, based on the flourishing state of the Library Society and

Bristol Institution. The *West of England Journal* contains articles on geology, zoology, archaeology, and physiology, as well as descriptions of fossils and Prichard's duly prominent ethnographic account of the Slavonic nations.[25] Notably, several articles attack theories of gradual development in nature, in line with Christian orthodoxy and in opposition to the rising theory of "gradualism" as proposed in Charles Lyell's recently published *Principles of Geology*. It soon became necessary to recruit authors from beyond Bristol.

Four issues of the *West of England Journal* were published, but by November 1835 Conybeare was in turmoil over the "expiring state of poor dear Mag." Could it be kept going until the upcoming Bristol meeting of the British Association for the Advancement of Science, at least? The embarrassment of a defunct scientific periodical would tarnish Bristol's pretensions to scientific eminence.[26] Alas, the journal's fifth issue of January 1836 contained Clark's bitter farewell editorial, in which he admitted the dryness and incompetence of many of its articles, notwithstanding some excellent contributions from the pens of eminent men. In its entirety, Clark acknowledged it unworthy of its dedication to Conybeare and Prichard. The short-lived *West of England Journal*, intended to showcase Bristol's intellectual prowess, demonstrated its indifference instead.

The Bristol Institution and Bristol College were in a precarious state throughout the 1830s, but Prichard gave up on neither.[27] But his fellow elite Bristolians seemed indifferent; it was as if having built the fine edifice of the BI, they considered their task accomplished. The younger generation of professionals and businessmen shied away from lecturing to the exclusive Phil & Lit or BI. Its sparse Reading Room and Museum were visited by a dwindling number of members. Meanwhile, Bristol College struggled to provide progressive education; its founders' dreams of creating a university were evaporating under the continual heat of Establishment ire. Churchman, conservative Prichard was in a quandary. It was obvious that to survive, the College needed more Anglican pupils.

The woes of the BI and the College throughout the 1830s were overshadowed by the nation's unabated social and political discontent, particularly in response to the new Poor Law with its Malthusian principles akin to Darwin's later "survival of the fittest." Amid reformist agitation, anticlericalism, general strikes, riots, shootings, and executions, the government and the Established Church stood shoulder to shoulder, though there were signs that the old conservative order would have to adapt.

The Establishment's grip on science was weakening somewhat, giving some rein to inspiring scientific thought. A younger generation of a few progressive BI members found themselves sitting on the fence; they were beginning more objectively to consider patterns in the natural world and gain insights into principles of natural development, opening themselves to attack for possible atheistic materialist and transmutationist notions. The Establishment, ever on the lookout for signs of unorthodox interpretations of nature, attempted to keep the younger generation in check.

One modern practical application of chemistry gained notoriety in the spring of 1835, no thanks to the Bristol Medical School. Murder never failed to attract interest, and a particularly notorious one led to the trial and prompt execution of Mary Ann Burdock. Suspicions about her sudden affluence had led to the exhumation of her deceased lodger's body and toxicological analysis of its stomach contents. William Herapath, joint lecturer in forensic medicine and toxicology at the Bristol Medical School, testified convincingly that the victim had been poisoned with yellow arsenic. His testimony greatly enhanced his and the school's reputations. This was a more satisfactory contribution to the new field of forensic chemistry, unlike Prichard's own brush with chemicals when the newspapers splashed "Poisoning at the Bristol Infirmary from Prussic Acid!!!" Prichard had to provide a deposition to the inquest on the body of the unfortunate, misdosed patient Mary Mabett.[28]

Brother and Daughter

The middle of the decade brought a family crisis. Tom had been silent over the winter of 1834 for good reason. He had barely survived a New Jersey winter in a home so inadequate that frostbite in both feet had caused a life-threatening infection. While thus bedridden in freezing conditions, he woke one morning to find his wife dead. It "was a most deplorable thing that two individuals residing together should be so helpless as not to be able to render the least assistance one to the other. You would hardly picture to yourself a more gloomy scene than a dark room with one of us dead in one bed, and the other a complete cripple in the next, with no one else in the house but an old nurse." Tom was brought back to Britain in July barely able to walk, "a helpless invalid, destitute and <u>alone</u>," as he described himself, a "wreck," as his niece observed. He divided his time between Ross and the Red Lodge. Kind and courteous Uncle Tom with his usual eager expression and piercing eagle eyes entertained the Prichard children with more tales. His adventurous, calamitous life was at a turning point; the problem now was what to do with him. Tom was found employment at a bank in Gloucester but soon threw that over, dismaying his father, who complained to Anna Prichard that "some difficulty presents how to dispose of Thomas. He talks of going to France, but whether this would be advisable or not I am quite at a loss to determine."

Tom returned from a short spell in France nearly recovered in health and full of stories about Bonapartist doings, but time weighed heavily on him. He returned to France in the spring of 1838 and stopped communicating. Meanwhile, his cousin Mary Wilkins, chronically depressed, went into a "decline." Tom died in August shortly after learning of Mary's death. Later family lore ascribed the misery of his life to being separated from Mary, who would not marry him on account of the Quaker ban on cousin marriage. Tom's situation was only hinted at when he was described as begging Prichard to cup or bleed him to relieve his head and "rigors," and then there was that need to "dispose" of him. His more candid niece remembered him as addicted to opium, first taken as a painkiller, but soon he could not be weaned from it. Boulogne had a reputation for being a safely distant location for the "remittance man" he had become. His brother Edward arranged the funeral and gravestone there.[29]

Anna and Prichard had other anxieties while mourning Tom and Mary Wilkins. Their daughter Mary had recently returned from a recuperative winter in Madeira, still with an ominous "cough." In 1839 she began married life with Jem's Oxford friend the Rev. William Henry Ley, first a schoolmaster in Hereford and then incumbent of Sellack Church, near Ross, much to her grandfather's pleasure. The Leys had two sons, but shortly after giving birth to a daughter, Mary died of consumption on November 25, 1844, and was buried in Sellack churchyard. Anna Prichard fostered the newborn for a few weeks until Prichard described his wife as "much indisposed by nursing the poor little infant, which she brought from the neighbourhood of Ross, our grandchild, which died yesterday morning."[30]

Henry Riley and the Bristol Zoological Society

Prichard's younger Infirmary colleague the physician Henry Riley fell afoul of Establishment opinion. His Paris education earned him suspicion of dabbling in Godless materialism, but he ameliorated it by marrying into a Tory family and becoming staunchly True Blue. His Bristol Institution lectures, however, revealed leanings toward so-called transcendental anatomy. Continental anatomists believed there were observable patterns of organization and development in plants and animals, and evidence of gradual change occurring over time. Riley's lectures represent early British consideration of French scientific and transcendental anatomy. The notion of gradualism in the sciences of anatomy and geology was akin to that of transmutation, a theory Riley was careful to criticize; transcendental anatomy and notions of gradualism and development were being discussed in Prichard's cherished Bristol Institution.[31]

Riley shared Prichard's commitment to reforming medical education, and he was involved in initiatives that "improved" Bristol, such as the subscription baths and the Bristol and Clifton Horticultural Society. Interested in anatomy, he became a founder in 1835 and secretary of the Bristol Zoological Society, another Bristol organization that nearly collapsed under the weight of Establishment oppression. It was meant to imitate the fashionable London Zoological Gardens, and if Liverpool already had a zoo, so must Bristol. It would both aid its elite citizens' scientific endeavors and serve as an instrument of edification and respectable entertainment for its lesser folk. Accordingly, a promenade through Bristol's zoological gardens would distract the populace from their rowdy gatherings, drinking, prize fights, and other entertainments. Morality would prevail among the grateful visitors. Irrespective of religion or party, Bristol's elite subscribed generously to the worthy Zoological Society. It was soon noticed, however, that as the only free day working-class Bristolians had to visit the zoo was a Sunday, the reformist subscribers planned to open it on the Sabbath. Crisis. Horrified evangelicals threatened to withdraw their subscriptions. They won, and the zoo was shut on Sundays, resulting in its near financial collapse toward the end of the 1830s.[32]

MD (Hon), Oxon

Penning anthropological contributions to the *West of England Journal* was more congenial to Prichard than lecturing and making unavoidable public speeches. What a momentous, nerve-racking, yet gratifying day was July 23, 1835, when he was honored, made a speech, and had a speech made about him at an assembly of about three hundred members of the medical profession gathered at the University of Oxford. The third annual meeting of the Provincial Medical and Surgical Association was a memorable conference packed full of medical and scientific demonstrations and lectures.

In the previous fifty years the university had grudgingly granted only one honorary MD, and that had been to the remarkable Dr. Edward Jenner. Now Prichard was receiving one, too—a bolt from the blue. Highly respected former professor of chemistry Dr. John Kidd wrote to Prichard in June with the news, and Dr. Charles Daubeny, Oxford chemist, botanist, and geologist, invited Prichard to be his guest. The day began with a formal breakfast at the Angel Inn, after which the members of the PMSA made their way to the museum, where for two hours the famous paleontologist and geological theorist Rev. Dr. William Buckland transfixed his audience with descriptions of paleontological phenomena using fossils from his collection: "With a good temper in his face, a gown on his shoulders, a wand in his hand, and a host of museum keys at his watch-chain, the professor urbanely greeted the crowd, took them at once to the cast of a portion of the vast megatherium, explained his own views of its structure and economy, . . . demonstrated the plesiosaurus, . . . described his volcanic theory of the earth's surface."[33] Buckland's was a hard act to follow.

In the afternoon the association gathered under the iconic classical rotunda of the Radcliffe Library. At the large round table in the center sat President Kidd, with Prichard on his left and the members and begowned professors on surrounding benches. As impressive as it must have seemed, it was soon marred by an unanticipated acoustic debacle: every little sound made by the large audience was amplified and echoed, rendering the speeches unintelligible. This boded ill for weak-voiced Prichard's performance. Dr. Kidd read the association's annual address, which included high praise of Prichard, after which "the President placed in the hands of Dr. Pritchard the parchment manuscript which constitutes the personal token of the honour conferred upon him. The presentation was loudly applauded." That parchment was the honorary MD (by diploma) of the University of Oxford conferred on him earlier in the day at convocation, amid even greater pomp and much Latin. He was appointed a member of the PMSA's council, as well. Instead of being elated, Prichard appeared rather pained at all the attention and flattery, then relieved to launch into his task, the reading of the annual retrospective address.[34]

Fortunately, Prichard's speech was later printed because it was not only inaudible but very, very long. Instead of conventionally plodding through recent medical and surgical achievements, he celebrated the demise of traditional and outmoded medicine and its supersession by a new spirit of "inductive philosophy." The medical theories of the past could now be relegated to the realms of historical detail. After reviewing the history of medicine at length, he did outline the year's progress, but so extended was his speech that he found himself skipping whole passages in order to cope with it. He managed to condemn homeopathy, praise the medicinal use of creosote, urge the collection of disease statistics, and call for a review of systems of quarantine and other treatment of contagious diseases. His "Retrospective Address," most valuable in welcoming in the new era of scientific medicine, was loudly applauded and followed by Sir Charles Bell's speech of thanks.[35]

More than two hundred medical men dined at the Star Hotel that evening, where Prichard and Dr. Carrick sat with Dr. Kidd. A vast number of toasts were drunk, speeches made, and thanks returned. When Prichard was toasted with three cheers, he returned his simple thanks, assuring the gathering that he would not make a speech as he had earlier trespassed so long on their attention. Several of his friends and Bristol medical brethren were there, wondering how Bristol might acquit itself at such a meeting in the future.[36] Prichard returned to Bristol the proud possessor of an MD (Hon), Oxon, with the full rights and privileges that he could not have obtained as a student and Dissenter before 1809. A fortnight later he boarded the steam packet to Dublin.

BAAS, Dublin, 1835

The fifth annual meeting of the British Association for the Advancement of Science required some careful reconnoitering because now that the nations' capitals and university cities had hosted it, Bristol was vying to be next. The six-day Dublin conference was even more exhausting than the PMSA meeting, as its many lectures were interspersed with excessive socializing. Prichard, Jem, and fellow Oxford student William Ley took lodgings on Harcourt Street in time for the start of the BAAS activities on August 10. Prichard found the meeting beneficial for the contacts he made with, for instance, Dr. William West, a member of council of the Royal Irish Academy, and archaeologist Dr. William Wilde.

Nearly two thousand people, "the rank and intellect of the metropolis," attended the first general meeting on Monday evening in the Rotunda. They learned hard; they played hard. All week there was a whirl of *conversaziones*, promenades, excursions, diversions, and discussions, as well as some fascinating lectures. For instance, on the afternoon of the August 11 there was a déjeuner at the zoological gardens followed by Dr. Dionysius Lardner's evening lecture on innovative "steam carriages." All over Dublin, the lions of science were not exactly prowling; Sir John Franklin was there, amiably chatting about his expeditions. Prichard endured public suppers, grand dinners, and breakfasts, including a breakfast at the College of Surgeons immediately followed by the Section E (Anatomy and Medicine) meeting in its anatomical theater. The Dublin Botanic Gardens hosted another déjeuner so well catered and elegant that many visitors skipped the lectures and spent the whole day there.[37]

The various sections reported on their proceedings to the general meeting, and there were some lectures such as one on tree-ring dating given by Charles Babbage, polymath and "father of the computer." As president of Section E, Prichard chaired most of its sessions. It seemed to be the least popular as its appeal was limited to a specialist, professional audience. At a final business meeting came the decision to hold the following year's meeting in Bristol, with Prichard as its treasurer.[38]

The lord lieutenant, Lord Mulgrave, in uniform resplendent with stars ablaze with diamonds, hosted a select and regally ceremonial dinner at Government House, Phoenix Park, on Thursday for about twenty-five guests of rank and fashion and some visiting savants, including Prichard. At the *beau finale* dinner in the imposing Trinity College Library, a memorable event unfolded. Suddenly clearing a spot among the guests, the Lord Mulgrave made a short speech in praise of Professor William Rowan Hamilton, the twenty-seven-year-old Irish mathematical genius. Then brandishing his sword, he commanded the embarrassed-looking professor to kneel and knighted him on the spot, complete with "Rise up, Sir William Rowan Hamilton!" Prichard had a lot to tell his family about his week in Dublin when the three weary travelers joined them summering at St Donat's Castle, Wales. At the BAAS Dublin, he had established fruitful relationships with Irish scientists, socialized with the famous, and collected some honorary memberships of Irish learned societies.[39]

Behind the scenes of that last planning meeting in Dublin, Prichard was discussed. Following the custom of other British societies, the BAAS council needed to elect a president for the ensuing year. It was an honorary position calculated to co-opt the prestige of some member of the aristocracy or remarkable professor. A witness to this meeting recounted:

> The ascendant party, Geologists and Physicists, named the Marquis of Lansdowne as President of the next meeting at Bristol. Others thought that Dr. J. C. Prichard, author of the Natural History of Man, and a resident, had a better claim. The Rev. Professor Robison of Armagh protested that he had never heard of Dr. Prichard, and could not tell in what department of science he was known. "That is not Dr. Prichard's fault!" cried half-a-dozen voices, among which, that of Dr. [Robert James] Graves, [a leader of the Irish medical community] was not the least indignant. But the nobleman prevailed over the founder of British Anthropology; and Lord Lansdowne became president of the Bristol Meeting.[40]

Lord Lansdowne's selection was not decisive, however. In November, Prichard replied to BAAS organizer Harcourt, dismissing several contenders for their tenuous connection to Bristol or their political bias, but he sang the praises of Lord Lansdowne like his life depended on it. Bristolians had a good opinion of the marquis.[41]

BAAS, Bristol, 1836

The British Association for the Advancement of Science was about to descend on Bristol. Not only would scientists from around the transatlantic world grace Bristol with their presence; some of them would visit the Red Lodge. Prichard's mother-in-law promised to provide a bed to "any German or outlandish professor he may wish to accommodate. This is all I can do for science which it has ever been my desire to promote."[42]

Organizing the BAAS meeting posed some problems, however, even with the support of several Bristolians with pretensions to liberality. The vexed question of the presidency had continued to preoccupy the organizers; not only was Lord Lansdowne not a member of the association, but as a Whig his appointment might alienate Bristol factions. Engineer Davies Gilbert was dismissed for not being Bristolian enough.[43] Conybeare was thought too excitable and Prichard "too tame," so they were appointed vice presidents, while Lansdowne accepted the presidency. "The good people of Bristol throw all their manufactories open to us & have subscribed £1600," reported geologist G. B. Greenough optimistically. Unfortunately, the lecture room at the BI held fewer than 350 people, so it would be necessary to impose the rule excluding ladies.[44]

The Bristol newspapers covered the BAAS meeting in several self-congratulatory columns; civic pride was heavily invested in its success. The Medicine and Anatomy Section's three papers "excited much attention." Prichard's "On the Treatment of Some Diseases of the Brain" advocated counterirritation as an effective form of treatment. He described the insertion of one to three rows of peas under the scalp, his favorite "Prichard issue," assuring his listeners it was not as severe a treatment as they might suppose. While it was contraindicated for maniacal or hysterical conditions, it was otherwise on a par with bleeding. Prichard's colleague Dr. Wallis testified to the merits of the procedure even on young children, and he claimed that of the one hundred cases he had witnessed, there had been only one failure. But what was most telling on this occasion was Prichard's prefatory speech, in which he regretted medicine's lack of progress in recent years. He seemed to approve of the recent "more precise" scientific approach to the study of disease at the level of tissue as in morbid anatomy but felt the practical application of new knowledge was still lacking. As in his Oxford MD speech of the previous year, Prichard placed himself at the threshold of scientific medicine and welcomed it in, despite its potential threat to religious orthodoxy.[45]

The Bristol BAAS meeting had the usual portion of social activities too. There was a very well-attended laying of the first stone of the stupendous Clifton Suspension Bridge, held at 7 a.m. so as not to interfere with the lectures of the day. Other pleasurable educational activities included excursions to a Mr. Miller's horticultural garden in Clifton and to Hanham and Keynsham, where the cuttings and tunnels for the new Great Western Railway had revealed some interesting geology. A voyage down the Avon to Portishead was accompanied by Conybeare's running commentary on the stratigraphy of the Avon Gorge. The steamer was on course for the islands of Flat Holm and Steep Holm, where the passengers could try their hand at geologizing. And, of course, there were several sumptuous dinners.[46]

Some personal accounts indicate the Bristol BAAS meeting was not a total success. Lord Lansdowne's absence attending his son's deathbed was regrettable; his friend the Irish poet and songwriter Thomas Moore, author of the wildly popular poem *Lalla Rookh*, attended to see, be seen, and gossip. Generally dismissive, he thought the balloon ascent was entertaining enough and the visit to the Bone Cave at Banwell interesting. The demonstration of a kite-propelled car was a bit of a damp squib, however, as the passenger was an overweight aristocrat and there was very little wind. Alarmingly, a man attempting to cross the gorge on a rail got stuck halfway across and was lucky to escape with his life. The Bristol Institution was jam packed and sweltering. After calling on Prichard, Moore went to a dull public meal and returned to a soiree at the Red Lodge, where a large party was assembled. Baron Charles Dupin was there, looking interesting but rather too theatrical in look and manner, while Babbage was evidently discontented with his brother Savants, who had produced an immense quantity of the ridiculous in their transactions that must be suppressed in future.[47]

The Dublin mathematical knight Hamilton more positively compared Dublin and Bristol: "This Meeting is inferior to the last in public buildings and public entertainment; but it is equal and perhaps superior in the presence of eminent men; for many are here who did not like to cross the Channel to Dublin."[48] One presentation at this meeting led Prichard to help make another Bristol "improvement." Bristolian Charles Bowles Fripp's lecture to the Statistical Section on the educational statistics of

Bristol highlighted the inadequacy of educational provision and the need to establish statistical societies to carry out social research. Collecting data was right up Prichard's alley.

The "Improving" Nature of the Bristol Statistical Society

Some new sciences required experimentation and refined observational apparatus, but the fields in which Prichard was most involved required the collection and analysis of information—Prichard's passion. From boyhood charts of kings and queens to vocabulary lists, he had always put great store in organizing facts. The number of tables included in his recent *Treatise on Insanity* illustrate this. Prichard was not alone in his faith in data. One enthusiast was the immensely popular biogeographer, ecologist, and naturalist of South America and Russia Alexander von Humboldt. Personal accounts of this Prussian scientific superstar refer to his obsession with gathering, measuring, and analyzing data in his quest to understand nature. Between 1814 and 1825 Prichard borrowed several of Humboldt's books from the Bristol Library. In European scientific practice, measurement and the application of mathematics were considered instrumental to discovering the laws governing both physical and social phenomena.

The BAAS Statistical Section had been established in 1833, partly owing to the encouragement of a liberal Anglican, progressive, reforming clique that included William Whewell, the scientist and historian and later philosopher of science with whom Prichard corresponded. As Prichard valued a statistical approach to comprehending epidemics, insanity, and humankind, he could see how it might be applied to understanding and improving Bristol too.[49]

A few weeks after the BAAS left the city, Prichard and some friends including Lant Carpenter, Symonds, Joseph Henry Jerrard, and William Tothill got together at the Bristol Institution to found the Bristol Statistical Society. Again, Lord Lansdowne was elected president, with the actual running of the society in the hands of its two vice presidents, one of whom was Prichard. The stated aim of the society was to systematically collect data on which to base rational inferences that would facilitate improvements in society, excluding party politics. One of its loyal members was Tory J. M. Gutch, the editor of *Felix Farley's Bristol Journal*, who energetically reported and promoted it in his newspaper. The Bristol Statistical Society met four times a year, with Prichard chairing its November annual general meetings. The members' £1 annual subscription funded an agent to carry out research and manage the publication of the society's *Proceedings*.

Not only did the Bristol Statistical Society aim to collect data for scientific purposes; it intended to study the ways of the poor to help reform their physical and social conditions sufficient to prevent radicalism. It inquired into the state of the working classes of Bristol, later adding data from commerce, the police, the coroner, and the city jail. Its 1838 report highlighted not its members' humane concern for their fellow citizens but the specter of bloody revolution should the poor be deprived of the means of leading civilized lives. Its fieldwork attempted to understand "the natives" so that they could be "improved." Eventually it pointed out the benefits of providing children from impoverished families an education *suited to their rank*. Statistics were a tool of social control. Henry Mayhew's *London Labour and the London Poor*, a book groundbreaking in its statistical approach, would cite Prichard in an attempt to classify "street-folk" anthropometrically.[50]

Like the BI, the Statistical Society was Anglican and Tory-dominated but not sectarian. It was affiliated with the national society and presented its findings to the Statistical Section of the BAAS, where again the conditions of the poor, their attendance at Sunday school, and the incidence of disease and crime were of prime concern. They offered to furnish the government with a sound basis on which to form policies that would obviate social unrest—not that they appeared to connect the wretched living conditions of the poor to wider economic issues such as industrialization. Statistical societies struggled to maintain the zeal of its members beyond the end of the 1830s. Perhaps being limited to the sterile collection of data was frustrating, especially as their findings were not evidently translated into beneficial legislation.[51] Prichard's efforts to find meaning through involvement in the Statistical Society evidenced his essentially humane outlook as well as his fears during a period characterized by a general desire to seek improvement in society while holding radicalism at bay.

Protégé William Benjamin Carpenter and Modern Science

With his explorations of order in the natural world, society, language, and the human mind, Prichard was a scientist in the decades just before the development of modern science. The early career of his young family friend William Benjamin Carpenter typifies science's mid-nineteenth-century transition.[52] He faced considerable cultural constraint. The Carpenters had been the Prichards' close friends since hardworking and deeply religious Unitarian Lant Carpenter brought his family to Bristol in 1817. Frequently at the Red Lodge, William and his brother became fascinated by science. They were apprenticed to John Estlin and attended the nearby Medical School.

Young Dr. Carpenter, with his Edinburgh MD in hand, turned out not to have a talent for building a private practice, nor could he eke out a living teaching at Bristol College and Bristol Medical School. Prichard seemed to see himself in Carpenter's yearning for a life in science, yet burdened by the reality of a physician's hard graft. He did what he could to support Carpenter in his choice of science, encouraging him to read his first paper, "The Unity of the Species," at the 1836 Bristol BAAS meeting. Carpenter's groundbreaking *Principles of General and Comparative Physiology* three years later determined his future. The book's supposed materialism brought the wrath of the Establishment down on his head. In defense, he maintained that propounding the laws of nature illustrates rather than denies the power of the Almighty. When he applied to join the staff of a new provincial college intended to be linked to the liberal London University, he cited Conybeare and Prichard's approval of the orthodoxy of his Bristol Institution lectures. Privately he was pessimistic:

> I fear that my religious opinions would be a serious obstacle to my receiving any office [at Liverpool College], since I know that the combination of religious with scientific instruction is especially aimed at. But ... I or any other Unitarian can make as much use of Science in explaining the foundation of <u>Natural</u> Religion, as the most orthodox Churchman, and that up to the point where Revelation commences, we entirely agree. No one can teach the truths of <u>Revealed</u> Religion from Science; but it is the duty of the Philosopher to show the accordance of these two departments of knowledge, and to teach such a mode of enquiry in Science as shall not clash with the indisputable truths of Revelation.

Carpenter also pointed out his agreement with the Rev. William Vernon Harcourt's 1839 BAAS speech establishing the principle that science must have freedom of inquiry. He had to look over his shoulder constantly: "I am myself doubtful how far it is desirable to be constantly dwelling upon <u>instances</u> of Creative Design <u>as such</u>, since I fear that the idea is thus apt to become trite;—and I think that the mind which has been trained to appreciate the value of <u>general laws,</u> is capable of erecting its notion of Design upon a much more extensive basis." As for politics, he proclaimed, "<u>Science is of no party</u>."[53] Three years later, his application to the University of Edinburgh was dismissed out of hand on the grounds of his Unitarianism.[54] Religious and political affiliation and personal opinions about religion and the natural world determined professional advancement. The Church intended to keep its grip on science.

Carpenter had been impressed by his youthful visit to Saint Vincent with John Estlin. Being steeped in his Unitarian community's commitment to the antislavery cause brought him further notoriety and a friendship with committed antislavery advocate Charles Darwin. He eventually gained appointments in London and became an eminent physiologist, invertebrate zoologist, and science educator. He maintained his commitment to demonstrating the original unity of the human species and, like Estlin, to the abolition and temperance movements. A star lecturer at the 1847 Oxford BAAS meeting, Carpenter's list of achievements filled an entire paragraph.[55]

Carpenter's views on the "species question" grew directly out of Prichard's work. He referred to his mentor in his *Principles of Human Physiology*, where he also noted that Prichard had coined the term "somatic death." Prichard and Carpenter did not agree on religion and politics, but they shared a desire to understand nature. Eventually, Carpenter admitted he "owed the foundation of whatever reputation he had achieved to Bristol and to Dr. Prichard, who had been his earliest friend and greatest teacher in scientific research and inquiry."[56] He had become the scientist Prichard had dreamed of being a generation earlier.

Illusive Oxford Professorships

Now entering his fifties Prichard enjoyed a national reputation and had an Oxford MD diploma on his wall, but to his regret, a desirable Oxford professorship had failed to materialize. He yearned for the intellectual atmosphere in which he felt most at home—the Oxford of his time there in 1809. With his friend Conybeare he joined Oxford's Ashmolean Society.[57] He sounded out or applied for Oxford professorships but in vain. Candidates already resident at the university had the inside track in any contest. Prichard's friend the influential autocratic bastion of evangelicalism and warden of Wadham College Benjamin Parsons Symons had got his hopes up about the professorship of Sanskrit, but it went to another. When Prichard was attempting to land a London appointment in April 1837, his father was "glad to find that the Drs journey to London has been satisfactory to him. I fancy him tempted to take up his residence in the Metropolis, & I can by no means wonder at such a choice; and if he should succeed in his application to the Lord Chancellor, I shall expect to hear of his forsaking Bristol. His interviews with Miss Aikin & Miss Martineau have not, I hope, had any tendency to connect him with their opinions-the latter in particular is with me an object of Odium Theologium, or Odium Politicum or some Odium."[58]

Prichard needed the backing of some Oxbridge professors and influential metropolitans. He must have encountered Harriet Martineau and Lucy Aikin with some trepidation, those independent feminist writers and forthright campaigners who dared to published on a wide range of topics, from history to mesmerism and insanity. Thomas Prichard was not alone in his disgust of their radical Unitarianism bordering on atheism, that cancer of the decade. Martineau was infamous for her *odium politicum* and freethinking, Whig soirees at her London home, where three Charleses—Babbage, Lyell, and young Darwin—could discuss species transmutation and mind dualism.[59] Tory Prichard had braved Miss Martineau's lions' den.

Prichard's most influential friends rallied around him in his 1842 attempt at an Oxford appointment. This time it was the Regius Professorship of Modern History, vacated by the sudden death of the famous Dr. Thomas Arnold. Despite the title, the post was not exclusive to historians of modern history, nor would it be necessary to reside in Oxford more than a few months each year. There were hardly any courses or examinable teaching of history there anyway. Arnold's predecessor had qualified for the post by marrying the daughter of the Duke of Marlborough and had gone years without delivering a lecture.

Prichard tried his best to secure this professorship. Oxford and Cambridge had been making some progress in broadening their curriculum beyond the classics, theology, and mathematics, but resistance continued.[60] He had made his views known at Oxford on the narrowness of its education, writing: "The change I most wish to see effected in Oxford is a great extension of the system of education. A man who takes a degree in the first class in literature ought to be acquainted with the languages & literature of the East—Sanskrit & Arabic, as well as with the Greek & Latin classics. I wonder that some acquaintance with modern sciences is not required."[61] With characteristic enthusiasm, Conybeare encouraged Prichard to apply. But he hesitated, first making a deferential approach to influential William Whewell. Prichard doubted his conception of history would be acceptable, particularly as it was founded on the Continental historians Jean-Pierre Abel-Rémusat, Julius Klaproth, the Schlegels, Karl Otfried Müller, and Carl Ritter's *Erdkunde*, and its scope was not confined to Europe and the classical world. This would challenge the Oxford view of history as an echo of the classics. What was Whewell's opinion of Prichard's prospects? Rumor had it that a particular young Oxford man who was not even a historian was a shoo-in.[62]

Whewell replied optimistically. After consulting William Buckland in Oxford, they laid out a strategy. Encouraged but still needing reassurance, Prichard described his view of history and its pedagogy to Whewell, beginning with the question: "But do you not think that ethnology belongs quite as much to modern as to ancient history?" He then enlarged upon the connection between world history and the fall of ancient civilizations and went on to imply one need go no further than his third edition of *Physical History* to see his dedication as a historian. Far from puffery was Prichard's confident claim that his work was deeply historical. If appointed, he would further academic reform at his alma mater by structuring the discipline of history education:

> I think I could make my method of surveying history of some use in Oxford where history is understood in as restricted a sense as is "*Science*" (Science there meaning Aristotelian studies and theology.) In a course of lectures on ethnology the moral history of nations & the history of their religion & literature forms an essential part and I should make a great point of giving [much wider extension?] to these subjects than I could do in a work on the merely physical hist. of Mankind, where they could only be introduced as they contingently bear on the principal questions.[63]

Applications flooded in, much to the annoyance of Prime Minister Sir Robert Peel, whose responsibility the appointment was. Several of the candidates already held other Oxford posts and were attempting to add to their number through a sort of professorial pluralism. Letters of support from the aspirants' colleges extolled their man's virtues with little concern for the actual subject of history.[64] The vice chancellor helpfully warned the chancellor, the Duke of Wellington, that one would-be professor was rumored to be a Whig.

While Conybeare was marshaling the support of influential men, Prichard's Ross friend Dr. Charles Atmore Ogilvie solicited the archbishop of Canterbury's endorsement of Prichard on the grounds of his scholarship, eminence, wide knowledge, and "zeal and energy, with which he has devoted his powers and attainments to the support and furtherance of the cause of true Religion." He pointed out that Prichard had studied at Oxford, and his MD (Hon), Oxon, meant he was a bona fide member of convocation.[65] To fellow geologist William Whewell, Buckland wrote confidentially about the candidates, but his choice was Prichard because he "like Arnold has a great subject in hand & if life be spared will work it onwards as he has begun— . . . Pritchard is a man in the same class as Hallam . . . whose name is known from China to Peru."[66] Whewell supplied a fulsome testimony to Prichard's historical works "considered throughout Europe as among the most learned and sound which have appeared in our time. . . . He is a man of genius, as well as of vast and varied erudition. . . . I conceive that if he has to deliver lectures, he will take his course, not at all in the way of a continuation of his predecessor's labours, but something original striking, and instructive. He will probably give the University a view of the results of the researches of Continental scholars such as will not in any other way come before the world." What more was there to say?

For good measure, Whewell sent a copy of his letter to Peel's ally the young William Ewart Gladstone, who quoted Whewell in his own recommendation to the prime minister, requesting to speak to him personally on the subject.[67] With the archbishop, Peel's Tory colleague, and the two most respected Tory scientists in England endorsing True Blue Prichard, his application to Peel, dated Oxford, July 23, 1842, seemed all but a formality. After listing his historical publications and supporters, including Baron Bunsen, Prichard made his pitch:

> It has been hinted to me that the professorship of history, vacant by the death of the late Dr Arnold, has not been filled up because no person has yet occurred who has been thought qualified to succeed to it. It will be long before a worthy successor of Dr Arnold shall be discovered and certainly nobody can be further than myself from entertaining for a moment the idea of making such a pretension, but should no person be proposed who is qualified by a long course of study, devoted to the subject, to give lectures on history and the sources of history before the university, I shall be willing to undertake to supply the deficiency for a time.
>
> The study of history, in connection with ethnography, and of the sources of history & literature in the different departments of mankind has been my favorite and I may say constant pursuit, during more than 30 years, and my works connected with those subjects have been sufficiently known to procure me a place in the Academy of Moral & Political Sciences in the National Institute of France and a doctor's degree (by diploma, not the commonly given honorary degree, but a

much more rare distinction) in the University of Oxford, where I was originally educated. . . .

The object of my works has not been merely archaeological, but to draw a philosophical comparison of the moral history, literature, mythology &c of different races, with a view to estimate the influence of various agencies physical, moral & political on the history of nations & of mankind. The same inquiries followed out with a somewhat more extensive plan, would if I mistake not, be a suitable addition to the somewhat restricted plans of historical studies hitherto followed in the University.[68]

By the time the archbishop's recommendation landed on Peel's desk, the post had been offered to someone who had not actually applied. John Antony Cramer, a university man more distinguished for the number of his appointments than for his reputation as a historian, got the job. In his letter of acceptance he candidly doubted he was suitable for the professorship as he specialized in ancient history and theology. No matter. Regius Professor Cramer gave nothing more than his inaugural lecture and resigned three years later to become dean of Carlisle.[69] Prichard had lost out to "one of their own." He was disappointed but would not give up.

In the spring of 1845, Prichard sounded out geologists Buckland and Daubeny on his chances of securing the vacant professorship of philology at Oxford, halfheartedly explaining: "I have often read papers or lectures on ethnological subjects—containing several views of philology which have been well received by large audiences at the Bristol Institution and I think I could lecture on philology (that is comparative philology as it is now called) well enough for the purposes of the new appointment. The subject might indeed be made to comprehend much connected with the train of my studies."[70] Receiving no encouragement, Prichard remained "out of the way" in Bristol. His attempts to enter academia came to an end.

Red Lodge Life

Family life for the Prichard children continued to include varied and stimulating activities, whether educational or recreational. Being Dr. Prichard's child was a source of anxiety as well as pride; the pressure was palpable. On one occasion when Jem was still a Bristol College pupil, his father was unavoidably absent from Bristol the evening he was scheduled to lecture at the Bristol Institution, so he sent Jem, spidery manuscript in hand, to read it in his stead to a large, appreciative audience.[71] Thomas Prichard had to plead for some lighter reading material for his grandsons, easier texts to translate, and an occasional break from study. They won prizes at Bristol College and crammed for scholarships, and even though they did not all become clergymen, they entered respectable professions. Augustin reminisced he had been relieved when he failed to gain an Oxford scholarship. Prichard the proud father wrote in 1837:

> Our boys, viz the three who are getting towards the size of men have all disposed of themselves. Augustin, the next after James has so strong a predilection for medicine or rather surgery that I could not persuade him to think of abandoning it. He has been about a year or rather more partly with Mr Estlin & in part at the Infirmary. He is so fond of the occupation that I thought it not right to do anything more than suggest a different course. The two next boys Constantine & Theodore have long set their hearts upon going to Oxford or Cambridge & from the application to study which they shew at present I am in hopes that they will both do well in an University career to which they must look not for accomplishments, but for the means of making their bread. The next boy after Theodore [Illtudus Thomas] is not yet old enough to go from home, & what he will be a few years hence we cannot tell.[72]

Prichard felt no need to mention his two surviving daughters, of course. Edith was still very young, and sweet, ailing Mary was at the time simply waiting to be married. Prichard's learned societies had no women members; only on special occasions might ladies be permitted to attend, and they would not dream of speaking publicly. There was neither higher education nor a profession in store for his daughters. Prichard did not disapprove of women's engaging in scholarship; he encouraged his cousin Charlotte Wilkins's studies by copying into her album a poem in "the oldest language in Europe" with its German translation, and he helped her to get her review of a German book published in the *Journal of the Geographical Society*, an exceptional occurrence. He also wrote a glowing letter of introduction to the editor of *Blackwood's Magazine* on behalf of the wife of an Irish friend, an experienced author who wanted to publish in an English periodical.[73]

Mary Prichard led a quiet life at the Red Lodge, sharing her parents' cares, occasionally traveling and keenly collecting mementos of famous visitors. In her very neat album there are poems of praise and blessing; Prichard's begins: "What words, dear Mary, shall I write upon thy spotless leaf? / A prayer that Heaven may grant of all its blessed gifts the chief."

Others contributed poetry in a similar vein. The evangelical stalwart Hannah More tersely commanded "Read the Scriptures / Clifton 1830." A few pasted-in entries represent the popular pastime of autograph collecting. Mirza Saleh Shirazi, a British-educated Persian who returned to Iran to become a newspaper publisher, public servant, and promoter of European technology, visited Prichard and the Infirmary on October 23, 1818, and presented Prichard's wife with his calling card. Other entries in the album are by distinguished visitors to the Red Lodge. The Ojibwe Kahkewāquonāby, a.k.a. the Rev. Peter Jones, Methodist, tribal chief, Indigenous rights campaigner, and translator on a speaking tour of Britain, must have fascinated Mary. Jones was ill at that time, and Prichard was his physician.[74]

Baron Charles Dupin, that Red Lodge guest during the 1836 BAAS meeting, wrote her a most fulsome entry:

> I feel most happy to have had that good fortune, as an observer of men and manners, to have lived for a week, in the middle of one of those truly british families, where virtue, peace and happiness are the moral example of life; where such treasurer of blessing are the domestic recompense of the high gifts of talent and Science. The eminence of these gifts seems at first overshaded, but very soon shine the more, as superior merit, shows itself in the unassuming characteristics of simple, noble and true genius. May long live and prosper, and continue the virtuous and learned lineage, the amiable, and gentle daughter of the kindest mother and a celebrated father! Such are the wishes of their most devoted friend.[75]

Another guest that day was classical philologist and literary critic August Wilhelm von Schlegel. When William Benjamin Carpenter's sister Mary, "a young lady of the greatest worth & highest intellectual endowments," was setting off for Germany, Prichard provided her with an introduction to him. Eighteen years later she took possession of the Red Lodge: "I entered the deserted house! Those stairs I had often in former years trodden with mingled feelings of respect & pleasing anticipation when going to visit Dr Pritchard, whose society I always esteemed a high privilege & intellectual treat. There I had been present at a grand soiree of men of high position in the Scientific world, assembled at the meeting of the British Association in 1836."[76] Carpenter established a reformatory school there and entered history as a pioneer in special education. She specialized in rehabilitating young girls who had fallen from the path of virtue, teaching them basic domestic skills and a sense of the Almighty before sending them off to be good servants.

Mary Prichard's album chronicles the family's social life too. After a page of hieroglyphics, there is a steady stream of contributions: poetry in 1834 by John Thelwall, whose abilities Prichard so admired; Baron Bunsen's German poem and blessings on the daughter of "my dear friend," November 12, 1838; a poem by linguist Vicomte Hersart de la Villemarqué; family members' greetings upon her safe return from Madeira; and a final, loving poem from her brother Theodore in 1841.[77]

After describing the Red Lodge and its "splendid drawing room," Baron Bunsen recorded his impression of the family he was visiting: "The whole family was collected, including the eldest son, who is tutor of Oriel college, mother and daughter very pleasing, and taking interest in the occupations and studies of the husband and father. After dinner we had some good singing and playing and we talked on till near midnight."[78] Prichard's friendship with Baron Bunsen continued. They spent some time together in his library discussing the latest philological publications he had acquired from American contacts. Prichard dedicated *Natural History of Man* to "his dear friend His Excellency the Chevalier Bunsen" on September 30, 1842, around the time Bunsen secured him a government appointment.

The younger Prichards must have been fascinated by one of their house guests, a young Turkish man who had just finished his education in France. "Edhem Bey, (the Turk's name) says he will knock down the slave market at Cairo, and build a large school house in its place." That was an understandable ambition as Ebrahim Edhem, later Pasha, a government minister and ambassador, had been enslaved before being adopted by the grand vizier.[79] The rather impetuous young Dr. William Budd, a future pioneer of epidemiology, came to the Red Lodge two or three times a week to play chess. Several close friends, like Dr. Symonds and some Bristol College students, had open invitations; otherwise, Prichard or his son would often send notes asking people whether they "will do us the pleasure of drinking tea with us tomorrow evg at eight o'clock?" Distinguished visitors were not the only people who took an interest in the Prichard children. Augustin described the atmosphere:

> In the large old oak drawing-room of the Red Lodge, many clever and learned men used to meet for two or three hours of intellectual conversation. The most intelligent and literary men among the inhabitants of this city, the masters of the old Bristol college, and on account of his book on the Physical History of Man my father's name was held in as much, if not more, esteem on the Continent than in England, any

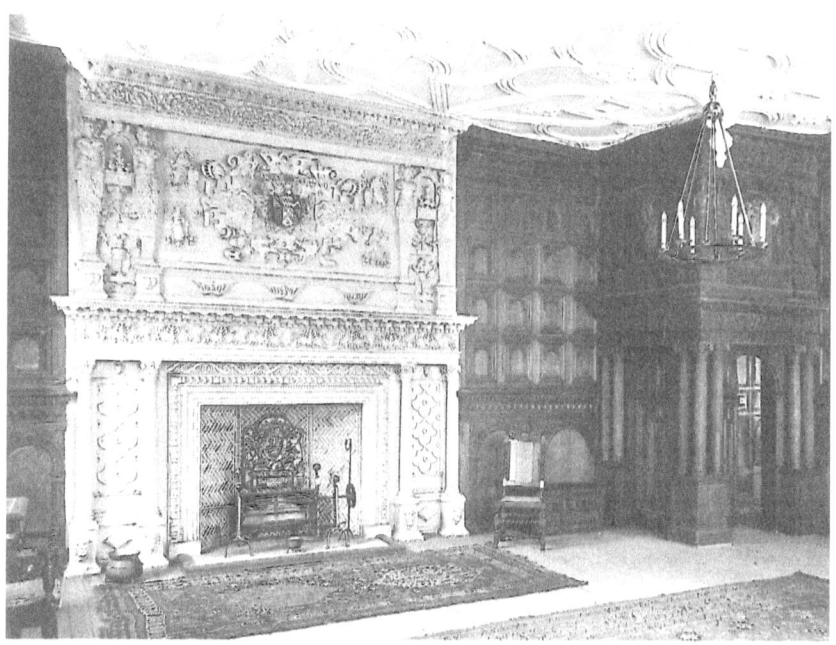

10. Imposing Tudor interior. The Great Oak Room, Red Lodge, Bristol. Photo by Derek Balmer. Courtesy of the author.

celebrity that was passing through or temporarily resident, formed the company invited according to the custom of the time to drink tea: they came about eight o'clock and dispersed soon after ten, and it was a matter sometimes of great interest, even to us boys, to be present.[80]

Bunsen had not exaggerated when he reported the fun and games in the Red Lodge. When Prichard complained of having difficulty hearing the sermons at St. Michael's Church, Jem composed a spoof "Church Service" booklet, to which the children all subscribed. It commemorated his fifty-ninth birthday and began "Patri dilectissimus."[81] For a considerable period the entire family were active reporters for the family newspaper, the *Red Lodge Intelligencer*, contributing their news, sketches, and creative writing. A swashbuckling drama set in nearby ancient Church Lane was written and performed by a cast comprising Jem, Gus, Con, and The. "Brothers well met! Whence wend ye here your way and whither?" opens the play, followed by a script packed with "thou," "dastardly," "who be it?," "steeds," "take that!," and references to despotic schoolmasters, ambrosial sweet shops, and a craven bully named John Wallis. A sword fight is clearly going well when The discovers that the exercise has given him a bit of an appetite, so the four brothers *exeunt omnes*, singing the praise of meat, bread, potatoes, and toasted cheese.[82]

Another family entertainment was the inhalation of laughing gas. Augustin described making it when he was an apprentice, collecting it in large bullock bladders fitted with a tube and cork. He and his brothers would sometimes administer it to family and friends with hilarious results. When it was to be exhibited, the performer was seated in the middle of the room, a bladderful was handed to him, and he was directed to breathe freely from it. Chaos generally ensued. A boy might rush about, aiming furious blows with his fists and trying to wrestle with anyone he could catch hold of. The girls, very rarely allowed to have it, would jump and dance and sing. The only after-effects were bruised knuckles from punching the walls.[83]

As for serious discussions at the Red Lodge, Prichard was knowledgeable about literature and the fine arts and could discuss them. He privately wrote his share of religious poetry and made translations from Greek and Hebrew literature as a pastime. In conversation, he preferred broad and decided views rather than hair-splitting distinctions but was never dogmatic or overbearing. Without condescension to the less well-informed, in an open and unassuming manner he would unroll a mass of information and ask his disputants a few questions that would somehow lead them to arrive at correct views rather than to suffer defeat. However, although he generally discussed topics without bias, he would sometimes for amusement play devil's advocate to draw out a fair analysis of a point. According to Dr. Symonds: "Everyone left his society impressed, as much by the modesty of the great man, as by the marvellous extent of his knowledge."[84]

Prichard's now international reputation and contacts with eminent scientists resulted in his steady accumulation of honorary memberships in learned institutions like the Académie Nationale de Médecine. He was elected member of the American Philosophical Society and a corresponding member of the Académie des Sciences Morales et Politiques, Institut de France.[85]

Prichard in Middle Life

Drs. Hodgkin and Symonds left the most searching descriptions of Prichard at the height of his career:

> Dr. Prichard was in stature rather below the middle height, and of rather slight make. He had light hair, and grey eyes, which, though somewhat small, were of singularly intelligent expression. The form

of his head was very fine; broad and prominent in the forehead, lofty and capacious in the crown. The countenance, to the most superficial observer, betokened deep thoughtfulness, with something of reserve and shyness, but blended with true kindliness. His voice was rather weak and low, but very distinct in articulation. His manners and deportment . . . were simple and unaffected;—and in general company he evidently spoke with effort or even reluctance, unless upon subjects of business or of scientific and literary interest.

Prichard's friends remarked that he had a prodigious memory and a tendency to collect and methodically arrange facts such that he could easily bring an immense amount of evidence to bear upon a particular point in a comprehensive if not very subtle way. He was particularly fond of tracing origins and causes. Prichard could achieve a lot in the three or more hours he studied before his working day began, and he was known to be highly focused on finishing whatever was needed. At other times he could develop trains of thought, be interrupted, and then return to the original argument unimpeded.[86]

Despite Thomas Prichard's initial negative impression of the Red Lodge, the family flourished there. Prichard himself was particularly proud of the magnificent oak-paneled drawing room. But after ten years of tenancy at £70 per annum, a large broadside and a newspaper advertisement announced that the Red Lodge was to be sold by auction on August 17, 1837. The agent particularly recommended its splendid Elizabethan carvings, which "being still in a high state of preservation is well worthy [of] the attention of any gentleman building in the antique style, as the whole might be easily removed." Prichard's offer of £1,050 was deemed an injustice to the reversionary legatees, so he stumped up another £50, and the Red Lodge was secured.[87]

Victoria Regina

With Victoria's accession in 1837 the momentum of reform quickened. The new young, virtuous monarch was the harbinger of regeneration. The decades of low national morale and threats of revolution would be tempered by generous helpings of civil pomp, expressions of loyalty, and growing national prosperity. Bristol itself was becoming a more pleasant place to live as well. Its civic institutions were better regulated since, in the wake of the Bristol riots and the Reform Act, the Municipal Reform Act of 1835 had forced reforms in local government. The Corporation's accounts were audited, and it was now compelled to provide its citizens with improved infrastructure, welfare, police, and other services, excluding education.

On the local economic front, the Corporation continued burdened with debt from the 1831 riot, and it failed to adequately regulate the all-important docks; the port was in decline. The new railway serving the city had the impediment of being uniquely wide-gauged; and bankruptcy had halted progress on the Clifton Suspension Bridge. But there were some thriving shipbuilding and small-scale manufacturing; the houses of Clifton were mostly built and the construction of the ostentatious Victoria Rooms was about to start. There were horse races on the Downs, balls at the Assembly Rooms and visits to the theater, the Bristol Zoological Gardens, bazaars, lectures, concerts, and the Bristol Institution's museum and gallery. The poor were as poor as ever, however, despite Bristol's plethora of charities and Sunday schools. When would the next epidemic begin?

Jem and His Younger Brothers

James Cowles Prichard Jr. shared his father's personality as well as name. He looked set to satisfy his father's wish for a brilliant Oxford career and church preferment. Jem was modest, confiding, unaffected, even tempered, amiable, and, unlike his father, disinclined to engage in disputes. His favorite studies were botany, philology (especially of Hebrew and Syriac), and theology, and he possessed great ability to compose in prose and verse. Jem wished to please his father, who "crammed" him successfully. At Oxford his intellectual gifts and superb ability to retain information were accompanied by what might have been considered the fault of reading too widely.[88]

From 1832 Jem was a scholar at Trinity College, won the Chancellor's Prize for Latin Verse in 1835, and was awarded a BA, first class, in classics in 1836. After a long period of preparation, in early 1838 he competed for one of the Oriel fellowships, an exacting process. Even finding out about Oriel vacancies was more a matter of whom one knew. There were various opposing factions. Jem had to pay the provost of Oriel an official visit to demonstrate that his attitude, beliefs, connections with existing fellows, financial position, and family background passed muster. He then had to compose several letters in Latin to the fellows and undergo their scrutiny in the common room and dining hall. Would he fit in? All this was even before the actual examination, conducted over four days during Easter week.[89]

The ordeal comprised both written and oral translations to and from Latin and Greek. The viva voce before the provost and fellows in the unfortunately named Tower brought the torture to a close. The following day, the provost's servant summoned Jem to Oriel to receive the congratulations of the fellows and attend a chapel service, at which he was granted a probationary fellowship. One of his competitors grudgingly described him as a compromise choice and "a very clever scholar of the superficial sort." While Jem was waiting to start his fellowship at Oxford, he was delighted to obtain a temporary post as a tutor to a family in the Lake District, especially as his brothers Con and The were allowed to join him there to carry on their studies under his supervision.[90]

Prichard was highly gratified by Jem's Oriel fellowship, but life in Oxford had its perils. The Oxford Movement was in full swing, centered on John Henry Newman and his associates at Jem's college. It had originated in a liberal reaction against the Established Church's abuses of wealth and privilege, especially in the Church of Ireland, but recently the whiff of popery among the Oxford Movement's adherents had become undeniable. Also called Tractarianism, this growing group of Anglicans was increasingly dissatisfied with the austerity of Anglicanism and attracted to some of the pre-Reformation ancient tenets and rituals of the Catholic Church. Eventually, its leader John Henry Newman converted to the Church of Rome and was later made a cardinal.

Jem was ordained at Hereford on July 4, 1841, and married William Ley's sister Emma Henrietta three days later, necessarily resigning his Oriel fellowship. After briefly holding the curacy of Madley in Herefordshire, he was granted the living of Mitcham, Surrey, the duties of which he undertook assiduously. Mitcham was in the gift of the Simpsons, the family of an Oxford acquaintance who had required assurances of Jem's sufficiently High Church leanings such as in favoring the celebration of saints' days. His education in the bosom of the Oxford Movement had had its effect. Unfortunately, the Mitcham post was insecure; he had to sign a bond requiring him to surrender it at one month's notice whenever young Richard Simpson wished to have it. Nor was it a sinecure; Prichard had to help Jem find private pupils to make ends meet. As it turned out, he soon had to resign Mitcham for quite another reason.[91]

The next few years were burdened with the deaths of two of Jem and Emma's three children and his constant illness, unrelieved by periods of recuperation in Barbados, sometimes at the Red Lodge, and in Madeira, that mecca of English consumptives. He surrendered his Mitcham curacy while Anna Prichard fostered their surviving child. In May 1848 and in poorer health than ever, he prepared his *Life of Hincmar* for the press, visited his childhood haunts in Bristol, and died at the Red Lodge on September 11.[92] Prichard and Anna would mourn the deaths of five of their children. As for Jem's younger brothers, their grandfather wrote proudly:

> Illtyd Prichard greatly distinguished himself & produced a beautiful latin translation of Gray's Elegy in a Country Church yard. The Drs boys seem to carry prizes for every thing they undertake, which must be very gratifying to their Parents, & I hope they will bear their honours as meekly as their Father bears his. Constantine has been highly honoured by his College, & preserves all the amiable simplicity of his character—he is a very interesting youth, & will some day be distinguished. He has abandoned the study of the law, and adopted that of Divinity, so that the coming generation will have more teachers than one of the name of Prichard. I hope his health will improve—he looks very delicate at present.[93]

Constantine's health never did improve, and Alboo (Albert Hermann) was then too young to attract Thomas Prichard's praise. Con's schoolmate and close friend Walter Bagehot described his "beautiful forehead and brow, so very intellectual and expressive; certes he is by far the best looking of the Prichards; only time can show whether he is the cleverest."[94]

During the 1830s, Prichard's sister Mary was worried about him, observing that "his mind was harassed and uncomfortable, and his letters very short."[95] There was no let-up in the causes of his anxiety. His considerable medical practice and expertise in psychological conditions required more and longer journeys to patients around the West Country and South Wales.[96] He attended meetings of scientific and medical organizations all over Britain and was deeply committed to local organizations, including Bristol College, Bristol Institution, and the Infirmary. His involvement in the regulation, professionalization, and institutional development of medicine and science, his various publications, and the honors bestowed on him betokened his eminence. There were private sorrows, but his family and visitors to the Red Lodge brought him pleasure. Although he was quietly making good progress on the five-volume third edition of *Physical History*, his recent publications on nervous conditions and insanity would soon lead him in a new direction.

12 · New Scientists, New Organizations, New Ideas

Developing British Anthropology, 1833–48

[Prichard] perhaps of all others merits the title
of founder of modern anthropology.
—E. B. Tylor, "Anthropology"

Having resigned from St. Peter's Hospital in 1832 and feeling more secure in his medical career, Prichard threw himself into a variety of projects. When not visiting patients or taking his turn at the Bristol Infirmary, he was organizing, overseeing, and promoting the Phil & Lit and Bristol College. By mid-decade he had published his books on Celtic linguistics and on insanity and was about to send to the press the first volume of a new edition of *Physical History*. This is where his heart was. Contemporary developments in British scientific culture allowed Prichard and his associates to make a start on creating the science of anthropology.

If Prichard wanted to see the "natural history of man" become an objective, humane, Christian, and successful human science, it would need organizing and promoting. He did this by getting involved in new scientific and medical associations, attending meetings, and giving lectures to cultivate relationships among men of science in Britain and abroad. His famous Red Lodge became a hub for scholars. There was a template for creating a science: found an association; elect prestigious officers; hold meetings; develop nomenclature and tenets; occupy dedicated rooms; and publish an official periodical and some definitive textbooks. It was an era of scientific disciplinary development.

British Society and Science

The Establishment kept a keen eye on several new sciences, intent they should have either clear Christian underpinnings or at least offer scientific evidence happily demonstrating the hand of God. The Almighty could not be left out of the equation. The press on both sides of the Atlantic monitored publications for signs of apostasy, finding medical men particularly prone to dallying in materialism. An American writer recognized the threat posed by young medical men flaunting materialist (naturalistic, Godless) notions concerning the workings of nature like those of Lawrence and some Continental researchers' "laughing at the old notion that men have souls to be saved." Few British scientists were bold enough to set Revelation aside in the face of both social and legal sanctions. The William Lawrence scandal of the 1820s served as a warning to any so-called freethinking, materialism-tainted natural philosophers.[1]

There was a rash of Continental revolutions in 1830. Paris in the early thirties was also a hotbed of scientific debate the fearful British Establishment associated with French political upheaval, as threatening to British social order as it had been in the 1790s. While young British gentlemen like the eager geologist Charles Lyell flocked to hear Parisian scientists lecturing on nature's self-development, back in Britain, the social and political detriments of Godless science became all too apparent when toward the middle of the decade radical views of nature became linked to the general reformism of the period. Lowlife "soapbox orators" and Chartist agitators keen to shake off elite Church and State control of society adapted evolutionary theories to call for equal opportunities throughout society, some proclaiming "nature's self-development" required no Creator, bringing the hegemony of the Church into question. Prichard and his father were horrified by these developments.

Whether pious or just cautious, British scientists bookended their writing with acknowledgment of the First Cause, God's initiating hand. The perils of holding proto-evolutionary views in the 1830s are typified by the case of Robert Grant, the radical comparative anatomy lecturer of the liberal new London University "sent to Coventry" for both his transformist views and reformist leanings. Prichard's protégé young physiologist William Benjamin Carpenter understood his employment depended on a clean bill of religious health. Robert Chambers later admitted his compilation of progressivist biological theories, *Vestiges*, had been written anonymously to protect the welfare of his children.[2] Charles Darwin would make himself chronically ill agonizing over his secret Godless evolutionary theories until *Origin*'s publication in 1859. Bearing early Victorian religious absolutism in mind allows clearer comprehension of the disciplinary and organizational development of British anthropology.

Before the development of individual fields of science, "natural philosophy" in Britain had few disciplinary boundaries until London, provincial, Oxbridge and Scottish coteries of men interested in the natural world started narrowing the focus of their efforts to, for example, geology or geography.

They promoted and professionalized their interests by founding national single-subject scientific societies and provincial general learned ones, the Bristol Institution being a case in point. As well as demonstrating the worth of their subject in lectures, at meetings and in the periodicals they published, they advertised their members' social worth by being generally exclusive—working-class men and any women need not apply. Gentlemen of science attained prominence, noted for their deep erudition in one subject, perhaps enhanced by what would now be considered polymathic breadth. Having gained their learned status, however, they tended to devote themselves to disseminating their knowledge in publications and elite institutional lectures rather than contributing to practical outcomes in industry or government.[3] Prichard was of this stamp.

In response to the development of sciences, "natural theologians" redoubled their efforts to preserve Britons from irreligious theorizing. In 1831 Archbishop of Dublin Richard Whately liberally opined that religion and science were independent of each other, nor should the former be used as a source of information for the latter. Oxford-educated clergyman-geologist William Buckland had to reassure the nation that as science served religion, theology had nothing to fear from geology. Especially sensitive was Prichard's science of God's chosen beings; its content needed scrutiny, not that anyone doubted his orthodoxy. An evangelical Quaker theologian remembering a satisfying meeting with Prichard in 1831 concluded that "enlightened science is the handmaiden of religion."[4]

Meanwhile, and notwithstanding palpable hostility, assertions of the mutability of species were becoming increasingly difficult for the Anglican Tory Establishment to repress despite a phalanx of British natural theologians' heroic efforts.[5] Evolutionary theory did suffer one famous setback in 1831when Étienne Geoffroy Saint-Hilaire's clear hypothesis of the evolution of species based on comparative anatomical and embryological research was put to the test: his comparison of a mummified to a living ibis indicated no morphological change had occurred in more than three thousand years. More acceptable to Prichard was Georges Cuvier's firm belief in the fixity of species. This contemporary French celebrity comparative anatomist held that so-called evolution had been nothing more than repeated catastrophic destructions and creations.[6] Around the transatlantic world general, medical, religious and scientific publications cited and paraphrased Prichard's anthropological books extensively and approvingly. Readers of the Baptist magazine *Church*, for instance, were assured they "may consult most safely the works of our excellent Dr. Pritchard on this subject." The

Société Ethnologique de Paris, a mixed group of Christian monogenists and the less orthodox, selected him as their first foreign corresponding member. Toward midcentury views started to change, however. When the *British Quarterly* reviewed American polygenists Josiah Nott and George Gliddon's *Types of Mankind* (1855), it had to defend Prichard from the book's accusations of cowardly adherence to Scripture.[7] Discoveries in geology, physiology, paleontology, and anatomy steadily undermined the integrity of Genesis even as, through much of the nineteenth century, writers continued to accommodate scientific evidence to Scripture.[8] British and American scientists carefully managed their scientific views until the later Darwinian revolution rendered religion less central and more of a private matter.

Returning to Prichard's era, science was all but absent from the English universities' restricted curriculum. A few of their professors, necessarily Anglicans and usually ordained, were devoted to the study of nature as proof of the existence of divine purpose. They lectured on this, fitting their students to become clergymen and gentlemen. The Bridgewater Treatises, an influential series of natural theological monographs, provided Oxbridge with a manifesto of Christian intellectual endeavor.[9] Aware that the University of Oxford was the safest religiously orthodox ground for him to cultivate his science of humankind, Prichard longed for a professorship there.

The Christian science that appealed to Prichard served Britain's ruling elite by preserving the status quo as it represented the perfect and comprehensible functioning of the world and human society. At the same time they evinced a certain repugnance to science and its association with lower-class, mundane industry and commerce flourishing in some developing northern towns. A man who needed to be trained to earn a living had no place at the English universities and in polite society, where education for financial gain was thought vulgar. Men of science emerging in the new industrial towns and at the Scottish universities were unembarrassed by synergies with "trade." London institutions with their utilitarian approach to science were different still; the science studied in the capital's medical schools, for instance, had clear, practical outcomes, and the reformist London University (est. 1826) and other metropolitan institutions were less wary of Continental and Edinburgh scientific ferment. While Oxbridge-inflected Christian science was non-utilitarian, stressing both divine design in nature and the gratification of the human mind, elsewhere in Britain, the story was different.[10]

Prichard and the Formation of Anthropology and Its Institutions

Prichard's involvement with scientists and their institutions helped him prepare and promote the third edition of *Physical History* and develop a British science of humankind. The most beneficial associations were the Aborigines' Protection Society, British Association for the Advancement of Science, the Geographical Society of London, and the Ethnological Society of London (ESL). On the Continent, where Hodgkin had earlier been involved in founding an anthropological society, and in America, those interested in the natural history of humankind were pursuing their research in a variety of ways, founding inspiring, rival societies. In London, the ESL was born out of the ethnological sectional meetings of the BAAS, the inspiration of the Aborigines' Protection Society and Thomas Hodgkin, Prichard, and their fellow enthusiasts' dedication to humanitarian causes and science.

The complex, multistranded early history of anthropology is prone to confusion and debate. Its structure varied from country to country, as it still does, and its nomenclature translates confusingly. The rather German term "anthropology" was used promiscuously among a variety of intellectual pursuits. In late eighteenth-century Germany it denoted both the anatomical and psychological study of human beings in various ways; an influential periodical on the subject of psychiatry and psychology from 1823 was titled *Zeitschrift für anthropologie*. At the start of the new century French philosopher Pierre Jean Georges Cabanis considered it a science of physical-mental relations, and French *anthropologie* was a form of human medicine. Theologically, it concerned the study of the mind/soul in relation to God or the anthropomorphic representation of God. Blumenbach applied the term to the study of human skulls. The Continental biological study of humankind that became known as anthropology was practiced mostly by medical men and considered one of the natural sciences. Prichard's single use of "anthropology" in *Physical History* (1836) indicates that at the time he considered it the strictly biological study of humankind. All in all, not only did the word possess multiple meanings, but as it bore no reference to human history, culture, and language, Prichard avoided it. In adopting the term "ethnology," the founders of the Ethnological Society of London in 1843 intended it to mean the study of humankind, both biological and cultural—as Prichard more succinctly defined it that year, the entire "history of nations."[11] The words "ethnology" and "ethnography" originate in German terms pertaining to the study of all humankind, Europeans included. A long-established Continental interest in the customs and manners of different nations broadened into a holistic study of all human culture eventually called ethnology. In the 1770s it signified "all peoples" or "one people" in a book including travelers' accounts and comparative linguistics. Gottfried Wilhelm Leibniz engaged in what is now called ethnolinguistics. In the 1780s Slovak Adam Kollar employed "ethnology" to mean the study of people's origins, language, and customs, while Italian linguist Adrien Balbi's 1826 work titled *Atlas ethnographique du globe* implied it as classificatory of languages.[12] Aware of how confusing and foreign these two "ethno-" words were, Prichard would have preferred to concoct a new term directly from the Greek. He allowed "ethnography" to slip into *Physical History* (1826) just once and into *Physical History* (1836) a few times and never prominently. By 1842 he managed to accept "ethnology" in the proposed efficient title of the ESL, and it became the British name of his science of humankind for several decades.

As to the fortunes of the term "anthropology," it became more strictly associated with racial classification and degeneration theory during the later nineteenth century before being again repurposed in the United States, Britain, and France as the umbrella term for the subdisciplines of biological anthropology, ethnography (describing a group's culture), and ethnology (comparing groups' cultures) and is associated with linguistics and archaeology. All in all, Prichard referred to his field of research variously as ethnology, ethnography, natural history of man, physical history of man, and physical history of mankind, with "history" not used in the modern sense. But as it was more widely known as ethnology in the 1840s, the term stuck to him even after its meaning shifted, causing some historians to misapprehend him as an ethnologist who conducted this narrower function within cultural anthropology.

Not only were "anthropology" and "ethnology" alien words to English speakers during the early decades of the nineteenth century, but English speakers did not much study or write about these subjects. Prichard's first, innovative publication, *The Physical History of Man* (1813), had presented mostly biological but also some cultural material to the extent that such information was available. Instead of focusing on either approach to the subject, he attempted to bring them together, and over the next three decades his research continued to combine biological and cultural-historical material.[13]

In Germany, France, Britain, the Netherlands, the United States, Italy, and Russia—the countries where anthropology developed—the conception and history of anthropology differ. In some countries the notion of human races came to dominate research. Initially, there had been little interest in classifying "races." That later nineteenth-century anthropological cul-de-sac can be traced back to speculations by the likes of French naturalist Buffon, philosopher Kant, and prolific German ethnologist Christoph Meiners, who would become resources for European and American polygenists and "race scientists." These rather single-issue theorists with great faith in anthropometrics dominated the biological study of humankind, identifying themselves as anthropologists. They founded anthropological societies with polygenetic tolerance, if not leanings, in Europe and America, and they clashed with the older monogenetic culture-, history-, and language-based societies. Prichard's lack of interest in ranking races and his focus on human culture, history, and language rendered him obsolete in the opinion of these dominant late-century biological anthropologists.[14]

A Mission Statement for Anthropology, the BAAS, June 1832

The founders of the British Association for the Advancement of Science in 1831 chose their title wisely. The Continental word "science" was gradually replacing "natural philosophy," "British" obviated regional rivalries; "advancement" promised progress; and even "association" suggested non-sectarianism and professionalism. Formed mainly by Oxbridge men wary of dominant, orthodoxically suspect London and Edinburgh science, the BAAS was an ideal platform for provincial scientists such as Prichard. It demonstrated that Britain was keeping up with rival Continental science while preserving natural theological hegemony over scientific ideas. But unlike the government-supported German association it emulated, British potential patrons and the government lacked interest in an organization offering little tangible economic benefit, instead preferring individual initiative to stimulate scientific progress. The gentlemen and clergymen scientists of the BAAS were left to their own devices.[15]

The year after attending the inaugural meeting of the BAAS in York, with growing optimism mixed with trepidation Prichard set out for the peripatetic organization's first annual meeting in Oxford. There the association's objectives were clarified: the promotion of the systematic acquisition of scientific knowledge, the spreading of this knowledge, the fostering of scientific discussion internationally, and the removal of impediments to scientific progress. To better develop and distinguish areas of scientific endeavor, they established different departments. Prichard's friend Conybeare's confident voice and orthodox status were doubly impressive when on June 23, 1832, he read Prichard's "A Comparative Review of Philological and Physical Researches as Applied to the History of the Human Species" to an audience of eminent scientists. Prichard staked out his claim for anthropology as a scientific discipline worthy of inclusion in the BAAS.

Prichard's "Comparative Review" asserted that comparative philology (linguistics) was actually a more useful research tool for the "natural history of man" than biology. After trying the patience of his audience by reviewing the history of linguistics and praising German scholars, he outlined the views of past eminent race theorists in order to dismiss race studies, claiming classifying humankind biologically was fruitless because physical characteristics do not correlate with languages and all humans are of the same species, according to the accepted definition of "species." Instead, dynamic language was the key, a reliable historical tool that could counter static, materialist polygenism. If two languages are related, their speakers are related: if all languages are related, all people are related. In short, philology allowed a deeper and truer investigation of the history of and relationships between human groups than the classification of skin color and skull shape. "Comparative Review" was meant to promote the study of humankind as a science and to counter polygenetic theorizing by steering research from human anatomy and physiology toward historical and comparative linguistics. This widely republished lecture also advertised his need for more data that would aid him in preparing a new edition of *Physical History*.[16]

Prichard's manifesto for a new science based on comparative historical linguistics rather than biology likely seemed a bit woolly to the dominant "hard" scientists of the BAAS. It managed to gain some status as the Ethnology Subsection of the Natural History Section, whose committee and proceedings were thoroughly Prichardian in nature. But being represented by some annual lectures at the BAAS was not enough; anthropology lacked the reifying credentials of having its own society and periodical like those of geology and geography. Prichard would support the founding of a society that would publish its members' research while preparing a more comprehensive textbook of anthropology. His close friend Thomas Hodgkin had the time, financial security, passion, and advantageous position in London to take the lead in this project.

Prichard and Dr. Hodgkin shared similar backgrounds and interests, but not personalities and lifestyles. Both were deeply influenced by the values of the Society of Friends, but Hodgkin retained his active adherence to their principals and rules. When a child he met a Mohawk chief whose story of the cruelty and injustice his nation had suffered deeply impressed him. Then, while serving as an aid to Quaker philanthropist and chemist William Allen, he developed the era's passion for reform, especially for the abolition of slavery and improvement of the welfare of colonial subjects. These interests led him to anthropology and Prichard.

Hodgkin's medical studies at Edinburgh a few years after Prichard were preoccupied with humanitarian projects such as a plan for "elevating" Indigenous peoples by educating and training them in Britain before returning them to their country to sow the seeds of Christian civilization. As for understanding the biological history of human beings, in his early career as curator of the Medical Museum at Guy's Hospital, he keenly accumulated a large collection of crania from around the world, and as demonstrator of morbid anatomy (pathology) there, he made himself a place in medical history by identifying the form of cancer that bears his name. He published on a range of subjects from medicine and anthropology to several types of social reform. He even testified as an expert on moral insanity in Edward Oxford's trial for the attempted assassination of the queen in 1840.[17]

Hodgkin and Prichard were humanitarians, but unlike Prichard, Hodgkin was a liberal campaigner. His gentlemanly refinement and the utmost modesty made him "a specimen of human greatness and goodness personified and combined."[18] Hodgkin supported the liberal London University and challenged professional discrimination against Dissenters like himself, reformist activism that marked him out for retribution. Following a contentious campaign about the welfare of Hudson Bay Indigenous peoples, in 1837 he was effectively dismissed from his position at Guy's in circumstances that coincided with a breakdown in his physical and mental health. Prichard advised recuperative foreign travel.[19]

Following a spell in France where he was involved in the founding of the Société Ethnologique de Paris, Hodgkin returned to London, ready for philanthropic action. With inherited wealth and unencumbered by family obligations, he had the security and leisure for a new career. Since the British abolition of slavery in 1833, Liberal and Quaker humanitarian activism tended to shift to the welfare of colonized peoples. Hodgkin believed that his youthful plan of "elevating" Indigenous peoples by civilizing and Christianizing them would better assure their survival, and in time, universal European cultural values would prevail. Meanwhile, the "natives" in question needed to be kept from extinction so especially their languages could be studied to elucidate the history of humankind. Prichard corresponded with Hodgkin and often visited his comfortable London home, a magnet for a diverse international network of distinguished guests who shared his interests in scientific medicine, antislavery, and the welfare of Indigenous peoples.

The foundation of the Ethnological Society of London followed a series of events propelled by the humanitarian zeal of evangelical Christian former antislavery activists. Economically inefficient slavery and the granting of "Companies" that sucked the wealth out of colonies were being superseded by colonization through emigration from Britain. A motley array of the poor, convicts, and adventurers were busily carving out a life for themselves in the colonies while the newly established Colonial Office struggled to formulate settlers' and Indigenous peoples' rights. It was the Wild West and all the other points of the compass. As more and more accounts emerged of the cruel and unjust treatment of Indigenous peoples, moralizing and Christianizing antislavery activists, women as well as men, were inspired to intervene.[20] Colonialism's "three C's," Christianity, commerce, and civilization, were fast becoming the pillars of Britain's empire, and these humane watchdogs agitated for laws that would ensure colonized populations would survive long enough to receive the benefits of the motherland's blessed C's. After a succession of minor commissions of inquiry into the situation, the Select Committee on Aborigines was set up in 1835 under the Parliamentary leadership of Thomas Fowell Buxton, the nineteenth century's evangelical reformer par excellence. Hodgkin took up a key role in it.

Hodgkin worked indefatigably for the Select Committee's influential members, such as Whig Sir George Grey, the strangely reformist evangelical Anglican Tory MP Baron Glenelg, and Buxton. Dramatic, grueling testimony filling the very long *Report from the Select Committee on Aborigines* (1836–37) essentially confirmed what Prichard had claimed in 1830: contact with civilization had corrupted and was in the process of exterminating Britain's colonized peoples.[21] The report noted that political-economic policies causing the colonized to starve were impeding their conversion to Christianity. Rather than pointing a finger at government, it conveniently laid blame at the door of white settlers, some of the dregs of British society, making enemies of the colonists to the detriment of future ameliorative initiatives.[22] There was an obvious, urgent need to address the injustices of colonial rule, yet few tangible reforms resulted. The *Report*'s more than one thousand pages of ethnological data did give Hodgkin a brilliant idea.

The Aborigines' Protection Society, London, 1837

Hodgkin's enthusiasm and crucial work for the parliamentary inquiry allowed him to build a network of correspondents and amass data on the plight of Indigenous peoples. So armed, he carried on his mission at the Society of Friends' Meetings for Sufferings and recruited Buxton, the writer on Inuit ethnology and agitator Dr. Richard King, William Allen, and several others to help him launch the Aborigines' Protection Society (APS) in 1837.[23] Hodgkin was especially keen to recruit eminent Dr. Prichard to its ranks. While pleased to learn about the new society and promising his support, Prichard regretfully felt of little use, writing to Hodgkin in the summer of 1838:

> I do not know any more honorable distinction than to be the acknowledged head & founder of so truly noble & philanthropic an institution. As there is a prevailing power benign & discriminating between right & wrong at the head of human affairs, I cannot doubt that such an undertaking will prosper and if such be the event, whole races of men in future ages of the world will have reason to remember you. I will not say as the cause of their preservation from ruin & extinction, because the best of men are only instruments [in] the hands of their maker & it is God who puts it into the heart of man to do every good work, but they will acknowledge you as the means under Providence of saving them from the lot which has befallen mammoths & mastodonts and as it is to be feared many human races also who have utterly perished thru the crimes or criminal negligence of their fellow-men.
>
> Nothing would afford me greater satisfaction than to contribute to the promotion of such a work if it were in my power. Can you suggest any means, or any thing that I could do? Living as I do out of the world, in association with almost none except patients & apothecaries I can do little more than go thro the routine of daily work, except the spending an hour or two, chiefly early in the morning, in indulging that scribbling habit which custom has rendered almost like the result of an in-born propensity.[24]

The humanitarian APS, like its inspirational antislavery movement, attracted some evangelical Anglicans as well as Dissenters. It aimed to "rescue and elevate the coloured races at large," assist in protecting the defenseless, and promote the advancement of "uncivilized" tribes in order to achieve justice and universal happiness in Christian civilization. This appealed to Prichard. He joined its committee, and when he moved to London he attended its annual general meeting.[25] He also benefited from the APS's policy of gaining support for its cause by publishing ethnographic material meant to cultivate empathy with Indigenous peoples and demonstrate their capacity for advancement. Less appealing to Prichard was the APS's modus operandi, patterned on the antislavery movement's rousing meetings, pamphlets, periodicals, and lobbying.[26]

Hodgkin took up Prichard's offer to help promote the objects of the APS. Their mutual friend, the Basque linguist, ethnologist, and explorer Antoine Thomson d'Abbadie was visiting London in May 1839, and Prichard, keen to discuss and check some of his previous observations on Africans, was invited to stay at Hodgkin's to meet d'Abbadie and attend the APS's first anniversary meeting at the popular Exeter Hall. Hodgkin felt the society needed Prichard's support in particular: "Though it is much to have the benevolent & religious rightly interested in this great cause there are many important points connected with it which render it essential that the scientific should give it prompt & powerful support. As there is no one in this country so likely to bring this about as thyself I cannot help greatly desiring that if not present thou wouldst favour us with a letter which might be read at the meeting, printed with the report & copied into various journals."[27]

Unable to attend, Prichard's heartfelt letter of support read to the meeting expressed his deep concern for the

> many whole tribes and families of men, who, without such interference, are doomed to be swept away from the face of the earth. Certainly there is no undertaking of the present time, that has a stronger claim on humanity, and even on the justice of enlightened men. For what a stigma will be placed on Christian and civilized nations, when it shall appear, that, by a selfish pursuit of their own advantage, they have destroyed and rooted out so many families and nations of their fellow creatures, and this, if not by actually murdering them, which indeed appears to be even now a practice very frequently pursued, by depriving them of the means of subsistence, and by tempting them to poison and ruin themselves.

Prichard continued dramatically that Cain's murder of Abel might very well have foretold this sorry story of civilized Christians' exercising a policy of extermination. Aside from its being a human tragedy, he predicted a great loss to science if this slaughter continued; the true physiological and psychological nature of humankind could not be elucidated if half the branches were lopped off the tree of humanity and replaced with grafts of a single stock, the more powerful (European) tribe. What could be understood from studying only Europeans? The psychological and physical aspects of all societies in different stages of development must be studied.

Prichard's APS statement underscores his broadening of the science of humankind that had in his BAAS speech seemed more language focused. Of course, he also urged the proper study of languages, aiming a jab at "the crude speculations of metaphysical writers, or even scholars, whose scope was limited to the classical languages of antiquity." Monboddo and even Adam Smith were his prime examples of "jejune," crude speculators. He concluded with the warning that the task of fathoming the true nature of humankind was in danger of being left incomplete "if whole families of languages should be rooted out and lost, as they are certainly doomed to be, unless preserved by the intervention of this truly philanthropic Society."[28] Hodgkin distributed offprints of it widely, pleased with eminent Prichard's endorsement.

Hodgkin kept up his correspondence and friendship with Prichard, providing him with anthropological material that so frequently came to hand, ensuring Prichard's continued support. He sent him some African hair samples and an introduction to a clergyman recently returned from Hudson's Bay who was willing to furnish Prichard with information about the Indigenous people of that region. A doctor fresh from witnessing the devastation settlers were wreaking on Australians and New Zealanders had an intriguing theory about the Polynesian origin of some Native American tribes. Another clergyman and a doctor recently arrived from South Africa agreed to answer Prichard's questions, while R. H. Schomburgk had just brought back a couple of interesting Indigenes of Guiana; would Prichard like to have portraits of them made or obtain any useful details?[29] Through Hodgkin and these missionaries' and doctors' early form of ethnographic fieldwork, Prichard gained access to the extra-European world.

Hodgkin's work for the APS and involvement in the American Colonization Society, a somewhat unpopular movement to ship its formerly enslaved and freeborn people of color to a new African colony named Liberia, made him a conduit of more anthropological data. Prichard made the most of his friend's contacts. For example, in 1838 the Colonization Society's project in Liberia allowed Prichard to ask for a portrait of a "Kroo" (Kru man) to be made, and he hoped to meet the visiting African in person in London. Hodgkin sent Prichard a grammar book of a South African language, to which he responded asking for specimens of other African languages to strengthen a theory he had been exploring. He then needed specimens of language for his comparative vocabulary of the Algonquian language family, and he wanted to verify the claim that the Chipewyans were physically distinct from their neighbors. Hodgkin offered to introduce Prichard to interesting travelers such as Jacob Samuel, "a learned Jew" who thinks "that he has discovered a positive remnant of the ten lost tribes. His proofs of this & his account of many other branches of the human family will I doubt not be interesting to thee." Hodgkin, the Colonization Society, the APS, traveling citizen fieldworkers, and exhibitions of "genuine" Indigenous people in the metropolis provided Prichard with valuable data. If only he were in London.[30]

The BAAS *Ethnological Queries* (1839)

With a keen eye on promotion, Hodgkin had another brilliant idea. There was nobody better able to garner support for the struggling APS than Prichard, if only he would make a "short & rousing appeal" on the society's behalf to the BAAS. Hodgkin would follow it up with a discussion and then summarize it at the general meeting. He would even prepare a press release to promote it in the national newspapers.[31] Prichard was frankly pessimistic about gaining any support at the BAAS, however. In his opinion, his science of humankind lacked the respect it deserved. He complained to an American correspondent: "I believe that ethnography & philology are objects of attention among the literary and scientific men in America in a much greater proportion than among the English. Certainly that observation applies to the French. In our British Association for the advancement of Science little or no attention is bestowed upon these objects, and even geographical knowledge is very little regarded. Every thing is swallowed up by geology and the makers anew of whole worlds think the parts of no consequence. Ichthyosauri are according to them much older than mankind and therefore more deserving of regard & curiosity."[32]

Prichard swallowed his envy of geology and treated the 1839 Birmingham meeting to a stirring speech, drawing a large audience of men and women. "On the Extinction of Human Races" stridently laments the extermination of fellow human beings, describes many examples of their annihilation along with the resulting loss of scientific data, and finishes by predicting the extinction of most tribes within a century. The Hottentots, once peaceable and inoffensive, wandering about in primitive simplicity, had been reduced to misery and destitution by conquerors undeserving of the name Christian. He attributed this devastation to the "relentless progress of civilisation.... Wherever Europeans have settled, their arrival has been the harbinger of extermination to native tribes," a point he had made in his article on the Guanches in 1830. Britain, the colonial power with all its resources and abilities, was morally responsible for obtaining whatever remaining data there was, Prichard emphasized. Furthermore, he believed the study of "pre-civilized" peoples would provide a window onto the remote past of humankind and prove its single origin. This call for support for the Aborigines' Protection Society was extensively reprinted, abstracted, and even translated and published in a German periodical.[33]

The prolonged discussion following Prichard's speech did not go smoothly. An American participant was rounded on for his country's persecution of Indians and enslaved people, and he brought a hornet's nest down on himself by proposing English spinsters should be married off to Indians. The audience roasted another American who barely managed to hold his ground. A phrenologist then attempted to hijack the discussion to claim his science as the legitimate key to understanding the natural history and mental qualities of the human races. At last, the discussion returned to the sufferings of so many human tribes and how these might be redressed.[34]

Hodgkin took to the floor to take the BAAS to task for being more interested in the preservation of endangered plants and animals than of humans. The association's attendees must have felt under siege that day, and not only by Hodgkin's and Prichard's going on about the plight of exploited "natives." The Birmingham meeting had nearly been called off as the city was in virtual lockdown, fearing more Chartist rioting. Some of the association's Christian Establishment grandees might have considered these APS reformists just a politer form of the leveling reformists outside. Attempting to put a scientific spin on the issue, Hodgkin asked the BAAS to sponsor the production and distribution of an ethnological questionnaire for sea captains, merchants, missionaries, and general travelers to use to observe and record data about Indigenous cultures thoroughly and accurately. Ethnology had not cut much of a figure at the BAAS previously, but on this occasion it made an impact.

Hodgkin's idea of an ethnological questionnaire was not novel; it had ancestors in the ancient historians' lines of inquiry and a thorough sixteenth-century questionnaire by Albrecht Meier. Hodgkin's sojourn among French students of humankind likely brought to his attention a similar one published by the Société des Observateurs de l'Homme at the beginning of the century, several human geography questionnaires produced from 1823 onward by the Société Géographie de Paris, and the Société Ethnologique de Paris's more recent one. Closer to home, Prichard's acquaintance Harriet Martineau had published *How to Observe: Morals and Manners* in 1838, arguably the first manual of sociological methodology. These questionnaires were a product of well-established natural historical observational practices. It was an era of questionnaires and scientific manuals.[35]

Prichard was more than comfortable with questionnaires and statistics; he had already compiled data on diseases, psychiatric conditions, languages, mythology, biblical chronology, and crania, and he was involved in the work of the Bristol Statistical Society. Now there was a prospect of having large-scale physical and cultural data accurately and systematically gathered, organized for expert analysis back in Britain. This would lead to a more scientific understanding of humankind and greater success in securing Indigenous peoples' human rights—a partnership between science and philanthropy. The BAAS allocated a moderate sum and appointed a committee to compile the questionnaire, though it was done almost entirely by Hodgkin and Prichard.[36]

In Prichard's Birmingham audience that day, young Charles Darwin listened with interest and became an inactive member of the new committee. With James Yates's help, Hodgkin drafted some questions and sent them to Prichard. This eventually stirred Prichard to send Hodgkin questions about physical characteristics, language, customs, and psychology, and he suggested more categories, keen that a standard list of words and translations of the Lord's Prayer should be obtained to make it easier to compare vocabulary and syntax. He then disapproved of Hodgkin's jumbled resulting draft and took over the task, revising, simplifying, and organizing the questionnaire and apologizing for any possible offense to his fellow committee members. The instructions for craniometrics being too complex to accomplish accurately, he suggested they should be replaced by a request for actual crania.[37] (He obviously had his crania collection in mind.) Prichard's range of questions again marks his conception of the science of humankind as based on physical, cultural, and linguistic observation.

Hodgkin consulted the rest of the committee about the content of the proposed questionnaire, except the phrenologically inclined Mr. Wiseman, ostensibly owing to some difficulties in addressing him and his interests. He pulled it all together at the eleventh hour, had it printed, and read the *Varieties of the Human Race, to be Addressed to Travellers and Others* at the September 1840 BAAS meeting. Its eighty-eight questions were introduced with an outline of the so-called *Ethnological Queries*' origin and purpose, pointing out Britain's premier position as a colonial power meant it ought not to be eclipsed by better material gathered by the Ethnological Society of Paris's questionnaire, the use of which he acknowledged.[38] The *Ethnological Queries*' ten sections cover physical descriptions, language, individual and family life, buildings and monuments, works of art, domestic animals, government and laws, geography and statistics, social relations, and religion. There are requests to note signs of population movements and mixture, acquire vocabulary lists, identify prevalent diseases, and explore the nature of religion.

Rather than relying on cobbled-together travelers' anecdotes and classical sources as Prichard had previously done, the *Ethnological Queries* aimed to facilitate the gathering of standardized cultural and biological data of greater accuracy and breadth.[39] For a few years BAAS minutes and reports note requests for its further funding. There was positive feedback from abroad and some articles were apparently based on it.[40] For years, Hodgkin diligently promoted it among travelers, merchants, missionaries, and colonial officials. This ancestral form of anthropological fieldwork continued to be done by men and women who may or may not have used the *Ethnological Queries* and who either sent their data back to centers of learning for analysis or published accounts that could be mined by anthropologists.

As the fourth decade of the century began, Prichard and his fellow anthropologists, with their publications, Ethnology Subsection presence at the BAAS, articles in its *Transactions*, and the *Queries*' codification of fieldwork, were making good progress in establishing a scientific discipline. But as the status of anthropology at the BAAS started to improve, it attracted the unwanted attentions of phrenologists and polygenists with their increasingly denigratory portrayals of Indigenous peoples. Charles Caldwell's research concluded that Africans were more closely related to the great apes "than to the highest varieties of his own species." His 1841 BAAS lecture called for the radical transformation of ethnological theory and methodology into an anatomical science, exactly what Prichard wished to avoid.[41] Polygenistic posturing was on the rise, trying to muscle in on the Ethnological Subsection of the BAAS.

Prichard recognized the association's usefulness in promoting his brand of anthropology, even if it was not always given its due, as he complained: "I found many subjects of interest at York, particularly in the new ethnological section. It is rather characteristic that they have made ethnology including the natural history and the psychological history of Mankind a subordinate department of Zoology."[42] At least it had managed to gain a seat at the bottom of the table of sciences.

The Ethnological Subsection of the BAAS and its *Ethnological Queries*, the social and political exigencies of the expanding British Empire, the Government Select Committee Report, and the Aborigines' Protection Society all stimulated the development of British anthropology. But after more than four years of effort, the APS had made little progress in improving the lot of oppressed Indigenous peoples. Recent legislation had been ineffective, unregulated colonial exploitation was on the increase, settler colonists were resentful of the do-gooding APS, and the British public were indifferent. To make matters worse, the APS and Prichard's dire warnings of entire Indigenous groups' impending demise seemed to have had the opposite effect of what he had desired, as it supported the counterargument of the inevitability of extinction. Investigating atrocities was sapping the APS's dwindling finances, diverting funding from the society's ethnological research. The society's gentlemen scientists were no campaigners like the other APS activists; they wanted to comprehend humankind scientifically and establish the unity of the human species. Some of them became less committed to the APS, turning instead to the more scientific atmosphere of the BAAS and its *Queries*.[43] Something had to change.

A Plan to Civilize Africa, London, 1839

The APS was not the only humanitarian organization in town in 1839. Hodgkin's co-activist Buxton became distracted by a government-backed scheme to "civilize" Africa, and Prichard gave it his support, impressed by the aims expressed in its title. The Society for the Extinction of the Slave Trade, and for the Civilization of Africa was founded in 1839 by Christians of various persuasions, including a strong Quaker element. Its members thought big, aiming to abolish the slave trade by cutting it off at its source. They would bring this about by Christianizing Africa in order to destroy idolatry and "return" Africans to pure monotheism, the civilizing effect of which would lead to the natural demise of slave trading. All that needed to be done was to encourage and finance Africans' own agricultural development as a replacement for slave exportation; establish trade in agricultural products for British manufactures; create written African languages; provide medical aid; support the government's expedition to the Niger; and keep anti–slave trade interest alive by, among other initiatives, publishing a fortnightly periodical called *Friends of Africa*.

The society's combination of commercial and Christian proselytizing greatly appealed to Bristolians. The Bristol Auxiliary's inaugural meeting was held in March 1841, attended by the bishop and with Tory merchants and bankers in control. Of its sixteen-strong committee, six members were clergymen, while the majority were merchants and bankers. Prichard joined the committee, undoubtedly in favor of its humane Christian mission and its potential as a source of ethnographic data. The society's Niger expedition ended in disaster, and the Society for the Extinction of the Slave Trade faded.[44]

The Ethnological Society of London, November 1843

Hodgkin and his associate Dr. Richard King realized anthropological research was starting to dominate the APS; its revised mission statement stressed it. Would it be worth forming an obviously scientific society solely for the study of humankind? Such a specialist society would attract men of more scientific inclination, and it would not be saddled with the APS's off-putting reputation for welcoming into its ranks campaigning reformist Dissenters and women. In more of a reorganization than a split from the APS, a new society was planned. Prichard's "natural history of man" was given a new name he was familiar with but did not often use; at least it had a satisfyingly scientific "-ology" suffix. The Ethnological Society of London would, like other scientific societies in the capital, be elite and exclude politics, religion, and women. This exclusivity soon conflicted with its need to maximize subscriptions.

The Ethnological Society of London's birth was protracted. From the start, Hodgkin and King solicited Prichard's support, initially by asking him to lend his name to the enterprise. After King issued its first *Prospectus* on July 20, 1842, canvassing for the new society began in earnest, using stationery embossed with the motto THE PROPER STUDY OF MANKIND IS MAN/ETHNOLOGICAL SOCIETY. They betrayed their APS leanings by warning that "the progress of commerce & colonization must in a short time so completely either exterminate or modify so many of the feeble, scattered, and imperfectly known tribes of mankind, that if the present period be neglected it will be [impossible] here after to pursue the subject of Ethnology with any prospect of success."[45] Formally constituted in November 1843, Hodgkin promoted the ESL by publishing an article on ethnology in a respected scientific journal, writing a lot of letters, and calling on Prichard's further aid. He also cleverly started linking his BAAS *Queries* correspondence with the ESL.[46] King and Hodgkin recruited widely among gentlemen who might be interested in attending the society's meetings held first at Hodgkin's, then at King's house in Sackville Street. The ESL's rooms, library, and museum space were finally established at 17 Savile Row in September 1847.

To disassociate itself from philanthropic organizations and lay claim to its scientific status, the byline of the ESL *Prospectus* proclaimed it "A Purely Scientific Society, for Investigating the Natural History of Civilized as Well as Uncivilized Man." It promised to promote the publication of systematic descriptions of human physical and cultural characteristics in an unbiased way and inquire into their causes. It would collect and disseminate useful facts, form a reference library and museum, fund projects, engage in correspondence with other societies and individuals around the world, promote the learning of Indigenous languages, and foster accurate data collecting to create a modern science based on sound methodology. King astutely stressed that the ESL would provide information beneficial to colonial administration, religion, and commerce.[47] The core assumption of the ESL was that its members would demonstrate scientifically the specific unity of humankind. Patterned on Prichard's research and with the aid of the *Ethnological Queries*, the Ethnological Society of London envisaged a global network of anthropologically trained informants. It hoped to attract members, appealing to national pride and philanthropic impulse as it created a science of humankind based on analysis of data supplied by "fieldworkers" worldwide. Its road ahead proved rocky.

The ESL was not the world's first anthropological society. The Société Ethnologique de Paris had been inspirational.[48] An older association, the short-lived Société des Observateurs de l'Homme, founded in 1799 by French naturalists, linguists, and geographers, as well as drawing up an ethnological questionnaire for travelers, published, formed a museum, and helped prepare an expedition to Australia. Importantly, the Observateurs had united the study of biological and cultural anthropology, just as Prichard had and the ESL hoped to do. Contacts between Russian scientists and the Geographical Society of London in the late 1830s may have included information about Russian efforts to establish ethnology as a science as well.[49] The founders of the ESL were aware of the philologically inclined American Ethnological Society, established in New York that same year. Hodgkin and King's canvassing letters implied the need to catch up with France and again stressed the ESL's role in preparing men to be involved in international commercial and colonial development.

A committee of a dozen or so ran the ESL, electing a president and four vice presidents. Hodgkin sent Prichard a copy of the rules in January 1844, asking for his approval and breaking the news that he had been made one of its vice presidents. The young society needed the luster of Prichard's name. It was not from lack of interest that Prichard missed learning about the Mandingos at the ESL's February 1844 meeting, and he was equally keen to see some Indigenous Americans and an Abyssinian traveler. When not visiting patients in Bristol and environs, Prichard was frustratingly preoccupied with his new duties as a metropolitan commissioner in lunacy.

Members read and discussed papers at the society's monthly meetings between November and June of each year, and they held an anniversary meeting each May. The ESL undertook to print and disseminate the ethnological material it accumulated; it published a periodical and offprints of its articles, and there was some coverage of its activities in the *Literary Gazette*, *The Athenaeum*, and the *Medical Times and Gazette*. The articles published in the first two volumes of the *Journal of the Ethnological Society of London* (1843–49) document members' interest in all aspects of anthropology.

ESL membership soon grew to more than 150 and included APS veterans, a handful of aristocrats, the archbishop of Dublin, some MPs and high-ranking military men, a sprinkling of clergymen and lawyers, some FRSs, quite a few "Esqs.," and a high proportion of MDs. Notwithstanding, the highly respectable geologist George Bellas Greenough warned a somewhat black-sheepish Dr. King of an existential threat to the society: aside from financial insecurity, its socially self-destructive policy was "the indiscriminate admission into the society of any one who chooses to offer himself. One or two black sheep are quite enough to contaminate an entire flock—surely we require some better guarantee for the respectability of those who may wish to join us than the signature of their names: the admission into our body of a single troublesome person, of any individual who has not the feelings or manners of a gentleman might prove fatal to the institution."[50] Greenough perceived a laddish element creeping in, attracted by the exotic subject. This less than "respectable" element would continue to grow and later in the century it peopled a rival anthropological society.

Richard King, Black Sheep

Prichard echoed Greenough's concerns about the ESL, always keen to keep his associations elite; he did not altogether approve of some of its members' views, but he might not have had Richard King in mind. Dr. King did have a habit of attracting negative adjectives, however. Often an awkward customer, he paid for it dearly. As ESL secretary, he corresponded, promoted the society, edited the *Journal*, and lectured at its meetings while writing books and articles, carrying on a medical practice, and getting involved in various projects that attracted notoriety along with a lot of bad press.

Born in 1810 the son of a London civil servant, King progressed through his medical training and obtained MDs by testimony from New York and Giessen, as opposed to attending university. At the time of his acquaintance with Prichard, King was secretary to the Statistical Society, held a few minor appointments, and was a practicing obstetrician. But it was an earlier adventure that shaped his life and reputation. King secured a post as medical officer, naturalist, and second in command to Sir George Back on his Royal Navy expedition down the Back River in northern Canada (1833–35). King prepared himself well for the journey, adopting the firm belief in the lightweight overland method of Arctic exploration. Perhaps he had read *Physical History* because he gathered ethnographical data on this expedition. At the time he was described as a "fine looking fellow," "resolute," and "just the man for the task," but King could also be impetuous, egotistical, overconfident, stubborn, and rudely blunt. Popular with the men under his command, he was distinctly less so with his superiors and the Admiralty. King blotted his copybook by publishing a critical account of the Back expedition, creating a scandal for which the authorities never forgave him. The Establishment *Athenaeum* was disgusted by King's tone of condemnation, vexation of spirit, and misconceived sense of grievance.

King published an ethnography of the "Esquimaux," and by employing Inuit knowledge of Arctic topography, he sketched out a remarkably accurate Arctic map and suggested a more successful strategy for exploration. His attempted contributions to Arctic science, annoying habit of making accurate predictions, and abrasive manner further alienated him from the government, the Geographical Society, and the Hudson's Bay Company. For instance, after *correctly* predicting that Sir John Franklin's 1845 expedition was being sent to its doom, he was again ignored when he *correctly* predicted where Franklin's lost expedition would be located. Attached to his detailed written justification of his Franklin rescue proposal of February 17, 1848, is Captain Ross's rebuttal, implying Franklin would be found anywhere other than the Great Fish River, as King had asserted. King's theories or initiatives seemed to warrant rejection on principle.[51]

While not at all Hodgkin and Prichard's type, King shared their commitment to the APS, ESL, BAAS, monogenism, and ethnology. They worked together effectively; the younger man praised Prichard and was as passionate about the success of the ESL as he was annoyingly correct about Arctic exploration. To Dr. King goes the credit of being an early ethnographic fieldworker who published his own firsthand research. His authentic experience among Indigenous peoples of the Arctic added a special dimension to the ESL that Prichard valued.

An Anthropological Network

There were synergies among the three organizations dedicated to studying and preserving endangered extra-Europeans. The ESL benefited from the international exposure of the BAAS and its publications; some of the

Ethnological Subsection's members were also active in the ESL. Several of the papers given at the BAAS Southampton meeting in 1846 were read on behalf of their presumably far-distant authors, one of whom was a woman.[52] Perhaps they had made use of the *Ethnological Queries*. The APS continued for a time to publish anthropological articles. It promoted its evangelically infused philanthropic mission, while the ESL justified its allied organization's efforts by establishing scientifically the fact of the single origin and unity of the human species.

Hodgkin was at the helm of two societies, in charge of the *Queries*, and a member of the Geographical Society. At the same time he continued pursuing his philanthropic goals he was a magnet for travelers from around the world, attracting data, extra-European artifacts, and crania. While enthusiastic members of the BAAS Subsection and the ESL were carrying out and publishing their Prichardian anthropological research, all Prichard could do was complain of being "so bound down by circumstances over which I have no control. . . . Be assured that it is owing to no want of inclination that I do not second you in all your undertakings connected with anthropology."[53] When not lamenting Bristol's remoteness, he complained to an American: "I am much gratified in learning that ethnological studies are pursued with great zeal by many of your countrymen. Here they are, except with a few, almost entirely neglected, and most of what is written of subjects connected with ethnology in this country is absurd and ridiculous."[54]

British anthropology developed in the context of the new scientific era and its institutions, gaining momentum toward midcentury. It was nourished by Prichard's publications and lectures and the activities of the APS, BAAS Ethnological Subsection, and the ESL. Prichard could keep abreast of the progress of his science abroad thanks to some early transnational exchanges of anthropological views through books in translation, reviews in periodicals, and the development of relationships among learned societies.

The *Ethnological Queries* became linked to the ESL and gave rise to successive anthropological questionnaires for more than a century. This society gradually made some progress in building an international network of anthropological observers, communicating with other learned societies and government and helping to shape anthropology's scientific methodology. It is ancestral to the Royal Anthropological Institute of Great Britain and Ireland. Hodgkin continued his management of the APS until his death in 1866, and the society continues its campaign today as Anti-Slavery International. Did Prichard, the ESL, and later Victorian anthropologists aid colonial exploitation? Historians have noted that anthropologists seemed to have benefited from the ethnological data they acquired from the colonies, while their esoteric digestions of this material were considered of minimal utility to colonial administration.[55]

Phreno-anthropology: A Fly in the Ointment

One major player in the field of anthropology, particularly in France and Britain, eventually faded from history. Phrenology, so disruptive to Prichard's science of the mind, also rivaled his anthropology, not to mention other human sciences; phreno-anthropology was hard to bear.[56] As well as obviously being based on cerebral anatomy, it drew on the ancient art of physiognomy, the estimation of a person's character through facial indicators, then enjoying a revival as a popularist study. Another physiognomy-inspired idea was the calibration of "facial angle"; it lent itself to ranking people, a practice encouraged by the success of Linnaeus's descriptive taxonomy and a growing belief in mathematics as key to understanding the world. Facial angle theory held that the more the forehead sloped backward, the less the cranial capacity—the lower the intelligence, the more "primitive" the person being evaluated. Satisfyingly calculable determinations of individuals' character and ability could be extended to whole nations. Yet another contributing factor was a passion for arranging hierarchies, inspired by the ancient notion of the Great Chain of Being and perhaps the rigid class system embedded in British and French society. Classifying and ranking, backed up by the biblical curse on Ham and his Black descendants, helped justify exploitation and slavery abroad. Phrenologists laid claim to this scientific territory.

As phrenology broadened into a way of understanding all humankind, British phrenologists started competing with Prichard's anthropology as early as the 1820s when they professed to reveal biological, psychological, and sociocultural truths. Prichardian research into human origins and the mechanisms of biological variation—matters of time and change—did not interest them. Phrenology was anatomically deterministic, as is evident in its doctrine of an individual's potential being fixed at birth by the relative conformations of the twenty-seven or so organs of the brain's impression on the shape of the skull. Phrenologists naturally looked unfavorably on the notion that external factors such as the environment or culture might be productive of human development.

Some phreno-anthropologists became dab hands at racial stereotyping, supplying evidence in support of European exceptionalism, polygenism, and racialism. They took to defining "national character"; the crania of whole "races" could reveal their fixed racial personality, ability, and potential, beyond which "progress" was not possible. Their anthropological articles generally found extra-Europeans' *innate* personalities and capabilities woefully lacking in positive characteristics; "savages" could not be civilized. One author stressed the only hope of meliorating the execrable personalities of the colonized lay in strong doses of Christianity and European rule. Phrenology made incursions on French anthropology; the Société Ethnologique de Paris's founder William Frédéric Edwards entertained it for a time, and physiologist François-Joseph-Victor Broussais lectured to audiences of three thousand in 1836, referring to "hopeless" Maoris, for instance.[57]

Phreno-anthropology fell on stony ground among the British scientific elite, by and large. Prichard did not deign to mention it in his anthropological publications, but phrenologists mentioned him. They stalked BAAS meetings, doing their best to win a place on platforms with Establishment men of science, and they organized among themselves ways to "expose" him. When a phrenological infiltrator into the Ethnological Subsection attempted to contribute a phrenological analysis of a Celtic skull during a post-lecture discussion, the chairman, Prichard's friend and follower Dr. Latham, called the meeting to order, reminding the participants that "phrenology was a prohibited subject!" The disgruntled phrenologist "could not learn the origin of this strange decree, but it is probably a sop to the antiphrenological tendencies of their president, Dr. Pritchard, and kindly designed to protect him from the possibility of the mortification of a face to face refutation of the vast deal of nonsense he has written on the subject." He further complained that the subsection's sister society, the ESL, was woefully mired in philology rather than engaged in the proper phrenological study of the brain. In open competition with anthropologists, phrenologists protested their exclusion from mainstream science. Privately they commented adversely on Prichard's skull.

During leading phrenologist George Combe's successful lecture tour of the United States, he examined Samuel George Morton's hundreds of skulls of Indigenous Americans and "a great many negroes." American skull traders included Morton, the proud possessor of race scientist Gliddon's ninety Egyptian and fifty African skulls. Dr. Morton was pleased to conclude that Native Americans are inferior to "Negroes," as he somewhat phrenologically determined the former to be ferocious, blood-thirsty, savage, and possessed of great self-esteem and independence, in other words, intolerant of enslavement. In African skull conformation, by contrast, he discerned docility and patience—ideal characteristics for enslavement.

Tenacious phreno-anthropologists gradually gained a foothold in British learned societies like the ESL, where their ideas threatened to divert Prichardian anthropology from its course. Improvements in print and illustration technology and in international communications allowed the efficient spread of a race-oriented biological anthropology, attracting men with hardening attitudes toward race, especially in colonial contexts. Their adoption of phrenology's seductively scientific craniometric contraptions, convincing imagery, and confident rhetoric paved the anthropometric way for later-century biological anthropology; for instance, head-focused and denigratory phrenology inspired descriptions of backward-sloping facial angles and the jutting jaws of "lower races."

Some younger ESL members in their London libraries may have wondered why they were laboring over obscure vocabularies when the key to understanding all humankind was sitting on the top of shoulders, ready to be calibrated. Articles in the Journal of the Ethnological Society of London began to have phrenological content; one author could claim that phrenology and ethnology were "intimately connected."[58] Now remembered as nothing more than a head-bump-feeling, fortune-telling, pseudo-scientific entertainment, phrenology was in its day a serious, challenging science whose practitioners contributed to the development of late nineteenth-century biological anthropology and race science. It just happened to be groundless.

Race Science à la Française

French biologists, aesthetic theorists, and phrenologists dominated the field of polygenism and race science throughout most of the nineteenth century, joined by American slavery apologists and British sympathizers eager to contribute their fair share of racialist elaborations. The foundations had been laid by seventeenth-century Isaac La Peyrère's pre-Adamism; later Petrus Camper's lessons for artists and the art of physiognomy were adapted for the purpose of ranking human groups. During the first decades of the nineteenth century French naturalist Georges Cuvier contributed by exploring physical differences, especially in the size of the brain. Joining in his race ranking and producing an array of negative descriptions of extra-Europeans were his polygenist compatriots such as vociferous naturalist Jean-Baptiste Bory de Saint-Vincent and the "two human species" claimant Julien-Joseph Virey.[59] These are just a selection of the participants in the polygeny versus monogeny debates plaguing Prichard's era and subsequently peaking during the regime of imperialist scientific racialism and race hygiene of late nineteenth-century France.

The members of the Société Ethnologique de Paris were not the only French students of humankind. Some Société de Géographie de Paris members adopted racial classifications of humankind that tended to be either polygenistic or rigidly hierarchically monogenistic. The Société Ethnologique attracted members of the Société de Phrénologie de Paris as well.[60] Société Ethnologique's William Frédéric Edwards, author of *Des caractères physiologiques des races humaines* (1829), was considered preeminent in the biological study of humankind. Like Prichard, he had published on Celtic linguistics in the early thirties, gaining expertise that allowed him to broaden his interests beyond growing race biology. Prichard made a few polite general references to Edwards's book in *Physical History*, perhaps avoiding it because of its stress on the fixity of races.

In the Société Ethnologique, Edwards hoped to unite biology, linguistics, history, and the study of culture. Like the BAAS *Queries*, the society's questionnaire for travelers focused predominantly on culture and language. But with its members variously committed to geography, phrenology, monogenism, polygenism, biological determinism, and race ranking, its progress and coherence suffered.[61]

Reflecting the growing popularity of French race science, by 1847 Société Ethnologique members could not agree whether theirs was a physical science or a historical-literary pursuit, as polygenists, monogenists, and hierarchical monogenists debated their points.[62] All in all, for decades French scientists of various sorts put a lot of effort into evaluating "the Other," arriving at conclusions that aided French colonialism and efforts to "civilize" its subjects. Much later in the century social and biological evolutionary ideas would manage to coexist uneasily with biological determinism, fostering racial classifying, scientific racialism, and theories of degeneration.[63]

The biological determinism and the predilection for hierarchizing infecting French human sciences fostered the idea of "the Other" that spread beyond its borders, undermining Prichard's humanitarian anthropology. Wary of French science and generally Francophobic, he was nevertheless drawn into a network of French contacts Hodgkin had cultivated during his time in Paris and through his leadership of the ESL and APS. In the 1840s Prichard met, corresponded and exchanged publications with, and wrote critical reviews of the publications of his Continental fellow scientists.

The Geographical Society of London and the Royal Society

Prichard thought anthropology had a claim on geography. Hodgkin, Greenough, Prichard, and several other members of the ESL were also members of the Geographical Society of London, just as there were geographers in the French Société Ethnologique de Paris. Prichard found its journal an ideal outlet for his articles and for promoting anthropology; he contributed articles to it and mined the society's well-stocked library for ethnographical material, keeping the society's librarian busy sending volume after volume to him in Bristol.

Founded in 1830 and "Royal" as of 1859, the Geographical Society of London was one of a raft of scientific societies created during this period. Cast in the scientific society mold, it was an elite, thinking man's club. Its members were of three social types: "men of high social standing," including several aristocrats; army and navy officers; and scientists. Among the latter and largest group were many fellows of the Royal Society. The character of the Geographical Society of London arguably became more seriously scientific, educational, and professional than the ESL.[64] Over a short, productive period, Prichard valued it as a source of international contacts and a treasure trove of anthropological literature.

From his earliest letter of May 8, 1838, Prichard frequently exploited the Geographical Society's secretary and fellow linguist Captain John Washington of the Royal Navy. He would borrow five or six books at a time, nor would he always promptly return them. Which volume of *Physical History* he was working on is evident; for instance, after apologizing for hoarding so many books, he admitted he needed seven more, especially one about Siberia. "I am greedy of all the information I can obtain respecting the continent of Asia." Prichard then requested regular shipments of half a dozen volumes of the *Journal of the Royal Asiatic Society* with a view to working through the entire series. In 1840 he wanted Klaproth's maps to help him prepare his own ethnographical maps, then he abruptly switched his requests to anything about the South Sea Islanders. Prichard put Washington to work collecting vocabulary and grammar samples from the regular flow of Native people being exhibited in London. If Washington could not organize portraits of the Mandingos, sketches and cranial measurements of them would suffice. Could he please obtain information about the visiting Ashanti princes?

Prichard reciprocated with an extensive comparative word list of several South Seas nations, a Cherokee newspaper, and advice on the BAAS paper Washington was preparing. He also refereed articles submitted by others, judging one book "superficial" and more appropriate for French dilettantes, and another simply "absurd." Prichard offered to write reviews of d'Abbadie and Müller, contributed the ethnological section to Washington's annual report on the progress of geography, helped with advice to travelers, and submitted and oversaw his cousin Charlotte Wilkins's review of a German book of travels published in the *Journal of the Geographical Society of London*. He also wrote an obituary of esteemed Blumenbach, a short puffing review of Morton's *Crania Americana*, and an abstract of Philipp Franz von Siebold's book about Japan. Prichard cleverly asked for his "Ethnology of High Asia" to appear in the journal well in advance of the same material being published in his book so readers would have had a chance to forget it and buy the book when it came out. He was keen on benefiting from any feedback as well.

As they became better acquainted, Prichard told Washington about the pleasant days spent with his friends Bunsen and Lepsius, who were busy getting to grips with hieroglyphics; his visit to Dr. Tweedie; books loaned him by the Marquis of Bute; and the correspondence and parcels of skulls and materials from American linguists Du Ponceau, Albert Gallatin, and John Pickering.[65] Prichard thanked Captain Washington and the other officers of the Geographical Society "for much help" in *Physical History*, and he presented a copy of *Eastern Origin* to Washington. But in early 1841 the captain resumed his career as a naval hydrographer, bringing their correspondence to an end.

Washington's less accommodating successor Julian R. Jackson loaned Prichard fewer books, and instead of asking him to write articles for the *Journal*, he more often asked him to referee other authors' submissions. Prichard had never bothered to seek election to the Geographical Society until W. R. Hamilton and G. B. Greenough supported his application on January 9, 1843. Four years later, when he was pressed about some confusion in returning a book, he snapped back: "When I subscribed & became a member of the Geographical Society it was for the sake of the Library & the Journal. I have been so much disappointed in the library, that I find my continuing a member of the Society useless, especially as the Journal is no longer given except on purchase, which I could effect without being a member. I shall therefore be obliged if you will erase my name from the list of members." His friend James Yates was also fed up. Prichard's resignation was not recorded, and this beneficial relationship ended.[66]

Even after Prichard moved to London, he was inactive in the elite, ancient Royal Society, although he had been appointed to the committee that judged the merits of papers submitted to it in the fields of anatomy, physiology, and natural history—fields of minor interest to the society. Perhaps the chance of hobnobbing with the heroes of science was less attractive than when he had attended William Herschel's and Humphry Davy's lectures four decades earlier. He did have the pleasure of supporting several of his friends' applications, including ones by Drs. Tweedie and Carpenter, and having "FRS" after his name was a social and professional mark of distinction.[67]

Some American Linguists

Prichard delighted in corresponding with men devoted to the study of Indigenous Americans. His correspondence with an avid student of their languages John Pickering began when an attendee of the Dublin BAAS's 1835 meeting wrote Prichard a glowing letter of introduction to him. He sent Pickering a copy of *Eastern Origin* and requested references to any work of scholarship on Indigenous Americans, as he was studying the relationships between the American languages for his final volume of *Physical History*. According to Pickering, little work had yet been done on individual languages and certainly not on the relationships between eastern and western tribes. Unfortunately, information about New World languages, not to mention cultures, was rather unreliable, but perhaps fellow philologist Peter Stephen Du Ponceau might be helpful. Prichard was pleased with the pamphlets, books, and periodicals that Pickering sent him and the prospect of making another American contact.[68]

Prichard admitted to Pickering that he was flattered by his election as honorary member of the American Oriental Society, and he predicted its counterpart in London and the new ESL would make strides in developing the natural history of humankind. But as for worthwhile books on linguistics, he could cite only his German friends Lepsius's Egyptian grammar book and Bunsen's forthcoming Egyptian history. Notwithstanding, he was optimistic that English-speaking scholars might break the monopoly of the Germans. Pickering appreciated the regard for American scholarship "so gracefully rendered by Dr. Prichard, who was so eminently qualified to judge, and whom he had always found just and true in opinion as he had been personally friendly in their long-continued correspondence."[69]

Prichard's correspondence with American scholars flourished from the mid-1830s onward. With Du Ponceau, the discussions ranged from the latest publications tracing affinities among languages to commiserating about their shared burden of defective eyesight. He described Prichard to ex-politician and linguist Albert Gallatin as "the best Philologist in the British dominions, & withal a most amiable man . . . as I judge from my correspondence with him & the report of those who know him."[70] Prichard sent Gallatin a long list of useful books, again, embarrassingly, almost all by Germans. They agreed that grammatical affinity among American languages indicated their common origin even though their vocabularies differed, and independent invention was unlikely to account for similar language structures, despite some fanciful German philologists' claims to the contrary. Prichard was sanguine for the success of one researcher's correlation of the languages of either side of the Bering Strait, and several others had recently claimed to have established American affinities with Asiatic languages. He evidently had been trying to tie the languages of the Americas to those of the Old World. Prichard, grateful for the gift of Gallatin's book on Indigenous Americans, promised to put it to good use in *Physical History*.[71]

This network of American scholars included linguist and diplomat William Brown Hodgson, with whom Prichard shared an interest in the Berber and "Foulah" (Fula) languages. And when George Gliddon, historian of Egypt and future champion of polygenism, came to Britain in 1845, he was pleased to bear a letter of introduction to Prichard.[72] At the height of his career, Prichard's relationships with such respected American scientists were a source of satisfaction.

British Organizational Anthropology, 1847

The anthropology pursued at the ESL was essentially more cultural, historical, and linguistic than biological, but later also archaeological. Its members were generally serious, Christian, monogenist, humane gentlemen. By no means was the ESL dogmatic, however; there was scope for some divergence in approach and opinion. The monogenist, diffusionist line nevertheless dominated in a descriptive historical linguistic activity conducted in the style of a science, an approach now called Prichardian ethnology.

The ESL's membership included men of impeccable reputation such as the geologist Greenough, anatomist Richard Owen, and surgeon and physiologist Sir Benjamin Collins Brodie. Among the society's liberal share of awkward customers were Robert Gordon Latham, "not exactly a nice person to see much of, though a good companion, and one overflowing with every sort of knowledge," and Richard King, another scientist who tended to rub people the wrong way.

As the internationally recognized, preeminent anthropologist of his day, a few months after settling in the capital, Prichard was elected president of the ESL, although his unrelenting Lunacy Commission duties would allow him to preside over only two of its meetings. He thoroughly approved of the society; it reified the science he had striven to create and would aid its further development. But after Prichard had served less than two years as president of the ESL, Hodgkin read his obituary to its meeting.[73]

In this initial phase of organized British anthropology Prichard and his contemporaries were just beginning to explore the scant, nonlinguistic elements of culture as more and more relevant data flowed into the country. This dynamic discipline had good prospects, to Prichard's mind, as he explained in his presidential address on June 22, 1847: "Ethnology refers to the past.... It derives information from the works of ancient historians, and still more extensively from the history of languages and their affiliations ... [and is aided by] anatomy, physiology, zoology, and physical geography.... Whole nations lie perhaps yet buried ... and with them may be found some relicts that may hereafter throw light upon their history." In adding archaeology to ethnology's remit, Prichard set out the encompassing nature of future Anglo-American anthropology.[74]

In a reprise of his ESL speech, Prichard's address to the Ethnological Subsection of the BAAS enthusiastically outlined what archaeology (a word whose modern meaning he was just getting used to) had to offer the science of humankind, and he pointed out that the new subdiscipline of paleontology (another new, French word) brought geology and ethnology together as the archaeology of the globe and its inhabitants. His BAAS audience that summer of 1847 was not well behaved, as sometimes happened: in a sign of troubles to come, it contained some not very friendly ethnologists, such as that outspoken linguist Dr. Latham, and the "Objector General" Mr. Crawfurd. At least there were a greater number and variety of anthropological papers given that year, several of them by foreigners.[75] Bunsen had cajoled the young German-born Friedrich Max Müller, philologist and Sanskrit scholar just establishing himself in Oxford, to present a paper. Chairman Prichard most chivalrously protected Max Müller from attacks by some members of the audience who were anti-German scholarship and anti-German anything: "Dr. Prichard was an excellent president and moderator, and though he had unruly spirits to deal with, he succeeded in keeping up a certain decorum among them."[76]

The overall success of Prichard's address to the BAAS Ethnological Subsection and of the meeting itself must have been gratifying, but anthropology showed no sign of becoming particularly fashionable or prestigious; members of the ESL did not proudly append "ESL" to their names. The society emphasized the scientific character of ethnological research, and its presence in the BAAS confirmed it. When Prichard described his science of humankind in 1847 and 1848 speeches, he played down its biological component—the very topic that interested the ESL's polygenistic foes, men whose views would harden into an increasingly pervasive negative approach to "the Other" at home and abroad, as had already happened in France.

Craniology and Archaeology

The new field of archaeology seemed to promise answers to the deep time questions exercising Prichard and his contemporaries. Excavations of "sepulchral remains" stimulated his interest in studying ancient human crania as he widened his search for conclusive, tangible evidence of the unity and single origin of the human species—evidence that his other types of research had failed conclusively to provide. He was typical in considering the skull the most informative part of the skeleton and frustrated by excavators' deplorable tendency to dig up and scatter the bones of ancient peoples, prizing artifacts to the neglect of human remains. Keen to be thorough and precise, when anatomist Richard Owen sent him an article on Danish archaeology that Prichard planned to insert in the Europe volume of *Physical History*, he asked Owen to check the accuracy of the drawing of the skulls. Traded, ill-documented crania frustrated him; he wanted to get his hands on as much clear and complete material as he could. To Owen he complained, "the Danes have museums appropriated to these remains of the antiquity of their country & it is a great pity that no collection has ever been made of the skulls found in the tumuli of this country, so that it is almost impossible to say what were the osteological or craniological characters of our Celtic forefathers or predecessors. I do not remember to have seen one skull in Sir R. Hoare's collection."[77]

In these early years of thrilling archaeological discoveries, passionate collector Prichard had been collecting crania, intending to publish an atlas of British modern and ancient crania, and perhaps of those the world over. He was grateful for Hodgkin's gift of some casts of crania, to which he reciprocated with an early British skull before greedily asking for Native American, "Esquimaux" (Inuit), and African crania in particular.[78] After John Pickering promised to send him some American specimens, Prichard's hunt for "genuine skulls" was printed in a Boston periodical.[79] Travelers sent him crania, and he traded with other collectors. When Prichard's son Theodore returned from Egypt, he delighted his father with a souvenir ancient Egyptian skull. The greatest proportion of crania in his collection was of ancient or modern Europeans and Africans. A few curiosities crept in, such as the skull of Napoleon's guard killed at Waterloo and a few specimens illustrating disease and mental conditions. After Prichard's death,

Augustin continued collecting, adding items such as "The Skull of a Kaffir killed whilst bravely holding his ground behind a rock at Debie Neck (between King William's Town & Fort White) during a skirmish by one of 'Catty's Rifles' in 1851. His gun & [illegible] are now in the possession of Col. Catty 46th Regt."

Prichard had meant to impress when he decided that the few illustrations in the Europe volume of *Physical History* would be of crania, accompanied by a detailed "Description of the Plates." Once he had completed *Physical History* and *Natural History* and was spending his days inspecting asylums and writing reports, he had little time to immerse himself in a taxing new anthropological project; acquiring data and producing convincing illustrations of skulls had to be done piecemeal, as opportunity allowed. He planned to further challenge the champions of polygenesis and phreno-anthropology on their own playing field. Engravings of crania might convincingly demonstrate the relatedness of nations more tangibly than the analysis of language. Prichard called for the formation of a national collection of skeletons, as the Danes had and as his friend Dr. Wilde was planning in Ireland.[80]

Prichard's contacts among pioneers of biological anthropology began to widen, just as it had among linguists. Professor Anders Adolph Retzius, Swedish anatomist, polygenist, and coiner of the skull proportion terms *dolichocephalic* and *brachycephalic*, was invited in the spring of 1847 to a dinner party at Prichard's home in London, where he was introduced to a few friends. In turn, Retzius introduced other visiting scientists to his London host. Upon returning to Sweden, they corresponded and traded crania, casts, pamphlets, and books. Prichard sent him Belgae skulls from Cirencester and Brigante ones from York, carefully pointing out their proportions, Retzius's particular focus. Aside from crania and casts, he sent the Swede a drawing of the skull of a "Bushman," an illustration for a paper he was writing on the South African nations.[81] Prichard stressed his own particular interest in grave goods and demonstrated his appreciation of archaeological theory when he asked whether certain excavations were "ante-metallurgical." His enthusiasm for his craniological collection was obvious when in March 1848 he asked John Phillips to get casts made of some ancient British skulls recently excavated in Yorkshire.[82] He stored his collection at the Red Lodge in Bristol and planned to publish some of Augustin's illustrations of them.

It appears that Prichard understood Retzius was a polygenist in the making, yet he could not let that stand in the way of their mutual interest in crania. Noticing that Retzius unfortunately emphasized the *differences* between nations, Prichard stressed that his own studies of crania demonstrated the common origins of different groups "for certain." He was always after evidence, following up with a probe: "We have not yet sufficient information as to the diversities which arise in the separated branches of the same race. . . . I should be glad to know in what precise anatomical variations the difference subsists." In his last letter to Retzius in the autumn of 1848, announcing another consignment of crania and discussing the archaeological evidence dating an ancient burial site, he mentioned his similar relationship with a Dr. John Thurnam. Prichard's comments to Retzius on British skulls were later translated and printed in Swedish and German periodicals. The Swede referred to Prichard often in his writing and published his obituary notice.[83]

When there was an issue related to biological anthropology, scientists knew who to call on. Eminent Irish surgeon Robert James Graves asked Prichard whether it was true the obliteration of the sagittal suture was characteristic of a particular tribe. He replied categorically that after examining his many "European" and "Negro" skulls, he had found heavy ossification resulting in suture obliteration irrespective of race.[84]

Whereas Prichard's growing interest in crania and the third edition of *Physical History*'s illustrations of them have been considered evidence of his shift toward biological anthropology that presumes interest in race ranking, evidence more clearly points to his goals being the preservation and description of crania and demonstration of the fallacy of the concept of race. This turned out not to be the case with Samuel George Morton. Prichard struck up a correspondence with the American craniologist, whose atlas *Crania Americana* amazed the scientific world and effectively promoted polygenetic, phrenological racialist theories. Their relationship turned out to be complex, demanding, and mutually beneficial.

Samuel George Morton's Scientific Racialism

The French started to face some stiff competition for preeminence in race science when Dr. Morton entered the field. Samuel George Morton is remembered as founder of American biological anthropology and its execrable product, scientific racialism. His inclination toward both polygenism and phrenology should have repelled Prichard, but Morton, circumspect to a fault, kept him initially unaware of his anathematic views. When Morton sent him some preprinted illustrations from his forthcoming *Crania Americana; or, A Comparative View of the Skulls of Various Aboriginal*

Nations of North and South America, Prichard was highly impressed. These engravings were so enviably superior to those in *Physical History* (1826) that Prichard displayed them at the Birmingham BAAS meeting and enthusiastically promoted Morton's project. Morton's letter notifying him of his election as corresponding member of the prestigious Academy of Natural Sciences of Philadelphia in 1838 was gratifying. Prichard rashly committed himself to *Crania Americana* without having seen its explanatory text.[85]

Morton had been busy measuring the capacity of crania, ranking humans in descending quality with superior Caucasians at the top, unsurprisingly for Americans in that era. His theories were destined for *Crania Americana*, along with George Combe's phrenological interpretations. For his part, Combe did not appreciate Morton's and other Americans' bending phrenology to their racialist ends. While Prichard would have despised both interpretations, it did not prevent him from accepting Morton's gift of a skull and making suggestions as they carried on corresponding. He reminded Morton that views of the base of the skull might enhance the illustrations, something relevant to his own work. And keeping in mind his own plans to publish a similar cranial atlas of Britain, he was more than a little apprehensive about the large investment Morton's project required.[86] If the American had intended to mislead Prichard by playing down his phrenological and racialist interests, Prichard repaid him by promoting *Crania Americana* as a work of anthropology divorced from negative associations and phrenology.

Prichard forwarded *Crania Americana*'s prospectus to the Geographical Society, assuring Morton he would "do what may be in my power to accelerate the acquaintance of my countrymen with your work, which will doubtless be appreciated both in this country and on the continent." He promised to have it ordered by libraries and publicized among all the principal scientific men of Britain and Europe at the upcoming BAAS meeting, and he suggested particular booksellers and scientists Morton should approach to secure notices and reviews. Prichard submitted a review of the projected work for publication in the Geographical Society's journal, and he later arranged for a friend to write a longer one for Forbes's *British and Foreign Medical Review*, the best such periodical in England. Notably, it effectively dismissed the phrenological content of *Crania Americana* while praising the anthropological.[87]

Wearing his phrenologist's hat, Morton was meanwhile cultivating the Combe brothers to enlist their support in promoting *Crania Americana* among British phrenologists. Upon discovering the British edition's dedication to phrenology's bête noir Prichard, George Combe took Morton to task over this undoubted slight:

> I am not gratified by learning that your English Edition is dedicated to Dr. Pritchard. He has an excellent Intellect, and a well balanced head, with one exception, a deficient organ of Conscientiousness. I speak from observing his development. In regard to Phrenology, he has shewn a lamentable defect of honest & fair dealing. A man of this kind is one who is a capital friend as long as it is his interest or inclination to be a friend; but no perfect reliance can be placed on his conduct where interest or inclination (vanity, for example, or ambition) dictate one course of action & duty another. He is much esteemed at Bristol, where he resides; and I hope no jealousy or other interested motive will render him unworthy of your regard. At the last meeting of the British Association, Dr. Pritchard asked money to procure specimens to enable him to illustrate the natural history of man. Mr. Hewett Watson asked him if he had examined the collection of national crania in the museum of the Phren: Socy of Edinh. when he was in that city. He answered No! Mr. Watson told him that he should use the materials within his reach before he asked for money to purchase more. Our collection is said to be the largest in Europe.[88]

Morton had been supping with the Devil. Combe had failed to appreciate the American's prime interest. Morton had invested heavily in *Crania Americana*, and while he cultivated the patronage of phrenologists, he was keener to make his mark among the scientific establishment with his new ideas about race. He attempted to mollify Combe:

> I ought also to have mentioned to you that I dedicated my work to Dr. Prichard first because of his long continued & most instructive Researches into the Physical Hist. of Mankind, altho' I have arrived at opposite conclusions from his array of facts. And in the second place, he has shewn a great interest for the success of my work in several letters addressed to me, & his communications to my friends; & Dr. Gibson informed me that Dr. Prichard took a roll of my plates to the British Association, & commended the then embryo book in strong terms to the attention of the learned men there convened. I had no idea, however, that he was so *hostile* to Phrenology as he has since been represented to me; which I very much regret; & trust you & I may both live to see him acknowledge his error.[89]

Combe and Morton never had the satisfaction of seeing Prichard repent. Prichard was surprised and flattered by the handsome dedication to him. Morton's clever claim that *Crania Americana* supported *Physical History* sealed Prichard's obligation to him: "I am most anxious to promote the interests of your work, which indeed on public grounds I ought to do.... If any other way of promoting the interest of your work occurs to me, be sure that I shall avail myself of it. But indeed it has no need of my aid or the patronage of any person at home or abroad. It is sure to make its way at all libraries under the management of enlightened persons."[90]

To another American Prichard wrote that *Crania Americana* "does credit to your country, being by far the most splendid work on ethnography yet published, if I am not mistaken, in any land. I hope the author will be rewarded for his labor and zeal better than I fear he would be in this country, where researches which have not an immediate bearing upon utility or upon some topic of popular interest are but indifferently recompensed."[91] Despite Prichard's poorly formed conscientiousness bump, he continued corresponding with Morton, sending him advice and copies of his own publications and making every effort to aid him, and he welcomed Morton's plan to produce *Crania Aegyptiaca*. Prichard no doubt deplored the text of *Crania Americana*, yet he promoted the atlas as an anthropological publication that would help him garner support for his own planned atlas of British crania. Morton's beautifully produced atlas, like the colored engravings Prichard had started including in his own publications, are prime examples of the convincing apparatus of the developing scientific profession.[92]

During his final years, Prichard collected, measured, analyzed, and wrote about human skulls, not to differentiate, rank, or determine intellectual capacity, but to describe peoples and discover the relationships among them. To his mind, lack of correlation of his three basic forms of crania with human groups stymied categorization, invalidating race ranking and polygenetic theory. In his last conversation with Hodgkin as they walked home from a meeting of the Ethnological Society, Prichard enthused about his projected atlas of crania that he apparently hoped would steal the march on the efforts of rival phrenologists and polygenists.[93]

Morton inspired polygenetic and racialist writers in antebellum America and for generations afterward. His contemporary Dr. Charles Caldwell, that belligerent Kentuckian medical educator, dabbler in phrenology, champion of polygenism, and race theorist, visited Britain in 1841, spoiling for a fight with Prichard. He planned to deliver a lecture at the BAAS Plymouth's "séance," where he hoped to "come into direct collision and conflict with the views of Dr. Pritchard." Caldwell was disappointed in his prey's absence and the time restriction that prevented him from blessing the BAAS with the full text of his "The Differences *in Full*, Internal and External, Bodily and Mental, between the Caucasian and the African Races." Caldwell claimed, "Prichard is a mass of error on that subject"; inferior races were destined for extinction. He was just as dismissive of Prichard's *A Treatise on Insanity*, which he considered lacking in science. Caldwell had another chance to tackle Prichard as he headed for Bristol to embark for America on the *Great Western*. He planned to have "a frank and courteous conversation, on the Subject of anthropology, which may possibly lead to a subsequent correspondence. At all events, should I meet him, I shall learn something of the tone, temper, and liberality or illiberality of his mind and opinions, and act accordingly."[94]

Caldwell was among a growing band of racialist theorizers openly challenging Prichard's anthropology. He vociferously claimed the "tameability" and inferior intelligence of Africans, which he considered "especially true as relates to the Bosehesemen, and other tribes of the Hottentot race. They and the Papuans are such miserable representatives of humanity, that it would puzzle a jury of naturalists to decide, to which they are most nearly allied, the genus Homo, or the genus Simia." Although he was certain that Africans were incapable of living independently, believing they must have masters to control their tendency to be "savage, wild, and indolent too," he nevertheless concluded American slavery was a great but unsolvable evil.[95] Caldwell claimed his *Thoughts on the Original Unity of Man* was based on sound foundations, unlike Prichard's publications:

> I have noticed and analyzed, perhaps with too much severity, the work of Dr. Pritchard, on the unity or diversity of man, I forget which. That writer, with all his learning (and he has an abundance of it) has not yet learnt the real difference between the African and the Caucasian. That difference is immeasurably greater than he admits or even suspects it to be. It is much greater than the difference in organization between the dog and the wolf; or between the fox and jackal. . . . Therefore radically and irredeemably, the African is an inferior race.[96]

Caldwell was fond of underlining. As hard as he worked to make creative use of phrenology and anthropology in support of his deplorable racialist theorizing, he could not hold a candle to the obnoxious views expressed by Morton's protégés Josiah Nott and George Gliddon. Nott condemned Prichard as cowardly for failing to come out against abolitionism, thus aiding the enemy in the race war to come.[97] Caldwell did not record whether Prichard had experienced the pleasure of his company in Bristol in back in 1841.

A few years after Prichard's death Joseph Barnard Davis and Dr. John Thurnam brought out *Crania Britannica*. Davis acknowledged that he had been inspired by Thomas Bateman's skull collection in 1849 and was taking up the mantle from Prichard, who in his concern for the preservation and study of British crania had intended to carry out the project himself. Its prospectus lists Thomas Hodgkin as a subscriber. Davis had swapped some skulls with Augustin Prichard that had been given to his father by Retzius; others he had obtained from Hodgkin. His initial plan to put an entirely phrenological slant on *Crania Britannica* had met with Thurnam's objections, so that it had been necessary to pacify Combe to keep him on board.[98] Like its inspiring American publication, *Crania Britannica* served both biological anthropology and phrenology, the former in its ascendancy and the latter in decline. Printed in parts between 1856 and 1865, it contains ethnographical descriptions as well as fine illustrations, a lot of craniometric figures, and twenty-eight references to Prichard.

Prichard was clearly proud of his role in creating the British discipline of anthropology. It was thriving, with its literature, society, theories, methodology, and relationships with other sciences, scientists, and their organizations. The Select Committee, Aborigines' Protection Society, *Ethnological Queries*, BAAS Ethnology Subsection, Ethnological Society of London, and Geographical Society of London had been instrumental to its development. Prichard's lectures and publications defining anthropology and decrying the plight of colonized peoples were milestones in its history, while his correspondence with scientists nationally and internationally and even tussles with phrenologists and collaboration with racialist polygenists had been rewarding. Looking to the future science of humankind, he called for the collection of archaeological remains and their preservation in museums and renewed efforts to prevent the further decimation of his fellow human beings.

Prichard's battle against polygenism was foundering, however, and it was becoming increasingly difficult to reconcile Scripture with what was day by day being revealed by the sciences he welcomed. The reformist and scientific societies Prichard supported had mixed futures in store. The BAAS would manage to keep British science safely Christian for a time and provide provincial scientists with an outlet for their work. Its Ethnological Subsection would be shifted among its sections until it became the Anthropology Section later in the century. The Geographical Society fared well, a reflection of British imperial expansion, while the ESL became a battleground for rival theories that seriously weakened it. The Aborigines' Protection Society, by contrast, was hardly successful in protecting the British Empire's Indigenous subjects. While it effectively gathered and shared evidence of settler colonists' injustices and atrocities, government and settlers alike more often considered the APS interfering. The government tried to benefit colonizers and the colonized alike, so rather than curtailing British colonial depredations, the APS accommodated itself to government policies.[99]

13 · Christian Humanitarian Anthropology

Publications, 1836–48, and Legacy

> Dr. Prichard's authority stood very high, and justly so, and his *Researches into the Physical History of Mankind* still remain unparalleled in ethnology.
> —Friedrich Max Müller, *My Autobiography*

The portraits of Raja Ram Mohan Roy's two attendants were dazzling, as Prichard had intended. They illustrate a greatly expanded edition of *Physical History*, "a good deal called for, & which he is at his leisure preparing under a new arrangement," his father boasted.[1] This encyclopedic five-volume third edition comprises one volume of biological anthropology followed by four of global ethnography. Realizing his previous arguments for monogenism did not stand on completely firm scientific ground, he seemed to want to convince his readers of the fallacy of polygenism by its sheer bulk of data of every kind. In this huge task, Prichard gathered whatever evidence he could find about every culture the world over in order not just to describe them physically but to present their geographical surroundings, history, migrations and interrelationships, languages, beliefs, customs, diseases, and psychology. In the course of the eleven years it took to complete *Physical History*'s final edition, Prichard maintained his international preeminence in the nascent science of anthropology and was variously appreciated and deprecated by his contemporaries and by following generations.

The 1830s had begun with Prichard's working on a variety of publications more or less simultaneously. His medical practice was flourishing, and he was widely engaged in the new world of institutional science and education. All along he kept in his sights the task of gathering further information in support of his theory of the unity and single origin of the human species, but instead of discrediting polygenism and phrenology, those unfounded notions were gaining popularity and acquiring some very vocal advocates, especially in France and the United States. In pursuing new lines of evidence to reinforce his argument for monogeny, he dropped some views expressed in the 1826 edition and modified others; for example, he revisited the idea that the environment played a role in stimulating biological change. Prichard hoped his science would support the abolition of slavery and force government to protect Indigenous peoples from colonial settlers' depredations. And in predicting a future when so many cultures had become extinct or "civilized" and Christianized, he wanted *Physical History* to serve as a resource for scientists. He found himself under an avalanche of ethnographical data. Then there was the increasingly vocal struggle between Scripture and some scientists' emboldened claims of nature's self-development to counter. Protégé and friend Francis William Newman challenged and exasperated him on this score:

> [The] doctor was driven to believe that Adam and Eve were black. He printed this as his earlier hypothesis. His pressure on me drew me into the study of the Zouavi (Numidian) tongues and brought me into much talk with him about his book when he was at his 3rd ed. He was in origin a Quaker, in development an Evangelical Churchman and stickler for as much Bibliolatry as he could accept. But he could <u>not</u> accept patriarchal longevity, while he regarded normal length of life to discriminate species. He managed to set up the doctrine that our genealogy of the ante diluvians was quite incomplete and the years from Adam to Noah quite uncertain. Already (1835) Geologists avowed that the Fossil Horse and Ass was not the same species as our Horse and Ass.
>
> When he opined all this, and declared it uncertain <u>how old</u> the Fossils might be, I was presumptuous enough to declare, that <u>if he gave time freely</u>, I could not see any serious difficulty in believing that asses, zebras and horses were all from a common stock, and the causes now separating them were of later origin.—This, in the name of <u>all the men of science</u> he repudiated as utterly impossible. But I went on to say, that since he held the interval of time between Adam & Noah to us of indefinite duration, surely that was his easiest mode of varying skin on the descendants of the original pair. The much talk which I had with him, carried me farther; viz. I said if once you doubt the strict guarantee of every bit of the book of Genesis as the work of the Holy Spirit, you will teach us to reconsider many historical probabilities, such as the distribution of animals over the world from Mount Ararat as their centre after Noah's flood, which Naturalists were already finding impossible. I think he could not deny it.

Newman made matters worse by pointing out the implausibility of the creation of a single human stock; rather, thousands of similar pairs of the same species must have been created, each tailored to their climate. He felt that the Mosaic account actually hampered rational consideration of evidence. As Prichard would not entertain multiple creations of several or a single human species, Newman decided further discussion was futile.[2]

This disagreement with Newman exemplifies the mounting challenge of reconciling Scripture and science. Prichard had tried to excuse discordance by variously pointing out errors on the part of biblical copyists; the use of figurative language in Genesis; the argument that reality had been different in the distant past; the Bible pertaining only to human history; the existence of miracles, and so on. Very early in his career he was among those who adopted the view that in Genesis a "day" was actually a period of time, albeit a far cry from Benoît de Maillet's Enlightenment assertion that time stretched back millions of years.[3] Faced with geological and archaeological evidence, he ended up allowing for unknown chiliads (millennia) of human history. Prichard struggled to account for the new evidence of development in nature. By the early 1830s, some of his younger contemporaries were already viewing his "bibliolatry" as a bit outdated and unscientific. But rather than merely objecting to new conceptions of the natural world, he called for further scientific research even as he started to retreat into citing biblical evidence more often.

The era's revolution in communications allowed Prichard to better carry out research from provincial Bristol. From the 1830s, not only did he travel more, including on the Continent, but he corresponded, met more national and international scientists, attended scientific and medical conferences, and gained access to foreign literature. The resources of the metropole, such as the Geographical Society and Royal Asiatic Society, became easier to exploit; he tasked others with fetching particular books and often took the long journey to the capital himself.[4]

Of course, residence in London or Oxford would have made researching, publishing, and promoting his work easier. Recent advances in print technology had decreased costs, but his readership was limited, and it could sometimes be a struggle to obtain reviews. Prichard advised a would-be anthropologist: "The subject not being a popular one you can not expect a rapid sale. My books were very slow at first and it was nearly 20 years before I gained a moderate remuneration for my work. Nor indeed have I ever been half repaid, except indirectly, viz thru my profession, in which some of my books were serviceable to me."[5] While his scientific tomes undoubtedly enhanced his reputation as a physician, they did not sell themselves; he had to cultivate the support of publishers, journal editors, and influential fellow scientists. There was some financial risk too. Prichard offered others patronage and advice. Dr. Morton and his *Crania Americana* is a case in point:

> The profit or loss of an author depends much on his booksellers. . . . I have access to one or two of the periodicals and shall use my best interest in these quarters. Do you know any thing of Professor Robert Graves of Dublin. He has the command of the Dublin medical press & could serve your work more in Dublin & in Ireland generally than any other individual known to me. I think it would be worth your while to send him a copy of the book. I will mention it to him. . . . He is fond of alluding to subjects connected with the physical history of human races in his lectures & has the Dublin scientific journal at his control as well as great interest in all that is going on in the literary & scientific circles in Ireland. . . . My Friend Dr Hodgkin . . . is particularly interested in the subject of ethnography, as connected with his philanthropic exertions for the protection of aboriginal races. He has access to very large numbers of persons engaged in similar pursuits. . . . It would be worth while for you to write to him & request him to notice your publication on the common grounds of the interest which it is calculated to excite. You are welcome to use my name to him in any way.[6]

Physical History, Third Edition (1836–47)

The third edition of *Physical History* further refines the structure of Prichardian anthropology. He adopted the terms "ethnology" and "ethnography" as generally synonymous with "the natural history of man," and in employing the phrase "science of ethnology" in the later volumes, he asserted his topic's scientific credentials. Lest any readers doubt his primacy in the broad science of humankind, he pointed out that the "comparative physiology and psychology of different races of men had never been made expressly the subject of inquiry, until the publication of my work."[7]

The two previous editions of *Physical History* had been countered by a raft of publications promulgating polygenesis, which Prichard was determined to sink. He devoted the entire first volume to biological exposition; it sets out his methodology, presents a somewhat better-organized text, and includes new sections on "psychic unity" and sacred history. From infinitely varying, uncorrelatable, and therefore evidentially invalid superficial human physical characteristics, Prichard shifted focus inward to the skeleton, physiology, language, and the mind. He concluded that the overwhelming universal congruity in human structure, physiology, and psychology establishes specific unity. The first volume attracted several reviews, and extracts appeared in journals.

Physical History's four huge ethnographic volumes are on Africa (1837), Europe (1841), Asia (1844), and Oceania and America (1847). They present an enormous mass of material and seize every opportunity to point out evidence of migrations and linguistic affinities supporting arguments for humankind's global diffusion and the relatedness of all peoples. He shifted some nationalities from European to Asiatic and adopted a general descriptive template: geography, history, physical type, and language, supplemented with accounts of religious and other cultural practices.

In developing these volumes, Prichard regularly rehearsed and recycled materials from them elsewhere. At the Bristol Phil & Lit he read "before a very numerous assembly of members and their friends, 'An Essay on the Native Races of America, with some general Observations on the Varieties of the Human Skull.'" After dividing the two American continents into eleven great nations and pointing out their common origin in the far northwest, he compared American and Asiatic crania, entertaining his rapt audience with specimens illustrating the three basic forms of skull: European, narrow-elongated, and broad-faced. As for his outline of American languages, he cited the works of his personal correspondents.[8] This hugely popular lecture publicized his books and supported the Phil & Lit.

A portrait of the bishop of Abyssinia recycled from the 1826 edition introduces readers to the second volume, *Researches into the Physical Ethnography of the African Races*. Much more had been learned about Africa since 1826. Prichard divided the continent into Atlantica, Highlands of Central Africa, and Lowlands, further subdividing them as he dealt with individual nations. As well as its beautiful illustrations, the volume contains tables of languages. Because so many peoples were yet to be visited or studied, at times he could do little more than list them.[9]

"I am now about sending to the press a third & thick volume of my new edition of Researches into the Physical Hist. of Mankind comprising the results of all that I have been able to collect on the history, philology &c of the European & Asiatic nations," Prichard was relieved to write in early 1840.[10] It was so thick it had to be split into two separate volumes that take readers on a tour of the continents. Europe presented a particular opportunity: the Indo-European language family did not correlate with the variations in physical characteristics typical of its nations. He considered some Continental authors' similar works on the nations of Europe in this era of growing European nationalism that inspired research into its distant past. While occupied with this volume he earnestly collected crania, both to illustrate it and to further his campaign against phrenology and polygenism using their enthusiasts' own weapon—the human skull.[11]

There were two more mountainous volumes to come. In 1843 he complained the much-delayed volume 4 "has cost me immense labor, much more than any former undertaking, and I shall be very glad when it is brought to a close."[12] *Researches into the History of the Asiatic Nations* opens with Persia and travels eastward to India, then around the Georgian, Caucasian, Great Tartary and Hyperborean (Siberian), Chinese, Indo-Chinese, and Syro-Arabian nations. It concludes with sections on the relationships among these different nations and some of their psychological and physical characteristics, and there are appendixes on the "Gipseys" and the Berber and Hausa languages. Among its few colored plates is the one of Ram Mohan Roy's two servants. The accompanying tinted ethnographic map, owing much to Alexander von Humboldt's recent publication on Russia, outlines the nations of Asia.[13]

Prichard could tackle the subject of his final volume with greater confidence than he had done in 1826. In exploring the cultures of Oceania and the Americas, he acknowledged his debt to American philologists, writing to Gallatin: "It seems to me almost presumptuous to ask you to accept a book, the best part of which is taken from your own writings." He also corresponded with J. K. E. Buschmann, a linguist of Native American languages, acknowledging his debt to him and his associate Wilhelm von Humboldt. Another correspondent was South American explorer and ethnologist Robert Hermann Schomburgk.[14]

Prichard's views on the varieties of Indigenous Oceanians evolved with each edition of *Physical History*. Benefiting from new research, he divided Oceania into three "groupes": Oceanic (Polynesians), Oceanic Negroes (Papuans), and Alfourus or Alforians (Australians). The peoples whose languages are related to that of the Malays he denoted Maylo-Polynesians, referring to the work of Wilhelm von Humboldt. As for Franz Bopp's view that Malayan is descended from Sanskrit, clearly with the single origin of languages in mind, Prichard felt they more likely shared a common ancestral language. The second half of volume 5 comprises a general description of and comparisons between Indigenous Americans and Asians, outlines the divisions and subdivisions of North and South American peoples, and provides some general observations on their history, physical characteristics, and psychology.[15] That linguistic data predominates in this volume reflects the material available at the time.

Physical History's "Race" and Developing Theories

Some of Prichard's readers might have been keener to learn about foreign customs and extreme physical variations found among far-flung humankind than about *similarities* in physiology, religious beliefs, psychology, and language. They also might have expected to find the volume on European nations illustrated with the "ideal" European physical type—a "Caucasian" or a classical Greek visage of upright facial angle, elevated forehead, and skin as white as the marble statue from which it was drawn. Prichard had a strategy to counter what he might have perceived as developing racialism.

He asked James Yates to help him obtain an accurate lithograph: "I have some idea of trying to get for a frontispiece to my new volume a coloured portrait of Rammohun Roy. Ram Mohan Roy was a very dark Brahman & the existence of such a complexion in the Brahman race is a fact of importance to my argument." He had previously observed that the skin of the more "civilized," elite members of a population became lighter in hue, but here was evidence to the contrary. Was it possible that European whiteness was the result of sudden accidental variation instead of the workings of civilization? Ram Mohan Roy's portrait riveted readers' attention on a "specimen of skin approaching to black in a tribe of the Indo-European stock" and contrasts it to his "civilized" state; this Brahmin's rather European features proved the futility of forming racial boundaries like those touted by polygenists. While Prichard labored to describe individual aspects of the human body in every possible way, inventing anthropological nomenclature for the purpose, he remained adamantly against solid racial categories, writing that "no particular figure is a permanent characteristic of any one race."[16]

Prichard had further surprises for readers inclined to Eurocentrism, as he explained to Hodgkin: "I am now writing when a little time falls to my lot, on the history of the nations of Asia & Europe in which I shall endeavour to show that their races long were & probably would have remained but for the communication of external aids, in a state of society as barbarous as that of the most savage Africans."[17] His chapter on psychic unity gave him an opportunity to demonstrate a glimmer of what is now termed cultural relativism when he noted the criteria for beauty were not universal. He was no doubt aware of the philosopher Gottfried Herder's discussion of this tenet of modern anthropology, which warns against evaluating the beliefs and customs of one society using the values of another.

Prichard encouraged readers to engage in self-reflection in several other instances. He pointed out that both ancient and modern Europeans were

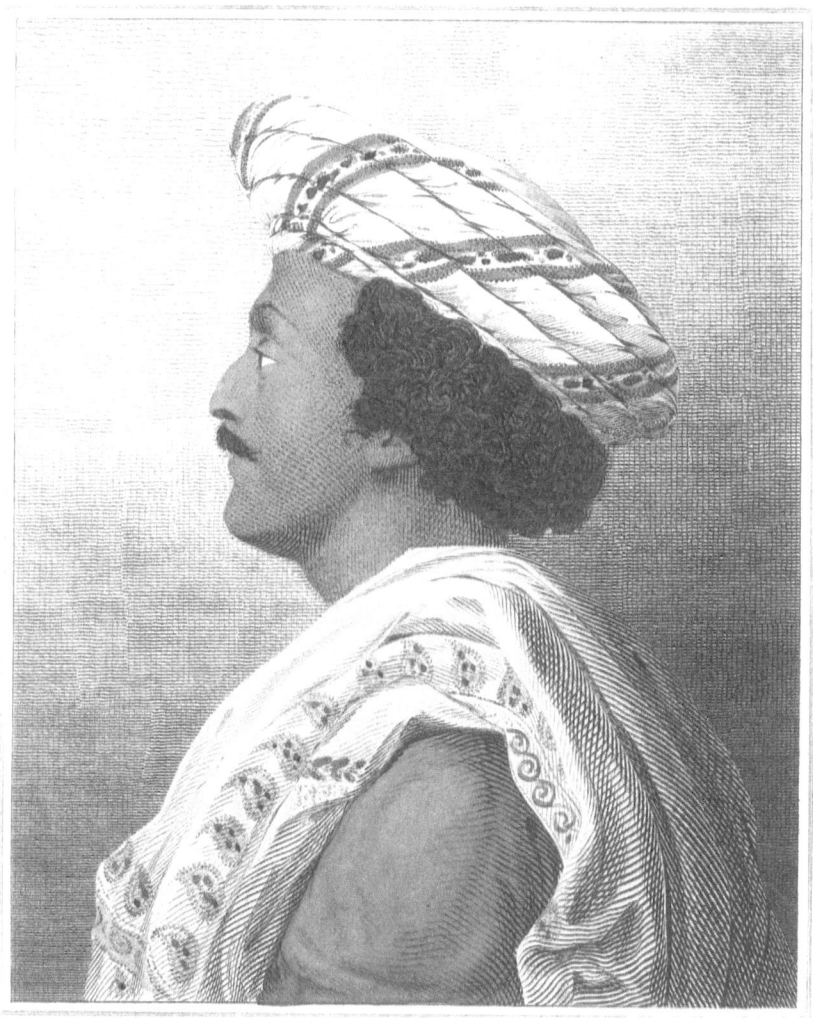

11. Theory. "A portrait of Rammohun Roy, affording an example of very dark complexion in a Brahman of undoubtedly pure race: a specimen of colour approaching to black in a tribe of the Indo-European stock." Colored frontispiece, *Researches into the Physical History of Mankind*, vol. 3 (1841).

subject to being superstitious, and ancient European cultures must have been on a level with those of the most primitive of contemporary extra-Europeans. Further, just as disparate peoples share similar religious beliefs and customs, cultures must have been independently developed around the world, rather than having been disseminated from a surmised original cradle. Within all populations there is a wide range of intelligence,

European included. He maintained that climate and social factors rather than capability inhibit societies from attaining the level of European civilization. Later anthropologists would for a time adopt his criterion of humanity the capacity to be Christianized. While the Christian monogenetic element of Prichard's anthropology would eventually become obsolete, his introduction of comparative psychology, the notion of psychic unity, and a degree of cultural relativism qualifies him as a contributor to early anthropological theory.

The successive editions of *Physical History* track Prichard's shifting views on the causes of human variation. As his readers would have expected, he named and described his now seven principal varieties of humankind. He continued to stress, however, these varieties' lack of clear and consistent characteristics; for instance, two physically similar populations might not share the same type of language. To further stress the invalidity of race categories, he created a new taxon "permanent varieties" to support his argument.[18] He again applied his tried and tested analogical argument to reiterate the specific unity of the human species based on its variations being no greater than within other species of animals. He even suggested that alterations in morphological traits could occur within the limits of history. Notably, his better use of new geographies such as Ritter's *Erdkunde* led him to reconsider the effects of "external circumstances" on human form; he now allowed climate somehow to stimulate biological development, and he drew less attention to his previously favored interbreeding and congenital causes of variation. Development could be improving or degenerating.

Prichard's qualified shift toward environmentalism, an idea associated with liberal and antislavery views, led him to reconsider Lamarck's theory of the inheritance of acquired characteristics. Although he suggested that there are biological mechanisms by which heritable changes occur and mentioned congenital change, he avoided explaining how the environment actually brings about change in human structure, writing that determining the causes "is an inquiry of secondary importance in reference to the principal object of this part of my work. The primary question is, whether any and what deviations have actually taken place in the physical characteristics of particular tribes within the period of time to which the evidence of history reaches back."[19] Prichard was apparently concerned that his previous theories of heredity had played into the hands of polygenists. More reassuring was geographers' greater evidence of migrations, a point which countered the polygenetic notion of populations being created for specific locations. The migration of humans out of biblical lands eventually covered the entire world. Notably, his opinion of European civilization had further deteriorated, exacerbated by his study of psychology and insanity and an awareness of atrocities carried out by "civilized" Europeans.

Prichard was obviously proud of his new chapter on the universal quality of mental faculties. It complemented his physiological evidence of the unity of the human species. His recently published *Treatise on Insanity* showed an appreciation of Gall and Spurzheim's theory of the mind, the entire emotive and instinctive system. There Prichard suggested that moral insanity, for example, is a lesion in the emotional structure of the mind. Importantly, this nonphysical structure, the psychical character that unites mind and soul, is the same among all human beings. To demonstrate psychic unity, the "common psychical nature or a common mind," he gathered evidence on extra-Europeans' religious beliefs and moral sentiments; his criteria were the potential for intellectual development and the aforementioned receptivity to Christianity. Prichard's exploration of the nature of the human mind thus united his psychology and anthropology. The term "psychic unity" became an element in anthropological theory later in the century, its invention attributed to others.[20]

African ethnographic material supplied Prichard with abundant evidence of psychic and therefore specific unity. First reminding his readers that Africans were no more barbarous than ancient Europeans had been, he pointed out their possession of "natural religion." Despite the trappings of fetishes, idols, and sacrificing, they believed in a supreme being, though they worshipped through mediators in the form of objects, lesser gods, and so on, and some believed in metempsychosis, or the transmigration of the soul after death. Africans prayed, had a priesthood and rituals, and seemed to believe in the immortality of the soul and divine retribution. They clearly possessed the universal human traits of having religious beliefs and the desire to "improve," as they were able to accept the Christian faith. Instead of entertaining his readers with accounts of strange superstitions or "debased" religious practices, Prichard drew their attention to similarities among cultures. His practice of comparative psychology sets aside superfluous cultural and superficial physical differences and instead recognizes the universality of humankind's nonphysical mind and soul.

In discussing religion as an aspect of cultural development, Prichard summoned an array of evidence. He admitted that it was debatable whether psychic unity as manifested in monotheistic religious belief was the result of original unity or the natural product of the human mind. He had previously considered monotheism as a God-given universal human trait, which among some peoples had degenerated in stages to polytheism. But while this religious "degeneration" was taking place, other aspects of culture were apparently developing, implying social evolutionary progress. Disconcertingly, God must have created Adam and Eve in a primitive state. Volume 4's concluding chapter is noncommittal on the question of degeneration or progress in religious development. He mused that shamanism "might be termed the religion of nature, if the most degraded and barbarised state of humanity were really the original and natural one. It is that form of superstition which is congenial to mankind, when they have long lost, or have as yet not gained by art and skill, a power over the physical elements."[21]

The third edition's reference to Scripture is more overt where the evolution of language and religion is discussed. Prichard drew on German Romantic philology's association of language structure and philosophical potential, the mental quality of its speakers. He did not seem to consider himself at all biased, as he speculated that unlike other languages that had evolved from the simple to complex and abstract, that of the "Shemites" was from its origin uniquely fitted to express higher-level concepts. Thus the people who nurtured the religion of the Bible had never experienced a primitive state of mind, nor had Christianity evolved as other religions had. As for the biblical account of the confusion of languages at the Tower of Babel, Prichard found "no difficulty in admitting such an event as supernatural in an age when so many events must have happened which were out of the present course of nature. But may not the habit of language-making, if I may use such an expression, which we trace in its active working in the first ages, and which afterwards ceased for ever to exist or operate, sufficiently account for the diversification of human idioms?"[22]

Prichard's appendix "Note on the Biblical Chronology" grapples with geologists' incontrovertible demonstration of the greater than biblical age of the earth. How could the huge timescale necessary for variations in physical form and dispersal of human groups around the world be reconciled with that of the Bible? A contemporary theory called "pre-adamism" posited the existence of human populations before the Creation, but as this left the door open to polygenetic argument, it did not appeal to Prichard. In *Egyptian Mythology* (1819) he had reconciled scriptural and the longer Egyptian historical chronologies by pointing out technical errors in the latter. The relatively short biblical chronology, however, disconcertingly left insufficient time for the development of human physical variation. Prichard explained this away by suggesting nature might have operated differently in the past.

Further discrepancies between Scripture and evidence needed tackling. Philosophers and historians had long attempted to fathom the duration of all history and humanity's place in it. Prichard pointed out that biblical history provides an accurate chronology only as far back as the mid-tenth century BCE; beyond that it was not possible to know how much time had elapsed between the Creation and the Deluge. The time span between the Deluge and the establishment of nations in the biblical lands apparently required some adjustment as human error had crept in: some of the earliest chronologists had been inaccurate, or had simply omitted periods of time in which there were no events relevant to human history. Similarly, as the longevity of the Patriarchs of the ten generations before the Deluge is not a fact independently supported in Scripture, it can be discounted as the exaggeration of later copyists. Prichard massaged sacred history and patently longer human history into accord without impugning Scripture itself.[23]

Prichard took every opportunity to trace more consistently the descent of and relationships among peoples. He reported recent discoveries such as intrepid Captain Alexander Burns's description in the *Bengal Literary Journal* of some newly discovered peoples of the Hindu Kush. Prichard enthused about it to American linguist Du Ponceau in 1839: "The curiosity of the matter is that they speak the Sanskrit more purely, as it would appear probable from a few specimens of their idiom, than any of the nations of Hindustan and they are a fair, red or light haired people, like the ancient Germans. I shall put all that I can collect respecting them into my next volume and we shall probably know much about them when Burnes returns from his present expedition."[24] What could be more germane to his theory of Indo-European migrations than this ancient language being spoken by Germanic-looking people? His global exploration of language greatly swelled the third edition.

Every scientific discipline spawns neologisms. Examples of Prichard's fondness for new terminology are "stenobregmatic" for skull shape, "palaetaphia" for ancient human remains, and "xanthous" for skin color. He was surprised that his friend Bunsen had used "Turanian" to classify Asian languages and was aggrieved that the great Alexander von Humboldt had neglected to acknowledge *Physical History*:

> If you will look into the 1st vol. of my book, you will find Turanian used as a distinctive epithet for a form of the skull and for the people who are characterised by it, viz the nations of High Asia. I proposed it there as a substitute for Mongolian, thinking that name improper,

for a reason given. Since my first volume was published the name of Turanian has been used by several German and other foreign physiologists in the same sense. One of these is, I think, Retzius of Stockholm. In the first volume of Kosmos you will see that Humboldt thinks the name of *Iranian* which I used instead of *Caucasian* preferable to *Caucasian*. . . . Neither he nor any body else has mentioned that the name was used by me.[25]

Physical History briefly concludes with a reminder that the principal object of the book is to determine whether humankind's physical and psychological characteristics are fixed or transmutable. He was confident that volume one demonstrates human specific unity based on morphological and biological criteria. Any variation he attributed to environmental influences affecting physical characteristics that "in a long course of time" distinguish the entire group. The four ethnographical volumes provide historical, geographical, linguistic, and whatever cultural evidence of human unity he could find.

The complexity of Prichard's arguments and his adjustments to them exposed him to criticism. With each edition of *Physical History* he amended his interpretation of the scope of the Flood, for instance, until he finally gave up and offered his readers a choice of two biblically sound versions. Whereas he had at first shortened Egyptian chronology to conform to biblical chronology, at the end of his career the evidence of geology forced him to lengthen biblical chronology to accommodate the obviously greater length of time needed for variation in human form. Instead of continuing to stress that biological change happened congenitally and spontaneously, he ended up suggesting change was somehow stimulated by the environment. Overall, unsuccessful in conclusively proving monogenism on biological grounds, the third edition turns to the idea of psychic unity, historical linguistics, and any other historical evidence he could muster.

In the spring of 1841, when volume 3 of *Physical History* was being published, volume 1 was being translated into German by Rudolf Wagner, professor of medicine at Erlangen University. He was well qualified for the task, as his own 1831 book was based largely on Prichard's *Physical History*. He completed the project in 1848. Prichard was delighted with this translator, writing to him to thank him for some preliminary and insightful observations on *Physical History*. In this letter he explained his original motivation for dedicating his life to anthropology. Beyond merely demonstrating the single origin and species of humankind, he was greatly concerned to preserve the civil liberties of all peoples.[26] This was written the same year he published a book calling for the protection of the civil liberties of the insane. Clearly horrified by the havoc Europeans were causing around the world and questioning the blessings of civilization, Prichard became less reticent to express his support for humanitarian causes. His volumes were his campaign banners.

The Natural History of Man (1843)

In an age of new sciences, educated Britons developed an appetite for comprehensible accounts of scientific subjects and for information about the world beyond Britain where so many of their compatriots were settling or serving the expanding British Empire. Traveling showmen were making good money charging eager audiences for the sight of Egyptian antiquities and thrilling dioramas. Prichard had taken his family to see a "human zoo" of Native Americans *en costume* in Paris, but he had always been reticent to lower the tone of his science, communicating with only the most educated reader. He did not get involved with institutions catering to the working classes such as the Mechanics' Institute until with Hodgkin he offered to edit a series of safely Christian popularizing anthropological publications for the Society for the Diffusion of Useful Knowledge. This plan to further the goals of the APS stalled.[27]

Prichard could reflect on his achievements. He had been known and respected for nearly three decades as the very model of a Christian man of science, admired for his phenomenal dedication and diligence. But by focusing on proving the unity of the human species had he made as much progress as his campaigning friend Hodgkin in preserving the lives and cultures of his fellow human beings and vanquishing the institution of slavery? Convinced that attracting a wider audience to his views would be beneficial, Prichard stepped up his efforts.

That wider audience was not particularly receptive. Social and political exigencies seemed to be steering them from curiosity about foreign peoples toward antipathy. Perhaps Prichard could counter this growing destructive view of "the Other." He greatly shortened and simplified *Physical History*, publishing *The Natural History of Man* (1843) as a single chunky, attractive volume. It took his readers on a journey around foreign parts, administering mild and reassuring doses of expected biblicism while arguing against rising polygenetic racialism and materialist evolutionary ideas. This handsome book was fit to be read at any middle-class Victorian fireside, and while no early coffee-table volume, its beautiful illustrations were a thrilling feature. In the style of the time, it came out in ten parts before being released as a single, handsomely gold-tooled and cloth-bound volume. He justified going down-market to an American correspondent, writing that it

> is a work which I have been induced by the solicitation of a bookseller to publish, on the subject of my former researches, in a more condensed form, as a kind of popular abridgment. It is a very imperfect work, and contains but a brief outline of general ethnography. Some parts, especially the earlier portion, are brought up more nearly to the present state of knowledge than the early and corresponding parts of my researches, and the plates are new. These things have given my new book some interest, and the sale of it has been considerable.[28]

Prichard took this opportunity to honor his well-connected friend Baron von Bunsen and perhaps to thank him for facilitating his appointment as a metropolitan commissioner in lunacy:

> But I wish very much to have the honor of connecting some of my books with your name by a public testimony of my respect, expressed in a dedication. I hope you will permit this & tell me whether I shall dedicate to you the remaining vols. of this work, Professor Blumenbach being deceased, or the new popular book which Baillière is now publishing for me. I shall desire Mr Baillière to send you the numbers already out that you may see what sort of a book it is likely to be. It is not worthy of having your name connected with it but I hope it will not be considered as a flimsy or altogether unscientific publication. But of its desert I am not an unprejudiced judge & when you have looked at it, I shall be obliged if you will tell me whether I may dedicate it to you. It is published in Paris in French, translated by a very able man M. Roulin, who is I believe, secretary to the Institute.[29]

After further correspondence about dedicating both the English and French editions to Bunsen, the longer of two fulsome versions was agreed.[30]

Until nearly midcentury, scientific books were generally unillustrated beyond the occasional monochrome frontispiece and a few figures. *Physical History* had been in the vanguard of illustrated science publishing, but it was trumped by *Natural History*. It is hard to imagine how impressive were its forty steel engravings, thirty-six of them colored, and a remarkable ninety on wood. The steam press lowered the cost of attractively illustrated literature of all kinds and steam transport made distribution cheaper. Information started spreading both globally and somewhat more democratically; the *Illustrated London News* had recently been founded. For many of *Natural*

History's readers, it would have been their first opportunity to see images of people from around the world, sympathetically posed to underscore Prichard's monogenetic message.

Natural History's illustrations were meant to strengthen his argument. Prichard often selected Europeanized images of extra-Europeans, some of which would be adapted to illustrate newspaper reports on colonial affairs. From full-page colored plates, dignified fellow humans in distinctly European poses often look directly at the viewer, as boldly and confidently as their hand-painted colors. A Papuan holds an implement like a general grasping the hilt of his sword in a bold, full-length portrait. Jan Tzatzoe, a "Kafir of the Amakosas Tribe," in his embroidered, brass-buttoned military uniform, arms folded in a three-quarter-turn, half-length, somewhat Napoleonic portrait, was undoubtedly officer material fit to serve the coming empire. A thoughtful Benguela woman with well-dressed hair and fine gold drop earrings is distinguishable from one of Queen Victoria's ladies-in-waiting only by the color of her skin. The occupant of one plate seems to tell the reader that while his skin may be Black, he is a Christian and a bishop, deserving every respect. A pair of less fully clad brave hunters are about to set off, and there is an affecting domestic scene in which some tidily dressed Korean fishermen are smoking their pipes and playing a board game while a woman nearby is teaching her toddler to walk.

As an Aleutian Islander draws attention to her gold cross, she reassures her Christian viewers that missionaries have been earning their sponsorship. The several illustrations of Indigenous Americans engraved from George Catlin's famous paintings were intriguing (though depicted with rather luridly red skin), while members of a recently massacred tribe in the poignantly titled "The Last of the Charruas" remind readers of Prichard and the APS's campaign against genocide. Following Blumenbach's example, he had selected portraits of high achievers, according to European values, to demonstrate that all humans possess equal potential. While these images cashed in on and fostered a growing fascination with viewing the exotic Other, Prichard intended them to foster empathy. The cultural content of *Natural History*'s illustrations is notable.[31]

Prichard did not stop at embellishing *Natural History* with affecting imagery. Encouraged by Bunsen, he felt he could improve on another author's outdated ethnographic maps and fill a gap in the market. He brought out *Six Ethnographical Maps* in 1843 and a separate coffee-table folio of *Natural History* and *Physical History*'s colored plates the following year. The set of board-bound, colored maps sold for the considerable sum

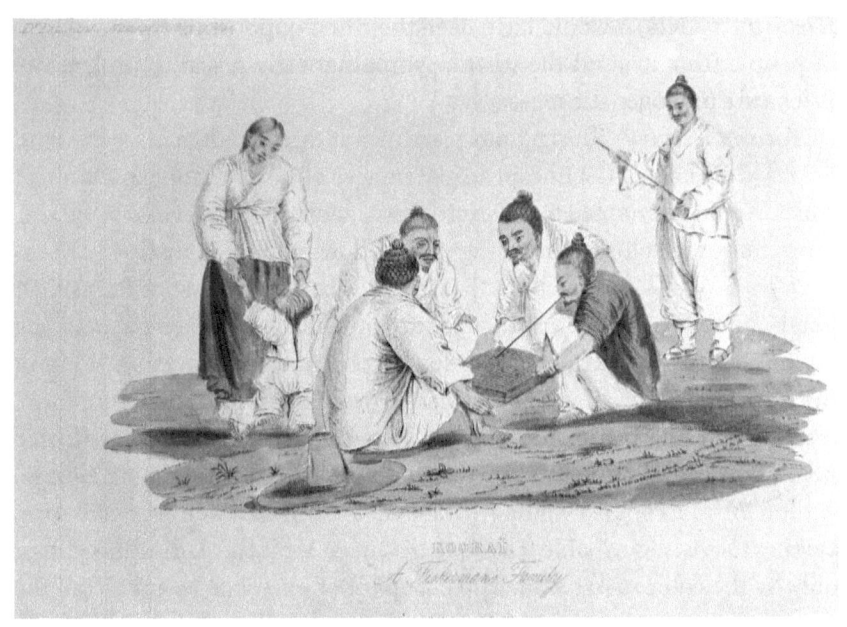

12. Culture. "Kooraï: A Fisherman's Family." Colored plate, *Natural History of Man* (1843).

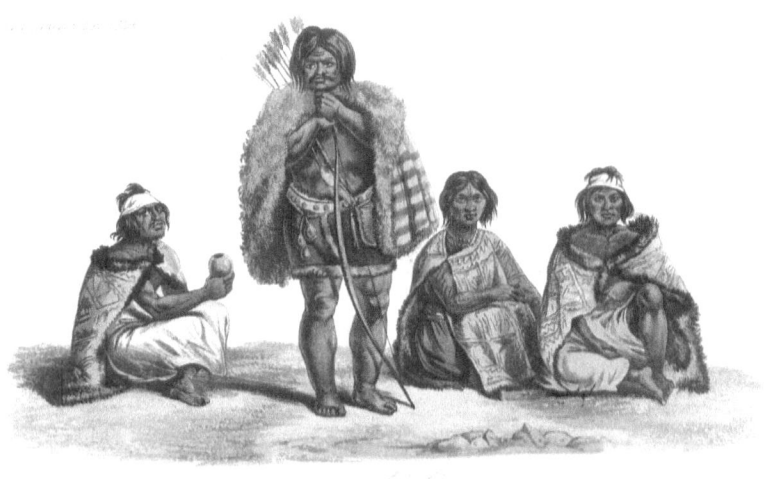

13. A warning. "The Last of the Charruas." Colored plate, *Natural History of Man* (1843).

of £1, 4 shillings, or could be purchased folded and bound into the back of *Natural History*. Prichard was concerned about their accuracy at a time when new information was constantly coming to his attention; for instance, he was anxious to get his hands on Klaproth's *Tableau d'Asie*, praised by Humboldt. While the plates seem at least partially hand-detailed in colored inks by factory boys, the practice until late in the century, the maps appear to be an example of early chromolithography. Anxious about the print quality, he pressed his publisher Hippolyte Baillière, a specialist medical and scientific publisher: "I have done Africa. It must be very carefully coloured according to the enclosed directions. The map will look very ugly unless the colour is put on very *light* in very light shades. Please to let me have a proof of the maps already sent before they are struck off. They may require some last corrections."[32] Prichard's illustrations and maps mark the modern era of scientific publishing and the revolution in print technology: scientific publications would increasingly feature tables, atlases, diagrams, and colored illustrations.[33]

Prichard began *Natural History* by explaining the motivation for his life's work had been to prove the unity of the human species and help secure the treatment of all people as human beings. He painted a lurid picture of those on the other side of the argument, men who thought it foolish for Parliament to attempt to protect the colonized as if they were on a par with Europeans, and who considered perpetual servitude or extinction their lot. They were not horrified as Prichard was by reports of settlers shooting Aboriginal Australians for dog food. He bitterly claimed contact with Europeans had rendered these oppressed peoples so miserably degraded that their intellectual capacities could not be fairly assessed, and he feared that the "ruder tribes" who could not be civilized "will at length be rooted out and exterminated in every country on the shores of which Europeans shall have set their feet."[34] He believed Christianizing these unfortunate peoples would save their souls, but he also realized that "civilizing" them might save their bodies but destroy their culture, a dilemma given Western civilization's detriments. This book brought his often-repeated warning of human extinctions from the audiences of learned societies to a somewhat wider readership. The Aborigines' Protection Society and the antislavery movement would have been delighted had he campaigned on their behalf so stridently.

Pointedly subtitled *Comprising Inquiries into the Modifying Influence of Physical and Moral Agencies on the Different Tribes of the Human Family*, Prichard's book marks a further shift from theories of heredity to those of the environment and behavior as drivers of human physical development.

He asks his readers: "He modifies the agencies of the elements upon himself; but do not these agencies also modify him?" Prichard condensed his biological anthropology into the first seventy-five pages. Otherwise, a section on "mixed races of men" appears notably among his analogical observations of plant and animal general variation, hybridity, and breeding. He thought he could score a point against growing racial denigration by revising Buffon's view that interbreeding improves the inferior breed; in nine pages, including a table and illustrations, he showed how intermarriages between the most dissimilar peoples actually produce *superior* offspring. The next sections describe and classify the varieties of humankind based on physical differences such as complexion and skeletal form. After thirty-three more sections describing nations individually, he included some general observations on matters such as human physiology.

Natural History outlines Prichard's unity and single-origin thesis, framed in the idiom of Scripture his new readers were used to and expected: "The Sacred Scriptures, whose testimony is received by all men of unclouded minds with implicit and reverential assent, declare that it pleased the Almighty Creator to make of one blood all the nations of the earth, and that all mankind are the offspring of common parents." There had been three great migrations from biblical lands, in which the two groups destined to become Asiatic and African experienced "gradual deviation," as opposed to "degeneration," albeit still implying that Europeans became the norm. After laying out his psychic unity argument, he explored the nature of instinctual behavior, concluding it could be acquired and then passed on to offspring as "instinctive hereditary propensities." This implies the existence of inherited differences in mental composition among peoples but as still mere variation within the species.[35]

The Natural History of Man was Prichard's final attempt to convince his readers of the evils of polygenism, religious skepticism and the decimation of colonial peoples. It attracted some criticism, both for his "bigoted and predetermined adherence to one opinion" and for having equivocated, or at least been overly cautious, in reaching conclusions. He felt guilty of neither. To his mind, the notion human specific unity is supported by evidence, and Scripture is a form of evidence. Another issue of more recent concern is the book's perplexing combination of antiracialist views and racialist expressions. The text is peppered here and there with what are now pejorative, xenophobic, racist expressions. Aside from his undeniable, typical Eurocentrism, his other public and private writing does not denigrate extra-Europeans. This deviation in tone may have been his clumsy adoption of a more popular mode of expression, an attempt to convey his monogenetic and humane message in terms his readers would find acceptable.[36]

While the publishing revolution fostered *Natural History*'s success, it had some disadvantages as far as the Establishment was concerned. Working people were gaining access to information allowing them to challenge the "natural order of society." For years a "People's Edition" of phrenologist Combe's *Constitution of Man* had been giving working-class autodidacts access to a materialist science of the mind while those cheap copies of Lawrence's banned book were proudly held aloft by anticlerical radical lecturers.[37] Unemployment and wage cuts were fueling Chartism, and the year of *Natural History*'s publication was one of a British general strike, riots, and shootings, more threatening than the 1830 Continental revolutions. Atheistic magazines and itinerant lecturers started regularly attacking natural theology and openly speaking about evolution, claiming that life needed no creator; religion was thus invalid, as was the hegemony of the Church. Written during this revolutionary era, *Natural History*'s more overtly Christian tenor than *Physical History* can be seen as a reaction to these dangerous times. It did still challenge attitudes and his government's destructive policies concerning the empire's colonized peoples.

The Natural History of Man went through three further editions between 1845 and 1855.[38] Along with the third edition of *Physical History*, they attracted many reviews in British, Irish, American, German, and French periodicals. The first volume of *Physical History* gained the most attention, but the whole set was often included in joint reviews, comparing it with books such as ones by Arthur James Johnes, Charles Hamilton Smith, and Louis Agassiz. Many reviewers approached their task as monogenists or Christian supporters. Some chose to seek flaws in his views; the opinions of northern U.S. reviewers differed from those of their southern counterparts, unsurprisingly. Among nearly one hundred reviews, some lavishly praised, some condemned, while others sought to add to Prichard's arguments. His vast research and erudition was generally acknowledged.[39]

Some of the reviews of Prichard's anthropology exemplify the changing times. The *British Quarterly* thought Prichard had answered the wrong questions: more apt would have been an explanation of why some races were so superior to others and how the eventual demise of the inferior ones would come about. In 1846 the *New Quarterly Review* wondered why the biological volume of *Physical History* had been conflated with four volumes of world ethnography, and implied that Prichard's obvious support of Mosaic history and humanitarian values was frankly unscientific. Several human species could have been separately created of such similar mold as to satisfy Prichard's definition of species. The reviewer went on to deem excessive the claim that human specific unity is "highly probable"; *possible* was more likely the case. Prichard's further faults were his shifting of the burden of proof onto the other side of the argument and "overdriving" language as a unifier when there was evidence of some peoples adopting other languages. The editor of this journal had to insert a footnote assuring readers that the *British Quarterly* was not endorsing this patently antimonogenetic proposition.[40]

Other reviews were more positive such as the one in the widely circulated *Athenaeum* that considered the work of "Dr. Prichard on the 'Natural History of Man' is not only a manual for the student of ethnography, but a favorite book with general readers." Henry Holland in the *Quarterly Review* could not resist bringing up Prichard's 1813 bold and "somewhat repugnant" original Black human skin theory, noting that his unverifiable view had been "abandoned by silent evasion." Prichard had nevertheless convinced Holland of the unity of the human species. William Benjamin Carpenter published an evaluation of Prichard's two works and his forty-page illustrated *Appendix to Natural History*. After suggesting that the definitive proof of the unity of the human species was every race's capability of being raised to "our level," Carpenter concluded the value of Prichard's thirty-seven years of effort was not his work on human unity but his assembling of a great storehouse of information. Prichard would have been better pleased to have been remembered for the former.[41]

Influence

Prichard was something of an intellectual celebrity who brought the extra-European world to a British and international readership. As well as the French and German translations of *Physical History* and *Natural History*, it was worth reprinting their "fourth editions" in the late 1850s. Authors recognizing the popularity of his topic paraphrased his publications extensively, acknowledged and unacknowledged. Physiology textbook writers such as John Bostock (1827), Herbert Mayo (1829), and Peter Mark Roget (1838) incorporated a great deal of Prichard's material into their chapters on "the varieties of man." His influence can be seen in publications such as an anonymous derivative volume of 1835 and more original texts such as Robert Chambers's famous *Vestiges* and William Cooke Taylor's *The Natural History of Society*. Prichard also influenced several French writers on anthropology such as Victor Courtet de l'Isle and Jean Louis de Quatrefages de Bréau and doyen of late nineteenth-century British anthropology E. B. Tylor. Toward the end of the century, fellow Briton and anthropologist John Beddoe made extensive uncredited use of Prichard's books.[42]

Prichard's younger friend and fellow member of the Ethnological Society of London Robert Gordon Latham attempted to step into Prichard's shoes. An Eton- and Cambridge-educated University of London professor of literature, he then qualified as a physician in preparation for a life in science. He lectured and wrote on anthropology, a firm Prichardian monogenist, using language as his weapon of choice at a time when it was losing out to "scientific" race studies. Prichard warmly supported Latham's application to join the Linnean Society.[43]

Latham became a bit of a stirrer, however. He published *The Natural History of the Varieties of Man* in 1850 and *Man and His Migrations* in 1851, in which a combination of linguistic and historical analysis led him to propose a whole new three-variety classification of humankind. But as his views were considered somewhat thin on evidence, rather obscurely justified, unevenly presented, and just so hard to follow, Prichard's were preferred. In 1857 Latham went on to publish a considerably enlarged edition of Prichard's *Eastern Origin* that earned excoriating reviews. More successfully, he organized the Great Exhibition's Ethnological Department, an acknowledged contribution to the development of anthropology. In a flight of vanity, Latham had a magazine illustration made of himself, Prichard, and Blumenbach representing the three greats of anthropology.[44]

Prichard's biogeography drew the attention of biologists and paleontologists studying the origin and distribution of life. They had already pointed out similarities between fossils and present-day species found in particular parts of the world. Why did individual, isolated land masses have their own characteristic fossil species? Prichard suggested there had been geographic centers of creation from which species spread to the extent to which they were capable. This was taken up by Edinburgh natural historian and geologist Professor Edward Forbes who developed a doctrine that conveniently did not specify how the first of a species in a particular location came into existence, and he admitted that it opposed the hypothesis of the evolution of all species from a single original form.

Another of Prichard's forays into biogeographical theory was that of localized postdiluvian creations. Comparative anatomist Richard Owen rejected it, instead alluding to a natural development of organic life as yet to be demonstrated, and in 1847 he published a translation of Oken's old

Lehrbuch der Naturphilosophie, scandalizing and intriguing the scientific world with its oblique but unmistakable natural developmental content and daring phrases such as "Man has not been created, but *developed*." Evolutionary thought was itself evolving from private murmurings about the mutability of species to views stimulated by Oken's book; open debate in Paris learned societies; von Humboldt's theory that the world is in a constantly dynamic state; reformist proclamations on the streets of Britain; Chambers's *Vestiges* bringing discussion of evolution into the polite drawing rooms of Britain; some forthright British lectures in progressive institutions; and finally Owen's 1849 public avowal of evolution.[45] Prichard stood firmly before these floodgates of evolutionary thought, posing religiously orthodox biogeographical hypotheses. Science would have to go on without him.

One reader interested in Prichard's work was Charles Darwin, no matter what he might have thought about the older man's religious bias. Upon hearing his 1839 BAAS speech, Darwin settled down, pencil in hand, to study the third edition of *Physical History*, and in the 1840s, long before he dared to bring out *Origin*, he was filling his secret notebooks with elaborations on what was being privately discussed by a new breed of scientists. He annotated *Physical History*'s third edition in obviously inverted syntax: "How like my Book this will be." By 1856 Darwin had extensively annotated and taken notes on *Natural History* and the five volumes of *Physical History*, twice going through its 1851 reprint. He intended to feature the development of the human species in his magnum opus.[46]

In their shared interest in human origin, Prichard and Darwin considered the migration of all species and the effects of geographical isolation. Darwin seemed unaware of Prichard's earlier limited evolutionary theorizing since he apparently confined himself to the third edition (although he noted the "old" edition), in which Prichard gave more scope to the environment as a stimulus to biological variation, obscuring his views in a plethora of detail. In Darwin's hundreds of annotations of Prichard's third edition, he noted issues such as Prichard's views on sexual selection, the benefits of dark skin in hot climates, and the relativity of beauty. He adopted some of these views, including animal breeding as a form of artificial selection. They both employed analogical reasoning; for instance, Darwin thought that as all pigeons could be traced back to the single ancestral rock dove, so might the original stock of human beings be discovered.

Aside from annotations in books as evidence of Prichard's influence on Darwin, there is the issue of Lawrence's serving as a conduit for Prichard's earlier, more evolutionary ideas. It is Lawrence's clearer version of Prichard's 1813 views plus his own materialist slant that survived unaltered to influence Darwin and later scientists. Through Darwin's study of Charles Lyell's *Principles of Geology*, he had also encountered some of Prichard's ideas.

Like Prichard, Darwin valued hard facts over speculation, and he attempted to out-Prichard Prichard in amassing data. In Darwin are traces of Prichard's views on the psychology of ethnic groups and the formation of dispositions and instincts. Darwin took up Prichard's call for research on susceptibility to particular diseases as a marker of species unity, and he privately mused on the older scientist's concept of "predisposition." Prichard had coined the term "permanent varieties" to signify the possession of new traits that "are propagated in the breed in perpetuity," and Darwin studied the work of and corresponded with Edward Blyth, who clearly acknowledged his reliance on Prichard, adopting "permanent variety" and renaming it "true variety." Permanent or true variety is speciation in all but name.

Privately unhampered by religion, Darwin was free to run with Prichard and Blyth's model of development, adding the crucial ingredient of natural selection, of course. Other Prichardian views directly or indirectly made their way into Darwin's work, such as the idea of domestication as a driver of change and the heritability of random or spontaneous variation. Many of the observations that Darwin garnered conveniently from Prichard were not entirely novel, however; Prichard had adapted them from previous authors such as Samuel Stanhope Smith's aesthetics in sexual selection, itself an Enlightenment idea. Prichard had synthesized these ideas into a resource that Darwin drew on. As *Origin* was nearing publication, Darwin's friend Lyell advised him to exclude humankind from it; his courage failed, and Darwin promised his publisher accordingly. The burning issue of the origin of humankind was expunged from *Origin*, but it continued to motivate him, as it had Prichard.[47]

Another of Darwin's annotations in *Physical History*'s third edition is "If I ever consider Man look over other & earlier Edition." He went on to consider humankind, but he did not leave handy annotated copies of Prichard's first two editions to prove he had consulted them. When Darwin finally tackled humankind in his *Descent of Man* (1871), there were more contemporary anthropologists he could call on; he referred to Prichard's third edition only fifteen times, concerning comparisons of crania and the relativity of beauty.[48]

In sum, Prichard was one of several scientists who anticipated aspects of evolutionary theory, though he failed to explain its exact biological mechanism. He could not entertain the transmutation of species, not only on the grounds of Christian doctrine but because it implied the possible existence of multiple human species, an idea that played into the hands of polygenists and placed humankind uncomfortably close to lesser species. Prichard's holding to species diffusion obviated the notion of species transmutation, anyway. Darwin valued Prichard for his many individual ideas but found little material on evolution in his later editions. About the unity of the human race, Darwin and Prichard were of one mind, as they were in their humanitarian and antislavery motivations.

While seeing the final volumes of *Physical History* and the editions of *Natural History* through publication and traveling around the country inspecting asylums, Prichard resumed researching human physical variation in support of his monogenetic campaign. He launched into collecting and studying crania for his next project, "Crania Britannica."[49] Progress on it was interrupted, however, by a call on Prichard's expertise; he was asked to contribute a chapter to a government-sponsored publication in which he would set out the authoritative definition of his science of humankind.

"Ethnology" in *The Admiralty Manual of Scientific Enquiry* (1849)

With the British Empire expanding rapidly, the Admiralty needed to systematize the collection of a wide variety of beneficial data. Sir John Herschel, in charge of compiling *A Manual of Scientific Enquiry Prepared for the Use of Her Majesty's Navy and Adapted for Travellers in General*, naturally asked Prichard to contribute a chapter on collecting anthropological data. Like the book's chapters on geography, geology, hydrography, and other topics, Prichard's "Ethnology" would aid Britain in acquiring high-quality, standardized scientific data. First published in 1849, the so-called *Admiralty Manual* was widely circulated and published in several editions. It indicated a growing tendency to focus on the differences between Europe and the rest of the world during this era of flourishing science and colonial expansion. Not unrelated to the BAAS *Queries*, "Ethnology" provides Prichard's guidelines for gathering both cultural and biological data—an early manual of anthropological fieldwork. It is considered ancestral to the Royal Anthropological Institute's long-running *Notes and Queries on Anthropology*.[50]

Prichard's *Admiralty Manual* chapter is significant in the history of British anthropology for its stress on acquiring accurate information through in situ observation; its definition of the Anglo-American discipline of anthropology as it is today; and its showing Prichard in didactic mode rather than as the passive anthologizer he is sometimes considered. In this last composition of his life, he noted anthropology's biological and cultural components equally. His broad definition of anthropology (still called ethnology, of course) was "all that relates to human beings, whether regarded as individuals or as members of communities." He then clearly subdivided it into the "physical history of man" and the "history of man as a social being." For the latter, Prichard provided a comprehensive list of psychological and cultural artifacts, from "sentiments" and beliefs to civil and religious institutions, customs, arts, literature, architecture, and commerce. He stressed that research into the origin and affinities of humankind must be of both aspects. Reflecting this division into physical and cultural components, he divided "Ethnology" into eight subsections about physical description, fifteen on cultural, and two on ethnographical methodology.[51]

The foundation of modern British cultural anthropology is typically traced to E. B. Tylor's definition of culture published around the time he was revising Prichard's *Admiralty Manual* chapter for the book's 1871 edition. Prichard's chapter had already defined culture in its anthropological sense, without using the word. This was hardly surprising, as before the 1860s the word "culture" pertained mostly to growing things or refinement of taste. His reading of Germans Adelung and Johann Severin Vater would have given him food for thought on the nature of human society and language, but he would not have considered adopting the German word *Kultur* on xenophobic principle. Rather Prichard compressed his previous cumbersome combinations of morals (emotions, beliefs, behavior), customs, manners, and habitudes into "history of man as a social being." Elsewhere, Tylor would shorten this to "culture," but here in 1871 he just slightly tweaked Prichard's text, and concluded with a new paragraph asking informants to provide specimens of everyday material culture and to record information directly in notebooks for ethnologists' use. He left Prichard's definition of anthropology and the structure of the chapter unaltered.[52]

For a few decades after Prichard's death, monogenist, historical and linguistic Prichardian cultural anthropology continued to hold sway in Britain, as exemplified by the publications of Carpenter, Bunsen, Latham, and Max Müller and the activities of the Ethnological Society of London and the BAAS Subsection. From Prichard's oeuvre and the subsequent editions of his *Admiralty Manual* chapter and its descendant RAI's *Notes and Queries*, there is some continuity with later anthropology through to the modern British discipline. Race science, making use of polygenetic theory and comparative anatomy continued to develop in a sort of rivalry to Prichardian anthropology, however, eventually overshadowing it for a period.[53]

Polygenism and Scientific Racialism Ascendant

At the start of the nineteenth century, European attitudes toward extra-Europeans were generally neutral. Prichard presumed humankind's basic equality. But despite his efforts to establish his "natural history of man" as a humane monogenetic science, by the 1830s he found himself sandwiched between a handful of mostly Continental polygenistic theorists and a rising international tide of contemporary ones; he committed himself to proving them wrong. The entanglement of anthropology with polygenetic theory and scientific racialism dominated anthropology during the second half of the nineteenth century, varying in inspiration from country to country. France's colonial exploits bred a thriving community of race scientists whereas in less colonially committed Germany its development was muted. Americans found polygenism and race science invaluable in arguing for the institution of slavery while growing British racialism reflected the exigencies of colonialism and failures in colonial policy and administration. Race scientists squandered their talents trying to prove the biological basis of the inequality Europeans were creating.

In 1843 Prichard congratulated the author of *Philological Proofs of the Original Unity and Recent Origin of the Human Race* for his Christian monogenism: "It is very satisfactory to me to observe that on the main question you arrive at the same conclusion with myself. I am the more pleased when I find a writer of great intelligence adopting this view, as I find that almost every foreigner who takes the question in hand or alludes to it, whether he be German, French or American, decides peremptorily on the other side or takes it as a thing granted & almost self evident that there are many distinct human races."[54]

There were quite a few of those foreign polygenists annoying Prichard during the 1840s. As the Atlantic world's premier monogenist, he was a target for a new breed of race scientists who gleefully pointed out how his philological anthropology and religious bias rendered his work patently unscientific. Even his mooting the theologically unsound theory of the single human species' three separate centers of creation had been counterproductive, playing into polygenists' hands. As Prichard adjusted his views on human physical variation with each edition of *Physical History*, he was struggling to counter rival race theories, and not just those of foreigners. Thomas Arnold's 1841 Oxford inaugural lecture proclaimed world history was driven by a favored race, the apotheosis of which was the British; less favored ones dwindled away. Critical articles appeared in periodicals like *Simmonds's Colonial Magazine and Foreign Miscellany*. In *The Natural History of the Human Species* (1848), Charles Hamilton Smith laid out the case for polygenism, calling the extinction of Indigenous populations a scientific inevitability. Imagine Prichard's consternation that same year when phreno-anthropologist Luke Burke published an article in a rival anthropological journal espousing the plurality of the human species divided into sixty-three races.[55]

A phalanx of Americans plumped for polygenism, Prichard's correspondent John Pickering among them, and his old phrenological foe Charles Caldwell continued to accuse him of prejudice, ignorance of the facts, and failure to prove universal equal intellectual potential. He turned the biblical tables on Prichard by pointing out the Deity's creation and then abandonment of the original pair of humans.[56] Some American polygenists generously larded their views with Scripture while others avoided it, preferring scientific-looking calibrated anatomical data on which their racial hierarchies were based. Particularly useful were pronouncements of general psychological traits founded on phrenological rhetoric.

Open season on Prichard continued. American race theorists accused him of cleverly manipulating facts in support of monogenism. John Howard Van Amringe's substantial *An Investigation of the Theories of the Natural History of Man, of Lawrence, Prichard and Others* (1848) asserted God's postdiluvian creation of four distinct species. Published mostly in the slaveholding Southern states, literature such as "The Diseases and Physical Peculiarities of the Negro Race" damned *Physical History* as "an abolition work" by an author "fearful the Bible will be invalidated." Another writer dubbed him a "teleological ethnologist."[57]

Prichard's polygenetic foes had more arguments up their sleeves. It was hard to counter the evidence that four thousand years ago Egyptians looked like nineteenth-century folk. When had all those spontaneous hereditary changes and environmental influences created varieties of humankind if, as the Bible claimed, human history spanned a mere six thousand years? Worryingly, one argument against the biological determinism of polygenism and phrenology, that of human variation being a natural process, supported the notion of transmutation. For instance, if the variation in color among humans had come about naturally over time, then an ape could very well have developed into a species of human being. Dragging the Bible into the debate again, Swiss American race scientist Louis Agassiz would assure his readers that the Bible pertained to and was for the guidance of white people only; clearly, all humans except Africans were of the same species. Finally, there could not have been human biological development; distinct races had been separately created, as the Bible itself explained.

To Prichard's eventual suggestion that there had been separate world centers of animal and plant creation, one American scientist argued the theory must apply to human beings as well. And was not the extinction of particular groups of humans that so grieved monogenists and humanitarians actually a natural event proving biological unfitness to survive? Another one of Prichard's arguments for monogenism was the existence of obviously fertile, vigorous "mixed-race" groups, a view that seemed to admit some doubt of human specific unity.[58]

At midcentury Prichardian anthropology seemed to be losing its appeal. Men with an interest in polygenetic theory started making inroads into British scientific institutions, the ESL included. Often from backgrounds in medicine and anatomy and interested in materialist phrenology and the latest ideas on race, this new breed of scientist favored a tangible, anatomical, race-fixated study of humankind. In 1847 the Ethnological Society of Paris tore itself apart over its approach to race studies and the issue of slavery, while the ESL's efforts to discriminate against polygenists in their ranks flagged. The science and scientific society so dear to Prichard were in danger of being perverted into the opposite of his intentions.

The notions of polygenism and "race" reflect the times in which they arose. Britain addressed social problems at home by exporting convicts, the poor, and adventurous citizens to compete with or exterminate the inhabitants of its new colonies as they exploited these countries' resources. Government policies of "protection" recently termed imperial humanitarianism, knowingly caused the dispossession, dislocation, deprivation of civil liberties, denigration of culture, and sometimes the extermination of colonized peoples. This seeped into British popular understanding, creating a hardening of attitudes toward those "indolent natives," ungrateful and reluctant to embrace the "three C's" of Christianity, commerce, and European civilization. Accounts of colonized people's violent resistance to subjugation and extermination had a greater negative impact on British attitudes than the outrages that had incited them. When they demonstrated a disinclination to embrace Europe's three C's, doubts arose as to whether they deserved or were capable of benefiting from such blessings. The government tried to balance competing interests, including those of the ESL, the APS, colonial administrations, and settler colonists to better manage the colonized. One initiative was a colonial administrator's 1840s program to "preserve" Aboriginal Australians by obliterating their culture and assimilating them into settler society.59

Prichard's impassioned BAAS speech of 1839 stressed the moral imperative of preserving endangered populations as well as the urgency of carrying out ethnographic research before their demise. This qualifies him as likely the first advocate of "salvage ethnology." In 1843 the newly formed ESL and Prichard in his *Natural History* condemned the decimation of Indigenous peoples by the "civilized." But colonialism, polygenism, and European exceptionalism were already embedding racism across the Atlantic world.

After Prichard's death his views continued to be assailed as untenable, laborious, teleological, self-contradictory, and unsubstantiated. Anatomist Robert Knox set out his explicitly racialist "race is everything" stance in *Races of Men* (1850), dismissing Prichard's science as "imperfect" and "antiquated." John Campbell's *Negro-mania: Being an Examination of the Falsely Assumed Equality of the Various Races of Men* (1851), P. A. Browne's *The Classification of Mankind by the Hair and Wool of Their Heads* (1849), and J. H. Van Evrie's *Negroes and Negro "Slavery": The First an Inferior Race, the Latter Its Normal Condition* (1853) need no explanation of their opposition to Prichard.60

Polygenism and race denigration fed off each other. In 1853 the French aristocrat Arthur de Gobineau published *Essai sur l'inégalité des races humaines* in four volumes, often citing or quoting Prichard and referring to the illustrations in *Natural History* as examples of the hopeless stupidity, the "scarce human form of these creatures," and the "utmost hideousness that the human form is capable of." Perhaps most infamous of all for its scientific pretentions and excoriation of Prichard's antiquated, unscientific biblicism was Nott and Gliddon's 1854 polygenistic compilation *Types of Mankind*, a milestone in the development of scientific racism.61 British, French, and American theorists competed in the race denigration stakes.

The Enlightenment desire to understand extra-Europeans as members of the single human family became overshadowed by a race science claiming human inequality.62 In 1863 a vociferous race-focused element founded the rival Anthropological Society of London, its members setting aside the Prichardian study of human history, culture, language, and the fluidity of human form in favor of the rigid and deterministic classification and ranking of "races." The ESL's "Ethnologicals" could not put on as interesting a show as the "Anthropologicals," with their measurements and images of objectified "natives." Whereas Prichard had argued that civilization, like domestication, could affect racial characteristics, the Anthropologicals claimed the reverse: race determined cultural and social achievement. The notion of white supremacy was gestating.[63]

In response to the gathering pace of American antislavery agitation, there were (mostly American) efforts to justify slavery while (mostly French) biologists devoted themselves to developing a coherent race science. Racialist propaganda was rife in Britain in the 1860s, persuasively peddled by the American Civil War Confederate government's agent provocateur members of the Anthropological Society and a sensationalizing press. The antiliberal Anthropologicals advised government on relevant policy.[64] Prichard would not have enjoyed attending British, French, and American anthropological society meetings later in the century when interest in history, language, and culture were supplanted for a season by biologically deterministic, phrenology-seasoned anthropology.

The popularity of the Anthropological Society of London was a sign of the times. The second British Reform Act's broadening the franchise among lower-class males threatened Establishment control of society. The growth of Irish Republican terrorism also brought back bitter memories of the 1798 Irish Rebellion and inspired an anti-Irish backlash, a feature of which was the long-lasting denigration of the inferior, uncivilizable "wild Irish race." In a fit of reactionary fervor, a Darwinian-supported notion now called "extinction discourse" further excused the decimation of Indigenous peoples: the weak were doomed to extinction anyway—the obverse of survival of the fittest. Charles Dickens felt free to say he looked forward to a time when all "savages" had become extinct if not civilized. There also arose a nightmare prediction of the preserved "unfit" of all kinds swamping society. Flourishing European nationalism championed racial purity, warning against "mixed blood" and fueling a preoccupation with teasing out racial differences and racial hierarchy.

Prichard's mentor Blumenbach had not been immune to the seduction of calibrating; he had chosen this validating activity to devise a "cranial index" expressing data as a percentage. But rather than using it to rank nations, he reflected standard Eurocentric value judgments concerning European skulls' obvious beauty, intellect, and indications of civilization. Retzius took up this fashion for calibrating in the 1840s, devising a "cephalic index" to classify the forms of human skulls and jaws. While phrenologist Combe weaponized his vocabulary, calling a Pawnee skull "villainously low," Prichard described skulls neutrally as "symmetrical" or "broad," and he did not rank. Disinclined to form evaluations based on cranial measurements, he merely described basic types of skulls across national boundaries. The fashion became otherwise.

Race-focused biological anthropology's clear-cut, scientific-looking methodology was appealing, and this model became useful to others. Anthropologists busied themselves gathering data essential to materializing or "biologizing" race into a science linking the intellect with racial types that encouraged speculation about the potential of extra-Europeans. Their use of craniology in this regard attracted the interest of psychiatrists who had their own Other to deal with in the form of the mentally ill and diverse. Degenerationist anthropometry took hold among psychiatrists and anthropologists. Why struggle to fathom the human mind and its ills when "facts" could be had with the aid of a pair of calipers and a pile of typological photographs?

Race scientists did not stop at investigating the exterior of the head. Parisian physician and transcendental biologist Étienne Serres studied the human brain and embryology for evidence of race, calling his polygenetic findings anthropology. Brilliant cerebral anatomist Pierre Paul Broca, atheist, inventor of anthropometric apparatus, theoretician of hybridity, and prolific author on these subjects, founded in 1859 the Société d'Anthropologie de Paris, an organization dedicated to race-focused biological anthropology. His contemporary Alphonse Bertillon cultivated the new field of criminology, employing biological anthropology, psychiatry, and old-time physiognomy- and phrenology-inspired craniometry to analyze the head and visage seeking indications of deviancy.

During the second half of the nineteenth century, a rash of new race scientists around Europe concocted ever more complex schema and apparatus to take measurements on which to base their claims of the existence and hierarchy of "races." Eventually, the tide of anthropometry turned as particularly Italian and German scientists tested its validity. In 1890 a Hungarian scientist's extensive research demonstrated the impossibility of arriving at a true classification of human types. Already weakened by the demise of its phrenological underpinnings, anthropometry's discreditation undermined race science as well.[65]

During these decades of race-dominated biological anthropology, the advocates of Prichardian anthropology were reduced to pleading for their monogenetic, historical linguistic discipline on humanitarian and Christian grounds. One defender writing during the troubled second half of the century was Scottish Canadian ethnologist and archaeologist Sir Daniel Wilson. When faced with unsettling geological evidence, he resorted to managing the Mosaic account, adopting Prichard's view of Scripture as pertaining to the doings of and guidance of humankind rather than being a manual of geology. And like Prichard, he took to comparing crania to demonstrate the fallacy of racial classification, concluding there was but a single human species. In 1857 Italy's first anthropologist and paleontologist Giustiniano Nicolucci earned himself the title "the Dr. Prichard of Italy" for his books promoting progressive, monogenetic thought and countering the repugnant American school of racial theory.[66]

Unfettered by religion and bolstered by race science, late Victorian biological anthropology eclipsed Prichardian anthropology for a time. It left a legacy in social Darwinism, Nordicism, racial hygiene, eugenics, national socialism, and white supremacy.[67] So discreditable was this phase to the subsequent generation of anthropologists, only reinvention could disassociate it from what should have never been.

Far from being an apologist for or harbinger of scientific racialism because he often described human varieties anachronistically as "races," Prichard attempted to invalidate the concept of "race." Further, he held that all varieties of the single human species have equal intellectual capacity and potential for development. His view of early humans gradually and peacefully migrating out of Africa and fishing their way around the continental coasts until their spread was global can be contrasted with a later anthropological theory of aggressive, male-centered struggles for territorial dominance, a view still evident in scholarship.[68] Prichardian anthropologists studied the affinities among peoples in terms of history, culture, language, and to a lesser extent biology, so unlike the contrastive tendency of later polygenetic and race-ranking biological anthropology.

Prichard supported the anti–slave trade and antislavery causes and the aims of the APS, speaking publicly in defense of the common humanity of all peoples, condemning the decimation of Indigenous populations and calling for measures to protect them from the "relentless progress of civilisation." A historian has recently noted Prichard's work as "wide-ranging, exhaustive and respectful in its treatment of far-flung peoples and their heritage. It was primarily descriptive rather than analytical, presenting facts, but rarely attempting to systematize or classify." Another credits him with having produced "the most exhaustive defence of racial unity ever published."[69]

Prichard's influence on anthropology was transnational and lasted for decades, but generally historians have Whiggishly tended to ignore both Prichardian anthropology for its Christian, monogenetic linguistic biases and the later nineteenth-century execrable race science that overshadowed it. When British anthropology started to reinvent itself toward the end of the century, a new generation described and compared cultures and more clearly sought to comprehend universal processes, social developmental stages, and the laws governing human society—the sort of analyses Prichard had attempted in his promulgation of psychic unity and the universality of religion, for instance. Monogenist Tylor and his fellow anthropologists attempted a degree of cultural relativism and were less often motivated to research human origins. They mined intellectual history, drawing on Scottish Enlightenment social evolutionary philosophy and the ethnology of the German Age of Reason. Studying culture, considering the Prichardian concept of psychic unity, and making use of new archaeological evidence and ethnographical data gathered by "citizen ethnologists," new generations of anthropologists created the modern science of humankind.

Another aspect of Prichard's anthropology detrimental to his status in the history of the discipline is that his research was essentially secondary rather than primary. Why had he not conducted his own fieldwork on the culture of a particular society, the rite de passage of twentieth-century anthropologists? Carrying out firsthand observation "in the field" was not totally unknown; Richard King, Robert Knox, and Willhelm von Humboldt had done so exceptionally. But during the first half of the nineteenth century, access to remoter parts of the world was severely limited, with little opportunity for a gentleman to travel beyond Europe. Having a medical practice and a large family to support, Prichard could only dream of roaming the wilds of America, amusing his family with the very idea of doing so.[70]

Prichard's anthropology attempted to replace the theorizing of past centuries with a scientific approach appropriate to his era. With a keen eye for accuracy and scientific credibility not always achieved, he adapted the scientific methodology of his era to create his own disciplined observational framework, whether for comparing languages, hair textures, or forms of worship, coining new terms. An *Athenaeum* article of 1851 described him as having inspired a new generation of researchers to take up the study of anthropology and to make more accurate observations of peoples around the world.[71] His books, articles, *Ethnological Queries*, and *Admiralty Manual* chapter were models of theory and methodology that unified the biological, cultural, and linguistic study of humankind, and he looked forward to the contribution archaeology would make to anthropology.

Nowadays anthropologists would not unreasonably feel Prichard had bitten off more than anyone could chew in attempting to produce an overarching anthropology combined with an ethnography of the entire globe while sitting snug in his Bristol home. And how could a scientist claim the classical historians and the Bible as factual? Where was his anthropology degree and professorship, and how could a provincial doctor be an anthropologist in his free time? Some have found it more attractive to identify with somewhat mythologized, more recent, better-documented milestone-makers such as E. B. Tylor, Bronisław Malinowski, or Franz Boas than a provincial doctor of so long ago. Prichard has thus been relegated to an apologetic footnote in the annals of anthropology's prehistory.

Prichard dreamed of seeing his subject studied at university; his Oxford professorship application claims it a type of world history suitable for academia. His posthumously published chapter "Ethnology" defined anthropology as encompassing both the biological and cultural study of humankind. He supported the scientific and humanitarian organizations that fostered the study of humankind, and his highly respected books, articles, and speeches laid the groundwork for anthropology's future development. Prichardian anthropology was valued throughout the rest of the century by those who appreciated its monogenetic, historical linguistic foundations and its vast store of ethnological material. At the 1847 BAAS meeting, Bunsen put Prichard's anthropological treatises on a par with those of Alexander von Humboldt's *Kosmos*, that paragon of nineteenth-century science,[72] and writing in 1901, linguist Max Müller remembered Prichard with wonder:

> Dr. Prichard's authority stood very high, and justly so, and his Researches into the Physical History of Mankind still remain unparalleled in ethnology. His careful weighing of facts and difficulties went out of fashion when the theory of evolution became popular, and every change from a flea to an elephant was explained by imperceptible degrees. He dealt chiefly with what was perceptible, with well-observed facts, and many of the facts which he marshalled so well, require even now, in these post-Darwinian days I should venture to say, renewed consideration. Like all great men, he was wonderfully humble, and allowed me to contradict him, who ought to have been proud to listen and to learn from him.[73]

14 · From the Red Lodge to Asylumdom

A New Career, 1839–45

> [Prichard's] ardent and unbounded love of science, his extreme liberality towards every nation under the sun, . . . his singleness of purpose.
> —William Gibson, *Rambles in Europe*

At the Red Lodge

Prichard kept up his reputation for having a multiplicity of projects on the go at the same time, from visiting patients to chairing meetings and corresponding widely. He even examined applicants for three Bristol life insurance companies.[1] He dealt with family matters and enjoyed having visitors, including friends Symonds, Carpenter, and Estlin, who would dine, play chess, and discuss matters from historical to historic. At fifty-three, Prichard was showing no sign of slowing down.

After a rather uncomfortable transatlantic voyage, William Gibson was determined to make the most of his year roaming around Europe. The University of Pennsylvania professor of surgery liked nothing better than chatting with fellow medical men and writing avalanches of description in his diary. It had been more than thirty years since he and Prichard had been students at Edinburgh, so he arrived at the Red Lodge, ready for a good catch-up—that is, when family members were not pumping their guest about America. He described Prichard as having an "expression uncommonly mild, open and benevolent; so much so, that almost any one would naturally inquire who he was. His hair is thin and scattering, and so white as to make him look older than he is, whereas, in former days, it was light chestnut, and so remarkably thick, bushy, and upright, as to form one of his striking characteristics. In dress he is singularly plain, simple and unostentatious, and, if in drab attire, might pass, readily, for a Quaker." Prichard seemed an extraordinary man in the guise of an ordinary one:

> Starchness and formality, however, make no ingredient in his composition. On the contrary he is very cheerful, sociable, frank, easy and unpretending, in his discourse and manners, and has so much

modesty, artlessness, and childlike simplicity, about him, that no one would be prepared to say, upon slight acquaintance, that he was any thing more than an ordinary, sensible, well-disposed man, however much they might be pleased, which they could not fail to be, with his benign and agreeable countenance. But it is impossible to be in his company long, and to hear him talk on any subject, without being strongly impressed with the depth and originality of his views, his sterling good sense and wisdom, his profound and varied information, his clear and luminous conceptions, his ardent and unbounded love of science, his extreme liberality towards every nation under the sun, his entire freedom from envy or jealousy of any description, and from professional rivalry and bitterness, his singleness of purpose, his goodness of heart, and his reverence for all the duties that belong to a Christian, an accountable being, and a man. Many of these thoughts crossed my mind during an evening spent with him, in long and close conversation, at a large literary party . . . , in after accompanying him home, and, finally, at his own house in Bristol.

Once the family got the American to themselves, the questions came thick and fast. Prichard clearly longed to do his own "ethnographical fieldwork," or perhaps he was just hankering after a boyish adventure:

He expressed great curiosity about [America]; asked a thousand questions concerning our great men, institutions, mighty rivers and lakes, organic remains, Indians, negroes, buffaloes; said how much pleasure it would give him to roam through our tangled brakes, and endless forests; to sweep over our vast and almost illimitable prairies; to scan our mighty mountains and cataracts, and to stand where the white man had scarcely ever stood before; at all which his handsome and accomplished wife, and their large and interesting family, of ten or twelve well-grown, comely, and most intelligent children, laughed immoderately—at the very idea of a man of his age, and large practice, and numerous avocations, laying aside such employments, and in sober seriousness, being so romantic and so enthusiastic, as to express, even, jocosely, such impossibilities.[2]

This image of Prichard the romantic adventurer would have startled more than just his doting family. When not entertaining visitors to the Red Lodge, he was himself a popular guest. The author John Sterling boasted to his mother in 1839: "A few evenings ago we went to Mr. Griffin's, and met there Dr. Prichard, the author of a well-known Book on the Races of Mankind, to which it stands in the same relation among English books as the Racing Calendar does to those of Horsekind. He is a very intelligent, accomplished person." Sterling thought otherwise about his fellow guest, the "great booby" and dean of Bristol. Prichard had a better line in epithets than that; he called one man falling foul of him not "a dull stupid asinine sot but a downright active preposterous fool."[3]

A steady stream of scientists and scholars visited the Red Lodge. Prichard had splashed out a considerable sum on Carl Ritter's multivolume *Erdkunde* and had adopted some of the Berlin professor of geography's views on, for instance, the relationship between geography and national character. Ritter was doing for geography what Prichard was for anthropology. Ritter realized Prichard valued his work, but when he arrived in Bristol in August 1841 on the new railway he was unprepared for the hospitality showered on him:

> Then I asked someone to guide me to Dr. Prichard's house on top of the hill, in order to pay him my visit. We agreed at once that I should dwell and live with him, he wanted to take care of everything, and in spite of my objections, he drove down to the inn himself and fetched my things; he treated me with untiring providence and love as his most intimate family friend. There was room enough, indeed, in his large, beautifully situated house, which dates back to the time of Queen Elizabeth; his wife, full of tenderness and goodness, told me that their son was now sitting his exams in Berlin. . . . Our profound friendship was sealed, and [Constantine] the younger son of the family, who was spending his holidays from Oxford here, became my steady companion. The intercourse with his father was very instructive for me because of his wide erudition and his knowledge of this country; he is the leading ethnographer in England—he gave me his "Physical history of man" as a gift; it is a famous book. In his doctor's coach he showed me to all the environs of Bristol and to the great Druid monuments in the neighbourhood—how magnificent the banks of the Wye and of Clifton Hill are!

Prichard soon packed Ritter off to his father and brother's in Ross via the hell of the iron-mining and copper-founding districts of South Wales. Once back in Bristol, Prichard treated him to an equally awesome sight of groundbreaking technology: down at the docks a vast iron ship, the SS *Great Britain*, was under construction. After some more fruitful scientific discussions, his guest was just as amazed at the speed of his rail journey back to London, accomplished in a mere four and a half hours. An altogether satisfying visit.⁴

Behind the scenes at the Red Lodge, family life was evolving. Prichard and Anna missed the children who had left home, one by one. Her mother reported:

> If you were now to call at the Red Lodge you would fancy it a "deserted Hall" for only the two younger children are there, Illtyd being at Hereford School Augustine in London and the rest at Oxford, with the exception of Theodore, who remains at home this Term to be under his Uncle John's care for the cure of his eyes. Only think of the privation he feels to be forbidden to read! Anna has a niece of the Doctor's staying there—Miss Mouline; whose brother is there also, for the advantage of the Bristol College. Albert has been very ill but is now nearly recovered.
>
> I sadly miss dear Mary Prichard's sweet smile and welcome whenever I enter the Red Lodge. She is however well and happy;—but, she is gone! Dear Mary Estlin and her papa—whom she follows like his shadow—are both well.⁵

Tended by Anna at the Red Lodge during her long final illness, Grandmother Estlin could follow the activities of the Prichard boys and saintly Mary; little "Dobbin" (Edith) was omitted. Edith Prichard merited only fleeting references in family lore. Her biography is that of a Victorian woman: she married Nicholas Pocock, one of Jem's Oxford friends, and died in 1919.⁶

Thomas Prichard also closely followed his grandchildren's progress and Prichard's struggles in Bristol on three fronts—the College, Institution, and Infirmary. As he reflected on his past life and contemplated death and his future state, he read his long-dead wife's diaries, full of pious thoughts. He was amused by what a conspicuous figure "Tommy" had played in her short life. After burning these diaries, he organized and stored a "multitude" of other family documents for his descendants to destroy.⁷

The Prichard family deeply felt the loss of their dearest friend. Con recalled the Rev. John Eden "godfather to all of us, & much beloved for his kindness, & simplicity, as well as respected for his knowledge & piety. He was a man of remarkable appearance, with white hair, very large bushy white eye brows, & a deep sonorous voice, in which he used to quote Latin poetry in the street."⁸

Aside from Eden, the Prichards were closest to the Estlins. Brother-in-law John Estlin shared Prichard's dedication to science and to creating a more humane world. As Bristol medical men, they supported the temperance movement and charitable provision of health services to the poor. A skilled ophthalmologist, Estlin had a large general practice and was appreciated for his successful charity eye dispensary. Another of his contributions to public health was his international distribution of a more potent smallpox vaccine in 1838–39, sourced from very near the spot Jenner had first obtained the matter for his vaccine in 1796. He published a thorough condemnation of mesmerism, phrenology, and homeopathy that pleased Prichard.

Estlin was a man of middle stature, pale, with a serious look in his face, extremely neat in his person and dress, and most methodical and punctual in all his affairs. The Prichard children relished visiting their uncle's natural history collection; one attraction was the bees entering the house through a channel in a window sill to busy themselves in their glass-fronted hive. In the garden they could gaze at his eagle, monkey, black bear, and box of snakes. One memorable day at Uncle John's they played with Chang and Eng, the famous "Siamese twins."[9]

Like Prichard, Estlin was active in medical associations, the Bristol Institution, and especially Bristol College. Unlike Prichard, he voted Whig and supported liberal causes such as nondenominational University College London and their friend Mary Carpenter's Ragged School. When not on the reformist stage, he was involved in national Unitarian affairs.[10] Once he had handed over his eye dispensary to Augustin Prichard, he and his daughter Mary Anne devoted themselves to doing good. They threw themselves into the antislavery movement like so many Unitarians did. In this they favored the Unitarian-inspired, provincial, more radical American Anti-Slavery Society, which demanded immediate abolition and promoted several other reforms such as women's equality, much to the disgust of most British middle-class, Anglican metropolitan abolitionists.

The Estlins promoted the charismatic Frederick Douglass's speaking tour of Britain; this American antislavery campaigner and man of color took the country by storm. At his sell-out Bristol lecture, he was mobbed by members of the audience clamoring to shake his hand. Estlin's widely circulated *A Brief Notice of American Slavery, and the Abolition Movement* (1846) was reprinted in 1851. Father and daughter continued tirelessly to campaign, correspond, and organize the national *Anti-Slavery Advocate*. When chairing an antislavery meeting at his home in 1855, Estlin suffered a fatal stroke.[11] As Unitarians and activists, the Estlins were most unlike conservative Prichard, but they shared a commitment to promoting the unity and dignity of the human species.

Wider Involvement

Middle-class Bristolians' entertainments in the early 1840s included watching kite-powered carriage demonstrations and tightrope walking across the Avon Gorge and attending recitals at the newly opened Victoria Rooms. There was a fascinating exhibition of the remarkable fossils discovered on the Downs, and they could marvel at the construction of the new railway linking Bristol and Gloucester. Bristol's science and learning continued muted, the polite and controlled activities of a conservative city more interested in appearing forward thinking. Prichard's own interests stayed focused on the wider world of knowledge: the sciences of origin, development, connection, and progress found in astronomy, natural history, geology, anatomy, and the study of humankind.

After eight years' involvement in the British Association for the Advancement of Science, he had made some progress increasing the status of anthropology and forming productive relationships, nationally and internationally. The BAAS held to its orthodox approach to science, had a fine reputation, and beneficially published its proceedings. At its 1839 Birmingham meeting, where Prichard delivered his famous speech "On the Extinction of Human Races," he renewed his friendship with the Irish physician William Wilde. Like Prichard, Wilde managed to combine a successful medical practice with researching human history. He was instrumental in developing Irish archaeology, about which he corresponded with Prichard on several occasions.[12]

Even while participating in the wider world of science, Prichard did not give up on "improving" Bristol. Its Statistical Society calibrated the evils of poverty, and its affluent members suggested solutions. He was among the city's elite gathered at the Guildhall on August 18, 1840, to found the Bristol Deaf and Dumb Institution, becoming a subscriber and member of its provisional council.[13] No longer would these disadvantaged children be outcasts. Prichard hoped such educational initiatives would combat poverty, maintain social order, and foster Christianity.

Prichard joined the newly formed Bristol Established Church Society and Book Association, a charity patronized by the bishop of Gloucester, Anglican clergymen, the mayor, and other worthy citizens. Its purpose was to disseminate books providing religious instruction and useful knowledge based on sound Church of England doctrine. They soon had a reading room and library of more than four hundred volumes, excluding books with a "popish" slant, of course. In the society's lectures, even the most practical subjects were approached from the perspective of Revealed Truth. This

Establishment effort to educate the "lower orders" was meant to counter those Radicals and possibly Chartists involved in the new Hall of Science opened in Broadmead, where the socialist Robert Owen came to speak in December 1840.

Prichard took to the Bristol Established Church Society with relish. The Tory press gleefully reported his seconding a resolution at its first anniversary meeting. His inspiring and entertaining Francophobe anecdote brought down the house. Prichard had been "told by a celebrated Frenchman, that in those parts of France where education was carried on, vice was the more prevalent; and when he (Dr. Prichard) expressed his surprise at that, his friend added, that the education in France was carried on unaccompanied by religion.—(Hear, hear) [Prichard told his audience that] putting intellectual acquirements into the hands of man without religious instruction, was like putting arms into the hands of savages.—(Hear)." Britain had escaped bloody revolution and owed the preservation of its glorious constitution and monarchy to its strong Anglican education. Prichard became one of the association's vice presidents and supported it with fundraising lectures on the "proof of original stock" in 1841 and the "natural history of man" in 1843.[14]

A New Career, August 23, 1842

While John Estlin continued his reformist activism, Prichard continued to publish supportive scientific books, articles, and speeches and keep up his involvement in learned societies. This commitment had begun at the Royal Medical Society of Edinburgh in 1805, a society that had recently elected him honorary member.[15] Involvement in organizations was time-consuming, however; he was still serving on the Bristol College Council at its last annual general meeting on February 25, 1841.[16] The following year, an opportunity from quite another quarter triggered a momentous decision. During the previous two decades the issues of insanity, the growing number of the insane, and the acknowledged need for proper asylum provision and management had become matters of national debate. With his considerable reputation as a mad-doctor, Prichard turned to laboring in the frustrating labyrinth of government to improve the lot of his suffering fellow human beings—or so he hoped.

Prichard's many encounters with insanity within his private circle and professionally made him the ideal person for a local government post. In 1824 the county of Gloucestershire appointed him Medical Visitor to its private madhouses, perhaps impressed by his recent publication on neuropsychiatric conditions. His reputation as a mad-doctor was thereby enhanced. Greater contact with asylum keepers supplied him with material for further research, and he committed his own patients to these madhouses. His Gloucestershire duties occupied him three or four days a year at 5 guineas per day plus personal and traveling expenses. He held this post until 1845.[17]

In 1842 rumors about Prichard's impending resignation from the Bristol Infirmary started circulating. Had he accepted a government appointment that would carry him away from the city? Young Dr. William Budd immediately started canvassing for election to Prichard's post, believing "public appointments and a good sum of fees will thus be thrown on the market. It will be hard if I do not get a slice of these good things . . . but this canvassing business is horribly fatiguing."[18] Prichard was disinclined to surrender his slice of good things, however. A deputation of eager partisans waited on him to learn his intentions, less concerned for the Infirmary and Prichard's welfare than eager to prevent opposition candidates from stealing a march on their protégés. Offended, Prichard advertised "he had not the slightest idea, nor had he remotely intimated a probability of a vacancy occurring in that valuable institution by a withdrawal of his services; and that, therefore, any canvass already commenced, or which might be persevered in, was quite unauthorised, if founded upon the prospect of his resignation."[19] The sharks continued to circle.

These rumors about Prichard's government post were not unfounded, but it was not a done deal in an age when who you were and who you knew trumped what you knew. His newly published *On the Different Forms of Insanity, in Relation to Jurisprudence* advertised his expertise on the subject and his potential as a bureaucrat, but his appointment as a metropolitan commissioner in lunacy owed at least as much to personal recommendation as to his suitability. His evangelical Tory credentials were crucial and his friend Baron Bunsen's social status instrumental. As a diplomat, Bunsen knew what to do. He approached Lord Ashley, MP, later the seventh Earl of Shaftesbury, the leader of the evangelical Tories in Britain, paragon of Victorian reformers, and architect of lunacy reform. Ashley duly suggested Prichard to the lord chancellor. Prichard wrote to Bunsen: "I can never sufficiently express my grateful sense of your kind & friendly interest in my behalf, which has succeeded in obtaining for me the object of which I was so desirous."[20]

Prichard's appointment as metropolitan commissioner in lunacy in 1842 was prestigious, but it required frequent absences from Bristol and time-consuming research, analysis, and report-writing on which future legislation would be based. As he began his duties he was also writing another volume of *Physical History*, preparing *Natural History*, and carrying on his private medical practice. How might he adjust his Bristol obligations to fit around a national career? Prichard attempted to hang on to his private practice, but it proved impracticable. Perhaps his son Augustin, newly qualified and just settling in Bristol, might take over some of his patients.

Reluctant to resign from the Infirmary, Prichard attempted to get his workload decreased by proposing the creation of the posts of assistant physician and surgeon, possibly having Augustin in mind. This came at a particularly fractious period for the faculty. As ever, there had been some recent internal disputes leading to the usual acrimonious newspaper correspondence, with senior physician Prichard appearing to be the author of a letter from which he later disassociated himself. Tempers ran high when he published a jab at Infirmary pupils' education provision, maintaining that his previous clinical lectures had been discontinued owing to poor attendance. His colleagues countered by publicly disagreeing with his call for assistants.[21] After over a year of debate, the committee announced new rules in January 1843, including one that limited faculty tenure to twenty years and another requiring the faculty to provide lectures. Prichard's call for assistants was ignored. Affronted, on June 7 he sent in his letter of resignation, solely on account of the assistant physician issue. Absent is the polite language called for on such an occasion, nor did he respond to the board's letter of thanks and his appointment as honorary physician. His twenty-seven years at the Infirmary came to an acrimonious end.[22]

A Medical Son, a Military Son

At least there was a new Dr. Prichard in town who could take on his father's private practice. Prichard had been as disappointed in Augustin's choice of a medical career as Thomas Prichard had been about Prichard's rejection of a business career back in 1802. Worse still was the young MD's desire to practice as a less socially prestigious surgeon. Augustin dug in his heels. After his intensive school life at Bristol College and given his keenness to "serve his time" with Uncle Estlin, Prichard had attempted to dissuade the stubborn would-be medic with a trick. One of his patients had strangled a cat in order to dislodge its jaws from the thumb of his servant. These things happen. Having then become concerned to know whether the cat was rabid, the man turned up at the Red Lodge demanding a feline autopsy. Instead of admitting it would not provide the required assurance, Prichard suggested that a stomach full of odd objects would indicate hydrophobia. Augustin was solemnly "shown down into the kitchen, where I found the cloth laid as if for my supper, with a dinner knife and fork and the cat" and told to perform the postmortem. It was negative; he dressed the servant's wounded thumb and received no fee.[23]

Not put off by his father, Augustin completed his apprenticeship, was a pupil at the Infirmary, and attended the Bristol Medical School. After studying at St. Bartholomew's Hospital, London, under Sir William Lawrence and qualifying to practice as a surgeon, Augustin continued his education abroad, armed with an itinerary/study permit courtesy of their houseguest Professor Ritter. He gained his MD from Berlin before studying further in Vienna and Paris.[24]

In October 1842 Augustin began practice, well supplied with his father's introductions to medical colleagues and patients, and soon he was signing certificates committing patients to asylums. He acquired a reputation for his excellent operative skills honed at his uncle Estlin's Eye Dispensary and was widely known for and published on surgery at either end of the patient—cataract procedures and lithotomy. Augustin lectured at the Bristol Medical School and became a surgeon to the Bristol Infirmary, as his son later did. Like his uncle Estlin, he was greatly interested in furthering scientific medicine through microscopy. In 1849 he described the Bristol Medico-Chirurgical Society's investigations into tiny fungus-like objects found in cholera patients' excretions, surrounding water and atmosphere, but that was as far as their identification of the cholera bacillus went.[25]

Augustin was tall, handsome, industrious, well read in the classics, devoted to sketching, a pioneer of photography, fond of joking, a rigid disciplinarian, and a staunch Tory. In 1845 he married Mary Sibellah Ley, his sister's sister-in-law, and in 1853 they moved out of the Red Lodge. Augustin contributed to ophthalmology by inventing numerous instruments, and he was a pioneer in enucleating injured eyes for the prevention of sympathetic ophthalmia. He was also famously wary of the use of anesthetics. His eminence was marked by being elected one of the first vice presidents of the Ophthalmological Society of the United Kingdom.[26]

Among Augustin's more than seventy publications are his two professional and personal memoirs containing several passages about his father. He shared his father's interest in collecting crania, lecturing and publishing on them at the Bristol Institution and the Zoological Society of London, and finally preserving the collection for donation to the Bristol Museum.[27] He also shared his father's passion for putting things in order; he arranged the family archives, a few items of which his physician son Edgar Albert preserved. Augustin's death on January 29, 1898, attracted a host of eulogies from friends, colleagues, and former students. Perhaps his father would have been proud of him after all.

Around the time Augustin was settling in to medical practice at the Red Lodge, another young Prichard was eager to fly the nest. Illtudus Thomas, "Illty" or "Hillty," had been a prize-winning student at a Hereford school before attending Rugby, but Oxford and life as a parish priest held no attractions. Illty might have consulted Augustin about how to handle their father. "It was by no means Dr. Prichard's wish that his son should go to India, but the young man's mind has become so firmly set on the idea, that his father is now anxious to further his wishes," explained an acquaintance. Prichard found himself running around London looking for strings to pull. He called on a former patient, retired lieutenant governor of Bombay Mountstuart Elphinstone, and secured the support of his Estlin relative (the banker Vincent Stuckey) and the chairman of the Metropolitan Commissioners in Lunacy, Lord Ashley. Illty was so keen to risk his neck in India he was satisfied with a rather lowly cadetship. He passed his examination and set sail for India on *The Monarch* in July 1845 to join the Fifteenth Regiment Bengal Native Infantry. He was soon promoted to lieutenant, saw action, and was awarded a medal.[28]

Illty and his first cousin Mary Moline married in Karachi in 1849, and they had at least three children. His subsequent careers were in the law as a "pleader" in the High Court of Agra, as the successful editor of the *Delhi Gazette*, and as the author of several books and articles on India, including *The Mutinies in Rajpootana* (1860). His "three-decker" novel *How to Manage It* was a very un-Prichardian publication. Illtudus was called to the Bar in 1865, and during a four-year period in Britain he wrote extensively, lectured, and campaigned on Indian affairs. He died of jaundice in Dehradun in the Himalayas in 1874.[29]

Psychiatry and Asylumdom Beckons

With professional and family ties binding him to Bristol, Prichard might have wondered if he had made the right decision in accepting the post of metropolitan commissioner in lunacy.[30] What had he let himself in for? He started out optimistically enough:

> I trust that the time is nearly drawn to a close, when lunatic asylums are to be prisons. They have been such long enough. If I live a few years longer, I trust that I shall see them the most comfortable places that men bereft of reason can inhabit. In particular their inmates must

not be shut up & deprived of exercise in the open air, but every means must be used to keep them in exercise & abroad as much as possible, in gardens, fields & the most pleasant exercising grounds that can be contrived. They can always be got to cultivate their own garden & grounds & thereby spare that which the public will be called upon to provide & that they must provide.[31]

Prichard envisaged asylums, whether private or public, transformed from eighteenth-century institutions of neglect, physical restraint, and punitive control into "hospitals" employing "non-restraint" and benignly intended behavioral conditioning. Once asylums were no longer prisons, asylum keepers were doctors, warders were nurses, and inmates became patients. As for the curability of insanity, eighteenth-century rationalism had suggested that insanity might be curable, not by medication, but by social and psychological means, including separating the insane from the pernicious causes of their affliction. This idea already advocated by Philippe Pinel on the Continent was adopted at The Retreat, York, where in 1813 Dr. Tuke published his system of care and treatment of the insane that optimistically relied on encouraging patients to behave properly. He called his method "moral treatment," with "moral" meaning social or behavioral. Moral treatment made further progress when Dr. John Conolly took charge of London's mammoth Hanwell County Asylum, already known for its occupationally therapeutic employment of patients. There he also set out a policy of "non-restraint," substituting the restraint of violent patients with periods of isolation. Prichard admired Dr. Conolly's paradigmatic asylum management, thanking one of his patients for a copy of "a report of Dr Conolly's treatment of Insane People. I am acquainted with the merits of his place, of the excellence of which I am convinced. Indeed I have seen the good results of its adoption in the Gloucester Asylum. Dr Conolly deserves the thanks of the medical profession for having suggested a great improvement in the management of very troublesome & distressing cases and for having removed from them one of the sources of opprobrium and reproach. I have no doubt that the milder method which he recommends will be universally followed."[32]

Asylumdom boomed. Over the years, Prichard committed many patients to privately run asylums near Bristol and kept in touch with them and their families.[33] But a separate category of "sufferer" needed special consideration:

> Harmless, quiet, congenital idiots are not the persons for an asylum, unless when they are destitute of domestic protection. If left to the

mercy of parish officers & farmed out, they are infinitely worse treated than in a proper asylum. . . . There are about 16,000 pauper lunatics in England & Wales & the greater number of them are now treated in a way disgraceful to the country. It is not always right to suffer idiots to roam at large about the land. I remember seeing a dumb, female idiot in Herefordshire, a most disgusting object, who was said to have borne two or three bastard infants, begotten nobody knew by whom.[34]

Prichard must have been gratified to have been instrumental in the call for separate asylum provision for the incurable cases that required the shelter of an asylum, believing these should be segregated from the insane and humanely treated. Conditions for the insane and incurables were no better in the United States at this time; in 1843 the prison reformer Dorothea Dix addressed the Massachusetts legislature on the subject of the insane being neglected and indiscriminately confined with criminals. Her efforts spurred the organization of state hospitals for the insane.[35] Prichard hoped that insanity would become better understood; medical specialists using proper scientific methods would develop effective treatments for it; the insane and mentally challenged would be humanely accommodated; and society would be thus "improved."

Asylumdom soon faced insurmountable challenges. There was the question of who should and should not be confined in asylums, for one thing. It was apparent that the substitution of mechanical restraint by seclusion was leading to the deprivation of patients' civil liberties and actually causing deleterious psychological effects. Moral treatment itself implied insanity was not medically treatable, throwing into question any medical model of care, and it was so labor-intensive that poor in county asylums had little or no access to it, or it was inappropriate for their particular condition.[36] Moral treatment degraded into mere "moral management," the modus operandi of costly, overcrowded, featureless warehouses of neglected humanity. By midcentury the focus of public asylums rapidly descended into the maintenance of patients and balancing of accounts as opposed to rehabilitation or cure. The asylum population was steadily rising in an atmosphere of therapeutic nihilism, until by the end of the century asylums had become essentially custodial.[37]

The Lunacy Commission and Lunacy Legislation

Asylum provision and regulation had started to become one of the Age of Improvement's targets years before Prichard's involvement in the Lunacy Commission. The 1808 County Asylums Act requiring counties to establish asylums for the insane poor was generally ignored by local governments, except for a few public asylums funded by local taxation or charity. Counties' individual, rather haphazard private asylum inspection regimes became a matter of concern. The Lunacy Commission proper dates back to the so-called Madhouse Act of 1828. Called the Metropolitan Commissioners in Lunacy, it was charged with inspecting private asylums in the London area. As the number of pauper lunatics grew steadily, asylum provision attracted public criticism. In 1833 the British Emancipation Act established the personal freedom of enslaved people abroad, while the following year the Poor Law Amendment Act incarcerated British paupers and subjected them to forced labor. Once Poor Law legislation settled into place, reformers returned to asylum provision and regulation.

The Metropolitan Lunacy Commission was drawn into advising on new legislation and policies to better enforce the creation and regulation of county asylums. After research by commissioners who had faith in the power of statistics or the evangelical desire to do good works on earth, the remit of the metropolitan commissioners was extended to the entire country. This required an increase in the number of specialist legal and medical commissioners, leading to Prichard's appointment on August 23, 1842.

As well as carrying out biannual inspections of all madhouses and asylums, the commissioners were tasked with compiling the *Report of the Metropolitan Commissioners in Lunacy to the Lord Chancellor* for 1844. Prichard threw himself into gathering data for and contributing to the nearly three-hundred-page report, a task that suited him better than inspecting asylums.[38] He likely drafted its section on medical therapeutics, which implied that there was a medical solution to mental disorders, though its general approval of alternative therapies conflicted with advocacy of physiological interventions. The *Report* tackled legal and administrative issues, provided advice on good practice such as the early admission of the insane, implicitly linked moral treatment to improved rates of cure and recommended new legislation.

The 1844 report became the basis of the tandem County Asylums Act and Lunacy Act of 1845, so-called Shaftesbury's Act, which made county asylums compulsory and required them to employ a medical officer. County governments provided the buildings, but the task of organizing and policing these new asylums and formulating protocols was left in the hands of philanthropists and legal and medical commissioners like Prichard.

Shaftesbury's Act was fiercely opposed in the House of Commons. MPs pointed out the inadequacies and arrogance of the former commissioners and the proposed extravagant remuneration of the future ones. Also up in arms were those involved in local subscription asylums, the newly formed watchdog Alleged Lunatics' Friend Society and the county governments who would have to foot the bill. In professional circles there was cautious optimism, nevertheless. This legislation effectively integrated the new profession of psychiatry into the apparatus of the state, as similar legislation had done in France in 1838. Britain now had a national system for the regulation of both private and public asylums.[39]

Being a Commissioner in Lunacy

During his first two years as a commissioner, Prichard had spent approximately one-fifth of his time researching the *Report* and traveling on inspection circuits, staying at each asylum and private madhouse for a day or less, depending on location and the number of patients examined. He had made fewer visits than his colleagues, and these were mostly to the counties surrounding Bristol. He did, however, manage to inspect and report glowingly on the famously elite, discreet Ticehurst Asylum.[40]

Prichard continued to be called on to testify in individual legal determinations of insanity as he had done in the case of the Earl of Kingston. At a Clifton hotel in 1844, he deposed as both an expert witness and the personal physician of a Mr. Edward Thomas, a gentleman possessing considerable landed property in the West Indies. A writ of de lunatico inquirendo certified his incompetence to manage his affairs, in this apparent case of early dementia. Prichard also provided evidence in a suit against Dr. Samuel Ashwell, accused of securing a will in his favor worth £25,000 from "a sick lady," Mrs. Eliza Lomi, in the absence of her husband.[41]

Aside from legislation fostering the rise of asylumdom, an independent organization was founded to represent the new profession of asylum medical officers, an initiative foundational to the discipline of psychiatry. In 1841 Prichard's friend Dr. Hitch, the innovative superintendent of Gloucester Asylum, founded the Association of Medical Officers of Asylums and Hospitals for the Insane, the first specialist psychiatric association. It met annually at different asylums to share knowledge supporting progressive methods of asylum management, in particular medical and moral treatment, and including nonrestraint. Its members collected data to add to the understanding of mental disorders but hardly engaged in campaigning. Prichard was among its earliest members, attending its 1844 York meeting, at which he was asked to communicate with the chairman of the Lunacy Commission on behalf of the association.[42]

Shaftesbury's Act restructured the Lunacy Commission and required its officers to be on duty at its London office frequently. This meant Prichard had to give up his private practice and other medical posts and move to London. He would finally live in the metropolis, associate with fellow scholars, and exploit the libraries of some of the nation's great institutions. The Prichards started packing.

As Prichard would be based in the capital, it became expedient to become an LRCP, a licentiate of the Royal College of Physicians, the qualification David Davies had criticized him for lacking decades earlier. Prichard traveled to London to be examined by its elite Oxbridge MD officers at their imposing Greek Revival–style edifice in Trafalgar Square. In its meeting chamber with several marble busts looking on, the examiners fired questions at him that would have reduced any newly qualified physician to a nervous wreck. Part 1, "En Parte Physiologica," began with, "Describe the functions of the various cerebral nerves." Five more questions were followed by the task of translating a classical Greek medical text into Latin and then a Latin paragraph into English. Prichard must have enjoyed the next part, perhaps quoting his own publications: "Mention the various forms of mental derangement and the difference between delirium and mania." After translating a passage by Hippocrates from Greek to Latin and rendering a Latin description of the symptoms of apoplexy into English, the final "In Parte Pathologica" was a doddle; after all, his friend and patient Dr. Richard Bright had identified and named the disease in question. Yet more translations completed his "ordeal."[43] With thirty-four years of medical practice and mastery of Greek and Latin, being examined alongside young hopefuls at the Royal College of Physicians must have been more irritating than challenging. He paid his £15 fee, received a handsome certificate, and could now append "LRCP" to his name.[44] Prichard was prepared for his new London post.

Then there was a hitch. As the new legislation reduced the number of commissioners, he was dropped for lack of seniority. Even when a vacancy immediately arose, the ambivalent chairman of the commission was neither perfectly candid nor wholehearted in his endorsement of Prichard. Lord Ashley "implored the Chancellor to appoint Dr Prichard [because] the success of the Commission will depend, humanly speaking, on the character of its officers. We must have the best men in every sense of the word; men, who can speak with authority to the skillful and experienced persons with whom they will be always in contact, & sometimes in collision." Privately, however, he felt that "Prichard has a reputation, & is by far the superior one of the remaining former commissioners, and as being one of them, we cannot pass him over, because he had some fitness. But he wants capacity as a Visitor of Asylums." On August 27, 1845, he was sworn in by three fellow commissioners in Bath. Ashley was relieved but continued to worry about mild-mannered Prichard's effectiveness as an asylum inspector.[45]

Thomas Prichard and Family Matters

During the early 1840s Prichard's relationship with his elderly father continued intense. He had leeched and medicated him through countless illnesses over the years; every time Thomas Prichard wrote predicting his own imminent demise, his son would annotate this doom and gloom with a comment such as "My father lived another twenty years." But in 1842, having missed his father's seventy-seventh birthday celebration, Prichard could no longer put off dealing with the urgent issue of his father's spiritual welfare. Respectfully he urged his baptism, claiming he did this "with no motive but an earnest wish for your entire safety and happiness." The old man snapped back that he had never found evidence that Christ intended "water-baptism" as a permanent rule; on the contrary, it appeared that Christ baptized with the Holy Ghost and with fire. He thought he had experienced his fair share of trials, did not believe in priestly mediation between himself and his Savior, and trusted his sins would be pardoned. In other words: not a chance.[46]

The following summer, confined to his home in Ross, unbaptized Thomas Prichard was preparing to meet his savior. In one of his last conversations with his sister, the lifelong Quaker reaffirmed his disbelief in water baptism, as being a Christian needed no outward rite.[47] Prichard and Anna, having just returned to Bristol on "pressing business," were not present at his death on August 21, 1843. His grandson-in-law the Rev. William Henry Ley wrote a loving memoir of him for the *Red Lodge Intelligencer*, and his grandson Constantine described him equally endearingly. They remembered the frail yet mentally vigorous old man and his wonderful home, blessed with happy and peaceful family visits from old and young alike. He had fine, noble features, an aquiline nose, and lively hazel eyes. He wore a brown wig and a "quaker's coat" under his jacket, a wrapper around his neck, and a brown silk cap. His religious beliefs shaped his "grace and refinement of manner, joined with a benevolence, the expression of which pervaded his words and actions. . . . His varied reading made his conversation instructive & intellectual, but the impression left most strongly on the mind in recollection of him is that of unaffected piety, elegance & cultivation of mind, & gentleness combined with elevation of character." He was remembered as having an unselfish, caring, liberal, generous character. Thomas Prichard especially loved being in the company of children, entertaining them at his table and playing their favorite game of Conglomeration, involving impromptu poetry composition. When not engaged in religious study and reflection, he devoted himself to pleasing and helping others, whether feeding the children treats, helping some poor protégé, pointing out meaningful passages from books, planning games, amusements and excursions, or giving gifts. He was known to say, "The greatest pleasure in having money is to give it."[48]

Thomas Prichard had been a pillar of the community, and not just as a partner in Ross Old Bank. For forty-three years he led a life free from actively earning a living. His support for the local school had been greatly valued,[49] and although he was a Quaker, his evangelicalism had ensured a positive relationship with some of the local clergy. His only publications seem to be a pious poem printed anonymously in a Hereford newspaper and a pamphlet of thirty pages weighing in on the Quaker doctrinal controversies of the period.[50] On August 27, 1843, the residents of the town filled the Ross Meeting House to pay their respects before his interment in its burial ground. In 1859 Con described his grandfather's life and death, inserted a few of his ancestors' love letters, and laid down his pen after completing the memoir his father had begun in 1847.

Thomas Prichard had the posthumous pleasure of making his son richer. Prichard had inherited a significant sum in 1817, and an 1820 inheritance approached £25,000, enough to buy twenty-two Red Lodges. His share of his father's estate and his own investments should have made him feel more secure, but he still had to support his sons at Oxford and in their early careers. His sister Mary Moline's life also changed. Like Prichard, she had been very close to her father, spending a few months with him every year. After his death and her children had grown, her ties to the West Country weakened. She died in 1868 and, like Prichard, left many descendants.[51]

"I have too many irons in the fire & am a good deal over done," Prichard admitted in early 1844.[52] Amid a multiplicity of obligations, projects, and family concerns, he still hoped to see Bristol become a place of cultural excellence. In a speech he urged the Bristol Medical School to erect a new building worthy of its high standing, and he joined a committee to organize a monument in the Bristol Cathedral to his friend Robert Southey, son of Bristol, poet, and defender of the faith.[53] After thirty-five years in Bristol, however, the poor were just as unhealthy and the insane paupers in St. Peter's just as miserable; the Bristol meetings of the BAAS and PMSA had not noticeably improved the city's reputation for science and medicine; his precious Bristol College had succumbed to Anglican hostility; the Bristol Institution was all but moribund; and his relations with his Infirmary colleagues had hit rock bottom. Prichard's children gave him little to look forward to. Augustin and Edith seemed in rude health, but Jem and Con had tuberculosis, and it had recently taken Mary; Alboo was having fits; soldier Illty was facing danger in India; and The's mental state was precarious.

In London Prichard would be able to contribute to improving the welfare of the insane. He would also get more closely involved in the development of the Ethnological Society of London, keeping it from the clutches of the polygenetic rabble. When official duties allowed, he would pursue his anthropological research and associate with learned men. At nearly sixty years of age, he took the plunge, exchanging his life as a Bristol physician for that of a well-paid government official. Prichard removed his family to London, leaving the Red Lodge to Augustin.

15 · Public Service and Private Misery

Living in London, 1845–48

> My fathers later letters . . . are full of expressions of anxiety
> & dejection—scarcely any without them. But it did not
> prevent him from doing a great deal of work.
> —Constantine Estlin Prichard to Augustin Prichard, January 18, 1860

Number 1, Woburn Place, on the north side of Russell Square, Bloomsbury, was a highly respectable address for the new commissioner in lunacy. From temporary lodgings at 39 Bernard Street the Prichards moved into their freshly redecorated home. Russell Square had been one of the Duke of Bedford's rapidly constructed building developments of about 1804; in its central garden designed by Humphry Repton, residents of the surrounding homes could promenade along curving, tidy paths bordered with shrubs, shaded by lime trees and graced by the duke's commemorative statue. One corner of the square faced Montague House, the home of the British Museum, then undergoing major reconstruction; its great library beckoned.[1] Nearby, the huge Corinthian columns of Nicholas Hawksmoor's neoclassical St. George's Church guarded the spiritual well-being of its affluent parishioners, while almost in sight of the Prichards' new home was the charity Foundling Hospital, storehouse of London's abandoned children.

Woburn Place had been decided on in a bit of a rush, as Prichard's duties started immediately. Anna supervised the unpacking and furnishing of their home, sending to Mitcham vicarage for Jem and Emma's furniture and to Bristol for the unfortunate couple's child and her own teenagers. Christmas 1845 found the family settled in the heart of London. Prichard began a brief period of overwork, frustration, and sorrow.[2]

London Life

Prichard's Lunacy Commission duties immediately occupied far more of his time than he had bargained for, but whenever possible he enjoyed the company of men of science at the capital's learned societies and accepted and extended invitations to dine. The Prichards did not neglect their Bristol friends and relatives; they invited Mary Anne Estlin and Walter Bagehot to join them on an excursion to Hampton Court, returning to London by boat. On that hot day in May 1846, Walter noticed ominously how considerably older than his mother Jem looked.[3] John Estlin was in London engaged in some stressful Unitarian business at the time, and he and his daughter were greatly occupied with antislavery campaigning.

Estlin brought the famous American abolitionist William Lloyd Garrison to breakfast at Woburn Place in the late summer of 1846. He and Frederick Douglass were on a nineteen-month antislavery lecture tour of Britain. It was a valuable opportunity to meet the tireless campaigner and learn about the remarkable Frederick Douglass, who, with his masterful oratory and best-selling autobiography, was living proof of Prichard's claim that all people could achieve the intellectual heights of Europeans. While the Estlins were antislavery activists, Prichard continued his scientific refutations of polygenism. The following year he helped Estlin get a pamphlet printed about the celebrated American and his noble campaign.[4]

One Woburn Place hosted scientists and travelers from near and far, Prichard's friend and fellow linguist Baron Bunsen among them. Thomas Hodgkin, with his Aborigines' Protection Society contacts, was a magnet to doctors, travelers, campaigners, and scientists—anyone from near or far with a compelling story to tell.[5] They would soon find their way to tea or a soiree at Woburn Place too. Prichard kept up his acquaintance with Sir Alexander Morison, mad-doctor and physician to Bethlehem Hospital and elsewhere; they visited private patients together to sign committals and attended meetings of the Ethnological Society. Morison had had a long struggle to achieve professional recognition and financial security, but by the 1840s, like Prichard, he was eminent in his field. He valued his relationship with Prichard.[6]

London's several learned societies, such as the Geographical Society, the Royal Society, the Royal Asiatic Society, and the new Ethnological Society provided further opportunities for Prichard to socialize. Less beneficial was his membership of the Athenaeum Club, a place for dining and making contacts, but no scholarly haven. Its library contained several of Prichard's books, and its popular *Athenaeum* was a journal worth reading. The *Athenaeum* rarely published notices of his publications, despite his best efforts with its editor.[7] The number of Prichard's memberships grew. He had been elected honorary member of the American Ethnological Society, and his connection with the American Oriental Society had likely been arranged by his correspondent John Pickering. Prichard and Hodgkin were made honorary members of the Bombay Branch of the Royal Asiatic Society on December 11, 1845.[8] He now found himself connected to more than enough scientists and their societies.

Lunacy Commission Duties

On Prichard's first day at the Lunacy Commission's Spring Gardens office, he and his former metropolitan commissioners discovered just how much the 1845 act had increased their obligations and duties. Of the eleven commissioners in lunacy, five were unremunerated laymen, three medical, and three legal. Junior member Prichard was the best qualified medical commissioner, being the only specialist in psychological medicine. His annual salary was an impressively upper-middle-class £1,500, plus 30 shillings per day on circuit plus expenses. Pairs of commissioners were charged with inspecting asylums at least once a year, provincial licensed houses twice, and metropolitan licensed houses, excluding ancient Bethlem Hospital, at least four times. Also within their jurisdiction were some workhouses and prisons, where their task was to identify lunatics and order their transfer to asylums.

The country was divided into inspection circuits, and it was a fortunate pair of commissioners who could visit several asylums in close proximity. Hanwell County Lunatic Asylum, a huge state-of-the-art facility built for the London insane, needed two pairs of commissioners to manage the examination of nearly a thousand patients in a single day. At the other end of the scale, even "single lunatics" kept in lodgings under the supervision of an attendant had to be inspected. At each institution the commissioners had to write a pro forma report in its visitors' book, running through patients' statistics, incidents of mechanical restraint, cleanliness, diet, and opportunities to engage in beneficial work and leisure activities and attend worship (Lord Ashley's favorite). Back at the office, there were tasks such as the licensing of asylums within the metropolitan district, examining provincial licenses, submitting semi-annual and annual reports to the lord chancellor, writing scores of special reports, and dealing with correspondence. Lord Ashley confided in his diary that "the duties and labour will far exceed our calculations." He was right. As Prichard's friends had feared, the post of commissioner in lunacy was a poison chalice.[9]

Prichard crisscrossed the nation in all weathers by carriage or in those so-called flying cars, leaving him little leisure for anthropology; he had to apologize for submitting a hastily written paper, adding, "I have had very little time for composing it, having lately returned from a journey in the North of England, where I have been engaged in my official duty, as Commissioner in Lunacy." In his first five months in the post, he traveled 2,052 miles, made 102 visits, and saw 4,624 patients. Over one three-month period, he was on the road thirty-four days. He averaged eighty inspection days per year, at almost sixty miles per day, often in carriages bumping over country roads. The commissioners complained among themselves about their inspection tours, an unpleasant task, especially in winter. A colleague on a circuit of six cities grumbled, "I hear nothing—I see nothing, but tunnels and railroads—madmen and chambermaids. No other things interest me—and I have no escapes or perils to speak of. I am sick of travelling." Prichard attended frequent meetings at the commission's office, wrote reams of reports, and suffered the slings and arrows of public criticism and scandals. Worst of all, he had to endure examining thousands of hopeless, miserable, neglected humans imprisoned and enduring every possible form of neglect.[10]

The Lunacy Commission employed an efficient and hardworking secretary. Its chairman Lord Ashley's sometimes overbearing, temperamental, and anxious outlook was highly colored by his conservative, evangelical background. His views were the commission's views, and unchallengeable. For example, he disapproved of family visits, inspections, or any activity on Sundays other than divine worship, making that day extremely dull for patients, especially as it was the only day most relatives were free to visit. The commission's requirements for asylum life were stultifying in their effect.

While Prichard shared Ashley's piety and no doubt respected his authority, he must have found his chairman's suspicion of medical opinion less acceptable. It was no secret that the presumed organic basis of mental "disease" remained elusive, and as the hope of discharging patients cured of insanity faded, other bases of the commission's success came to the fore, such as the humane containment of the insane and the efficient administration of asylums. The commissioners' task became the increasingly paternalistic application of central government rules; if asylums could be made to function without mechanical restraint, so much the better sense of control. The prospect of understanding insanity and restoring sufferers to health receded into the background.[11]

The commissioners had the power to recommend or even demand that asylums make improvements. They suggested patients be given increased opportunities and space for exercise and that asylum libraries provide light reading matter, while they condemned small rooms and inadequate bedding. Their instructions were not always carried out promptly, such as when the superintendent of Ticehurst private asylum took more than a year to discharge a lucrative patient the commissioners considered sane. The commissioners condemned St. Peter's Hospital, Bristol, as totally unfit to accommodate lunatics, a complaint made long before by its erstwhile physician Prichard. Following their previous criticisms, minimal improvements had been made, while the visiting magistrates had repeatedly failed to induce Bristol's Guardians of the Poor to provide a proper asylum elsewhere. The commissioners repeated their inspection and condemnation of St. Peter's on June 24, 1847, noting that the mortality rate was much higher than the national average, the wards and yards were "totally unfit for the purpose," the "present arrangement is utterly discreditable, and unless the corporation take measures for its amendment, the condition of the insane poor of Bristol will require the intervention of some higher authority." For good measure, their next report to Parliament featured St. Peter's as an exemplar of failure. Stony ground.[12]

Prichard was often in the company of his commission colleagues, including the laymen Lords Shaftesbury and Lyndhurst. Fellow medical commissioner John Robert Hume was a Waterloo veteran, a friend of the Duke of Wellington, and most famous for being lampooned in the reformist *Lancet* as a sinecurist and religious skeptic. The legal commissioner who accompanied Prichard on his last inspection could not have been more unlike him. As a young London lawyer, Brian Waller Procter mixed in literary circles, becoming a poet and writer publishing under the nom de plume Barry Cornwall. Proctor was famous for his library, collection of Old Masters, and generosity. The job had its perils too; R. W. S. Lutwidge later met an unhappy end, murdered by a patient in the course of an inspection.[13]

There was a lot of admin to be got through at the commission's office and weekly, monthly, and frequent special meetings to attend. At Prichard's first meeting, he and another colleague were tasked with preparing the 1846 *General Report* based upon data collected from 949 institutions. To standardize data collection, the commission produced forms containing a Prichardian nosology of mental conditions, including "moral insanity," ensuring *A Treatise on Insanity*'s influence on psychiatry for a few decades, as later writers on insanity tended to adopt the commission's classification.[14] When not actually on circuit, the commissioners also had to scrutinize license applications, examine plans, estimates, and accounts, and confer with magistrates and architects. Soon there was little time left to carry out an increasing number of special investigations. Prichard found himself mired in making troubleshooting inspections and compiling reports on asylums that had been the subject of general complaints or accusations involving individual patients.

Then there were the pros and cons of publicity. As insanity became less of a taboo subject during these reformist decades, asylums and insanity became topics of popular discussion. Accounts of abuse in asylums swirled in the press, particularly in the reformist *Lancet*; fear of wrongful incarceration grew, while shame and secrecy among the families of the insane continued unrelieved. Individuals and special interest groups lodged more and more complaints about asylums. Soon both commissioners and asylums were prime targets.

This was not Prichard's first exposure to negative publicity. One incident occurred at his friend George Gwinnett Bompas's Fishponds House Private Lunatic Asylum, Stapleton, where Prichard and Estlin had committed Maria Acland in 1838. She managed to smuggle out a letter painting a gruesome picture of asylum conditions, making accusations against both its owner and Prichard. As Gloucestershire Medical Visitor, he had inspected asylums run by medical officers who were his friends. One was Edward Long Fox, whose Northwoods Asylum had been severely criticized, while at Fishponds Asylum fifty incorrect certificates and evidence of neglect and cruelty were uncovered.[15]

Any relationships with asylum owners exposed the lunacy commissioners to accusations of corruption. This was an impossible situation. When Prichard and his fellow medical commissioners had previously been in practice, they had committed patients to asylums they now inspected, and they were members of the same societies and organizations as the asylum owners and officers whose behavior they now monitored.[16] At least private asylum owners themselves were ineligible for appointment to the commission. Still, some critics wondered whether the medical commissioners were less exacting than they should be.

Now that there was a body responsible for investigating complaints about asylums, accusations started flooding in from members of the public, journalists, and reformers. There were rumors of the wrongful committal of unwanted or errant wives, embarrassingly misbehaving offspring (mostly wayward daughters), rich ladies deprived of fortunes, alcoholics, and generally inconvenient family members. Who should be in asylums and why: The insane, the dangerous and insane, the incurable? To protect society, to protect the insane, to cure? Some thought the 1845 Lunacy Act would prevent abuses; others understood it was just the start of the struggle.[17] The name Haydock Lodge must have sent a shiver down Prichard's spine.

Haydock Lodge Asylum required repeated inspections in 1846. It was initially found damp and overcrowded in places; the commissioners' next inspection noted the problems diminishing, a rather laissez-faire response that did not satisfy Thomas Wakely, *The Lancet*'s champion of medical reform. This private pauper lunatic asylum was alleged to be nothing more than a business venture in collusion with the local Poor Law officers in which overcrowded, undernourished, and ill-treated paupers from around the country were stored and dying like flies. The commission launched a special investigation involving Prichard and three other commissioners spending several days examining Haydock Lodge and its 393 patients, questioning twenty-three witnesses under oath. The saga reached government, precipitating a full-blown scandal, investigation, and House of Commons debate. As one of the commissioners who had produced rather pat reports, Prichard was in the eye of the storm.[18]

There was more to come. One special report concerned a woman's alleged unlawful detainment, and Prichard and Procter had to compile another one on Warwick Union Workhouse. Commissioners William George Campbell and Prichard had particular difficulties in their repeated inspections and spot checks on Gate Helmsley Retreat, York, about which they produced a twenty-four-page report on abuses there. The proprietor of the asylum was ill and had left his wife in charge; the matron lied to the commissioners; and the patients were underfed and lacked adequate bedding. When the commissioners showed they did have a tooth or two by revoking Gate Helmsley's license, the press had a field day, castigating them for initially taking the word of a mere matron. Concerning the death of a patient in Lincoln Asylum, Prichard and his legal colleague William James Mylne took statements from eleven witnesses before writing their report containing six findings.[19] It was one report after another.

The overworked Lunacy Commission came into conflict with the legal profession over determining criminal responsibility. Within government, the two separate bodies controlling the lives of "lunatics" were also at odds; the lord chancellor who oversaw commissions in lunacy on individuals clashed with the commissioners. When greater flexibility in the conduct of de lunatico inquirendos started to occur, such as when they interpreted inability to manage one's own affairs and deviant behavior as symptomatic of insanity, the boundary with immorality became blurred.[20]

Prichard must have been ambivalent about a new society seemingly dedicated to attacking the Lunacy Commission. In 1845 a former asylum patient advertised for people to join him in fighting for better treatment of the insane. The Alleged Lunatics' Friend Society (ALFS) is considered the first mental health campaign organization. It aimed to prevent illegal incarceration, improve asylum conditions, develop aftercare for the discharged, and destigmatize insanity—a tall order. The society decried the separation of the mentally ill from their families and doctors' tendency to ignore what the insane said, hence their further demands that the insane have access to information and a say in their own care. Most threatening to the medical and legal professions was the ALFS's questioning of the very definition of insanity; where did eccentricity and immorality end and insanity begin? The ALFS rooted out cases of illegal committals, constantly agitating, petitioning, lecturing, launching legal challenges, and becoming something of a watchdog over/thorn in the side of/unofficial investigative assistant to the Lunacy Commission. They even criticized the system of moral treatment so valued by Prichard and the new wave of psychiatric physicians and asylum superintendents, claiming moral treatment crushed a sufferer's spirit with its infantilizing reeducation and behavioral training.

The ALFS and its rather mixed bag of adherents came in for a lot of criticism, especially as it lacked the patronage of the middle and upper classes, who feared association with stigmatizing insanity. The society bombarded the Lunacy Commission with suggestions, and a few reformist MP members of the ALFS presented bills to Parliament in 1847 and 1848 that would improve the function of the commission. This campaign group, the press, the public, and the government kept the commissioners on their toes. *The Further Report of the Commissioners in Lunacy* of 1847 is a case in point. Prichard's substantial role in compiling this report, with its stress on maintaining a medical approach to the care of the insane, was noted by asylum reformers.[21]

The care and treatment of the insane was one of the era's prime objects of reform and improvement. Parliamentary reports, successive legislation, the Lunacy Commission, the scandals, the ALFS, the Association of Medical Officers of Asylums, and Prichard's and his fellow alienists' literature on insanity and its jurisprudence all contributed to the development of British asylumdom and the discipline of psychiatry. Prichard hoped the Lunacy Commission would be the instrument by which the welfare of his insane fellow human beings would be improved, just as he hoped his anthropology would benefit Britain's colonized subjects.

The reality of Prichard's life as a commissioner was that his good name became linked with controversies over the definition, rights, care, and control of the insane. He spent a large proportion of his time traveling, rooting out misconduct and abuse. He seemed distressed by his endless examinations of so many incurables and warehoused souls deprived of training and amusement, battered, cold, underfed, untreated, and humiliated. He found human beings under restraint and in one asylum stored in small cupboards. It was exhausting. Did he wonder whether his efforts were worthwhile? Putting on a brave face, he wrote to the American psychiatrist Amariah Brigham in 1848: "Your countrymen seem to be improving rapidly in every thing. We have many drag-chains in this country, and get on slowly, but still surely."[22] In public he grappled with the drag-chains of legislation and public opinion: in private there were other struggles.

"Sickness and Sorrow Have Been Our Lot"

A few months after the Prichards settled in London, Anna's sister Caroline's letter was consolatory: "I am glad that your visit to Selluck is over I know that it must have been a very painful one to you. I hope that the Dr's spirits will get better."[23] While the Haydock Lodge scandal was calling Prichard's reputation into question, he had other reasons to be out of spirits that summer of 1846. Their visit to their son-in-law at Sellack vicarage meant a visit to their daughter Mary Ley's grave. It was also the day they surrendered her baby, whom they had been fostering. Jem's baby daughter had recently died after being brought back from Madeira, where he had been attempting seasonal relief from his relentlessly debilitating tuberculosis. With the peaceful River Wye meandering nearby, Sellack churchyard held another grave to stand over and contemplate God's will. There was little prospect of Prichard's spirits ever mending.

The stigma of insanity ran deep, a topic of discussion best avoided. Even his superior at the Lunacy Commission Lord Ashley had shamefully stashed his epileptic son in lodgings abroad. Both men could understand a later campaigner's letter attributing lack of progress in mental health reform to prejudice. Insanity

> is treated by modern society more as a crime than an affliction. Like the lepers of old, all intimate union is a disgrace. . . . The wisest shrink from acknowledging that insanity exists in any members of a family; how they will excuse it, find reasons for it— . . . "He or she never recovered from a fall." . . . How often has an unhappy young man who had over read or over drank himself at the university, been sent to a house of confinement a considerable distance from home, that the report of his insanity might not injure his sister's or his brother's marriage in hope

or in expectation.... I do not know what ought to be, but I am quite sure the time is very far distant when it will be, that the deep-rooted feeling among poor and rich should disappear; that insanity existing in a man's family, even remotely, is not an obstacle to the settlement of his children, and in some sort his disgrace.[24]

Prejudice among both poor and rich endured; Lord Ashley was no exception.

While Prichard had become quite successful at molding two of his sons into scholar-clergymen, his fourth surviving son proved a challenge. Theodore Joseph had done well at Bristol College, progressing to Oriel College, Oxford, in December 1836 after his father secured special dispensation for underaged admission by asserting his son's studies were highly advanced.[25] It took The several years to gain his degree, as he had two long leaves of absence, the first of which was on account of a "dangerous illness," although he was not consumptive like siblings Jem, Mary, and Con. The second was occasioned by his accompanying his consumptive cousin Roger on his fatal trip to Alexandria. On The's return in 1844, a family friend noticed: "Dr Prichard and all his family were up at Oxford, where I called upon them. Theodore Prichard has just returned from Egypt, bringing with him lots of drawings &c, I think him very much improved in manners."[26]

The became a demy at Magdalen, and after gaining his BA in classics, second class, in December 1844, he continued studying, doubtless for a fellowship or ordination that would please his father. Instead of being satisfied with The's progress, at the end of a bleak February 1846 Prichard found himself back at Sellack Church, quietly burying him. The family memorial tablet in the church bears the young man's name, dates, and inscription: "Apud Dominum misericordia, et copiosa apud Eum redemptio"—"with the Lord, there is mercy/pity and redemption." Anna described the tragedy to a friend:

> We have indeed received a very heavy shock,—when I last saw you I was trembling for the life of my youngest boy [Albert Hermann, prone to convulsions]—poor Theodore was then well—A week or two afterwards he became deprest and unwell—and went into the country and likewise to Oxford to pay his brother a visit and then returned to us—but he did not get better here, and we hoped a change into the country would benefit him—and he had only left us a very few days, and was just settled in some pleasant lodgings in the neighbourhood of Gloucester when he died—It has been a great grief to me, not to have been with him. Sickness and sorrow have been our lot since we have been here.[27]

In 1953 Prichard's grandson Theodore Innes Pocock's account of his uncle The was quite different: "He overworked at Oxford, went out of his mind & in a year or two died in Gloucester asylum. That is all that my mother knew, I think: But through Uncle Con's family it came out that he took his own life."[28] His brother-in-law William Ley conducted Theodore's burial on March 7, 1846, in the plot that would receive his mother, Uncle Edward, and father. Years later Constantine confirmed to Augustin:

> Indeed, altho' as a family we have had a good many distresses, deaths & the like in the last ten years, I do not feel, on looking back, that there is anything that we ought to wish otherwise than it was ordered, except one thing, poor The's death & its circumstances. All others, even the suddenness of my mother's, had alleviating points, and one can think of them with softened and even happy associations. In his case, there is more of pain. But it is useless to give way to this, and we must trust God's mercy that even it was (if not best, for this it is impossible to think) yet not an irremediable sorrow, as it seemed almost at first.[29]

Con also described Prichard's own depression, apparent since 1844: "My fathers later letters, during James' illness & his journeys in 1848, are full of expressions of anxiety & dejection—scarcely any without them. But it did not prevent him from doing a great deal of work."[30] Augustin recorded in his Family Chronicle: "1845 T.J.P. ill / 1846 Theodore died—Fcby 24."[31] That was the end of The.

Prichard's grief was compounded by the fear of the shame and suspicion suicide cast on relatives. While not prohibited in the Bible, later Christian doctrine condemned it. As the nineteenth century opened, outright hostility toward it waned as its association with the supernatural faded, but the bodies of those who died by suicide were still meted disrespectful public treatment, including prohibition of Christian burial. An 1823 law attempted to replace the lingering custom of burying suicide victims at a crossroads with burial in churchyards or cemeteries after dark and without a religious service. Some clergymen still refused to officiate. The law allowing the confiscation of the personal assets of those who had taken their own lives had already fallen into disuse but was repealed only in 1870.[32] Suicide remained illegal in the United Kingdom until 1961.

The's suicide threatened more than Prichard's professional standing. He had other children whose marriages and career prospects would have suffered from having a "deranged" brother who had taken his own life—double grounds for suspicion. Did insanity run in the family? The's mother was likely aware of his suicide. Paradoxically, her grief might have been somewhat tempered by the tragedy's occurring under the similarly shameful condition of insanity, as this was accepted as a mitigating circumstance in law regarding suicide. Coroners' verdicts on middle-class deaths by suicide were almost invariably that of self-murder while the mind was *temporarily* deranged, obviating sanctions and ameliorating relatives' reputation. But The's tragic death drew no public notice, nor was there an inquest, as required by law. When Prichard faced choosing between detriment to reputation and breaking the law, he chose the latter and compounded the misery of his final years.

By law, all deaths had to be recorded at the national General Register Office, and details of inquests were kept in county records. Corroborating the family's account of The's death should have been straightforward. Instead, a tangle of conflicting information presented itself, starting with Theodore's obituary notices. They gave the place of death as Oxford, while the Sellack Church burial register stated Gloucester. The conflicting death dates of February 24 and 25 were perhaps owing to the death's having occurred in the middle of the night. Although failure to register a death was a criminal offense, the name Theodore Joseph Prichard does not appear in the Register of Deaths. Instead, there is a Theodore James, gentleman, age twenty-five, who hanged himself on February 25, 1846, in Wotton, the location of Prichard's friend Samuel Hitch's Gloucester Lunatic Asylum. Was Anna's reference to her son's "pleasant lodgings in the neighbourhood of Gloucester" not quite the case? Rather than Hitch's asylum listing a Theodore James or Theodore Joseph Prichard, it recorded the admission of Mr. T. J. Richards on "June 16, 1845, a 24 year old temperate unmarried Divinity student whose first attack commenced two weeks previously & was caused by over study." The surname Prichard is derived from the Welsh Ap Richard, "son of Richard." This patient's insanity had started with general confusion and disposition to violence, and he suffered from simple mania with gay illusions and a tendency to mischief and violence, but with remissions and general good health. The week after T. J. Richard's admission, Gloucester Asylum's Day Book records a payment "for Mr. Prichard"—accidentally the correct name.

Did the patient T. J. Richards exist? His London address was not occupied by anyone named Richards, nor did the two "brothers" who signed the contract reside at the addresses they gave. There are no obituary notices or registration of the death of T. J. Richards during this period either. Uncharacteristically, the Gloucester newspapers did not cover the necessary inquest. One of the two medical men who signed T. J. Richards's medical certificate for admission could not be traced in Gloucestershire residential or the standard medical directories. Mr. Richards's name does not appear in the asylum's otherwise efficient accounts of payment, treatment, discharge, or death, nor do the Gloucestershire Court of Quarter Sessions archives contain the required legal documents.[33]

Gloucester Lunatic Asylum, safely distant from Bristol, Oxford, and London, was the ideal choice for The's confinement; Prichard knew the asylum and its physician Dr. Hitch very well. He had been a visitor and then inspector there for some time and had written about it positively. Hitch's observations and contribution of statistical information, including his patients' remarkably high recovery rate, were acknowledged in Prichard's book on insanity. Estlin had visited Hitch in 1842 also. Hitch corresponded with Prichard and stayed at the Red Lodge in 1845, when they were working on plans for the new county asylum for Somersetshire.[34]

About seven weeks after T. J. Richards's admission, the committee of the asylum granted Dr. Hitch permission to have a maximum of four private lunatics in his own separate residence, a situation that could account for Mr. Richards's disappearance from the asylum's records. Unfortunately, things got difficult for Hitch when the committee later rescinded that permission. He then sent several queries to the Lunacy Commission in London, asking advice about keeping individual patients. On December 29, 1845, Hitch was particularly concerned about a patient placed in lodgings on trial. He asked for advice on how to proceed with one such patient in his charge whom he thought unfit to be at large but whose family had refused to agree to having him returned to an asylum. Prichard had to sit through the meeting at which Hitch's letter was read and considered.[35] In "some pleasant lodgings in the neighbourhood of Gloucester" six weeks later, The was found hanging.

As a physician, asylum inspector, and author Prichard had long professional experience of the insane. But when it came to it, his desire for respectability prevailed. Like any other middle-class Victorian with a family member's state of mind to disguise, Prichard made special arrangements, such as The's leave of absence from university and a final out-of-the-way placement, and this is what had come of it.[36] Grieving and guilty, all he could do was carry on as usual. Walter Bagehot wrote that "Dr. & Mrs. Prichard have been at York but are returned, & were gone to Greenwich when I called this morning; they are certainly possessed of the faculty of locomotion."[37] Their whirlwind of activity did not blot out the memory of The's tragic end.

Somehow Prichard managed to pull together the fifth and final volume of *Physical History*, publishing it in 1847. Its huge mass of ethnographic data would be useful to future generations of anthropologists while a new edition of his popularizing *Natural History* attempted to counter growing polygenetic and inhumane racialist attitudes and destructive government policies. The reprint of *Different Forms of Insanity* came out, an appropriate reminder of his eminence as an alienist. After preparing a lecture that would define his science of humankind, he would be free to start the new project he had been considering for some time. His collection of crania had been growing, and he planned to publish a "Crania Britannica."

Con

Now that Jem was being consumed by tuberculosis, tall, thin, solemn, hard-studying young Constantine seemed set to fulfill his father's aspirations, despite his similarly "delicate" health. He started promisingly as a Balliol College, Oxford, scholar in 1837, throwing himself into the classics and theology and numbering founders of the Oxford Movement among his friends and tutors. His close friend and fellow consumptive Henry Balston became Prichard's patient, but on a harsh January day in 1841, Con was one of Balston's pallbearers at his funeral in Magdalen College Chapel.[38] Con went on to gain a First in 1841, Balliol Fellowship from 1842, and MA and English Essay Prize in 1844. Upon ordination in 1847, he left Oxford to take up the vice principalship of Wells Theological College.[39]

Prichard soon wrote Con in Wells by way of congratulation: "I think I am not at all anxious about the number of my remaining days. The greatest happiness of my life and the blessing for which I hope I am most thankful is to have my children ματ άνθςωον what they ought to be." After encouraging Con to move on from Wells soon and praising Jem's plan to write a biography of Hincmar that would elucidate Carolingian civil and ecclesiastical history, Prichard admitted he feared for adolescent Alboo's health.[40] Perhaps in contemplating his own end and the future of his surviving sons, Prichard was drawn to the memory of his father and a duty owed him. He sifted through the family archives and started writing Thomas Prichard's biography.

A high-achieving scholar and composer of sacred poetry, Con continued to associate with the men of the Oxford Movement, agreeing to write one of John Henry Newman's *Lives of the Saints*. He married Mary Alice Seymour, the sister of an Oxford friend and niece of the Duke of Somerset, in 1854 and had at least five children. That year he became rector of South

Luffenham, Rutland, in the gift of Balliol.[41] He died there of tuberculosis in 1869. The dean of Salisbury remembered him as "a man who impressed every one who knew him with a sense of his pure and high-minded nature. Constantine, after spending many years of his life in the care of country parishes, passed away without leaving the mark which his many friends expected. Two small volumes of Commentaries on the Romans and some other Epistles, and an admirable paper on 'Theories of the Atonement,' in the *North British Review*, were evidences of the delicacy and skill with which he handled difficult themes."[42] Among others who remembered him, Oxford contemporary Lord Chief Justice John Duke Coleridge wrote: "Certainly this world has not turned its sunny side on him. What between health, and means, and afflictions never long absent, he has been sorely tried. I think you and I will agree that we have known no better man, and not many really abler, yet how little has the world heard of him!" Another Oxford friend started preparing Con's poems for publication, but lost all but a few of the manuscripts.[43]

Two Alberts

The year 1847 was one of constant activity. With another new honorary membership to his name, corresponding member of the Russian Geographical Society, Prichard and Anna attended the Oxford BAAS meeting in June, the guests of Dr. Joseph Arnould, Prichard's old university friend, at nearby Wallingford. The Oxford meeting was thronging. One star attraction was the remarkable Michael Faraday. On a raised platform under the rotunda of the Radcliffe Library, Faraday posed with all the grace of a Roman god. So rapt was the great crush of ladies and gentlemen by his seamlessly choreographed demonstrations of galvanism, they forgot to interrupt with applause.[44] At the Ethnological Subsection, meanwhile, Prichard faced a "host of literati," including his friends Bunsen, Henry Hallam, and Hodgkin, and started reading his lecture on ethnology's relation to other branches of science. One member of his audience made Prichard more apprehensive than usual: "Prince Albert has just been exhibiting himself here in the Ethnological Section of the Association. Dr. Prichard and Chevalier Bunsen, and Dr. Latham went off about Ethnology, languages, ancient Egypt, etc., which the Prince tried hard to look as if he understood, but did not succeed completely.... The doctor slid off the platform during the rush of Prince Albert to a neighbouring corner. Bunsen's speech was to a considerable extent an eulogism on the Doctor's Book. Ethnology is only a subsection of the British Association."[45]

The Molines and Uncle Alfred Estlin visited Woburn Place in February 1848 to dance the fashionable polka at Albert Hermann's birthday party.[46] Alboo turned out most unlike his siblings. He started off as Prichard would have desired, matriculating at Merton College, Oxford, in 1849 and gaining a BA in due course. He became librarian of his father's old haunt, the Bristol Library, for a few years, but being disliked, he was forced out. After a spell in India editing the *Poona Times*, he married Mary Schilling, returned to England, was ordained in the Church of England, and held three successive curacies. Unlike the rest of the family, Albert Hermann was a committed and active socialist and eventually a convert to Roman Catholicism. He died in London in 1912, leaving an estate of £25 and an unmarried only daughter.[47]

1848

London was on tenterhooks. The year 1848 was rocked by revolutions across Europe. Would Britain be next? Chartists marched and made political demands while the government vigorously quelled dissent, mobilizing troops, swearing in a gentlemen militia, and evacuating the queen from the capital. A grandson remembered Prichard as completely uninterested in politics. Prichard witnessed these events but turned inward to his disappointments and regrets, both personal and professional. He had lost his father's guiding hand. Jem and Con were seeking meaning through the Oxford Movement's spiritual reform and renewal. Prichard's daughter recalled of him that "towards the latter part [of his life] he became rapidly more and more of a Catholic in faith and practice."[48] He continued researching, publishing, lecturing, and fulfilling his never-ending Lunacy Commission duties, traveling, summer and winter, day and night, in all weather. Walter Bagehot's was the first alarm:

> By the way you have no doubt heard that Dr. Prichard has been rather seriously ill at Salisbury. Mr. Proctor came home without him & Constantine went down directly & West soon followed. They do not expect to be able to move him for some days, I believe, & he seems to have suffered a good deal though he is now better.... I am sorry to say that I have just heard an unfavourable account of Dr. P. He has not got at all better, they say, & I shd. fear he was rather worse if anything. Constantine came to town today to fetch Dr. Tweedie.[49]

Prichard realized he was dying. He dictated to Con parting messages to several people on his mind. He particularly wanted Estlin to know the depth of his feelings and his belief they might both enjoy eternal salvation, no matter their differences in regard to doctrine. His illness had been brought on by exposure to the cold in driving across Salisbury Plain on a winter's night on a circuit of asylum inspections. Having brought Prichard home to Woburn Place, on December 20, 1848, several distinguished medical men, including Benjamin Travers and his son and Drs. Tweedie, Lawrence, Hodgkin, and Latham, held a consultation on their patient. Their efforts were to no avail. A severe feverish attack "proved to be of a rheumatic gouty character, baffling all the efforts of medical skill, and terminating his life after much suffering, by pericarditis . . . and extensive suppuration of the knee joint" on December 22.[50]

Francis Newman candidly reported Prichard had treated himself too "heroically": "He did not trust the medical men there, & doctored *himself* by bleeding & opium, after which he never rallied. His son (a surgeon) & Dr Tweedie, I am told, both condemn the opium, as did the Salisbury practitioner: and *I* condemn the bleeding! alas! I do not joke. It is indeed a great loss. Poor Mrs Prichard in a few years has lost two sons, a daughter & a husband, & it is feared may sink under it, though in soul quite tranquil & sustained."[51]

Eleven years later, Anna's body joined Prichard's and The's in Sellack churchyard. Several of Prichard's possessions were scattered among his family: a grandfather clock, the seals that appear in his portrait, a pair of candlesticks, some of his books, his father's snuff box, a Spanish piece of eight, a precious watercolor of his firstborn Annie sitting under a tree in her grandfather's garden, some medical illustrations by his lost friend John Pole, a few silhouettes, a diary of a long-ago trip to France, and a two-volume manuscript biography of his father.[52]

Conclusion

An Estimate of his Merits.
—George Rolleston, "Address to the Department of Anthropology"

Thomas Hodgkin attempted to sum up Prichard's qualities in a single sentence: "High moral and religious principle, an affectionate disposition, and instinctive sentiment of delicacy, propriety, and consideration of the feelings of others, and retiring modesty and simplicity of deportment, as much distinguished and endeared him in the domestic and social relations of life, as his literary and scientific attainments elevated him to the eminence he held in public estimation; he furnished, indeed, a bright example of the scholar, the gentleman, and the Christian." Medical educator Sir William Osler more succinctly wrote in 1908: "What a wonderful man Prichard was!"[1]

For a few decades Prichard was remembered as a famously erudite and prolific writer of a broad range of scientific works based on diligently amassed evidence. He participated in the creation of the human sciences, an advocate of modern scientific method and a role model for scientists in a transitional period when the exploration of deep time was bearing fruit and religion was starting to loosen its grip on scientific thought. Biographical articles on him can be found in *Celebrities of the Century*, successive editions of *Encyclopaedia Britannica*, *A Critical Dictionary of English Literature*, *The Dictionary of National Biography*, the more recent *Dictionary of Scientific Biography*, and online resources. He has a place in the histories of several disciplines.[2]

Prichard considered Johann Friedrich Blumenbach the initiator of the science of anthropology, while his contemporaries credited Prichard with its advent, certainly in its broader conception. E. B. Tylor, the anthropologist who would take his turn at being the founder of the British discipline, later wrote in his *Encyclopaedia Britannica* article "Anthropology" that Prichard, "perhaps of all others[,] merits the title of founder of modern anthropology." Sir Arthur Keith qualified this as "founder of British Anthropology."[3] With a bit of British bias, evolutionary biologist George Rolleston told the BAAS in 1875 that Prichard has been called, and, I think, justly, the "father of modern anthropology." . . . I compare his works to those of Gibbon and Thirlwall, and say that they have attained and seem likely to maintain permanently a position and importance commensurate with that of the "stately and undecaying" productions of those great English historians. . . . Still his works remain, massive, impressive, enduring—much as the headlands along our southern coast stand out in the distance in their own grand outlines, whilst a close and minute inspection is necessary for the discernment of the forts and fosses added to them, indeed dug out of their substance in recent times. If we consider what the condition of the subject was when Prichard addressed himself to it, we shall be the better qualified to take and make an estimate of his merits.[4]

This last sentence underpins this biography.

Prichardian anthropology structured the Ethnological Society of London during its early decades. Its founders had intended the society to assemble sound historical, cultural, psychological, archaeological, linguistic, and biological evidence that would demonstrate the unity and single origin of humankind. But new social and political realities ushered in a later nineteenth-century period of sterile race science. When this gave way to a more modern form of the discipline, its new founders with new values obscured the anthropology of Prichard's era.

Prichard was just as much a humanitarian as a defender of the faith. His conservativism is apparent yet he had much in common with his liberal friends and relatives; he was remarkable in his essentially humane attitude toward all humankind, from Indigenous peoples on the other side of the globe to the mentally ill of Britain. He held respectability in high regard; his reticence to engage openly in the great reform movements of his era preserved his status as an unbiased, sober scientist. He was at his most direct when he became perhaps the first proponent of "salvage ethnology," passionately calling for the protection of Indigenous peoples from extinction, not just to secure materials for study, but because he upheld universal human worth. Prichard's science was his humanitarian campaign.

In shaping the study of language into a tool of anthropology, Prichard participated in transforming the philology of the previous century into an early form of anthropological linguistics. He is credited with introducing German comparative and historical linguistics into British scholarship and with being the first to demonstrate convincingly Celtic's membership of the Indo-European language family. Prichard is now considered one of the founders of modern Celtic linguistics. He distinguished the members of the Bantu language group, established that the North African languages are related to the Semitic, and devised some descriptive terminology.

Prichard's exploration of the nature of the human mind united his medicine, psychiatry, and anthropology. He produced more accurate descriptions of epilepsy and dementia, refined the nosology of psychiatric conditions, and was dedicated to benefiting sufferers from these conditions. He was involved in attempting to secure asylum patients' more humane treatment and civil rights and their fair treatment under the law. His concept of moral insanity was mostly well received by the medical profession even while it was distrusted or dismissed by the legal profession and the general public. Debated for decades internationally, it is ancestral to various psychiatric conditions.

As for Prichard's medical practice, to ask whether his form of therapeutics actually benefited his patients is to ask the wrong question. He practiced traditional humoral medicine because that was what medicine was, but he realized laboratory-based scientific medicine would revolutionize it. His rejection of innovative phrenology and mesmerism was based on the weakness of their scientific bases. Despite welcoming scientific medicine, the laboratory was not for the likes of Prichard; rather he confined his observations and experiments to his patients, for example, in transfusing blood. His efforts to contribute to science are better represented by his book on biological theory. For a few decades he was credited with having efficiently overturned the science-inhibiting notion of a vital principle, until scientific discoveries rendered the topic irrelevant.

Prichard, a dutiful son and loving and exacting father, lived at a time of political, economic, social, and religious turmoil, in the ferment of reformism and during a revolution in science and technology. Within the framework of his sincerely held beliefs he labored to improve the world using the tools at his disposal. Were he alive today, he would recognize with pride the scientific disciplines he had helped to create. He would also be surprised to learn that the story of his scientific and personal life has provided a window onto British science and society during the Age of Improvement.

Notes

Preface

1. For a recent exploration of Prichard's anthropology and psychiatry, see Augstein, *James Cowles Prichard's Anthropology*.
2. Thomas Kerslake (1812–91). Kerslake, *T. Kerslake's Catalogue*; Constantine Estlin Prichard to Shaw, June 15, 1849, Correspondence Collection, RGS. For Prichard's books subsequently transferred to the University of Bristol Medical School Library, see the older items marked "7," donated by his grandson J. E. Prichard in "Library of the Bristol Medico-Chirurgical Society Fortieth List"; Munby, *Formation of the Phillipps Library*, 72. The eleven volumes would have comprised research material, as Prichard's personal papers were retained by his family.
3. Personal communication, the Rev. Edward Cowles Prichard. Aside from letters in collections around the world, Prichard's collection of crania was displayed in the Anatomy Department of the University of Bristol, on permanent loan from the Bristol Museum, while its catalogue is in the Bristol Museum Archives, file 1642. His grandson Edgar Albert Prichard donated Prichard's portrait to the Bristol Museum, file 205. Prichard's diplomas and certificates of membership of institutions are in Bristol Archives, 16082 (1–10).
4. Constantine Estlin Prichard to Augustin Prichard, July 5, [1859], and July 13, [1859], Woods family private collection.
5. T[heodore] Pocock, "Account of the Centenary Celebration of the Death of James Cowles Prichard, Tuesday, December 22, 1948, Royal Anthropological Institute, London," Prichard family private collection.
6. "Bristoliana," *Bristol Times*, February 7, 1912.
7. Kenneth Lee Pike, 1967, in Vermeulen, *Before Boas*, 34. See also Lightman, "Introduction," 30–35.

Introduction

1. Joseph John Gurney (1788–1857). Braithwaite, *Memoirs of Joseph John Gurney*, 440.
2. Whewell to Gladstone, July 22, 1842, Gladstone Papers, vol. 274, ff. 161–62, BL, Add.MS. 44,359.
3. Prichard to Wagner, April 30, 1841, Cod. Ms. R. Wagner VI: Prichard, Manuscripts and Scientific Collections, Niedersächsische State and University Library.

Apologia

1. For the issue of "assassination by anachronism," see Darnell, "A Critical Paradigm."
2. What constitutes the academic discipline of anthropology differs confusingly among countries. In some, ethnology is a subject in the humanities, while anthropology is the separate, specifically biological study of humankind ranked among the sciences. British and American academia agree in considering "anthropology" the umbrella term covering the four subdisciplines of biological anthropology, sociocultural anthropology, linguistics, and archaeology. The word "ethnology" in English now refers to the study of cultures comparatively while "ethnography" is the description of a culture—both function within the realm of sociocultural anthropology. Anglo-American anthropology notably spans the humanities and science in the same way Prichard defined his science of ethnology. While he avoided the term "anthropology," what he actually did is currently termed "anthropology," not "ethnology." This is why this biography anachronistically refers to Prichard's discipline as anthropology. For a further discussion of this, see chapter 12.

1. Time and Place

1. Prichard, "A Memoir of the Late Thomas Prichard Esq. of Ross, Part 1, 1847," 1–3, Orton family private collection.
2. Prichard, "Memoir, Part 1," 123. The town is now known as Ross-on-Wye.
3. Mellor and Wright, *Kingsdown*, 18–24, 50–52.
4. Edward Harford (1720–1806); John Scandrett Harford the elder (1752–1815). Raistrick, *Quakers in Science and Industry*, 128, 146–51; Minchinton, "Bristol," 69–89, 82–84; Minchinton, *British Tinplate Industry*, 17, 20–24.
5. Quaker John Barnes lived on Paul Street, Kingsdown Parade, from at least 1793 to 1800. Sale of the Dwelling-House in the Tenure of John Barnes, *Felix Farley's Bristol Journal* (hereafter *FFBJ*), March 23, 1793, 3, and October 4, 1800, 2; *Matthews's New Bristol Directory* lists him as (Private) Latin teacher and accomptant; Wilkinson, "French Emigres in England," 313–15. Philip de Rosemond was educated at the Mazarin College, and in the 1790s his address was "French Academy, Marlborough-street," *Matthews's New Bristol Directory*, 71. Mordente's *Spanish Language* is in at least five editions, 1807–22. He later sought financial support from the Royal Literary Fund, London. Rollin, *Histoire Romaine*; Rollin, *Histoire ancienne des egyptiens*; Prichard, "Memoir, Part 1," 139.
6. Richard Durban, Advertisement of His Academy in College Green, *FFBJ*, January 4, 1794, 3. The school prepared pupils for "Trade, the Navy, the Army, and the University."
7. A. Prichard, *A Few Medical & Surgical Reminiscences*, 15.
8. Symonds, *Some Account*, 7, 9; A. Prichard, *A Few Medical & Surgical Reminiscences*, 15.

9. Prichard, "A Memoir of the Late Thomas Prichard Esq. of Ross, Part 2, 1847–," 411, Gee family private collection.
10. Prichard, "Memoir, Part 1," 143.
11. Prichard, "Memoir, Part 1," 145–47.
12. A. Prichard, *A Few Medical & Surgical Reminiscences*, 6–7.
13. Beeson, *Bristol in 1807*, 189.
14. Hodgkin, "Obituary," 184; Symonds, *Some Account*, 7.
15. Blaise Castle Estate was landscaped by iconic Humphry Repton. Woolrich, "American in Gloucestershire," 185–89; Prichard, "Memoir, Part 1," 139–41.
16. "The Establishment" refers to the combined religious and social elite of Britain and their predominant beliefs and values, especially considering the nation's state religion, Anglican Protestantism, or the Church of England, otherwise called the Established Church.
17. The number of Bristol Quakers decreased from 636 to about 400 between 1830 and 1900. Sturge, *Some Recollections*, 48–49.
18. Sturge, *Some Recollections*, 17–20. Sturge thought Bristol's only great scientist was Prichard, confirmed by McDade, "'Particular Spirit of Enterprise,'" 285–86.
19. [Silliman], *Journal of Travels in England*, 2:162.
20. Richardson, "Eighteenth-Century British Slave Trade," 58, cited in Morgan, "Economic Development of Bristol." Bristol's share of the British slave trade in 1742 was 42 percent, in 1773–77, 10 percent; by 1807 it was a mere 1 percent.
21. Thomas Clarkson (1760–1846); John Prior Estlin (1747–1817). Marshall, *Anti-Slave Trade Movement*, 1–6.
22. John Baker Holroyd, Earl of Sheffield (1735–1821). Marshall, *Anti-Slave Trade Movement*, 7–21.
23. Evan Baillie (1741–1835), Whig MP (1802–12), and Charles Bragge Bathurst (1754–1831), Tory MP (1796–1812). Marshall, *Anti-Slave Trade Movement*, 21–26.
24. Atkinson, "Early Example of the Decline," 72.
25. Raistrick, *Quakers in Science and Industry*, 128, 148–49.
26. Minchinton, "Bristol," 85–86, 73–79.
27. E. Shiercliff, *The Bristol and Hotwell Guide, Containing an Account of the Ancient and Present State of that Opulent City* (Bristol: Bulgin and Rosser, 1805), in Beeson, *Bristol in 1807*, 19–22.
28. [Silliman], *Journal of Travels in England*, 2:155–56.
29. Julius Caesar Ibbetson et al., *A Picturesque Guide to Bath, Bristol Hotwells, the River Avon and the Adjacent Country* (London, 1773), in Beeson, *Bristol in 1807*, 12–13.
30. James P. Malcolm, *First Impressions or Sketches from Art and Nature. Animate and Inanimate* (London: Longman, 1807), in Beeson, *Bristol in 1807*, 10.
31. *New Bristol Guide* (1804), in Beeson, *Bristol in 1807*, 118.
32. Ibbetson et al., *Picturesque Guide to Bath*, 15–16.
33. McIntyre, "Mineral Water Trade," 2–10.

34. Latimer, *Annals of Bristol*, 71; [Silliman], *Journal of Travels in England*, 2:149–50.
35. Beeson, *Bristol in 1807*, 26–27; Latimer, *Annals of Bristol*, 71–72. For Andrew Carrick's description of the Hotwells in 1789 and 1816, see *Bristol Times*, October 18, 1862.
36. [Silliman], *Journal of Travels in England*, 2:152.
37. Ibbetson, *A Picturesque Guide to Bath, Bristol Hotwells*, in Beeson, *Bristol in 1807*, 28–29, 31–32, 64–67.
38. Malcolm, *First Impressions*, 200–201. Robert Southey (1774-1843). [Robert Southey], *Letters from England; by Don Manuel Alvarez Espriella* (London: Printed for Longman, Hurst, Rees and Orme, 1808), in Beeson, *Bristol in 1807*, 178.
39. Simond, *Journal of a Tour*, 17.
40. Shiercliff, *Bristol and Hotwell Guide*, 132–33.
41. *FFBJ*, January 10, 1807, in Beeson, *Bristol in 1807*, 134–35, 137.
42. *Bristol Gazette*, September 3, 1807, in Beeson, *Bristol in 1807*, 135. See also Bettey, *St James's Fair*.
43. [Silliman], *Journal of Travels in England*, 2:160.
44. George Weare Braikenridge, *Bristoliana*, in Beeson, *Bristol in 1807*, 136. A drawing of St. James's Fair indicates that the "Flying Coaches" and "Ups & downs" were a four-car wooden Ferris wheel and a roundabout/merry-go-round.
45. Latimer, *Annals of Bristol*, 5; Beeson, *Bristol in 1807*, 137–39.
46. Latimer, *Annals of Bristol*, 25–26; Beeson, *Bristol in 1807*, 139.
47. At this time, a Whig was generally a "liberal" or "reformer," committed to modernizing the system of Church and State and believing that power should be in the hands of propertied citizens through Parliament; a Tory was a "conservative" upholder of the status quo, excluding Dissenters, for instance, and championing the power of the monarchy and Established Church. It should be noted that the ruling elite's will to reform can be traced to expediency: repurposing themselves as pious reformers to avert their heads ending up on pikes, as had happened in France.
48. Dresser, "Protestants, Catholics, and Jews," 96–97. Dissenting Protestants, including Quakers and Unitarians, gained their full civil rights in 1828; Roman Catholics in 1829; Jews in 1858. See also Dresser, *Bristol*.
49. Samuel Taylor Coleridge (1772–1834). Lamoine, *Literature and Politics*, 150–51.
50. For Bristol scientists Thomas Beddoes and Humphry Davy, see chapter 2.
51. Hannah More (1745–1835). Crossley Evans, *Hannah More*, 1–5.
52. M. Jones, *Hannah More*, 134–35.
53. Crossley Evans, *Hannah More*, 6–12. Horace Walpole (1717–97). See also Stott, *Hannah More*.
54. Sturge, *Some Recollections*, 16.
55. But by the 1820s the Corporation had fallen into the hands of Tories allied with some "West India Whigs," carefully excluding liberal values. See Barry, "Bristol Pride," 25–47.
56. M. Harrison, "'To Raise and Dare Resentment,'" 558.

57. P. D. Jones, "Bristol Bridge Riot," 75–87.
58. P. D. Jones, "Bristol Bridge Riot," 89–91.
59. M. Harrison, "'To Raise and Dare Resentment,'" 578–79.
60. Latimer, *Annals of Bristol*, 20–21, 6–8. On a single night in 1803, press-gangs rounded up upward of two hundred men. A mob of Bristolians attempted to rescue them at Rownham Dock when a boy was killed in the fray.
61. Poole, "Documents in Focus," 2–6.
62. Prichard, "Memoir, Part 1," 283.
63. Malpass, *Bristol Dock Company*, 8, 20–23.
64. Prichard, "Memoir, Part 1," 145.
65. Obituary of Thomas Prichard, *FFBJ*, March 3, 1798, 3. Edward Prichard's marginalia: "I have heard my Father say all the Property in the house at Ross belonged to him & complain much of the distribution of it wch took place, which He had not the firmness or probably the inclination at the time to resist." Prichard, "Memoir, Part 1," 141.
66. Prichard, "Memoir, Part 1," 147–49.
67. Prichard, "Memoir, Part 1," 149.
68. Pontneddfechan, a village in the Brecon Beacons.
69. Prichard, "Memoir, Part 1," 151–53.
70. Samuel Dyer (1747–1809). Obituary of Samuel Dyer, *Bristol Mirror, Late Bonner and Middleton's Bristol Journal* (hereinafter *Bristol Mirror*), February 11, 1809, 3; "Samuel Dyer in Dictionary of Quaker Biography," London Society of Friends (hereafter LSF); Prichard, "Memoir, Part 1," 179, 267: "S. Dyer received rents for my father in Bristol, viz Ground rents of Prichard Street and other places in St Pauls." Dyer and Thomas Prichard corresponded about traveling on the Quaker ministry and Quaker affairs in 1800.
71. Prichard, "Memoir, Part 1," 181–91.
72. Prichard, "Memoir, Part 1," 201–3.
73. Prichard, Sale of 47 Park Street, *FFBJ*, April 26, 1800, 2. The Prichards had been living on Park Street for a few years in a substantial home built just before 1790, facing Great George Street and with a walled garden to the rear.
74. Prichard, "Memoir, Part 1," 281; Thomas Prichard Jr. to James Cowles Prichard, January 28, 1800, Birthday Book of the Prichard Family, property of the Fedden family. While in Bath James received from his brother Tom this letter, almost entirely devoted to their livestock and plans to consume it.
75. Prichard, "Memoir, Part 1," 153–57.
76. Rev. James Mills (d. 1834). Prichard, "Memoir, Part 1," 61.
77. Hodgson, *Society of Friends*, 29–57.
78. Prichard, "Memoir, Part 1," 167.
79. Prichard, "Memoir, Part 1," 179. Socinianism, a doctrine that professed adherence to Christian Scripture but denied the divinity of Christ and was naturally antitrinitarian, could not have been more abhorrent to Prichard.
80. Bristol street directories usually titled *Matthews's*, 1775–1809; Turpentine-distillery Business, *FFBJ*, May 30, 1761, 3; Obituary of John Cross, *FFBJ*, December 9, 1809, 3; Obituary of John Brent Cross, *FFBJ*, June 14, 1845, 8; John Brent

Cross, Letter to Richard Smith, July 13, 1831, Bristol Infirmary Biographical Memoirs (hereafter BIBM), vol. 11, 1813–17, 504–6, BA, 35893/36/k_i; Partnership of John Brent Cross, John Penrose and Edward Prichard, *FFBJ*, October 31, 1812, 2. Margaretta Cross (d. December 18, 1819, aged sixty-eight or sixty-nine) was sister of Samuel Love, minor canon of Bristol Cathedral; John Brent Cross (bapt. March 14, 1784). John, a chemist and druggist of 114 Redcliffe Street, was for a time in partnership with Prichard's brother Edward.
81. Prichard, "Memoir, Part 1," 157.
82. Prichard, "Memoir, Part 1," 169–75.
83. Prichard, "Memoir, Part 1," 287–91.
84. Prichard, "Memoir, Part 1," 3–5.
85. Prichard, "Memoir, Part 1," 7–9.
86. Prichard, "Memoir, Part 1," 9–21.
87. Prichard, "Memoir, Part 1," 23–25.
88. Prichard, "Memoir, Part 1," 27.
89. Richard Reynolds (1735–1816). Prichard, "Memoir, Part 1," 45–49; extracts from correspondence and a poem by members of the Cowles families, 1711–61, are on pp. 63–87.
90. Prichard, "Memoir, Part 1," 59; Commonplace Book of John Walker of Arnos Grove, Enfield Local Studies and Archives, GB053M/3.
91. Owen, *Life of Robert Owen*, 93–94; Mason, *Story of Southgate*, 61–62.
92. Prichard, "Memoir, Part 1," 61–63.
93. Prichard, "Memoir, Part 1," 87–89.
94. Prichard, "Memoir, Part 1," 25, 51–55.
95. Prichard, "Memoir, Part 1," 43–45, 137.
96. Prichard, "Memoir, Part 1," 122–23.
97. Prichard, "Memoir, Part 1," 95, 91–101.
98. Prichard, "Memoir, Part 1," 93.
99. Prichard, "Memoir, Part 1," 129.
100. Prichard, "Memoir, Part 1," 95–97.
101. Prichard, "Memoir, Part 1," 109–11.
102. Prichard, "Memoir, Part 1," 113–23. This includes more information about the Morgan and Reece families and property, including the Morgan descendants named White and Southall.
103. Prichard, "Memoir, Part 1," 125–27.

2. "A Studious Turn of Mind"

1. Poskett, *Horizons*, 1–30.
2. The inspiring science of the period is covered more fully in chapter 6.
3. Prichard, "Memoir, Part 1," 291–93.
4. Hodgkin, "Obituary," 184.
5. Parkinson, *Hospital Pupil*, 6–23.
6. Parkinson, *Hospital Pupil*, 25–58. It has been suggested that English society at this time did not value medical training in a physician, as training was associated with lower-class manual activities. Education in the classics was thought

superior to medical education as it prepared the physician to associate with (and charge high fees to) middle- and upper-class patients. The University of Oxford did allow Dissenters to attend but not gain a degree.

7. Singer and Holloway, "Early Medical Education," 9–10.
8. Fissell, "Physic of Charity," 33. In Bristol in 1800 there were thirty apothecaries, forty-five surgeons, and twenty MDs. See also Loudon, *Medical Care*; and Digby, *Making a Medical Living*.
9. "Prof. Frank's 'Travels in France and England'"; Newman, Rolleston, and Select Committee in Chitnis, "Edinburgh Professoriate," 274.
10. Herman Boerhaave (1668–1738). Singer and Holloway, "Early Medical Education," 1–2.
11. [Oxonian], *Observations on Medical Reform*, 420.
12. Whalley, "Vindication of the University."
13. Chitnis, "Edinburgh Professoriate," 275.
14. Prichard, "Memoir, Part 1," 291–93.
15. Edward and Tom were bound to Francis Fisher, Merchant, Orchard Street, Bristol, November 4, 1807, no duration specified. Bristol Apprentice Register, 1802–1819, n.p., BA, 05055(9); Prichard, "Memoir, Part 1," 299–301.
16. Wilkinson, "Nelson in Ross."
17. Edward Davies (1756–1831). "Celtic Davies" was author of *Celtic Researches*, a significant publication in the history of ethnology to which both James and his father subscribed, and another famous work on the mythology of the Druids. Prichard explained that Davies had been invited to meet the Prichards.
18. Prichard, "Memoir, Part 1," 305–7.
19. Aunt Newman's widower later destroyed all his wife's correspondence with Thomas Prichard, much to Prichard's regret.
20. Bristol Library Society Register, BCL, B7470–73. Between August 9, 1802, and June 20, 1803, Prichard borrowed C. N. S. Sonnini de Manoncourt, *Travels in Upper and Lower Egypt*, 1799; Jean Racine, *Oeuvres*, 1723; James Bruce, *Travels to Discover*, 1790; and other travel books. Between the start of 1803 and his leaving Bristol the following June, he read Thucydides, *De Bello Peloponnesiaco*, 1731; John Smith, *Galic Antiquities Consisting of a History of the Druids, Particularly Those of Caledonia*, 1780; and William Tooke, *History of Russia*, 1800.
21. The phrases surrounded by virgules imply Prichard's negative opinion of Pole. Prichard, "Memoir, Part 1," 295–98.
22. Wofinden, "Public Health in Bristol," 124–25.
23. Wedmore, *Thomas Pole*, 1–31; Medical Society of London, Ordinary Meetings Minutes, vol. 3, September 28, 1795–December 17, 1804, Medical Society of London Archives, WC, SA/MSL/D/2/1/3.
24. Inkster, "Public Lecture."
25. Pole, *Prospectus of a Course*, 1–6, 10–19. These lectures were advertised in the Bristol press in the autumn of 1802. Pole used the word "science" in its modern sense as Prichard would do in *Physical History*, 1813. William Whewell is credited with introducing "scientist" to Britain in 1830.

26. Thomas Pole, Report on the Amount of Rain in Bristol during the Last Ten Months of 1803, *FFBJ*, January 7, 1804, 3.
27. Griscom, *Year in Europe*, 167. Dr. Pole is described as a person of celebrity and of "much private worth."
28. McKenzie, "Social Activities," 87; Rowntree and Binns, *History of the Adult School Movement*, 12–14.
29. Wedmore, *Thomas Pole*, 31–32; Thomas Pole, "Memoir of the Life and Last Illness of John Pole," n.d., LSF, Box Q.
30. Prichard, "Memoir, Part 1," 315–19.
31. Bristol Library Society Register, BCL, B7472. During the summer of 1803 James borrowed Baron D. V. Denon, *Travels in Upper and Lower Egypt*, 1803; Thomas James Mathias, *Pursuits of Literature*, 1798; F. C. Hornemann, *Journal of Travels from Cairo to Mourzouk, in 1797–8*, 1802; John Barrow, *Account of Travels into the Interior of South Africa in 1797–9*, 1801–4; and J. L. E. Reynier, *State of Egypt after the Battle of Heliopolis*, 1802.
32. Prichard, "Memoir, Part 1," 321–23. Pope must have been entertaining the Prichards with stories of Edinburgh University lectures by the famous chemist Dr. Joseph Black (1728–99).
33. Simmons, *Medical Register for the Year 1779*, 109; Lambeth Palace, Muniment Book V 1802–1808, Lambeth Palace Library, London, FI/v, f.38v; J. G. Galt, "Letters Testimonial," 16; London Friends' Institute, *Biographical Catalogue*, 526–27; Hawson, "Robert Pope, M.D."; Robert Pope, Registered Copy Wills, NA, PROB/1735; "Dr. Pope and the Highwayman"; Peacock, "Memoirs of Percy Bysshe Shelley," 100; Childe-Pemberton, *Romance of Princess Amelia*, 190, 193, 194, 195; Aspinall, *King George IV*, 414, 419, 452. Robert Pope was born in Wilton, Wiltshire in 1748. There were only thirteen such degrees granted between 1800 and 1848. Dr. Pope discontinued another doctor's cupping, leeches, blisterings, and bleedings of Princess Amelia in favor of warm baths and powders.
34. Hodgkin, "Obituary," 184–85. This passage appears to have been communicated by William Tothill's son.
35. William Tothill (1760–1842). "Death of Mr William Tothill," *Western Daily Press*, December 3, 1875, 2.
36. Bristol Library Society Register, BCL, B7473; Prichard, "Memoir, Part 1," 325–27. James borrowed M. M. Clifford, *Egypt: A Poem, Descriptive of its Inhabitants*, 1802; and Henry Kett, *Elements of General Knowledge*, 1803.
37. Symonds, *James Cowles Prichard*, 7.
38. Symonds, *James Cowles Prichard*, 8; Cameron, "Richard Bright at Guy's," 267; General Entry of Pupils, 1805–1813, Wills Library, Guy's Hospital Medical School.
39. Lawrence, "Entrepreneurs and Private Enterprise," 191–92.
40. "Medical Education in 18th Century Hospitals," 40, 36, 38, 28.
41. William Babbington (1756–1833); William Allen (1770–1843). N. Colley, "Medical Chemistry at Guy's Hospital," 155–57; Payne, "William Babbington (1756–1833)"; Babbington and Curry, *Outlines of a Course of Lectures*, 1811.

42. James Curry (d. 1819). Bettany, "John Haighton (1755–1823)." See also "Notes from lectures in physiology given by John Haighton, 1801, 1810," 2 vols., WC, MSS.2663–64; Munk, *Roll of the Royal College*, 2; Curry, *Examination of the Prejudices*.
43. Cameron, "Richard Bright at Guy's," 263–64; Lawrence, "'Desirous of Improvements,'" 91.
44. William Charles Wells (1757–1817). W. D. Foster, "William Charles Wells Physician"; [Lister], Obituary of William Charles Wells.
45. Frederick William Herschel (1738–1822). Kofoid, "American Pioneer in Science," 80. Historians of science consider Wells's essay on dew an example of the ideal scientific approach, and Charles Darwin eventually acknowledged Wells had prior claim to being one of the proposers of the theory of organic evolution through natural selection, albeit in a limited form; Shryock, "Strange Case of Wells' Theory"; Journal Book of the Royal Society, vol. 38 (January 13, 1803–November 20, 1805), 524, and vol. 40 (November 10, 1808–November 21, 1811), 227, Royal Society of London Archives.
46. Thomas Turner (1756–1830); William Lister (1756–1830); Henry Cline (1750–1827). Munk, *Roll of the Royal College*, 26; T. B. H., "William Lister, M.D."; Birch, *Gentleman's Magazine*; Payne, "John Birch (1745–1815)," 64–65; Parsons, *History of St. Thomas's Hospital*, 1–36; Rhodes, "Mr. Cline's Surgical Lectures"; Bettany, "Sir Astley Paston Cooper (1768–1841)," 137–39; Lawrence, "Entrepreneurs and Private Enterprise," 172.
47. Newman to Ann (Prichard) Newman, n.d., c. October 1805, Henry Newman Letter Book 2/6, LSF, Strongroom 1, case 101.
48. Bristol Library Society Register, BCL, B7475–76. Between April and August 1805, James concentrated on reading mostly histories: F.-M. A. Voltaire, *Oeuvres completes*, 1784; J. H. Zschoche, *History of the Invasion of Switzerland*, 1803; Edward Gibbon, *History of the Decline and Fall of the Roman Empire*, 1776–88; Richard Colley Wellesley, *Notes Relative to the Late Transactions in the Marhatta Empire*, 1804; and A. J. P. Segur, *Les femmes: Leur condition et leur influence dans l'ordre social chez différentes peuples anciens et modernes*, 1803.

3. MD, Edin

1. [Silliman], *Journal of Travels in England*, 3:203–4.
2. Prichard, "Memoir, Part 1," 329–33.
3. Prichard, "Memoir, Part 1," 339–43.
4. Prichard, "Memoir, Part 1," 345–49.
5. Prichard, "Memoir, Part 1," 337–39.
6. Prichard, "Memoir, Part 1," 357.
7. Prichard, "Memoir, Part 1," 353–55.
8. Simond, *Journal of a Tour*, 495–98.
9. For Scottish Enlightenment influence on medical education at the University of Edinburgh, see Chitnis, "Edinburgh Professoriate"; and Lawrence, "Medicine and Culture."

10. William Cullen (1710–90); Joseph Black (1728–99); James Hutton (1726–97); John Leslie (1766–1832). Holland, *Recollections of Past Life*, 85–86.
11. Dugald Stewart (1753–1828). Burke, "Kirk and Causality in Edinburgh," 340–54.
12. Chitnis, "Edinburgh Professoriate," 259–71, 321–23. See also Rosner, *Medical Education*.
13. Jefferson to Stewart, June 23, 1789, in Horn, *Short History of the University*, 64.
14. Jenkinson, "Role of Medical Societies," 253–75; Jenkinson, "Medical Societies and the Scottish Enlightenment," 69–84.
15. Morrell, "University of Edinburgh," 158, 159.
16. Morrell, "Medicine and Science," 41–48.
17. Sweet and Waterston, "Robert Jameson's Approach," 82.
18. Abraham Gottlob Werner (1749–1817); Robert Jameson (1794–1854); John Playfair (1748–1819). Flinn, "James Hutton and Robert Jameson," 256; Chitnis, "Edinburgh Professoriate," 212–24. Much later Jameson abandoned Wernerianism for Huttonian theory. He may have been a secret adherent of Lamarckian evolutionary theory too.
19. Morrell, "University of Edinburgh," 160–61.
20. Morrell, "University of Edinburgh," 164, 166.
21. Morrell, "Medicine and Science," 40–43.
22. Morrell, "University of Edinburgh," 164.
23. Kaufman, *Medical Teaching in Edinburgh*, 27.
24. Tyson, "Cumbrian Medical Student," 201.
25. [Silliman], *Journal of Travels in England*, 3:207.
26. "Lodging Houses," 70.
27. John Davy, unpublished manuscript quoted in Smith, "History of Nitrous Oxide," 349.
28. Tyson, "Cumbrian Medical Student," 202–3.
29. [Silliman], *Journal of Travels in England*, 3:204.
30. Chitnis, "Edinburgh Professoriate," 324–41.
31. Chitnis, "Edinburgh Professoriate," 310–17.
32. "Prof. Frank's 'Travels in France and England,'" 331–32.
33. Tyson, "Cumbrian Medical Student," 202–3.
34. Jones and Gemmill, "Notebook of Robley Dunglison." See also chapter 5 for clinical practice and therapeutics in Bristol.
35. Y., "Account of Medical Education," 306.
36. Johnson, *Guide for Gentlemen*. For those wanting degrees, the first year should include anatomy, institutions of medicine, infirmary, and materia medica; second year, chemistry, clinical lectures, infirmary, practice of medicine; and third year, anatomy, botany, midwifery, practice of medicine, and infirmary. Moral philosophy, natural philosophy, and mathematics are also recommended. Professor Hamilton generously praised his own course and condemned his enemies' courses.
37. University of Edinburgh, "Matriculation Register, 1804–1816," 1805, Heritage Collections, UE, IN1/ADS/STA/3.

38. Thomas Charles Hope (1766–1844). Clow and Clow, *The Chemical Revolution*, 599, in Chitnis, "Edinburgh Professoriate," 181; Bower, *Edinburgh Student's Guide*, 42–44.
39. Morrell, "Practical Chemistry," 70. The RMS bought its own chemistry apparatus.
40. "Biographical: Dr. Thomas Charles Hope," 158–59. See also Chitnis, "Edinburgh Professoriate," 180–87.
41. [Brown], *Notice of the Life and Character*; Christison, *General Diffusion of Knowledge*; Steven, *History of the High School*, 164; "Late Professor Christison," 186–87.
42. John Davy quoted in Smith, "History of Nitrous Oxide," 349.
43. Prichard was elected Ordinary Member of the RMS on November 8, 1805; Royal Medical Society of Edinburgh, *General List of Members* (1823), 52. He was elected Honorary Member of the RMS on April 2, 1841. Royal Medical Society of Edinburgh, *General List of Members* (1850), 74; Kaufman, *Medical Teaching in Edinburgh*, 153–57; Royal Medical Society of Edinburgh, Certificate of James Cowles Prichard as an Extraordinary Member of the Royal Medical Society of Edinburgh, May 1808, BA, 16082(1)a.
44. Prichard, "Memoir, Part 1," 369–71.
45. Prichard, "Memoir, Part 1," 363–65. The "cave of Trophonius" refers at its most moderate to a passage in Aristophanes' *Clouds* meaning "to sustain a fright." At its harshest, it likens Edinburgh culture to one of horror and obscenity bringing about insanity.
46. Thomas Hancock (1783–1849). Prichard, "Memoir, Part 1," 365–67.
47. Prichard, "Memoir, Part 1," 367.
48. Prichard, "Memoir, Part 1," 367–69.
49. Royal Medical Society, Minute Book, Oct. 18, 1805–April 26, 1811, RMSE.
50. "University of Edinburgh (List of Medical Classes for 1806–7)," 506; Tyson, "Cumbrian Medical Student"; *Post-Office Annual Directory*, 84; Hope, Class List for Courses in Chemistry, 1806–1826, Special Collections, UE, lists Prichard as "October 28, 1807, ticket no. 199, James Cowles Prichard, Herefordsh., Drummond St. 15 Fowell."
51. Dabit Deus his quoque finem: "God will put an end to these troubles as well" (Virgil); Prichard, "Memoir, Part 1," 375–77.
52. University of Edinburgh Matriculation Register 1804–1816, Discipuli 1806; James Gregory, Class List of the Students Attending the Lectures on the Practice of Medicine, in the University of Edinburgh, 1790/1–1811/12, Heritage Collections, UE, EUA, CA14.
53. Select Committee II, 87, in Chitnis, "Edinburgh Professoriate," 304. See also Barfoot, "James Gregory"; and [P. Gregory], *Records of the Family*, 63, 65.
54. Bettany, *Eminent Doctors*, 106; "Biographical Notice of the Late Dr. Gregory," 426.
55. Lawrence, "Edinburgh Medical School," 269.
56. James Hamilton the younger (1767–1839). James Hamilton, Lists of Students Attending the Lectures on Obstetrics, 1802–1810, UEL, EUA, CA14; Johnson,

Guide for Gentlemen, 26–32; Young, "James Hamilton (1767–1839)," 62–67; Simpson, "History of the Chair," 494–96; Obituary of James Hamilton, 102.

57. Prichard, "Memoir, Part 1," 377–81.
58. University of Edinburgh, Minutes of Senatus Academicus, vol. 2, July 31, 1790–December 19, 1811, 440–42, Heritage Collections, UE, EUA, IN/GOV/SEN/MIN/II.
59. "University of Edinburgh (List of Medical Classes for 1807-8)," 498–99. Prichard's last year at Edinburgh began with Dr. Rutherford lecturing on clinical cases at the Infirmary. University of Edinburgh Matriculation Register, 1804–1816, Discipuli 1807.
60. Alexander Monro Tertius (1773–1859). Ashworth, "Charles Darwin as a Student," 98.
61. Lawrence, "Edinburgh Medical School," 265–66.
62. Johnson, *A Guide for Gentlemen*, 5–10.
63. John Barclay (1758–1826). Grant, *Story of the University*, 2:390–91.
64. Herman Boerhaave (1668–1738); John Brown (1735–88). Lawrence, "The Edinburgh Medical School," 62.
65. Andrew Duncan (1744–1828). Huie, *Harveian Oration*, 5–20.
66. Bower, *Edinburgh Student's Guide*, 54–63; Duncan, *Reports of the Practice*, 33–38; Prichard, "Letter in Testimony to the Qualification of Andrew Duncan, Jun," in Duncan, *Additional Testimonials*, 24–25.
67. Daniel Rutherford (1749–1819). Grant, *Story of the University*, 2:382–84; Weeks, "Daniel Rutherford," 101–7.
68. James Home (1760–1844). Chitnis, "Edinburgh Professoriate," 293–94.
69. Dugald Stewart's moral philosophy course and his *Elements of the Philosophy of the Human Mind* (1792) were the essential resources at the University of Edinburgh on the subject of insanity. Prichard borrowed this book from the Bristol Library in 1814 and again in 1828. See also chapter 8.
70. Ritchie, "Double Centenary," 30–37.
71. For Prichard's student anthropological compositions, see chapter 6.
72. "Biography of the Late Professor Jameson," 574.
73. See especially Chitnis, "Edinburgh Professoriate," 197–207.
74. Hodgkin, "Obituary," 186.
75. Royal Medical Society, Minute Book, Oct. 18, 1805–April 26, 1811; Royal Medical Society, Annual Lists of Subjects of Dissertations 1797–98 to 1820–21, year 1807-8, no. 19, and year 1808-9, no. 9; J[ames] C[owles] Prichard, *Of the Varieties of the Human Race*, no. 3, 87–133; and *Virulent Gonorrhoea*, no. 3, 171–88, RMSE.
76. Royal Medical Society, Minute Book, Oct. 18, 1805–April 26, 1811; Royal Medical Society, Apparatus Committee, Minute Book, May 7, 1796–June 3, 1829, RMSE.
77. Royal Medical Society, Minute Book, Oct. 18, 1805–April 26, 1811.
78. [W. Carpenter], "[Oration at the] Centenary," 85–86, in which he lists the RMS's great scientific events, including Prichard's *Physical History of Man*; Royal Medical Society of Edinburgh, *Dissertations by Eminent Members*.

79. Thomas Hancock (1783–1849). Finsbury Dispensary, Monthly Minutes March 25, 1808–April 27, 1814, June 2, 1808, L5.11, Finsbury Library (which houses many other documents about Hancock's association with the dispensary); Annals, vol. 18 (1807–1811), f. 117, Royal College of Physicians of London Archives; Guardian Society for the Preservation of Public Morals, *Eighth Report*, [4].
80. Hancock, "On Lunatic Asylums," *Belfast Monthly Magazine* 4 (January 31, 1810): 1–3; (March 31, 1810): 162–66; (May 31, 1810): 344–47; Hancock, "Dr. Hancock's Account of the Asylum for Lunatics, at York," *Belfast Monthly Magazine* 8 (April 30, 1812): 256–60; Hancock, *Researches into the Laws*, 340, 342, 346–47; Hancock, *Laws and Progress*; May, *Memoir of Samuel Joseph May*; Hancock, *Essay on Instinct*, 420f; Journal Book of the Royal Society, vol. 45 (February 8, 1827–April 29, 1830), 433, Royal Society of London Archives; London Friends' Institute, *Biographical Catalogue*, 329–31.
81. See chapter 14.
82. Joseph Arnould (1786–1859). Justices of the Peace, Berkshire, Justices Roll 1801–1895, Berkshire Record Office, Reading, Q/JL1; "Death of Joseph Arnould, Esq., M.D.," *Reading Mercury, Oxford Gazette*, June 18, 1859, 4.
83. Despatches, Officers, and Individuals, 1818, Colonial Office, Barbados, Original Correspondence, NA, CO28/87, no. 36, fol. 36; Biographical Sketch of Renn Hamden, 177; "Election for the Borough of Lyme Regis and Charmouth," *Barbados Globe and Colonial Advocate*, August 31, 1837, 2; Obituary of Renn Hamden, *Liberal*, May 12, 1852, 2.
84. Kenneth Francis Mackenzie (1751–1831). Prichard, *De generis*, copy in the Royal College of Surgeons of England, London.
85. "Obituary: Death of an Eminent Scottish Physician," *New York Herald*, August 12, 1862, 5; Mackenzie, "Analysis of Compact Feldspar" and others; Holland to Holland, April 7, 1811, NLS, Acc. 7515; [Lennox], *Three Years with the Duke*, 225–26; Mackenzie, *Notes on Haiti*, iv.
86. Mackenzie, *Practical Observations*; Burial of Patrick Mackenzie, April 10, 1823, Burial Register, St. Anne, Westminster, Westminster Public Library.
87. Prichard, "Memoir, Part 1," 385.
88. University of Edinburgh Medical Faculty, Minutes of the Proceedings of the Medical Faculty, April 30, 1798–May 1811, Heritage Collections, UE, EUA, IN1/ACA/MED.
89. "Questions Proposed to a Candidate," 340–42.
90. Holland to Holland, July 22, 1811, Sir Henry Holland, Letters to His Father, NLS, Acc. 7515.
91. Prichard, "Memoir, Part 1," 385–89.
92. University of Edinburgh, Minutes of Senatus Academicus, vol. 2, 385–89; Holland to Holland, June 24, 1811, Sir Henry Holland, Letters to His Father, NLS, Acc. 7515. The newly created Dr. Holland estimated the cost of printing his thesis would be £7, especially as he had to give copies to the professors, ten to the library, and two each to his fellow students. See also Morrell, "University of Edinburgh," 169.

93. Y., "Account of Medical Education," 303–6; "Exposition of the Present State," 501.
94. University of Edinburgh Medical Faculty, Minutes of the Proceedings of the Medical Faculty, April 30, 1798–May 1811, 468.
95. Holland to Holland, July 1, 1811, Sir Henry Holland, Letters to His Father, NLS, Acc. 7515.
96. Record of University of Edinburgh Laureations and Degrees, 1585–1809, Heritage Collections, UE, EUA, IN1/ADS/STA/1/1. The page is titled "Formula Sponsionis Candidatis deferri solita qui sunt ex eorum Secta quos Angli Quakers vocant."
97. "Graduations at Edinburgh," 507–8; Certificate of Degree of Doctor of Medicine from the University of Edinburgh Granted to James Cowles Prichard, June 24, 1808 (Sealed, signed by the principal and nineteen professors), BA, 16082 (1)b; University of Edinburgh, Minutes of Senatus Academicus, vol. 2, 468–69. Among the thirty-seven students who graduated MD on the same day, twelve were from England or Wales, while Scotland accounted for eight, Ireland eleven, the Caribbean four, and America two.
98. Holland to Holland, July 1, 1811, Sir Henry Holland, Letters to His Father, NLS, Acc. 7515.
99. Prichard, "Memoir, Part 1," 389–91.
100. Prichard, "Memoir, Part 1," 393–95.
101. Samuel Prichard sold out of the agreement and emigrated to a log cabin on the Wabash, Illinois, where he died of fever.
102. Prichard, "Memoir, Part 1," 397–99, 401.
103. "John Hudson (1773–1843)"; Venn, *Alumni Cantabrigienses*, 196. Prichard is listed as admitted pensioner, tutor Mr. Hudson, and did not graduate in Ball and Venn, *Admissions to Trinity College*, 56. He matriculated February 18, 1809, at Trinity College, University of Cambridge, Matriculations, December 17, 1751–May 24, 1823, University of Cambridge Archives, Matr. 4.
104. Slee, "Oxford Idea," 62–63.
105. Stephen, *Lectures in the History of France*, vol. 1, 1851, vi–viii, in Roach, "Victorian Universities," 133; Slee, "Oxford Idea," 64.
106. Foster, *Alumni Oxonienses*, 1152.
107. Society of Friends, Bristol, Men's Monthly Meeting Minutes 1801–9, August 4, 1809, BA, SF/A1/19; St James Bristol, Baptisms and Burials, January 1, 1797–December 27, 1812, 153, BA, P/st, H./R1 (i). Some historians have anachronistically and mistakenly concluded that Prichard converted to Anglicanism in order to gain admittance to the English universities.
108. Hodgkin, "Obituary," 187.
109. Stafford, "Religion and the Doctrine," 381, 384.
110. Medical Society of London, Ordinary Meeting, Minute Book No. 5.
111. Lord Grenville (1759–1834). "Lord Grenville," 708–12; Cross to Smith, July 13, 1831, BIBM, 11:504–6, 4.
112. Prichard to Daubeny, June 22, 1835, Papers of Charles Daubeny, Magdalen College Library, UO, F26/C1/36.

4. Citizen, Husband, Gentleman

1. Henry Hunt (1773-1835). Beeson, *Bristol in 1807*, 115.
2. Latimer, *Annals of Bristol*, 35, 38-39.
3. Latimer, *Annals of Bristol*, 36-47.
4. Beeson, *Bristol in 1807*, 116.
5. Poole, "To Be a Bristolian," 76-95.
6. M. Harrison, "'To Raise and Dare Resentment,'" 557-85.
7. L. Colley, "Apotheosis of George III," 102-12.
8. Powell, *Bristol Commercial Rooms*, 13-18.
9. Annual subscriptions paid by J. C. Prichard 1811-22, Bristol Commercial Rooms Share Register, BCL, B20732.
10. Simond, *Journal of a Tour*, 18.
11. Sturge, *Some Recollections*, 29-30.
12. The Green Album, c. 1829-1838, Orton family private collection; Beeson, *Bristol in 1807*, 37.
13. Sturge, *Some Recollections*, 34.
14. Bristol Library Society, Subscription Book, 1773-1872, BCL, B7530, 7532; Bristol Library Register, BCL, B7481; *Edward Sheircliffe's Catalogue*, in Hapgood, *Friends to Literature*, 3.
15. Bristol Library Society, Minute Book of the Annual General Meeting, BA, 32079/153, f. 90, also in Hapgood, *Friends to Literature*, 12-13.
16. Kaufman, "John Peace to William Wordsworth," 193-99.
17. Bristol Library Society, Subscription Book 1773-1872, 62. At first Prichard borrowed books on his father's ticket, but in 1803 Thomas Prichard transferred his membership to his son, who in turn transferred it to his friend John Brent Cross upon leaving his studies with Dr. Pole. On settling back in Bristol, he resubscribed to the Library Society on May 28, 1810, and ended his membership on March 3, 1846, having moved to London.
18. Maria Edgeworth (1768-1849). Hare, *Life and Letters*, 19.
19. Hapgood, *Friends to Literature*, 7-9. Membership peaked at nearly three hundred in the 1810s; Shiercliff, Bristol and Hotwell Guide, in Beeson, *Bristol in 1807*, 133.
20. Seyer, *Outline of Proposals*; Bristol Library Society, Minute Books of Committee, 1807-1856, 2 vols., BA, 32079/LS/M/4-5, lists Prichard as attending 287 meetings between 1812 and 1835; Bristol Library Society, General Meeting Book, December 2, 1772-March 28, 1870, BA, 32079/LS/M/1; Bristol Library Registers, BCL, B7485-87. The Bristol Central Library's register of books borrowed tracks Prichard's interests over the years. Carter, Notice of the Bristol Library Society Annual Dinner at 4 o'clock on April 18, 1814; General Meeting of the Bristol Library Society, August 14, 1815, FFBJ, July 30, 1814, 3; Seyer, *Outline of Proposals*.
21. "Rev. Samuel Seyer," 471-72.
22. "Mr. John Peace," 577-78; [Peace], *Axiomata Pacis*. Prichard was Peace's physician.

23. Hapgood, *Friends to Literature*, 22–23. Prichard's son Albert Hermann succeeded John Peace as librarian in 1855, and in the same year the library moved to a wing of Bishop's College, followed by amalgamation with the Bristol Institution in new premises at the top of Park Street. In 1906 it became the foundation of the Public Library in College Green.
24. As well as *T. Kerslake's Catalogue* of his books, Prichard's grandson J. E. Prichard donated many medical books to a medical society; from there they were given to the Medical School of the University of Bristol. The pre-1848 books on the donation list are likely to have been Prichard's. "Library of the Bristol Medico-Chirurgical Society Twenty-Eighth List"; "Library of the Bristol Medico-Chirurgical Society Fortieth List."
25. Byron, *English Bards and Scottish Reviews* (1809), in Beeson, *Bristol in 1807*, 117.
26. Sturge, *Some Recollections*, 21–23.
27. James Sadler (1753–1828). Penny, *Up, Up and Away!*, 9–10.
28. Latimer, *Annals of Bristol*, 41.
29. Sturge, *Some Recollections*, 25–26.
30. John Wesley (1703–91). Elliott-Binns, *Early Evangelicals*, 333–37.
31. By obtaining temporary dispensations, Dissenters were sometimes exempted from signing the oath to the Established Church and allowed to serve in local government.
32. John Ryland (1753–1825) and Robert Hall (1764–1831). Ryland, *Pastoral Memorials*, 34, for Prichard being called in consultation to the death bed of this influential Baptist minister in 1824; R. Hall, *Works of Robert Hall*, 6:111, for Prichard being called in consultation shortly before Hall's death in 1831, and 133–34, for a long extract of a letter from Prichard to Dr. Frederick Thackeray of Cambridge, outlining the findings of Hall's postmortem; J. Foster, *Life and Correspondence*, 75, 96–98, for the similar case of another Baptist minister, the Rev. William Anderson (1784–1833): "Dr. P. attended him most assiduously, with all the kind anxiety of an affectionate friend." Hall had previously written that he had been acquainted with Prichard, "for whose qualities I have a high esteem, while I am amazed at his attainments, and his prodigious *faculty* of attaining."
33. Hickey, *History of the Old Chapel*.
34. Prichard, "Memoir, Part 1," 395.
35. Prichard, "Memoir, Part 1," 411–13; Society of Friends, Bristol, Men's Monthly Meeting Minutes, 1810–18, September 25, 1810, BA, SF/A1/21.
36. John Prior Estlin (1747–1817), minister of Lewin's Mead Unitarian Chapel, 1770–1817; Robert Southey was Bristol-born and late in life was Prichard's friend. Hobhouse, *Recollections*, 2; Cottle, *Robert Southey and Bristol*, 2–3.
37. O. Griffiths, "Side Lights," 126–29.
38. Latimer, *Annals of Bristol*, 35.
39. Latimer, *Annals of Bristol*, 36–37.
40. Latimer, *Annals of Bristol*, 33.
41. Living, *Bristol's Gas Supply*, 2–3.

42. Latimer, *Annals of Bristol*, 45–46.
43. Latimer, *Annals of Bristol*, 53.
44. Marriage of James Cowles Prichard and Anna Maria Estlin on Thursday, February 28, 1811, FFBJ, March 2, 1811, 3; Bristol Diocesan Registry, Marriage License Register, January 1804-June 1827, BA, EP/J/3/3/8.
45. Prichard, "Memoir, Part 1," 417–19.
46. *Second Annual Report of the Bristol Infant School*, 7; Birthday Book; Will of James Cowles Prichard, proved February 5, 1849, under £10,000, NA, PROB 11/2088/255.
47. Prichard, "Memoir, Part 1," 425.
48. Prichard, "Memoir, Part 1," 427–29.
49. Obituary of Anna Maria Prichard, 1812–19, FFBJ, June 5, 1819, 3. Anna Maria Prichard died May 29, 1819, and was first buried in the Unitarian Cemetery, then reinterred in Anglican Redland Green Chapel graveyard.
50. Prichard, "Memoir, Part 1," 449–51.
51. Certificate of City of Bristol, The Oath of a Burgess, Register Book of Burgesses No. 17, 263, also inserted between 208 and 209, Birthday Book.
52. Richard Hart Davis (1766–1842); Henry Hunt (1733–1838). Latimer, *Annals of Bristol*, 50–53; Williams, *Parliamentary History of the County*, 129–30. "Plumping" means giving both votes to the same candidate. Prichard voted for the conservative candidates in the Parliamentary elections of 1812, 1818, 1832, 1835, 1837, and 1841; he did not vote in 1820 and 1830, Bristol Poll Books, BCL. While a loyal "King and Country" Tory, Prichard maintained the dignity of a physician and did not join the local militia and ride about on horseback, as mistakenly recorded in Augstein, *James Cowles Prichard's Anthropology*, 11.
53. Edward Protheroe (1774–1856). Latimer, *Annals of Bristol*, 51–53.
54. [Morgan], *Hints towards the Formation*, with several in BCL; Prudent Man's Friend Society, Report of a Meeting, December 22, 1812, *Bristol Mercury*, January 4, 1813, 2; Latimer, *Annals of Bristol*, 53–54, 69–70. A native of Bristol, Quaker Richard Reynolds (1735–1816) made a huge fortune as an industrialist in Coalbrookdale before returning to Bristol, where his philanthropy exceeded £200,000.
55. Hole, *Early History*, 256–60.
56. A reference to an unnamed infant. Susanna (Bishop) Estlin (1760–1842). Prichard, "Memoir, Part 1," 451–53.
57. B. and O. Smith, Advertisement for the Sale by Auction of 39 College Green, FFBJ, October 10, 1812, 2; Alfred Estlin, Advertisement for Sale of Let of 39 College-Green, FFBJ, April 29, 1820, 3. The Prichards left 39 College Green in 1820, perhaps because of creeping commercialization of the neighborhood. The house was destroyed by enemy action on the night of November 24, 1940.
58. Prichard, "Memoir, Part 1," 457–59.
59. Latimer, *Annals of Bristol*, 54.
60. Birthday Book. Augustin and his children contributed to this large volume, but he also pasted in some of his grandfather's and father's letters and some

family artwork. Augustin wrote in it: "Having recently found, among some old papers, this short but very interesting account of family events in 1814, in my mother's handwriting, I think for two or three reasons that it ought to be preserved in our birthday book, & accordingly I transcribe it—Jan 30. 1892 A.P." Anna Maria's account of family life, her husband's efforts, and current affairs is copied onto pages 179–82 and used in this passage. See chapter 6 for Prichard's early anthropological publications.

61. Latimer, *Annals of Bristol*, 59–60.
62. See chapter 5.
63. "Comedies of Aristophanes."
64. James Cowles Prichard, Advertisement for a Course of Medical Lectures Commencing March 8, 1814, *Bristol Mirror*, February 26, 1814, 3; James Cowles Prichard, Advertisement for a Course of Medical Lectures Commencing November 6, 1815, *FFBJ*, October 7, 1815, 3. See also chapter 5.
65. John Cave et al., Petition to James Fowler, Mayor, *Bristol Mirror*, July 2, 1814, 2. The petition had the involvement of major Tory Establishment figures such as the prominent clergymen Thomas Biddulph and Samuel Seyer but also the Dissenter John Ryland. As for politicians, there were the Fripps, Thomas Castle, and Charles Elton; Prichard's fellow medical men included John Edmond Stock, his former teacher Dr. Pole, and Reforming Whig Dr. Edward Kentish. But Prichard's name is not on Letter to the Mayor, *FFBJ*, May 10, 1823, 3.
66. "Slave Trade," *Bristol Mirror*, July 9, 1814, 3; Notice concerning the Suppression of Slave Trade Petition, *Bristol Mirror*, July 16, 1814, 3; "Slave Trade," *Bristol Mercury*, July 18, 1814, 3.
67. Bartholomew Barry, "Education of the Poor [Appeal for Donations]," *FFBJ*, February 22, 1812; *Annual Report of the National Society*, 5.
68. "Bristol Diocesan Society, for the Education of the Poor in the Principles of the Established Church," *FFBJ*, January 22, 1814, 3.
69. Prichard to Susan Lewis, November 3 and December 27, 1815, Bundle of letters, Prichard Family, Records of Rev. Theodore Innes Pocock, BA, 46875/Co/3.
70. Latimer, *Annals of Bristol*, 62–63.
71. Marriage of Mary Prichard and Robert Moline, September 28, 1814, *Bristol Gazette and Public Advertiser* (hereafter *Bristol Gazette*), October 13, 1814, 3; Green Album; Marriage of Edward Prichard and Rebecca Merrick, November 28, 1814, *Bristol Gazette*, December 22, 1814, 3. The ceremony took place at the Friends' Meeting House, Manchester, indicating that Edward was still a Quaker; Prichard, "Memoir, Part 1," 457–59.
72. See chapter 5.
73. Edward Colston (1636–1721). "Colston's Anniversary," *Bristol Mirror*, November 18, 1815, 3; Dolphin Society, *Bristol Mirror*, November 16, 1816, 3; "Colston's Anniversary [November 13, 1820, at the White Lion]," *Bristol Mirror*, November 18, 1820, 3. Prichard attended six annual meetings of the Dolphin Society between 1815 and 1842, according to its newspaper reports.

74. Prichard, "Remarks on the Treatment of Epilepsy," Bristol, July 8, 1815; its positive review and abstract appeared in *London Medical and Physical Journal* 34 (December 1815): 517-19. See also chapter 8.
75. Francis Prichard (November 5, 1814–February 3, 1817). Prichard, "Memoir, Part 2," 48-49.
76. Prichard, "Remarks on the Older Floetz Strata," 20.
77. Prichard, "Geological Observations." This geological description of his travels and the aquatic fossils he collected on high mountains is signed Bristol, September 15, 1815. Gilby, "Geological Description"; Gilby, "Geological Observations."
78. Homo, "XL. On Jameson's *Preface*"; "Townsend's 'Character of Moses,'" attributed to Prichard on circumstantial evidence.
79. William Hall Gilby (1793-1835); Georges Cuvier (1769-1832), French naturalist influential in establishing the fields of paleontology and comparative anatomy; Buffon (1707-78), highly influential French naturalist who theorized on geological history and evolution. Prichard, "[Letter to Alexander Tilloch] On the Cosmogony of Moses," 285-88; Sloan, "Evolutionary Thought before Darwin." Cuvier, *Essay on the Theory of the Earth*, avoided confrontation with Genesis, popularized geology, and went through several editions from 1813 to 1827. See also chapter 6.
80. Prichard, "[Letter to Alexander Tilloch] On the Cosmogony of Moses," 289-90.
81. Prichard, "[Letter to Alexander Tilloch] On the Cosmogony of Moses; in Reply to F. E——s," August 1816, and six more until Prichard, "[Letter to Alexander Tilloch] On the Cosmogony of Moses," December 1816.
82. [Prichard], "'The Character of Moses,'" attributed to Prichard on circumstantial evidence.
83. The thirty-six books Prichard borrowed from the Bristol Library in 1814 and 1815 pertain to what he was publishing, such as George Campbell, *A Dissertation on Miracles*, 1762; Joseph Townsend, *The Character of Moses*, 1813-15, borrowed three times; Alexander Michaelis, *Commentaries on the Laws of Moses*, 1814; John Playfair, *Illustrations of the Huttonian Theory of the Earth*, 1802; Robert Jameson, *Mineralogy of the Scottish Isles*, 1800; John Pinkerton, *Petrology: A Treatise on Rocks*, 1811. Several were on literature, such as Luis de Camoens, *Lusiad*, 1776, and on history, such as William Coxe, *Memoirs of the Kings of Spain of the House of Bourbon*, 1813. Others indicate his steady accumulation of ethnographical material: H.-B. de Saussure, *Voyages dans les Alpes*, 1779-96; Leopold von Buch, *Travels through Norway and Lapland*, 1813; F. H. A. von Humboldt, *Personal Narrative of Travels*, 1814-29; and general science, as Humphry Davy, *Elements of Agricultural Chemistry*, 1813, and Carl Linnaeus, *General System of Nature*, 1806; Bristol Library Registers, BCL, B7485-87.
84. Iolo Morganwc (1747-1826). Prichard to Williams, February 2, 1815, Iolo Morganwg Manuscripts, NLW, MS. 21,282E; Prichard to Williams, January 17, 1815, Miscellaneous Papers in the hand of Edward Williams, NLW, MS. 13159A.

Prichard encouraged Williams's son to gather and preserve his deceased father's manuscripts. See Estlin to Williams, July 24, 1828. NLW, MS.21,272E, letter 171.
85. See chapter 10.
86. [Prichard], "Origin of Pagan Idolatry," 387. Authorship attributed to Prichard in Charles Abraham Elton to Henry Hallam, December 24 [unclear 1818 postmark], Papers of Henry Hallam, vol. 2, ff. 131-32, Christ Church Library, Oxford. A mis-transcription of the topic of this review led to successive obituarists' and bibliographers' erroneous reference to Prichard as the author of an unknown work titled "*Faln* and Schlegel."
87. "Origin and Antiquity of the Zodiac," 387. For an account of its impact on conflicting scientific and religious thinking of the time, see Buchwald and Josefowicz, *Zodiac of Paris*.

5. "Sharpening Their Wits"

1. "Hints to Young Practitioners," *Edinburgh Medical and Surgical Journal* 5 (1809): 335-39, in Fissell, "Physic of Charity," 67-68.
2. A Trustee to the Infirmary, *House-Committee*, 14.
3. John Edmonds Stock (1774-1835); John King (d. 1846, aged eighty). William Budd to Richard Budd, September 5, 1842, Budd Family, WC, MS.5153/A/3-37; "Stock" section of BIBM, vol. 9, 1810-1813, 72, BA, 35893/36/i; Maby, "Life and Letters of John King," BCL, B.28573; Cross to Smith, July 13, 1831, BIBM, 11:504-6. *Matthews's Bristol Directories* lists the Medical Institution on Broad Quay until 1812.
4. Cross to Smith, July 13, 1831. Internal evidence indicates that Prichard was the physician who distributed this circular in 1811. Joseph Storrs Fry, George Fisher Jr., and John Brent Cross, Printed Circular concerning a Dispensary Established by James Cowles Prichard on January 8, 1811, Seeking Subscriptions (Bristol: J. M. Gutch, n.d.), in BIBM, 11:568-70.
5. An advertisement for Prichard's Dispensary appeared in *Bristol Mercury*, January 6, 1812, 3; a news story in FFBJ, January 4, 1812, 3, announces its establishment; and another advertisement listing it as "lately established" is in *Bristol Gazette*, February 27, 1812, 3. Prichard's brother-in-law John Estlin got involved in seeing Prichard's patients with eye complaints, but when the dispensary was suspended, he established his own.
6. *Arrowsmith's Dictionary of Bristol*, 323.
7. Chisholm, "On the Statistical Pathology," 281.
8. Prichard, "Memoir, Part 1," 423.
9. St. Peter's Hospital, Announcement by the Court of St. Peter's Hospital, June 13, 1811, FFBJ, July 27, 1811, 3; St. Peter's Hospital, Announcement of the Election of James Cowles Prichard and Henry Hawes Fox, August 8, 1811, *Bristol Mirror*, August 17, 1811, 3; Johnson, *Transactions of the Corporation*, 104-11.
10. Bristol Corporation of the Poor, *Bye-Laws, Rules, and Regulations*, 19-22.
11. Prichard, *History of the Epidemic Fever*, 9-11. St. Peter's Hospital was destroyed by enemy action in 1940.

12. James Johnson (1764–1844). Johnson, *Address to the Inhabitants of Bristol*, 35–49.
13. Henry Hawes Fox (1788–1851). Fox, Letter to the Subscribers of the Bristol Infirmary, FFBJ, September 8, 1810, 3.
14. Prichard, *History of the Epidemic Fever*, 9–10.
15. Prichard, *History of the Epidemic Fever*, 11–12.
16. *Arrowsmith's Dictionary of Bristol*, 324. Eventually, a former prison on the outskirts of the city was repurposed as a supplementary poorhouse.
17. For a history of the struggle to force Bristol to establish a lunatic asylum, see Smith, "Lunatic Asylum."
18. Prichard, *A History of Epidemic Fever*, 334, f. 31, claiming Bristol Infirmary had long ignored the rule excluding fever patients.
19. Loudon, "Origins and Growth," 323–29, 334–36, 341.
20. Clifton Dispensary, *Formation of the Clifton Dispensary* (printed for the Committee by W. Collard, 1812), 1–3, BA, 16071(1); BIBM, 11:561–85; A Parishioner, Letter to the Editor against the Proposed Clifton Dispensary, *Bristol Mercury*, November 2, 1812, 3; Z., "To the Printers of the *Bristol Gazette* [against the Proposed Clifton Dispensary]," *Bristol Gazette*, November 5, 1812, 3. For the histories of the Clifton and other Bristol Dispensaries, see Whitfield, *Dispensaries*.
21. Chisholm, "On the Statistical Pathology," 66–73; Chisholm, "Extract of a Letter," 456–58; Resignation of Dr. Colin Chisholm, *Bristol Mercury*, November 10, 1817, 3; "Biographical Sketch of the Late Dr. Chisholm," 428; Hosack, "Memoir of the Life," 394–402, containing a comprehensive bibliography; Obituary of Colin Chisholm, 647–48. Chisholm, a native of Inverness-shire, served as an army surgeon throughout the Revolutionary War, eventually rising to the rank of inspector general of ordnance hospitals in the Windward Islands in 1797. Pensioned, he practiced in Clifton and wrote scientific essays, dying in London in 1825.
22. Dr. William Gilby (d. 1840, aged eighty-three). Obituary of William Gilby, *Bristol Mirror*, November 21, 1840, 3. For William Hall Gilby and Prichard's geology, see chapter 4.
23. Report of the First Annual Meeting of the Clifton Dispensary, FFBJ, January 15, 1814, 1; Junius, "To the Physicians and Surgeons of the Clifton Dispensary," FFBJ, January 22, 1814, 3. Prichard and Chisholm's nosology was based on the taxonomic approach of François Boissier de Sauvages de Lacroix (1706–67).
24. Prichard, "Concerning the REPORT of the CLIFTON DISPENSARY, TO THE EDITOR," FFBJ, February 5, 1814, 3.
25. Saunders, *History of the United Bristol Hospitals*, 78; Perry, *Voluntary Medical Institutions*, 16–17; Wofinden, "Public Health in Bristol," 125–26. More than forty years after its inception, a Clifton Dispensary physician reported to a government commission on the "Sanitary Condition of Bristol and Clifton" that the mortality rate in the Hotwells district per thousand was double that of the residents at the top of the hill. The average room in Hotwells was occupied by six to ten people and was unventilated and without water or sanitation. After

the formation of the National Health Service in 1948 the Clifton Dispensary remained a charity.

26. *State of the Bristol Dispensaries*, 1–2.
27. John Newman, Benjamin Spencer, and Fran[ci]s C. Bowles, "[Smallpox Inoculation at the] Bristol Dispensary, Jan. 5, 1802," FFBJ, January 9, 1802, 3.
28. Perry, *Voluntary Medical Institutions*, 7–8; *State of the Bristol Dispensaries*, 1–2; Saunders, *History of the United Bristol Hospitals*, 77–78. See also BIBM, vols. 2, 3, and 14, BA.
29. Edward Kentish (1763–1832). Obituary of Edward Kentish, *Bristol Mirror*, December 8, 1832, 3.
30. Barry, "Bristol Pride," 33–34.
31. For histories of the Infirmary, see Munro Smith, *History of the Bristol Royal Infirmary*; Perry, *Voluntary Medical Institutions*; and the Infirmary's archives in the BA.
32. Pritchard [*sic*], Advertised Letter to the Subscribers of the Bristol Infirmary, FFBJ, September 1, 1810, 3.
33. Andrew Carrick (1767–1837). Report of the Election of Physician to the Bristol Infirmary, September 20, 1810, FFBJ, September 22, 1810, 3; Bristol Infirmary General Board Book Commencing Jany. 1st 1800, 244, BA, 35893 c; "Obituary Notice of Daniel Wait, (d. 1813)," FFBJ, September 4, 1813, 3; Prichard, "To the Subscribers to the Bristol Infirmary," FFBJ, September 22, 1810, 3. Wait was an influential Tory politician, former mayor, and poor law governor.
34. Prichard, "To the Subscribers to the Bristol Infirmary," FFBJ, March 16, 1811, 3; letters by Drs. Stock, Dyer (1758–1833), Bernard, and Porter in the same location.
35. Richard Smith in BIBM, vol. 5, 1784–1789, 652, BA, 35893/36/e_i.
36. Prichard, Advertisement for a Course of Medical Lectures, FFBJ, February 19, 1814, 3. This was repeated in the following week and in a similar advertisement in the *Bristol Mirror*, February 26, 1814, 3, for lectures commencing March 8.
37. Prichard, Advertisement for a Course of Medical Lectures, FFBJ, October 7, 1815, 3. This was repeated in the following week and in the *Bristol Gazette*, October 12, 1815, and *Bristol Mirror*, October 14, 1815; Munro Smith, *History of the Bristol Royal Infirmary*, 367–71; Bowles and Smith, Announcement of a Course; Cross, "Early Medical Teaching in Bristol."
38. Munro Smith, *History of the Bristol Royal Infirmary*, 125–27; Richard Smith in BIBM, 5:654.
39. J. J. Palmer, Letter to the Subscribers of the Bristol Infirmary, FFBJ, February 24, 1816, 3.
40. "To the Subscribers of the Bristol Infirmary," FFBJ, February 7, 1816, 3; BIBM, 5:656. Richard Smith ascribed authorship of A Subscriber to Dr. Stock.
41. Fair Play, Letter to the Subscribers to the Bristol Infirmary, FFBJ, February 24, 1816, 3; BIBM, 5:656, 658.
42. Another Subscriber, Letter to the Subscribers to the Bristol Infirmary, FFBJ, February 24, 1816, 3; BIBM, 5:660; Prichard, Printed Letter Seeking Support in the Election to the Bristol Infirmary, February 29, 1816, in BIBM, 11:4; A

Trustee, "To the Editor," *FFBJ*, February 24, 1816, 3; Q, "To Mr. Printer," *Bristol Mercury*, February 26, 1816, 3.
43. Candidus [James Cowles Prichard], "To the Editor of the *Bristol Mirror*," *Bristol Mirror*, April 6, 1816, 3; Prichard, "To the Subscribers to the Bristol Infirmary," *FFBJ*, February 24, 1816.
44. Thomas Stock (1768–1838); Thomas Sanders (d. August 30, 1854, aged eighty-five). "Thomas Stock, Esq," 215; "The Late Mr. Stock," *FFBJ*, May 12, 1838, 3; "Death of Thomas Sanders, Esq.," *Bristol Times and FFBJ*, September 2, 1854, 8; "The Late Thomas Sanders, Esq.," *Bristol Times and FFBJ*, September 9, 1854, 5; Society of Friends, Friars Burial Ground, 1808–1946, BA, SF/R2/1(h). Prichard became the Stock family physician.
45. "Election of Two Physicians to the Infirmary," *FFBJ*, March 2, 1816, 2; Bristol Infirmary General Board Book, 244–47; [Millard], "T. W. Dyer, M.D.," 278. Prichard's relative Richard Reynolds wrote in his diary for February 18, "Red'd lrs from my Son & Thos. Pritchard," and for February 29, "Went in a Coach & voted for Drs. Fox & Prichard to be Drs. at Infirmary," Diary for the year 1816, the Rathbone Papers, Sydney Jones Library, University of Liverpool Library, IV.3.3. Dr. Dyer never managed to obtain the post of infirmary physician.
46. Munro Smith, *History of the Bristol Royal Infirmary*, 138–43, 148–49, 161–62.
47. Alford, "Bristol Infirmary," 166.
48. Bristol Infirmary, *State of the Infirmary, 1816*; Munro Smith, *History of the Bristol Royal Infirmary*, 316, 199.
49. Bristol Infirmary, *Rules Confirmed by the Subscribers*, 21.
50. Alford, "Bristol Infirmary," 166–68; Bristol Infirmary, *Rules Confirmed by the Subscribers*, 22–26; Bristol Infirmary, *Proposed Rules*, 32–35; Munro Smith, *History of the Bristol Royal Infirmary*, 36, 299–300, 482. By 1824 the secretary's salary was £150 per annum and the matron's £50 per annum.
51. Alford, "Bristol Infirmary," 166.
52. Prichard, "Reminiscences of the Bristol Royal Infirmary," 198–99.
53. Munro Smith, *History of the Bristol Royal Infirmary*, 51–53, 197–99.
54. Carrick, *Observations*, 19; Bristol Infirmary, *Report of the Special Committee*, 2–3; Bristol Infirmary, *Proposed Rules*, 31.
55. Perry, *Bristol Royal Infirmary*, 16; Bristol Infirmary, *Proceedings in Relation to a Proposed Extension*. Prichard's signature does not appear on this address seeking an increase in the number of medical pupils for the purpose of facilitating cooperation between the Infirmary and Medical School. The Bristol Royal Infirmary Archives, BA, contain scores of manuscript and printed testimonial letters by Prichard singly or jointly with colleagues on behalf of their former pupils' applications for appointments and qualifications.
56. [J. C. Prichard and J. E. Stock, "Advertisement of] Medical Lectures," *FFBJ*, October 5, 1816, 3.
57. Stock to Richard Smith, September 28, 1816, BIBM, 9:84; [John Edmonds Stock and James Cowles Prichard], Medical Lectures, October 14, 1816, BIBM, 11:544; [Stock and Prichard], *Syllabus of a Course of Lectures* (Bristol: J. M. Gutch, Printer, [1816]), in BIBM, 11:546. No opposition is recorded in the minutes

of the weekly committee, although any adverse comments might have been reported by one of its members, John Bishop Estlin. Bristol Infirmary Weekly Committee Book, 1814-1820, 144-46, BA, 35983/2 e; Perry, "British Hospitals," 281; "Report of the Adjourned Meeting of the Trustees of the Bristol Infirmary," *FFBJ*, January 21, 1843, 2.

58. Munro Smith, *History of the Bristol Royal Infirmary*, 285. Prichard wrote to Richard Smith offering to save the library money by selling it his unwanted copies of the *Philosophical Transactions*, Prichard to Smith, n.d., BIBM, 11:562.
59. Smith, *An Address*, 7; Munro Smith, *History of the Bristol Royal Infirmary*, 378-81; A. Prichard, *Bristol Medical School*; [Parker], *Schola Medicinae Bristol*.
60. Alford, "Bristol Infirmary," 190; Munro Smith, *History of the Bristol Royal Infirmary*, 207-13.
61. Alford, "Bristol Infirmary," 190-91; Munro Smith, *History of the Bristol Royal Infirmary*, 210-14.
62. Munro Smith, *History of the Bristol Royal Infirmary*, 213.
63. Munro Smith, *History of the Bristol Royal Infirmary*, 280-81.
64. Frederick Leman on behalf of Prichard, Form Letter to Richard Smith requesting a consultation, February 3, 1827, and Prichard to Smith, December 10, 1822, BIBM, 11:556; Bristol Infirmary, *Rules Confirmed by the Subscribers*, 8-9.
65. Bristol Infirmary, *Proposed Rules*, 7, 28.
66. Bristol Infirmary, *Rules for the Government*, 17-18.
67. Alford, "Bristol Infirmary," 176-78.
68. R[obert] Stock, Advertisement, *FFBJ*, August 1, 1829, 3, in which Prichard, seven other doctors, and four surgeons endorse Stock's method of cupping; A. Prichard, *A Few Medical & Surgical Reminiscences*.
69. Munro Smith, *History of the Bristol Royal Infirmary*, 54-55; Alford, "Bristol Infirmary," 189.
70. Alford, "Bristol Infirmary," 178-79. For a fuller discussion of the medical philosophy of the era, see chapter 9.
71. William Swayne (1790-1825). Smith, *History of the Bristol Royal Infirmary*, 173; Alford, "Bristol Infirmary," 169-70.
72. Munro Smith, *History of the Bristol Royal Infirmary*, 220-21. It took a further eight years for a new prison to be built.
73. Munro Smith, *History of the Bristol Royal Infirmary*, 201.
74. For example, Prichard, Testimonial letter on behalf of James Barrington Prowse, *FFBJ*, October 10, 1840, 3; "Distressing and Fatal Accident at the Bristol Infirmary," *FFBJ*, February 25, 1826, 3.
75. Alford, "Bristol Infirmary," 170-72; Munro Smith, *History of the Bristol Royal Infirmary*, 179-80.
76. Alford, "Bristol Infirmary," 172-74; Munro Smith, *History of the Bristol Royal Infirmary*, 180-82.
77. Alford, "Bristol Infirmary," 174-76; A. Prichard, *A Few Medical & Surgical Reminiscences*, 26.
78. George Wallis (1787-1869). Munro Smith, *History of the Bristol Royal Infirmary*, 301-2, 441-44.

79. John Howell (1777-1857). Munro Smith, *History of the Bristol Royal Infirmary*, 302-3, 441-44.
80. Henry Riley (1797-1848). Munro Smith, *History of the Bristol Royal Infirmary*, 303-4.
81. Richard Smith Jr. (1772-1843). Neale, *Medical Progress in Bristol*, 6.
82. Richard Smith, Visitors to Mr. Richard Smith's Museum (1828-1838), BA, 35893/36; Alford, "Bristol Infirmary," 179-82; Munro Smith, *History of the Bristol Royal Infirmary*, 464-65; BIBM, vol. 6, 1789-1801, 441-506, BA, 35893/36/f.
83. Obituary of Richard Smith; A. Prichard, *A Few Medical & Surgical Reminiscences*, 21-25. For the Phil & Lit, see chapter 9.
84. William Hetling (1772-1837). Alford, "Bristol Infirmary," 183-84; Munro Smith, *History of the Bristol Royal Infirmary*, 188-91.
85. Richard Lowe (1780-1850). Munro Smith, *History of the Bristol Royal Infirmary*, 191; Alford, "Bristol Infirmary," 184-86. Staunch Tory Lowe signed the 1829 anti-Catholic petition. His long tenure as surgeon gave impetus to the committee's establishing the rule limiting length of service.
86. Henry Daniel (1783-1859). Alford, "Bristol Infirmary," 186-87; Munro Smith, *History of the Bristol Royal Infirmary*, 191-92.
87. Nathaniel Smith (1782-1869). Munro Smith, *History of the Bristol Royal Infirmary*, 194-95; Alford, "Bristol Infirmary," 187-88.
88. Thomas Shute (d. 1816). Munro Smith, *History of the Bristol Royal Infirmary*, 194.
89. Bristol Infirmary, Report by the Committee of Enquiry, 6; Munro Smith, *History of the Bristol Royal Infirmary*, 167; Prichard to the Surgeons of the Bristol Infirmary, BIBM, 11:564.
90. Munro Smith, *History of the Bristol Royal Infirmary*, 196, 223.
91. Bristol Infirmary Weekly Committee Book, 1820-1828, 306-19, Bristol Royal Infirmary Archives, BA, 35983/2 f; Richard Smith, Account of which hospitals were asked about the rights of their medical officers, BIBM, 9:844; Prichard to Smith, [1835], BIBM, 9:912; Prichard, Reasons Why the Faculty Ought Not to Be Entirely Excluded from the Committee, BIBM, 9:838-39; Bristol Infirmary General Board Book, 61-62, 95-106.
92. Carrick, *Observations Submitted to the Trustees*.
93. Poem in BIBM, 11:469, and in Munro Smith, *History of the Bristol Royal Infirmary*, 469.
94. Marmion, *Bristol Eye Hospital*, 42-45. Thomas Prichard was a subscriber for many years. Estlin remained one of the Dispensary's surgeons until the 1850s, by which time some sixty thousand patients had been treated. Prichard's son Augustin and his grandson Arthur William also worked there as it expanded into larger premises on Orchard Street with inpatient facilities and a teaching program.
95. Bristol Refuge Society, *First Report*.
96. List of the First 111 Members of the Medical Reading Society, inserted in Minute Book, October 1, 1879-August 4, 1909, Archives of the Medical Reading Society, Bristol.

97. Medical Reading Society, *Rules of the Medical Reading Society*; L. Griffiths, *Medical Reading Society*; [A. Prichard], "Obituary—Crosby Leonard," 352; List of the First 111 Members; Frampton, "Science in the Nineteenth-Century Periodical." Prichard's son Augustin and grandson Arthur William were also members.
98. Munro Smith, "Notes on Some Bristol Medical Societies," 274–76; Bristol Medical and Surgical Association, A Collection Pertaining to the Bristol Medical & Surgical Society, 462–539, in BIBM, vol. 14, BA, 35893/36/g_i.
99. Bristol Infirmary General Board Book, 319–20.

6. The Single Origin of Humankind

1. Hodgkin, "Obituary," 186.
2. Prichard, *Researches into the Physical History of Man*, ii. "Mosaic records" refers to the sacred writings of the Mosaic period, starting with Moses receiving the Ten Commandments and ending with the crucifixion of Christ, a span of 1,500 years. For a preliminary discussion of the inspiration of science in Prichard's youth, see chapter 2.
3. Absolutism and inhibition were more strictly the case in Britain than on the Continent, where biological naturalistic theories, including autogenesis, were discussed in scientific circles more freely, for which see Rupke, "Origins of Racism," 238–39.
4. For the Christian intellectual tradition in theories of humankind, see Keel, "Blumenbach's Race Science."
5. Charles White (1728–1813); Julien-Joseph Virey (1775–1846). The opposing terms "monogenism" and "polygenism" were first used by J. C. Nott and G. R. Gliddon in *Indigenous Races of the Earth* (Philadelphia, 1857) but are used here anachronistically for the sake of economy.
6. For the vital role of extra-European contact and extra-European science in the Scientific Revolution, see Poskett, *Horizons*.
7. For an account of an early form of cultural anthropology arising among German speakers in the second half of the eighteenth century, see Vermeulen, "Origins and Institutionalization."
8. Montesquieu (1689–1755); Isaac La Peyrère (1596–1676); Immanuel Kant (1724–1804).
9. For early race hypotheses, see Livingstone, *Adam's Ancestors*, 27–39; and Stock, "'Almost a Separate Race.'"
10. Georges-Louis Leclerc, Comte de Buffon (1707–88); Johann Reinhold Forster (1729–98); Johann Gottfried von Herder (1744–1803). Niekerk, "Buffon, Blumenbach, Lichtenberg."
11. Edward Long (1734–1813); Charles White (1728–1813); Petrus Camper (1722–89); Samuel Thomas von Soemmerring (1755–1830); Samuel Stanhope Smith (1751–1819). Long, *History of Jamaica*; White, *Account of the Regular Gradation*; Camper, *Verhandeling van Petrus Camper*; von Soemmerring, *Vom Baue des menschlichen Körpers*; Smith, *Essay on the Causes*.
12. Carl Linnaeus (1707–78); Pierre Louis Maupertuis (1698–1759); Georges-Louis Leclerc, Comte de Buffon (1707–88).

13. William Paley (1743–1805). Paley, *Natural Theology*.
14. Conlin, *Evolution and the Victorians*, 32–45.
15. Erasmus Darwin (1731–1802). Darwin, *Zoonomia*. For the history of early international evolutionary thought, see Poskett, *Horizons*; and for an outline of the history of the transformism debate, see Sloan, "Evolutionary Thought before Darwin."
16. Johann Friedrich Blumenbach (1752–1840). Prichard, "Memoir, Part 2," 209–10; Augstein, *James Cowles Prichard's Anthropology*, 80–85; Prichard to Washington, May 23, [1840], RGS. The most often used translations of Blumenbach's work by Thomas Bendysche, 1865, a member of the polygenesis-leaning Anthropological Society of London, have been proven mistranslated to give the appearance of ethnocentrism and racism, for which see Michael, "Nuance Lost in Translation."
17. Scott, *Lady of the Lake*; Hodgkin, "Obituary," 185–86.
18. Henry Home, Lord Kames (1696–1782); James Burnett, Lord Monboddo (c. 1714–99). Kames, *Sketches*; Monboddo, *Of the Origin*; Greene, *Death of Adam*, 208–18.
19. Prichard, *Researches into the Physical History of Man*, 4.
20. Prichard, *Researches into the Physical History of Man*, ii–iii.
21. Dugald Stewart (1753–1828). James Bridges, Notes from Mr. [Dugald] Stewart's Lectures on Moral Philosophy, Read in the University of Edinburgh Winter 1801–2, UE, Dc.5.88; John Borthwick, Notes from a Course of Lectures on Moral Philosophy Delivered by Dugald Stewart, December 1, 1806–April 1808–May 24, 1809, UE, Gen. 843.
22. [William Dansey], Lectures on Natural History by Professor [Robert] Jameson, [1816 or 1817], fols. 118–23, UE, MSS Dc.3.33–34. Jameson's lectures also dealt with temperament and national character, a topic Prichard took up much later in life.
23. University of Edinburgh Library [Borrowers' (Students)] Receipt Books, November 17, 1804–March 25, 1805, March 27, 1806–December 29, 1807, UE, Da. 2.36, 37. For instance, he borrowed Peter Simon Pallas, *Spicilegica Zoologica*, 1767; Antonio Herrera y Tordesillas, *Novus orbis*, 1622; and Adam Smith, *The Theory of Moral Sentiments*, 1761. In 1805 he also borrowed le Sage, *Aventures de Don Chérubin de la Ronda*, 1783; and in 1807 de Lesseps, *Travels in Kamtchatka*, 1790; Mitford, *History of Greece*, 1789–97; and Locke, *Essay concerning the Human Understanding*, 1795.
24. Royal Medical Society, Index to the Dissertations, RMSE. As well as the RMS dissertations cited in this chapter, examples of MD dissertations are Richard Duncan Mackintosh, *De hominum varietatibus earumque causis*, 1799; John Taylor, *De hominum varietatibus*, 1806; and Robert Eveleigh Taylor, *De hominum varietatibus*, 1800. MD theses written after Prichard's include John Stephenson, *De humani generis varietatibus*, 1817, which contains references to Prichard's *Physical History*.
25. Prichard, "Of the Varieties," Royal Medical Society Dissertations, ff. 87–89, RMSE.

26. Prichard, "Of the Varieties," ff. 90–93.
27. Prichard, "Of the Varieties," ff. 97–98.
28. Prichard, "Of the Varieties," ff. 98–110.
29. Prichard, "Of the Varieties," ff. 110–33.
30. Prichard, *De generis*.
31. Gottfried Wilhelm Leibniz (1646–1716), philosopher, mathematician, and German historian; Sir William Jones (1746–94).
32. Jean Baptiste Chevalier de Lamarck (1744–1829). Lamarck, *Philosophie zoologique*.
33. Prichard, *Researches into the Physical History of Man*, 10.
34. Stocking, "From Chronology to Ethnology," xxiv–xliii, and see cxix–cxliv for an annotated list of *Physical History*'s sources.
35. Prichard, *Researches into the Physical History of Man*, 243–44.
36. Prichard, *Researches into the Physical History of Man*, 247–48.
37. Prichard, *Researches into the Physical History of Man*, 318–472. For Jones on language structure as ethnological evidence of the unity of humankind, and Prichard's use of Jones and the *Asiatick Researches*, see Simpson, "Historicizing Humans in Colonial India."
38. Prichard, *Researches into the Physical History of Man*, iii–iv.
39. Francis Bacon (1561–1626), called "the father of empiricism," stressed that scientific knowledge should be based solely on inductive reasoning and disciplined observation of natural phenomena.
40. *Researches into the Physical History of Man* contains reference to Leibniz on race as cited in Blumenbach; using French and English translations, he referred to cartographer and explorer Carsten Niebuhr (1733–1815) on the Middle East and India, cited in Buchanan, *Journey from Madras*; Prussian biologist and zoologist Peter Simon Pallas (1741–1811), who worked in Siberia and Crimea; and articles in the late eighteenth-century Saint Petersburg *Acta academiae scientiarum imperialis Petropolitanae*. Prichard's access to modern German linguistics and ethnologies was initially limited to translations, as he did not start learning German until 1814. He borrowed no books from the Bristol Library in German before 1814, nor were there any in German in his known personal library. The second edition of *Physical History* refers to some early German ethnologies, especially ones on Siberia. The third edition, vol. 3, 1841, has many references to Niebuhr, mostly concerning his interpretations of the ancient historians, many references to German linguists, and two to Leibniz. Prichard privately acknowledged the preeminence of German linguists.
41. Stocking, "From Chronology to Ethnology," xliii–lxix.
42. Prichard, *Researches into the Physical History of Man*, 174–94.
43. Prichard, *Researches into the Physical History of Man*, 194–204, 37–40. See also Livingstone, *The Preadamite*, 14–18.
44. Prichard, *Researches into the Physical History of Man*, 46–65.
45. Prichard, *Researches into the Physical History of Man*, 66–84.
46. Prichard, *Researches into the Physical History of Man*, 41–42; Staum, *Labeling People*, 26–28; Schiebinger, *Nature's Body*, 133–34; Darwin, *Descent of Man*.

Prichard might have had in mind Blumenbach's statement in *Handbuch* that Europeans have the most beautiful form of face and skull "according to the European concepts of beauty." For evaluating Blumenbach's (and, by association, Prichard's) views on beauty based on the complex physiognomic aesthetics of the period, see Ritter, "Natural Equality and Racial Systematics"; and Marino, "At the Roots," 11.

47. Prichard, *Researches into the Physical History of Man*, 208–32. See also Bynum, "Time's Noblest Offspring," 103.
48. Prichard, *Researches into the Physical History of Man*, 133–55.
49. Prichard, *Researches into the Physical History of Man*, 233–39. See also Kidd, *Forging of Races*.
50. Prichard, *Researches into the Physical History of Man*, 155.
51. Prichard, *Researches into the Physical History of Man*, 247–48.
52. Prichard, *Researches into the Physical History of Man*, 247, 243–317.
53. Sera-Shriar, *Making of British Anthropology*, 46–49.
54. Prichard, *Researches into the Physical History of Man*, 247–48, 318–472, 320.
55. Prichard, *Researches into the Physical History of Man*, 423–69, 471–72.
56. Prichard, *Researches into the Physical History of Man*, 473–525.
57. Prichard, *Researches into the Physical History of Man*, 526–34. For Prichard's *Eastern Origin* (1831), see chapter 10.
58. Prichard, *Researches into the Physical History of Man*, 536–46. Although since childhood Celtic history and language had fired his imagination, he devoted only eight pages to the Celts, based almost entirely on the classics. This would be rectified later.
59. Prichard, *Researches into the Physical History of Man*, 547–54.
60. Prichard, *Researches into the Physical History of Man*, 554–58.
61. "History of the Firm," 455; Mortimer, "Quaker Printers, 1750–1850," 113.
62. [Bostock], "Prichard's 'Researches,'" 127–34; "Prichard's 'Researches,'" 89–106, 266–75.
63. "Dr. Prichard—Physical History of Mankind,'" *British Critic*; "Dr. Pritchard on the 'Physical History of Man,'" *Annals of Philosophy*; "Pritchard's 'Physical History of Man,'" *Literary and Statistical Magazine*.
64. Lawrence, *Lectures on Physiology*.
65. William Lawrence (1783–1867). Bynum, "Time's Noblest Offspring," 122–63; Wells, "Sir William Lawrence," 319–61; Stinson, *Role of Sir William Lawrence*, 16, 20, 22, 25; Lawrence to Hone, c. 1821, BL, MSS. 40120; Lawrence to Glynn, president of Bridewell and Bethlem, April 16, 1832, Archives, Royal College of Surgeons of England, London, MS. Addit. 194; Prichard, *Researches into the Physical History of Mankind*, 2nd ed., 1:vi; Goodfield-Toulmin, "Blasphemy and Biology," 9–18. Lawrence's friendship with Prichard seems to have dated from Prichard's early visits to relatives in Cirencester, Lawrence's hometown and where he had been apprenticed. They exchanged signed copies of their books. Prichard later sent his son Augustin to study ophthalmology with this by then highly successful pillar of society. Augustin was impressed with the kind, if sometimes acid-tongued, physician. A copy of Prichard's *Physical*

History, 1826, inscribed to William Lawrence is in the Medical College Library, St. Bartholomew's Hospital, London; A. Prichard, *A Few Medical & Surgical Reminiscences*, 35–36.

66. William Elford Leach (1791-1836). Mackenzie et al., Letter of proposal of James Cowles Prichard as member of the Linnean Society, proposed March 2, 1813, elected May 4, 1813, signed the Obligation and admitted November 16, 1813, resigned by letter April 20, 1823, because of remoteness and "I derive no advantage" (Archives of the Linnean Society of London). The subscription was 1 guinea per annum. The society possessed his *Physical History*, 1813.
67. List of Papers Read before the Public Meetings of the Philosophical and Literary Society, from its Commencement to 26th May 1836, Nos. 3, 40, 44, 50, 32079, BA.
68. Advertisement for *Physical History*, FFBJ, November 25, 1826, 3.
69. Prichard, *Researches into the Physical History of Mankind*, 2nd ed., 1:[iii], v–vii.
70. Prichard, *Researches into the Physical History of Mankind*, 2nd ed., 2:562–66.
71. Stocking, "From Chronology to Ethnology," lxv–lxvi.
72. Prichard, *Researches into the Physical History of Mankind*, 2nd ed., 2:525–58, 549.
73. Prichard, *Researches into the Physical History of Mankind*, 2nd ed., 2:532, 536, 545, 548–49, 575; Schiebinger, *Nature's Body*, 138.
74. Alexander von Humboldt (1769–1853); Augustin Pyramus de Candolle (1778–1841); Robert Brown (1773–1853). Augstein, *James Cowles Prichard's Anthropology*, 79, 112; Prichard, *Researches into the Physical History of Mankind*, 2nd ed., 1:3, 7, 27, 40.
75. Prichard, *Researches into the Physical History of Mankind*, 2nd ed., 1:83–89. The geological theory of catastrophism opposed that of uniformitarianism, the latter proposing gradual change.
76. Prichard, *Researches into the Physical History of Mankind*, 2nd ed., 1:81–83.
77. Prichard, *Researches into the Physical History of Mankind*, 2nd ed., 1:138–91, 173–74, 238–39.
78. Prichard, *Researches into the Physical History of Mankind*, 2nd ed., 2:584–91. Later, he tended to avoid the word "race"; his posthumous chapter in the *Manual of Scientific Enquiry*, "Ethnology," 426, uses "the several tribes of the human family."
79. Between 1815 and 1825 Prichard borrowed about 150 books from the Bristol Library on travel and world history, some several times, such as Elphinstone, *Account of the Kingdom of Caubul*, 1815; and Jablonski's *Pantheon Aegyptiorum*, 1750–1752, Bristol Library Register, BCL, B.7486–500.
80. Prichard, *Researches into the Physical History of Mankind*, 2nd ed., 1:531–44.
81. Prichard, *Researches into the Physical History of Mankind*, 2nd ed., 2:592–606.
82. Prichard, *Researches into the Physical History of Mankind*, 2nd ed., 2:606–23.

83. "On the Physical History," 112-44; "Dr. Prichard—Physical History of Mankind," *British Critic*, 33-61.
84. Heusinger, "Anthropologie." August Wilhelm Schlegel described Prichard as "paradoxical, but erudite" and not always up-to-date in his knowledge. (The porcupine skin story dates back to 1731.) Schlegel to von Humboldt, May 19, 1823, in Augstein, *James Cowles Prichard's Anthropology*, 65-66, 111-15.
85. Charles Caldwell (1772-1853). Caldwell, *Thoughts on the Original Unity*; "Caldwell on the Unity of the Human Race." Caldwell was accused of denying biblical truth and serving the interest of slavers and exterminators of Indians in [Bronson], Review of *Thoughts on the Original Unity*.
86. Wallace to Poulton, June 13, 1897, 3-4, Poulton Papers, UO; see also Oldroyd, *Darwinian Impacts*, 301. Poulton, "Remarkable Anticipation of Modern Views," 278-96, was reasonably considered by Darwin's son in Darwin, *More Letters*, 43-44, to be an exaggeration of Prichard's achievement.
87. Zirkle, "Natural Selection," 104-6; Prichard, *Researches into the Physical History of Mankind*, 2nd ed., 2:581.
88. Desmond and Moore, *Darwin's Sacred Cause*, xvii; Moore and Desmond, "Introduction," xi-lxvi.
89. [W. Carpenter], "Ethnology." See chapters 12, 13, and 8 herein, respectively.

7. Epidemics, History, and Mythology

1. Mary Prichard (December 6, 1816-November 25, 1844).
2. Hobhouse to Hobhouse, January 15, [1817], Broughton Papers, BL, BM Add. MS. 36460, ff. 1-2.
3. Ellen Laetitia Estlin to Anna Maria Prichard, August 11, 1817, Birthday Book, 165-70; [Barbauld], "Memoir of the Late Rev. John Prior Estlin."
4. Raison and Goldie, *Servant Girl Princess Caraboo*, one of several books and a feature film on this hoax; Bird's portrait of her is in the Bristol Museum and Art Gallery.
5. Advertisement for freight and passengers on the *Columbia*, *Bristol Gazette*, October 22, 1818, 3.
6. Prichard, Letter to John Haythorne, Mayor, concerning Typhus Fever, *FFBJ*, November 22, 1817, 3.
7. Editorial concerning a Letter from a Correspondent Regarding James Cowles Prichard's Letter on Typhus Fever, *Bristol Gazette*, November 27, 1817, 3; a letter in qualified support of Prichard appeared in the *Bristol Mercury*, November 24, 1817, 3.
8. Prichard, Letter to the Editor concerning Cases of Typhus in Bristol, *FFBJ*, December 6, 1817, 3.
9. Chisholm, "Typhus Fever, to the Editor, Park-Street, Dec. 1, 1817," *FFBJ*, December 6, 1817, 4.
10. Prichard, "Cases of Typhus Fever," 413-16. "Typhus" was a term applied to fevers of indeterminate origin during this period before the bacteriological revolution and redefinition of typhus and typhoid.
11. Critical Analysis of James Cowles Prichard's "Cases."

12. Percival, *Practical Observations*, 4, 33.
13. [Morgan], *Appeal to the Good Sense*. Prichard's letter dated January 29, 1819, is on 30–31.
14. Advertisement for Prichard's *History of the Epidemic Fever*, FFBJ, March 4, 1820, 2. Prichard's successor at St. Peter's and the Infirmary, William Budd (1811–80) noticed cases of typhoid occurring among thirteen families sharing the same well on Richmond Terrace, Clifton, and with his many similar observations from 1839 onward, he is credited with recognizing the mechanism of contagion and is considered a pioneer of public health, Moorhead, "William Budd and Typhoid Fever."
15. Prichard, *History of the Epidemic Fever*, 1–7, 31.
16. Prichard, *History of the Epidemic Fever*, 8–43.
17. Prichard, *History of the Epidemic Fever*, 32–43.
18. Prichard, *History of the Epidemic Fever*, 45–46.
19. Prichard, *History of the Epidemic Fever*, 47–49.
20. Prichard, *History of the Epidemic Fever*, 51–52, 73.
21. Prichard, *History of the Epidemic Fever*, 53–56.
22. Prichard, *History of the Epidemic Fever*, 56–62.
23. Prichard, *History of the Epidemic Fever*, 63–73.
24. Prichard, *History of the Epidemic Fever*, 74–76.
25. Prichard, *History of the Epidemic Fever*, 81–87.
26. Prichard, *History of the Epidemic Fever*, 88–89.
27. Prichard, *History of the Epidemic Fever*, 90–95.
28. Prichard, *History of the Epidemic Fever*, 98–101.
29. Prichard, *History of the Epidemic Fever*, 106–12.
30. For the 1832 cholera epidemic and establishment of the Board of Health, see chapter 10.
31. J., Review and Notice of Twenty-Four Works on Fever; "Epidemic Fever"; "Prichard on Epidemic Fever"; Critical Analysis of the Review; "Dr. Prichard on Epidemic Fever"; "Dr. Prichard on Fever."
32. Latimer, *Annals of Bristol*, 68–69.
33. John Loudon McAdam (1756–1836). Latimer, *Annals of Bristol*, 63–65, 75–76, 84.
34. Williams, "Bristol in the General Elections," 175, 182; Latimer, *Annals of Bristol*, 82.
35. Latimer, *Annals of Bristol*, 82–83.
36. Latimer, *Annals of Bristol*, 84–85.
37. Johannes von Mueller (1752–1809). Prichard to Fardon, received July 7, 1806, Gibson IV.141, Archives and Manuscripts, Society of Friends Library; Gruetter, *Johannes von Müllers Begegnung mit England*, 204–6; [Account for *An Universal History*], Divide Ledger No. 6, entries beginning May 9, 1818, MS 1393, Longman Group Archive, Special Collections, University of Reading. Four American editions were each published in four volumes in Boston between 1831 and 1882.

38. Mueller, *Universal History*, 344; Review of the English Translation of Johannes von Muller's *Universal History*, 150; [Taylor], "Muller's *Universal History*," 234; Morgan, *Critical Bibliography of German Literature*, 344.
39. Prichard to Retzius, May 2, 1847, and Prichard to Retzius, Saturday, n.d., Kungliga Vetenskapsakademien Biblioteket, Stockholm.
40. Griscom, *Year in Europe*, 121. John Griscom (1774–1852) and Prichard maintained their acquaintance, corresponding until at least 1831, when Prichard informed Griscom that he had been elected an honorary member of the Phil & Lit.
41. Edward Bird (1772–1819). "Edward Bird, Esq. R. A."; Latimer, *Annals of Bristol*, 86–87.
42. Mueller, *Universal History* (1818), 1:344.
43. Prichard, "Memoir, Part 2," 84.
44. Prichard requested the purchase of and extensively borrowed travel books from the Bristol Library; Bruce, *Travels to Discover*, 2:464–65, Bristol Library Society Register, BCL, B7489–96; Prichard, *Egyptian Mythology*, i–ii.
45. Prichard, *Analysis of the Egyptian Mythology* (1819); [Prichard], "Analysis of the Egyptian Mythology," 90–97 (attribution on internal evidence); Griscom, *Memoir of John Griscom*, 374.
46. Jablonski, *Pantheon Aegyptiorum*. Prichard borrowed this book from the Bristol Library six times between January 1817 and March 1819 and again in 1824. Bristol Library Society Register, BCL, B7489–93.
47. Prichard, *Egyptian Mythology*, iii–v. The introduction of cross-cultural studies is often attributed to E. B. Tylor.
48. For the influence of William Jones, Jacob Bryant, Friedrich Schlegel, John David Michaelis, and German Higher Criticism and Romanticism on Prichard's *Egyptian Mythology*, see Augstein, *James Cowles Prichard's Anthropology*, 183–209.
49. Prichard, *Egyptian Mythology*, vi–vii, and the 138-page separate section titled "A Critical Examination of the Remains of Egyptian Chronology."
50. "Analysis of the Egyptian Mythology"; "Prichard's Analysis of Egyptian Mythology"; "Prichard on the Egyptian Mythology."
51. Conybeare and Phillips, *Outlines of the Geology*, xxxix; Creuzer, [Georg Friedrich] (1771–1858). Creuzer, *Religions de l'antiquité*. Anglican geologist priest Conybeare and his friend Prichard shared a desire to use science to demonstrate biblical truth, for which see chapter 9. The French translator's notes supplementing Georg Friedrich Creuzer's *Symbolik und mythologie der alten volker, besonders der Griechen* cited Prichard twenty-two times.
52. Karl Otfried Müller (1797–1840). Müller, Review of James Cowles Prichard's *An Analysis of the Egyptian Mythology*; [Wheaton], "Egyptian Antiquities."
53. Thomas Young (1773–1829); Jean-François Champollion (1790–1832); Rasmus Rask (1792–1832). Champollion, *Apercu des Resultats*; Rask, *Den gamle Ægyptiske tidsregning*; Prichard to Schlegel, June 30, 1842, Manuscripts, Sächsische State Library, Dresden, Mscr. Dresd.e90.XIX, Bd.17, nr.50; Prichard, *Egyptian Mythology* (1838). Prichard's *Egyptian Mythology* was translated as *Darstellung*

der Ägyptischen Mythologie, 1837 and reviewed in several German periodicals such as Georgii, "Prichard, *Darstellung der Ägyptischen Mythologie*."
54. [Cullimore], "Trinity of the Gentiles," 328, 332; Wilkinson, *Manners and Customs*, 402; Gruppe, *Geschichte der klassischen Mythologie*, 133, 140, 141, 143; W. Dawson, *Who Was Who in Egyptology*, 237–38.
55. Henry Bright (1784–1869). Williams, "Bristol in the General Elections," 198–201; Latimer, *Annals of Bristol*, 87–89, 92.
56. Rubinstein, "End of 'Old Corruption.'"
57. Latimer, *Annals of Bristol*, 92–95.
58. Prichard, "Memoir, Part 2," 69–71; Prichard to the British and Foreign Bible Society, February 1, 1821, Archives of the British and Foreign Bible Society, London (in this letter Prichard is annoyed at being reminded to send them Joseph Cowles's £200 legacy). The Green Album records the births and deaths of Edward's children and his wife's death. "Obituary of Joseph Cowles," *Bath Chronicle*, March 16, 1820, 3: "At his house in Kingsmead-terrace, Joseph Cowles, esq, aged 67, formerly of Pontypool; a gentleman, whose singularity of manners whilst taking the air en carriage, attracted such general observation."
59. Munro Smith, *History of the Bristol Royal Infirmary*, 215.
60. Munro Smith, *History of the Bristol Royal Infirmary*, 216–20.
61. Munro Smith, *History of the Bristol Royal Infirmary*, 220. Horwood's skeleton has recently been claimed by his relatives.
62. Advertisement of 12 Berkeley Square, FFBJ, March 11, 1820, 2; Parish of St. Augustine-the-Less, Bristol, Church Rate Book, BA, P.St_Aug/ChW/2/a; Prichard, "Memoir, Part 2," 81.
63. Prichard, "Memoir, Part 2," 81–83, 86.
64. Advertisement for *History of Epidemic Fever* and *Treatise on Diseases of the Nervous System*, FFBJ, November 16, 1822, 2. For the latter book, see chapter 8.
65. "Living Authors, Natives of Bristol," 221.
66. Munro Smith, *History of the Bristol Royal Infirmary*, 226–28.
67. John Eden (d. 1840, aged seventy-eight). Munro Smith, *History of the Bristol Royal Infirmary*, 229–34. For Eden, see chapter 14; for the Phil & Lit, see chapter 9.

8. Nervous Diseases

1. Stewart, *Elements of the Philosophy of the Human Mind*, 3 vols. and several editions.
2. Thomas Arnold (1742–1816); Thomas Beddoes (1760–1808). Arnold, *Observations*; Beddoes, *Hygeia*. For the sake of economy of expression, "psychiatry" and related terms are used anachronistically throughout; French- and English-speaking mad-doctors, alienists, or physicians of the insane resisted the German word *psychiatrie* until nearly the end of the nineteenth century.
3. For a social history of the psychiatric profession at this time, see Suzuki, *Madness at Home*. For a concise general history of psychiatry, see Bynum, "Psychiatry in Its Historical Context," 11–38.

4. Goldstein, *Console and Classify*, 49–59.
5. Goldstein, *Console and Classify*, 1–5, 200–210.
6. Wallace and Gach, *History of Psychiatry*, 354–55.
7. Franz Josef Gall (1758–1828); Franz Anton Mesmer (1734–1815). Mora, "History of Psychiatry," 23–26.
8. Benjamin Rush (1746–1813). Rush, *Medical Inquiries and Observations*.
9. Philippe Pinel (1745–1826), considered the founder of modern psychiatry, established moral treatment, a psychological rather than generally punitive approach to the care of the insane. Among Pinel's nosography of insanity is *manie sans délire*, a form of insanity that Prichard would clarify and elaborate, calling it "moral insanity." Pinel's landmark book *Traité Médico-philosophique sur l'aliénation mentale ou la manie* (1801) was translated as *A Treatise on Insanity* (1806), Kendler, "Philippe Pinel," 2667–72. Jean-Étienne Dominique Esquirol (1772–1840). For Pinel, Esquirol, and moral treatment, see also Goldstein, *Console and Classify*.
10. Prichard, *Treatise on Diseases*, v–ix.
11. Prichard, *Treatise on Diseases*, 39–55.
12. Prichard, *Treatise on Diseases*, 7–8.
13. Prichard, *Treatise on Diseases*, 40, 43.
14. Prichard, *Treatise on Diseases*, 371–76; Prichard, *Analysis of the Egyptian Mythology* (1819), 296.
15. Prichard, *Treatise on Diseases*, 375–81. George Combe had already discussed religion as a cause of insanity in 1818, and George Man Burrows would do so in 1828.
16. Prichard, *Treatise on Diseases*, 45–55.
17. Prichard, *Treatise on Diseases*, 58–81.
18. Prichard, *Treatise on Diseases*, 85–112.
19. Prichard, *Treatise on Diseases*, 113–32.
20. Prichard, *Treatise on Diseases*, 132–38.
21. Prichard, *Treatise on Diseases*, 139–40.
22. Prichard, *Treatise on Diseases*, 141–214.
23. Prichard, *Treatise on Diseases*, 215–344.
24. Prichard, *Treatise on Diseases*, 345–84.
25. Prichard, *Treatise on Diseases*, 385–425.
26. Prichard, *Treatise on Diseases*, 381–82.
27. "Prichard on the Diseases of the Nervous System," 130–42; [Combe], "Dr Pritchard and Phrenology," 48, 54.
28. Notice of *Treatise on Diseases*, 87; "Prichard and Georget," 115–53, pertaining to Prichard only; "Dr. Prichard on Diseases of the Nervous System," *London Medical and Physical Journal*; "Dr. Prichard on Diseases of the Nervous System," *Medico-Chirurgical Review*; "Treatise on Diseases," *Medico-Chirurgical Review*; "Prichard on Diseases of the Nervous System," *American Medical Recorder*; V., "Prichard—'Diseases of the Nervous System,'" 58–73; "J. C. Prichard's 'Treatise on Diseases,'" 524, suggested that it should be translated into German; "Treatise on Diseases," *Medicinische-chriurgische Zeitung*; Review

of *A Treatise on Diseases*, *Göttingische gelehrte Anzeigen*; "Beobachtungen uber die Beziehung," 243–51, translation of *Treatise on Diseases*, 14–22; Review of *A Treatise on Diseases*, *Annali universali di medicina*.

29. Gregory, *Elements*, 1825, and in 1828, 1835, and 1836 editions; see also Cooke, *History and Method of Cure*, 1823; Good, *Study of Medicine*, 1825; Graham, *Modern Domestic Medicine*, 1835; Hooper, *Lexicon Medicum*; Romberg, *Manual of the Nervous Diseases*; Sieveking, *On Epilepsy*, 1858. As for Prichard's antiphlogistic bloodletting, Sieveking represents the growing mid-century condemnation of earlier therapeutics such as Prichard's, writing that it "ought to be eschewed"; e.g., Reynolds, *Epilepsy*, 1861; Gowers, *Epilepsy*, 1881; Baker Brown, *On the Curability*, 1866.

30. Hunter and Macalpine, *Three Hundred Years*, 838, prefatory to an extract from Prichard, *Treatise on Insanity* (1835), 839–42; Hunter, "Status Epilepticus," 165; Aigner and Mulder, "Myoclonus," 600–615; Temkin, *"Falling Sickness,"* 249, 256–57, 260, 265, 278, 286, 289.

31. "Paralysis," 926–27; "Dr. Prichard's Pathology," *Anderson's Quarterly Journal of the Medical Sciences*, 300; "Osservazione sulla paralisia," 442–44; "Observations sur les altérations," *Archives générales de médecine*, 273–74; "Observations sur les altérations," *Journal complémentaire*, 283.

32. John Conolly (1794–1866), *Enquiry concerning Indications of Insanity*, in Suzuki, *Madness at Home*; Prichard to Bunsen, July 26, New York, Manuscripts and Archives, New York Academy of Medicine, New York, MS1307.

33. Alexander Tweedie (1794–1884); Sir John Forbes (1787–1861). Tweedie, *System of Practical Medicine*, 5 vols., 1840–41, and 2nd American ed. in 3 vols., 1842; the American edition is *Cyclopaedia of Practical Medicine*, revised by Robley Dunglison, 1845, and four further printings; Obituary of Dr. Alexander Tweedie, 1101; Jenner, Memoir of Alexander Tweedie, Royal College of Physicians of London Archives, MS1300.

34. Prichard, "Delirium."

35. Samuel Thomas Soemmering (1755–1830). Prichard, "Temperament"; [Combe], "Cyclopaedia of Practical Medicine."

36. Prichard, "Soundness and Unsoundness of Mind," 54.

37. Prichard, "Somnambulism and Animal Magnetism." For mesmerists' criticisms, see Colquhoun, *Hints on Animal Magnetism*, 43–47; Braid, *Neurypnology*, vii, 7, 10; for Prichard's *Vital Principle*, see chapter 10; for scholarly histories of the topic, see Winter, *Mesmerized*; Palfreman, "Mesmerism and the English Medical Profession"; and Lanska and Lanska, "Franz Anton Mesmer."

38. Prichard, "Memoir, Part 2," 276.

39. Cheyne, *English Malady* (1733) in Fischer-Homberger, "Hypochondriasis of the Eighteenth Century," 391–92. Cheyne pointed out inciting English conditions: "The moisture of our air, . . . the rankness and fertility of our soil, the richness and heaviness of our food, the wealth and abundance of the inhabitants (from their universal trade) the inactivity and sedentary occupations of the better sort (among whom this evil mostly rages) and the humour of living in great,

populous and consequently unhealthy towns." For a history of the condition, see also Berrios, "Hypochondriasis."
40. Fischer-Homberger, "Hypochondriasis of the Eighteenth Century," 392–98.
41. Prichard, "Hypochondriasis," 552–57. Also preprinted as *A Treatise on Hypochondriasis*.
42. "Insanity" was printed as a pamphlet, *Della Pazzia* (1839), from his translated article "Della Pazzia," *Enciclopedia della medicina pratica* (1839); "Cyclopaedia of Practical Medicine," 27.
43. Prichard, "Insanity," offprinted as *Treatise on Insanity*; [Symonds], Review of "Insanity."
44. Bynum, "Psychiatry in Its Historical Context"; Eghigian, *From Madness to Mental Health*, 94–104.
45. Examples of new diagnoses based on mental physiology appear in James Davey's *On the Nature and Proximate Cause of Insanity*, 1853, derived from the *First Principles of Medicine* by Archibald Billing, 1830s to 1860s editions, and in the notion of disordered brain function propounded in the 1850s. Despite this new approach, the descriptive language of humoralism lasted throughout the century. See Jansson, *From Melancholia to Depression*, 41, 53, 64–65, 70–71.
46. Samuel Tuke (1784–1857). Prichard to Tuke, July 22, 1834, in Hack Tuke, *Prichard and Symonds*, 14.
47. Prichard, *Treatise on Insanity* (all citations to 1835 ed.); Berrios, *History of Mental Symptoms*.
48. Prichard, *Treatise on Insanity*, 26–79.
49. Prichard, *Treatise on Insanity*, 12–26.
50. Prichard, *Treatise on Insanity*, 83–99.
51. Prichard, *Treatise on Insanity*, 99–111.
52. Prichard, *Treatise on Insanity*, 146, 126–56. For an analysis of this section, see Andrews, "'Of the Termination of Insanity.'"
53. Prichard, *Treatise on Insanity*, 173–76. Recent research confirming the greater prevalence of insanity among developed societies was a topic of discussion in Horatio Clare, "Is Psychiatry Working?" BBC Radio 4, January 20–February 24, 2023.
54. Prichard, *Treatise on Insanity*, 177–249.
55. Prichard, *Treatise on Insanity*, 250–79.
56. Tuke, *Description of The Retreat*, 1813; Prichard, *Treatise on Insanity*, 279–305.
57. Prichard, *Treatise on Insanity*, 306–27.
58. Prichard, *Treatise on Insanity*, 328–51.
59. Johann Christoph Hoffbauer (1766–1827). Hoffbauer, *Die psychologie*; Prichard, *Treatise on Insanity*, 352–70.
60. Prichard, *Treatise on Insanity*, 370–80.
61. Prichard, *Treatise on Insanity*, 380–84, 22–23.
62. Prichard, *Treatise on Insanity*, 397–99. The term "irresistible impulse" is still in use, if more in popular literature than psychiatry.
63. Prichard, *Treatise on Insanity*, 398–99.

64. Prichard, *Treatise on Insanity*, 399–401.
65. Prichard, *Treatise on Insanity*, 405–83. For Prichard's lectures at the Bristol Phil & Lit on the combined subjects of phrenology and mesmerism, reflecting phrenologists' growing interest in mesmerism as their focus on phrenology started to dissipate, see Dr. Prichard: Observations on the Evidence of Phrenology, *Bristol Gazette*, January 8, 1835, 4.
66. Johann Christian August Heinroth (1773–1843). For an extract from Heinroth's 1818 textbook, see Eghigian, *From Madness to Mental Health*, 105–10.
67. Christian Friedrich Nasse (1778–1851); Carl Wigand Maximilian Jacobi (1775–1858). Prichard, *Treatise on Insanity*, 234, 247–49.
68. François-Emmanuel Fodéré (1764–1835); Joseph Guislain (1797–1860); Pierre Laromiguière (1756–1837); Étienne-Jean Georget (1795–1828). For discussions of Prichard's position relative to other theorists outlined in the following three paragraphs, see especially Bynum, "Psychiatry in Its Historical Context"; Augstein, *James Cowles Prichard's Anthropology*; and Berrios, *History of Mental Symptoms*, 103–5, 164, 426–27.
69. "Dr. Prichard on Insanity," *Medico-Chirurgical Review*; Review of *A Treatise on Insanity*, 78; "Prichard on Insanity," *Lancet*; "Dr. Prichard on Insanity," *Medical Quarterly Review*, 32; Esquirol, *Des maladies mentales*, 5, 82. Hack Tuke, *Prichard and Symonds*, 18, states Esquirol had written to Prichard expressing his debt to him.
70. Leidesdorf, "Sandon und die folie affective," 1187; Bonfigli, "Ulteriore considerazione sull'argomento"; "Ueber die Arten," 275; Leupoldt, *Lehrbuch der psychiatrie*.
71. Translated from Heinrich, "Kritische Abhandlung," 501–7, 514, 524–26, 539.
72. J. M. Galt, *Treatment of Insanity*, 282–88; [Conolly], *Familiar Views of Lunacy*. An example of antiphrenology is Michie, *Challenge to Phrenologists*, containing an extract from Prichard's *Treatise*, 465–74 on pages 203–9. For high praise, see [Conolly?], "Prichard . . . on Insanity." The history of psychiatry during this period and Prichard's contributions to it can be found in works by Richard Hunter and Ada MacAlpine, Erwin H. Ackerknecht, Henry E. Sigerist, Garrison Fielding, German E. Berrios, and Andrew T. Scull, in dictionaries and encyclopedias of science and psychiatry, and several PhD dissertations. For the clearest disentanglement of the various meanings of moral insanity, see Whitlock, "Prichard and the Concept," 72–79.
73. Schaeffer, Review of Prichard's *A Treatise on Insanity*, 137–43; "Prichard on Insanity," *Boston Medical and Surgical Journal*, 288; Prichard, *Om Sindssygdommene*; Review of *Om Sindssygdommene*, *Bibliothek for Læger*; Review of *Om Sindssygdommene*, *Journal for Litteratur og Kunst*.
74. Prichard, *Treatise on Insanity* (Philadelphia: E. L. Carey and A. Hart, 1837) and (Philadelphia: Haswell, Barrington, and Haswell, 1837); Earle, "Psychologic Medicine," 275–77; Dain, *Concepts of Insanity*, 74–75.
75. Bynum, "Theory and Practice in British Psychiatry," 83–76; Duncan, "On Insanity," 180; Bucknill and Hack Tuke, *Manual of Psychological Medicine*; Blandford, *Insanity and Its Treatment*, 139, 298–310.

76. Johann Spurzheim (1776–1832); Johann Caspar Lavater (1741–1801). Wallace and Gach, *History of Psychiatry*, 355–56; Staum, *Labeling People*, 30–35.
77. George Combe (1788–1858); Archbishop Richard Whately (1787–1863). Combe, *Essay on the Constitution of Man*; Papers of George Combe, NLS.
78. George Combe, Copy of a Letter to Thomas Murray, April 27, 1838, Private Letter Book, March 6, 1838–December 5, 1844, Papers of George Combe, NLS, MS.7388, ff. 31, 32; Wrobel, "Orthodoxy and Respectability," 38–39; George Combe, Copy of a letter to Watson, March 10, 1838, Private Letter Book, March 6, 1838–December 5, 1844, Papers of George Combe, NLS, MS. 7388, ff. 9–12; Cooter, "Cultural Meaning of Popular Science," 6–28; Bynum, "Time's Noblest Offspring," 196.
79. John Gordon (1786–1818); Peter Mark Roget (1779–1869). Gordon, "Doctrines of Gall"; Roget, *Treatises on Physiology*.
80. Amariah Brigham (1798–1849). Brigham to Combe, January 29, 1839, Papers of George Combe, NLS, MS.7249, ff. 91, 92.
81. Simpson to Combe, April 26, 1837, Papers of George Combe, NLS, MS.7244, ff. 5, 6; Combe, "Dr. Prichard and Phrenology." There were anti-Prichard remarks in at least a dozen articles in the three periodicals between 1834 and 1845.
82. Barlow to Combe, April 23, 1834, Papers of George Combe, NLS, MS.7232, ff. 29, 30.
83. Combe to Prichard, July 22, 1836, Private Letter Book, May 14, 1836–3d March 1838, Papers of George Combe, NLS, MS. 7387, f. 82; Prichard to Combe, October 10, 1836, Papers of George Combe, NLS, MS. 7241, ff. 16–17.
84. Williams, *Physical and the Moral*, 182–87, 190–92; Staum, *Labeling People*, 64–82, 163–65; Parssinen, "Popular Science and Society," 12–14; Cooter, "Cultural Meaning of Popular Science," 3. See also Kaufman, *Edinburgh Phrenological Society*.
85. Prichard to Johnes, July 24, 1843, Glansevern Collection, 3837, NLW.
86. Lord Matthew Hale (1609–76); Thomas Erskine, Baron Erskine (1750–1823); John Singleton, Baron Lyndhurst (1772–1863). Prichard, *On the Different Forms* (all citations to the 1842 edition), [v]–17.
87. Prichard, *On the Different Forms*, 30–63.
88. Prichard, *On the Different Forms*, 161–202.
89. Prichard, *On the Different Forms*, 202–43.
90. Review of *On the Different Forms*, *Athenaeum*; "Prichard, Winslow, Crichton, Rumball &c," 81–87; Review of *On the Different Forms, London Medical Gazette*; [Harris?], "Plea of Insanity."
91. [Taylor], "On MacNaughten's Trial"; Romeyn and Beck, *Elements of Medical Jurisprudence*; Wharton, *Treatise on Mental Unsoundness*; Weiss, "American Forensic Psychiatry Begins," 3–19.
92. For the history of moral insanity under the law, see Hayward, "Murder and Madness"; and Eigen, *Unconscious Crime*. For explorations of the concept of moral insanity's contribution to the formation of psychiatry and the rise of

the psychiatric legal expert, see D. Jones, "Moral Insanity" and Lewinstein, "Historical Development of Insanity."

93. Prichard, "Observations on the Connexions of Insanity," 323–24, reprinted with editor's criticisms in the *Phrenological Journal*, abstracted in *American Journal of the Medical Sciences, Schmidt's Jahrbücher der in-und ausländischen gesammten medicin, Lancet, Medical Times, Annales de la chirurgie française et étrangère, Annali universali di medicina, Filiatre-sebezio: Giornale delle scienze mediche*, and abstracted with criticism in *Zeitschrift fur phrenologie*; Augstein, *James Cowles Prichard's Anthropology*, 35.

94. Prichard, *Treatise on Insanity*, 191–92, 196.

95. McCartney, "Facts, Opinions, and Possibilities"; Bachman, "'Furious Passions of the Celtic Race'"; Trotter, *Paranoid Modernism*; Ganz, "Carrying On"; Smith, "Madness of Ahab"; Rosen, *Madness in Society*, 243; Henderson, "Epidemiology of Alzheimer's Disease," 3; Wood, *Passion and Pathology*.

96. See chapter 15 for Prichard's service as a commissioner in lunacy and the Alleged Lunatics' Friend Society's views of asylumdom.

97. Henry Maudsley (1835–1918). Mann, *Manual of Psychological Medicine*, 47, 107–18; Prichard is referred to on almost every page of Hughes, "Moral (Affective) Insanity-Psycho-Sensory Insanity"; Hack Tuke, *Prichard and Symonds*, 12; Hack Tuke, *Dictionary of Psychological Medicine*; Hack Tuke, *Chapters in the History*, 454–55; extract from *Treatise on Insanity* in Goshen, *Documentary History of Psychiatry*, 133–55; Bynum, "Psychiatry in Its Historical Context"; Wallace and Gach, *History of Psychiatry*.

98. Williams, *Physical and the Moral*, 246–48. In *Descent of Man*, 1871, Darwin refers to his proto-eugenicist cousin Francis Galton's (1822–1911) call for stemming the deterioration in society through managed corrective human breeding. Moore and Desmond, "Introduction," xlvi, liv, 152–72.

99. Dain, *Concepts of Insanity*, 74–75.

100. Boyer, "Religion, 'Moral Insanity,'" 70–78.

101. McCallum, *Personality and Dangerousness*, 4, 28–29. Horatio Clare in his 2023 six-part BBC 4 Radio series "Does Psychiatry Work?" points out a trend toward "social therapy" and concludes that "psychiatry is waiting for its next evolution."

102. Foucault, *Histoire de la folie*; Bynum, "Psychiatry in Its Historical Context," 29. Histories of psychiatry vary in content and interpretation greatly, especially as they have tended to be written with presentist and progressivist attitudes toward the subject. For discussion of this, see Beveridge, "Reading about . . . the History of Psychiatry."

9. "Irksome Things"

1. Prichard, "Memoir, Part 2," 90–95. The books were by Michaelis and Griesbach.
2. Poole, "To Be a Bristolian."
3. Stephens and Roderick, "Nineteenth Century Educational Finance."
4. Neve, "Natural Philosophy, Medicine," 41–58. For Beddoes, see chapter 2.

5. *Report of the Council*, 10; Morris, *Class, Sect and Party*, 228–29; Clark, "Foundation and Early Years," ii.
6. "Bristol Institution," *FFBJ*, January 17, 1824, 4. By 1825 Prichard had subscribed the considerable sum of 25 guineas for a life membership in the Bristol Institution and was a member of its council. The Bristol Institution premises were later sold to the Freemasons, gutted by a World War II incendiary bomb, and rebuilt. For the architect and architecture of learned societies, see Watkin, *Life and Work of C. R. Cockrell*, 49, 96, 136, 145–46, 249, pl. 35; "Bristol Philosophical and Literary Institution," *FFBJ*, November 30, 1822, 2–3.
7. For histories of the Bristol Institution upon which these paragraphs are based, see Symonds, *Our Institution and Its Studies*; Neve, "Natural Philosophy, Medicine"; Neve, "Science in a Commercial City." For contents of the library, museum, officers, members, and debts, see Bristol Institution, *Proceedings of the Twenty-Third Annual Meeting, Report of the Proceedings of the Institution, Report of the Provisional Committee*, and *Proceedings of the Annual Meeting*; along with extensive archival material such as the Minutes of the Philosophical and Literary Society of the Bristol Institution at BA.
8. Richard Bright Sr. (1754–1840); Richard Bright Jr. (1789–1858), physician and discoverer of Bright's Disease, wrote that in about 1815 Prichard and Estlin saved his life. Richard Bright Jr. to Augustin Prichard, June 15, 1855, Estlin Papers, BA. John Scandrett Harford the younger (1785–1866).
9. Martineau, Biographical Memoranda, Harris Manchester College, UO, MS. J. Martineau 13, Wykes 11/117–43.
10. William Daniel Conybeare (1787–1857). Personal communication from Anita Bacci, Accademia dei Fisiocritici, Siena, letter, 1974; "Bristol Philosophical and Literary Society," *FFBJ*, January 10, 1824, 3.
11. Mary Anning (1799–1847). Taylor and Torrens, "Saleswoman to a New Science."
12. "Literary and Philosophical Society annexed to the Bristol Institution," *FFBJ*, March 27, 1824, 3; Prichard, "Essay on the Origin of the Various Species of Vegetables," lecture abstract, *FFBJ*, February 28, 1824, 3; and in Philosophical and Literary Society, Minutes of the Proceedings, Records of the Bristol Institution, 38–39, 44–48, BA, 32079(142); Prichard, "On the Origin and Distinction of Plants and Animals," lecture abstract, *FFBJ*, March 27, 1824, 3.
13. Prichard, "A Collection of Abraxean Stones, Deposited in the Museum by B. H. Bright, Esq.," *FFBJ*, July 31, 1824, 3; Philosophical and Literary Society, Minutes of the Proceedings, Records of the Bristol Institution, 76, BA, 32079(142); Prichard, "Short Description of a Collection."
14. "Bristol Institution, [Remarks Made upon the Opening of a Egyptian Mummy]," *FFBJ*, December 11, 1824, 3.
15. The curator's talented son produced an accurate drawing of the mummy case for Prichard's lecture. So pleased was Prichard with the eleven-year-old's artwork, he presented him with a highly prized box of watercolors, a fond memory of the leading member of the Bristol School of Artists, W. J. Muller (1812–45). Prichard, "On the History of Mummies," a very long abstract of his lecture,

and "Bristol Institution," *FFBJ*, January 15, 1825, 4; Prichard, "Observations on Egyptian Mummies. Read 6th January, 1825," in Philoso. and Lit. Society Lectures, January 5, 1824–March 17, 1825, BA, 32079/PL/L/1; Prichard, "On the History of Mummies," Philosophical and Literary Society Annexed to the Bristol Institution, Minutes of the Proceedings, December 10, 1823–August 25, 1828, BA, 32079/PL/M/1.

16. Prichard, "Observations on the Races of People Who Inhabit the Northern Regions of Africa," lecture abstract, *FFBJ*, June 3, 1826, 4.

17. Prichard, "An Essay on the Native Races of America," *FFBJ*, December 30, 1826, 4.

18. "Philosophical and Literary Society," news clipping, n.d., BIBM, 11:647.

19. "Interlineal Translations"; Prichard, "Some Observations on Literal Interlineary Translations," lecture abstract, *FFBJ*, May 19, 1827, 3. Johann Spurzheim (1776–1832), "Bristol Institution, Lectures on Phrenology," *FFBJ*, January 27, 1827, 3; "Observations on the Evidence of Phrenology" and "An Outline of the History of Animal Magnetism," lectures, *Bristol Gazette*, January 8, 1835, 4; Prichard, "An Historical Account of the Most Remarkable Pestilences Which Have Afflicted Mankind in Different Ages," lecture abstract, *FFBJ*, October 20, 1827, 4; Prichard, "An Historical Account of the Most Remarkable Pestilences Which Have Afflicted Mankind in Different Ages—Part 2," lecture abstract, *FFBJ*, February 16, 1828, 4; Prichard and Hartnell, *Circular Announcing the Concluding Part of J. C. Prichard's Lecture on Pestilences*; Bristol Institution, Announcement of James Cowles Prichard's Lecture on the Vital Principle, *FFBJ*, November 22, 1828, 3. For phrenology and psychology, see chapter 8; for phrenology and anthropology, see chapters 12 and 13; for Prichard's publication on the biological doctrine of vitalism, see chapter 10.

20. Report of the Annual Meeting of the Bristol Institution, *Bristol Mercury*, February 18, 1828, 3.

21. Miller to De la Beche, November 12, 1829, De la Beche Papers, NMW, 84.20G.D.977.

22. Phillips to Harcourt, October 16, 1829, letter 11 in volume of letters from Phillips, Smith, Conybeare, 1821–1873, Harcourt Family, UO, MS. Eng. d. 3876.

23. Neve, "Natural Philosophy, Medicine," 124–34, 150, 158; Bristol Institution, *Proceedings of the Twenty-Third Annual Meeting*, 35, 38.

24. Prichard had borrowed Horace-Benedict De Saussure, *Voyages dans les Alpes*, 1779, from the Bristol Library, and in the month before the trip he borrowed William Cox, *Travels in Switzerland*, 1789, for Mont Blanc; Thomas Watkins, *Travels through Swisserland, Italy, Sicily*, 1792, for the Geneva Public Library and Chamonix; and Simond, *Journal of a Tour*, for the stand-offish behavior of English tourists who are not as high class as in the past, Bristol Library Register, BCL, B.7496. His personal copy of Richard Duppa's *Travels on the Continent*, 1829, was inscribed to him by the author, who had visited Mont Blanc in 1822.

25. Prichard and Prichard, "Journal of a Trip to France and Switzerland 1823," 1–4, Prichard family private collection.

26. Prichard and Prichard, "Journal of a Trip," 4–11.
27. Prichard and Prichard, "Journal of a Trip," 11–16.
28. Prichard and Prichard, "Journal of a Trip," 16–19.
29. Prichard and Prichard, "Journal of a Trip," 19–25.
30. Prichard and Prichard, "Journal of a Trip," 25–27.
31. Marc-Auguste Pictet (1752–1825); John Calvin (1509–64); Jean-Jacques Rousseau (1712–78). Prichard and Prichard, "Journal of a Trip," 25–28.
32. Prichard and Prichard, "Journal of a Trip," 28–31.
33. Prichard and Prichard, "Journal of a Trip," 32–35.
34. Prichard to John Arch, Bristol, February 18, 1824, WC, Autograph Letter File, 69099.
35. See chapter 8.
36. Prichard, "Memoir, Part 2," 98, 107.
37. *Prospectus of the Bristol and Clifton Oil Gas Company*, in BIBM, 11:532–33.
38. Conybeare to Harcourt, January 17, NY, volume of letters to William Vernon Harcourt, Harcourt Family, UO.
39. "Suffering Greeks," *FFBJ*, January 10, 1824, 2; "Cause of the Greeks," *FFBJ*, January 31, 1824, 2; Prichard, Seyer, and Elton, *Cause of the Greeks*.
40. Penn, "Philhellenism in England," 654–59. See also Zegger, "Greek Independence"; Prichard to Hodgkin, August 17, 1840, Hodgkin Family, WC, PP/HO/D/A.
41. Prichard, "Memoir, Part 2," 112–13.
42. Prichard, "Memoir, Part 2," 113–16.
43. See chapter 5.
44. Prichard, "Memoir, Part 2," 125.
45. [Prichard], "On the Genealogies."
46. Sanigar, "Notes concerning the Eden Family of Whitehall," n.d., BCL, B.19446; Eden, *Book of Psalms*, containing a memoir and portrait; Birthday Book, 124.
47. James Yates (1789–1871). Prichard to Yates, August 10, [1826], Oskar Diethelm Historical Library, New York Hospital–Cornell Medical Center; Obituary of James Yates; Yates, *Memorials of the Family*, 24–36.
48. Nathan Branwhite (1775–1857). Prichard to Branwhite, Berkeley Square, May 7, [1827], WC, Autograph Letter File, 56474. This portrait in oil by Branwhite, Bristol's leading portraitist, was in the possession of a grandson in the early twentieth century.
49. Prichard, "Memoir, Part 2," 121–43, 209.
50. [Prichard], "Biographical Notice of the Late Mr. William Swayne," reprinted in *Bristol Mirror*, September 3, 1825, 1. Authorship attributed to Prichard, BIBM, 11:852. See also chapter 5.
51. Obituary of Edward Rochemont Estlin; [James], "Memoir of John Bishop Estlin," 468; Munro Smith, *History of the Bristol Royal Infirmary*, 213.
52. Prichard, letter of recommendation for Edward Oxley's MD, St Andrews University, May 24, 1825, University Muniments, UY350; Prichard and Bernard, letter of recommendation for William Arundel Yeo's MD, St Andrews University, February 1, 1818, University Muniments, UY350.
53. Prichard, "Memoir, Part 2," 144, 145, 157.

54. D. Davies, *Letters on Medical Consultation*, 4.
55. D. Davies, *Letters on Medical Consultation*.
56. Holland to Holland, July 1, 1811, Sir Henry Holland Letters to His Father, NLS, Acc. 7515. Dr. Holland apparently overcame his doubts, published on his international travels, and became a society and royal physician, baronet, and father of a future viscount. See also chapter 5 for medical therapeutics as practiced at the Bristol Infirmary.
57. Rosenberg, "Therapeutic Revolution," 490; Youngson, *Scientific Revolution in Victorian Medicine*, 11–20. See chapter 3.
58. Rosenberg, "Therapeutic Revolution," 491–94; Jewson, "Medical Knowledge and the Patronage System," 372–78, 381–82.
59. Youngson, *Scientific Revolution in Victorian Medicine*, 23–24.
60. Rosenberg, "Therapeutic Revolution," 488–89; Jewson, "Medical Knowledge and the Patronage System," 371–72.
61. Prichard's commitment to bloodletting is discussed in chapter 5.
62. Prichard to Fardon, received July 7, 1806, LSF, Gibson IV, 141.
63. [J. Gregory], "Notes of the Lectures."
64. Welsh, *A Practical Treatise on the Efficacy of Bloodletting*.
65. Perry, "Observations on Blood-Letting," 115.
66. John Armstrong (1784–1829), *Facts and Observations*; Niebyl, "English Bloodletting Revolution," 471. For more examples of Prichard's therapeutics, see *History of the Epidemic Fever*, 56, and marginal notes in his copy now in the Medical School Library, UB; Prichard, "Clinical Lecture Delivered."
67. Prichard, "Successful Case of Transfusion of Blood," *Provincial Medical Journal* and *Retrospect of Practical Medicine and Surgery*, also reported in the foreign press, for example, *Journal de pharmacie et de chimie*, *Annali universali di medicina*, *Filiatre-sebezio: Giornale delle scienze mediche*, *Annales de la chirurgie française et étrangère*, *Österreichische medicinische Wochenschrift als Ergänzungsblatt*, and *Vierteljahrschrift für die praktische Heilkunde*. Equally experimental and unusually interventionist was Prichard, "Evacuation of Fluid," which was reprinted in *Retrospect of Practical Medicine and Surgery*, with abstracts in German periodicals such as *Jahrbücher der in-und ausländischen gesammten Medicin*.
68. Prichard to Huxtable, n.d. but between 1827 and 1845, Autograph File, Houghton Rare Book Library, Harvard University Library; Newman to Martineau, January 17, 1849, Letters from F. W. Newman to James Martineau, 1846–1892, Harris Manchester College, UO, MS. J. Martineau 4; Prichard, "Memoir, Part 2," 268–69, 365.
69. Prichard, "Memoir, Part 2," 276–77.
70. Toogood, *Reminiscences of a Medical Life*, 111.
71. Symonds, *Some Account*, 50.
72. Rathbone to Rathbone, September 23, [1846], Rathbone Papers, Special Collections Department, Sydney Jones Library, University of Liverpool, VII.1.209.
73. A. Prichard, *A Few Medical & Surgical Reminiscences*, 19–20.

74. Prichard, "Remarks on the Treatment of Paralysis"; Prichard, "Dr. Prichard on the Use of Issues," which was abstracted in Prichard, "Paralysis," "Dr. Prichard's Pathology," *Journal of Foreign Medical Science and Literature*; "Observations sur les altérations du système nerveux dans la chorée" (a French abstract of the *London Medical Repository* article), "On the Treatment of Hemiplegia," "Trattamento dell'emiplegia," "Treatment of Hemiplegia," and "Traitement de l'hémiplégie"; Pitschaft, "Miscellanen, rhapsodien und erfahrungen," 16; Bureaud Riofrey, "Retrospective Review of the Therapeutical Progress."
75. Toogood, "On the Advantages of Counter-Irritation," 519; Toogood, *Reminiscences of a Medical Life*, 6; Prichard's "On the Treatment of Some Diseases" was abstracted and translated in several English, Indian, American, French, and German medical journals.
76. Prichard, "Address Delivered at the Third Anniversary Meeting."
77. Youngson, *Scientific Revolution in Victorian Medicine*, 21–22, 9–11.
78. Alison, "Reflections on the Results." Change of type theory was effectively contradicted by Markham's *Bleeding and Change*.
79. Warner, "Therapeutic Explanation," 244–46.
80. Pellegrino, "Sociocultural Impact," 247; Rosenberg, "Therapeutic Revolution," 486–87; Risse, "Renaissance of Bloodletting," 4–5.
81. A. Prichard, *A Few Medical & Surgical Reminiscences*, 16.
82. William Williams to Taliesin Williams, March 4, 1843, Taliesin ab Iolo MSS, Williams, NLW, MS.21278E, T-W, letter 994.
83. Gibson, *Rambles in Europe*, 278–79.
84. A. Prichard, *Some Incidents*, 90–91.
85. Prichard to Rathbone, March 24, [1848], Menninger Foundation, O D Misc Box 2 Prichard, 1.
86. Richard Duppa (1770-1831). Duppa to Prichard, c.1826-1831, Birthday Book, 193.
87. Royal Society of London, *Record of the Royal Society*, 388; Certificates of Election and Candidature, Royal Society of London Archives, EC/1826/18.
88. Prichard, "Memoir, Part 2," 154–55.
89. Prichard, "Memoir, Part 2," 154–65.
90. Prichard, "Memoir, Part 2," 158–60, 170.
91. Prichard, "Memoir, Part 2," 163–64.

10. The Early Red Lodge Years

1. Prichard, "Memoir, Part 2," 173.
2. Sturge, *Reminiscences of My Life*, 30.
3. *The Red Lodge*, [1, 2]; Pritchard, "Bristol Archaeological Notes," 147, 148.
4. Barrington, *Life of Walter Bagehot*, 98–99.
5. Bagehot copy to Thomas Watson Bagehot, April 26, 1842, and c.1845/1846, St. John-Stevas family private collection.
6. Bagehot copy to Edith Stuckey Estlin Bagehot, May 2, 1842, St. John-Stevas family private collection.
7. Irvine, *Walter Bagehot*, 15.

8. Southey, *The Doctor*, 2:3, where Southey thanks Prichard for providing the Ossete etymology of the place-name Doncaster; 7:480–81, for Southey's praise of Prichard's *Physical History* for providing the philological proof of the unity of mankind and confirmation of the scriptural account; Mary Prichard's Album, Special Collections, University Library, UB, DM. 931.
9. Lant Carpenter (1780–1840); William Benjamin Carpenter (1813–85); Mary Carpenter (1807–77); James Martineau (1805–1900); William Herapath (1796–1868); John Foster (1770–1843); Robert Hall (1764–1831). J. Carpenter, *James Martineau*, 58–59; Drummond and Upton, *Life and Letters*, 1:48; 2:263.
10. Prichard, "Memoir, Part 2," 183–84, 215–17, 225.
11. Prichard, "Memoir, Part 2," 184–85, 192–93; Pollok, *Course of Time*. All the rage in 1828, this poem soon faded from the English literary canon.
12. Prichard, "Memoir, Part 2," 185–86.
13. Prichard, "Memoir, Part 2," 187–91.
14. Prichard, "Memoir, Part 2," 194–96; Bristol Library Register, BCL, B.7502–4.
15. "A Review of the Doctrines of Modern Physiologists Respecting a Vital Principle," no. 80, in List of Papers Read before the Public Meetings; Prichard, *Review of the Doctrine*, iii–viii.
16. Williams, *Physical and the Moral*, 46–54.
17. Joseph Priestly (1733–1804); John Hunter (1728–1803). Priestly, *Disquisitions Relating to Matter*. Prichard employed a lot of vitalist-laden terminology in this volume, such as "force," "power," and "constitution." For a discussion of reductionism versus materialism and Prichard's accommodation of these, see Knight, "Vital Flame," 5–6, 11–12.
18. Goodfield-Toulmin, "Some Aspects of English Physiology," 284–86.
19. Goodfield-Toulmin, "Some Aspects of English Physiology," 292–97.
20. See chapter 6 for a more detailed account of the Lawrence affair. For vitalism in medical philosophy, see especially Williams, *Physical and the Moral*.
21. Prichard, *Review of the Doctrine*, 22–26.
22. Prichard, *Review of the Doctrine*, 141–42; Goodfield-Toulmin, "Some Aspects of English Physiology," 295. See also T. Hall, *Ideas of Life*, 2:232–36.
23. Prichard, *Review of the Doctrine*, 143–91. See also chapter 8.
24. Prichard, *Review of the Doctrine*, 195–236.
25. T. Hall, *Ideas of Life and Matter*, 232–36.
26. John Joseph Gurney (1788–1847). Prichard, "Memoir, Part 2," 308.
27. "Dr Prichard on the Vital Principle"; "Prichard on a Vital Principle," *Eclectic Review*; "Prichard—On the Vital Principle," *British Critic*; Hy., Review of Prichard's Vital Principle, *Göttingische gelehrte Anzeigen*; [Symonds], Review of Prichard's Vital Principle, *Bath and Bristol Magazine*.
28. "Barclay and Prichard on the Principle of Life"; Rupke, *Richard Owen: Victorian Naturalist*, 311–12, 306–7, 309; Blakey, *History of the Philosophy of Mind*, 560–62, citing Prichard's belief in the distinctness of the mind.
29. Bostock, *An Elementary System of Physiology*, 405, 459, 531, 540, 745; Goodfield-Toulmin, "Some Aspects of English Physiology," 290, 304–6.
30. Prichard, "Memoir, Part 2," 205–7.

31. Prichard, "Memoir, Part 2," 209–10; Prichard, "To the Editor of *Felix Farley's Bristol Journal*," FFBJ, February 13, 1830, 3, reprinted in *Outline of the Plan*, 12–13; Miller to Henry Thomas De la Beche, November 12, 1829, De la Beche Papers, NMW, 84.20G.D.977.
32. O. Gregory, *Brief Memoir*, 214, 266–67.
33. J. Foster, *Letters from John Foster*, 17–18.
34. Roman Catholics would eventually emerge from the shadows of Bristol culture to establish their first church in 1843, St Mary on the Quay. Two years later a wealthy Jewish merchant was elected a Conservative member of the city council, whose non-Anglican members were in the majority. Dresser, "Protestants, Catholics, and Jews," 106–16.
35. John Champeny Swayne (c. 1786–1852). Prichard, "Bristol College [Notice of a Meeting of Subscribers]," FFBJ, November 19, 1829, 3; Historicus [James Cowles Prichard?], "Bristol College, To the Editor of the *Bristol Journal*," reprinted in FFBJ, November 14, 1829, 4; Estlin to Coates, November 3, 1829, Papers of the Society for the Diffusion of Useful Knowledge 26, UCL.
36. "Report of the Meeting of Subscribers to Bristol College," FFBJ, November 28, 1829, 3. The College was planned to have a capital of £15,000 raised in three hundred transferable shares. Prichard bought two. This report was printed as *Bristol College, for Classical and Scientific Education* (Bristol: n.p., 1829), bound in BIBM, 11:662.
37. *Prospectus of a College*.
38. Estlin to Coates, November 30, 1829, Papers of the Society for the Diffusion of Useful Knowledge 26, UCL.
39. Robert Gray, bishop of Bristol (1762–1834). Gray, "Circular Letter to the Clergy concerning the Establishment of Bristol College, December 4, 1829," *Bristol Mercury*, December 8, 1829, 3.
40. "Bristol College, Meeting to Appoint a Provisional Committee and Establish a Theological Lecture Fund," FFBJ, December 12, 1829, 2; *Bristol College Theological Lecture Fund*.
41. Prichard, "Memoir, Part 2," 213–14.
42. Estlin to Coates, January 8, 1830, Papers of the Society for the Diffusion of Useful Knowledge 27, UCL.
43. "Bristol College. To the Editor," FFBJ, December 5, 1829, 3; "Bristol College," FFBJ, December 12, 1829, 3, contains an editorial condemning the College, more negative letters, and a report of the December 10 meeting recounting the disruptions and complaints by several clergymen; A Member of the Royal College of Surgeons, *An Address to the Shareholders*.
44. [Bristol College Council], "Address of the Council of the Bristol College," FFBJ, December 26, 1829, 2.
45. Shackleton, Letter to the Council of Bristol College, FFBJ, January 30, 1830, 2; Prichard, "To the Editor of *Felix Farley's Bristol Journal* [Introducing the Rev WD Conybeare's Letter in Support of Bristol College]," FFBJ, March 20, 1830, 4.
46. Prichard, "To the Editor."

47. Estlin to Coates, March 13, 1830, Papers of the Society for the Diffusion of Useful Knowledge 27, UCL.
48. Estlin to Coates, May 2, 1830, Papers of the Society for the Diffusion of Useful Knowledge 27, UCL.
49. "Bristol College [Report of a Special Meeting, June 9, 1830]," *FFBJ*, June 12, 1830, 3; [Budd], *Memoir of the Rev. Henry Budd*, 266-67.
50. Joseph Henry Jerrard (1801-53), *Outline of the Plan*; "Opening of the Bristol College," *FFBJ*, January 22, 1831, 4; Carrick, *Address on the Opening*; Estlin to Coates, January 19, 1831, Papers of the Society for the Diffusion of Useful Knowledge 28, UCL.
51. Francis William Newman (1805-97). Newman to the editor of "Men of the Time," April 14, 1864, UCL, MS. Misc. 3N; Newman to the Council of London University College, June 1, 1846, College Correspondence RE: F. W. Newman, UCL, Mylne, J. W., 1846: June 4.
52. For attempts at professorships, see chapter 11. [Prichard], "On Oneirophantia & Daemonology"; Prichard, "Memoir, Part 2," 284-85, 232-33.
53. Bristol College, *Proceedings of the Fourth Annual Meeting*; "Bristol College Examination," *FFBJ*, July 11, 1835, 3; *Part of the Evidence Given by J.H. Jerrard, D.C.L.*
54. [Swayne], "In Memoriam," 8.
55. *Mathews's Annual Bristol Directory*, 1832, 277, and until 1841, 48-49, when the entry for Bristol College was greatly expanded to include detailed description of its curriculum; Jerrard to Coates, July 13, 1832, College Correspondence, Special Collections, UCL, 1833:2983; Jerrard to Coates, September 24, 1834, Papers of the Society for the Diffusion of Useful Knowledge 31, UCL.
56. Prichard to Clark, April 1834, Box 1, Letters to G. T. Clark, 1822-1847, G. T. Clark Manuscripts, NLW, letter 31.
57. John Sterling (1806-44). Estlin and Sterling, Memoranda for an Appeal for Bristol College, 1841, Estlin Papers, BA.
58. For discussion of Prichard's treatment of hemiplegia, see chapter 9. Prichard and Conybeare, Obituary Memoir of J. S. Miller, *FFBJ*, November 20, 1830, 4; Prichard, "Geography of Palestine."
59. John Addington Symonds (1807-71). Hack Tuke, *Prichard and Symonds in Especial Relation to Mental Science*, 29-57; "Obituary: John Addington Symonds," 268; "Some Famous Bristol Doctors"; A. Prichard, *A Few Medical & Surgical Reminiscences*, 28-30.
60. Prichard to John Griscom, June 19, 1830, property of the author; Bristol Library Register, BCL, B.7502-5.
61. [Prichard], "Remarks on the Poetry of the Hebrews." Its offprint, annotated by Lant Carpenter, "From the Author Dr Prichard May, 17.37.(9)," is in Dr Williams's Library, London.
62. P[richard], "Horae Africanae, No. 2," 737-43. the table of contents of this periodical gives the author as "Dr. Prichard"; P[richard], "Horae Africanae. No. 2," offprinted as *Horae Africanae. No. 2.—History of the Guanches*.
63. P[richard], "Horae Africanae," 477. By "civilization," Prichard meant "culture," as the latter term had not yet come into English usage in its anthropological

sense. Prichard used Gregorious's portrait as the frontispiece to the second edition of his *Physical History*.

64. Prichard, "Memoir, Part 2," 227–28.
65. Estlin to Brougham, April 29, 1830, Brougham Papers, UCL, 5161.
66. Large, *Radicalism in Bristol*, 10–11.
67. Anderson, "Cousin Marriage in Victorian England," 286–91. One of Prichard's children married a first cousin.
68. E. Prichard, *Observations on the Changes*; E. Prichard, *Reply to the Chapter*; E. Prichard, *Marriage with a Deceased Wife's Sister*; Society of Friends registers, parish registers, and Hereford newspapers used extensively in this account.
69. Prichard, "Memoir, Part 2," 233–45.
70. Prichard, "Memoir, Part 2," 175–76, 260–61; Russell, *Connection of Sacred and Profane*; [Prichard], "Chronology," in which he includes a short notice of the Danish linguist Rasmus Rask's *Den gamle Ægyptiske tidsregning*, 1829; Bristol Library Register, BCL, B.7506–7.
71. E. Davies, *Celtic Researches*, lxiii.
72. John Pinkerton (1758-1826). Horsman, "Origins of Racial Anglo-Saxonism," 387–98. For the extrapolation of ideas of race from philological studies of the European nations as discussed in encyclopedia articles in the decades around the turn of the nineteenth century and an analysis of Pinkerton's polygenism and anti-Celticism, see Stock, "'Almost a Separate Race.'"
73. Curtis, *Apes and Angels*, 19–20; M'Lauchlan, *Celtic Gleanings*, 167.
74. Franz Bopp (1791-1867). "To the Reverend William Daniel Conybeare, A.M. F.R.S. &c. Rector of Sully, and to Professor Jacob Grimm of the University of Goettingen, this Work is Inscribed, in Testimony of the High Respect and Regard of the Author," in Prichard, *Eastern Origin*, 1st ed., iii.
75. Prichard, *Eastern Origin*, 187.
76. Sir William Jones (1746-94). "Prichard on the Celtic Nations," *Eclectic Review*; [Garnett], "Prichard on the Celtic Nations."
77. Stanley, *Life and Correspondence*, 178.
78. "Origin and Affinity"; "Remarks on the Review of Dr. Prichard's Work."
79. Edward Burnett Tylor (1832-1917). Hack Tuke, *Prichard and Symonds*, 7.
80. Jacob Ludwig Karl Grimm (1785-1863). "Prichard, the Celtic Nations," in Grimm, *Kleinere schriften*, 5:122–25, 123, 259; Ebel, *Celtic Studies*, vi; Pott, *Etymologische forschungen*, 478; Lefmann, *Franz Bopp*, 224–25 (Bopp's copy of *Eastern Origin* is in Cornell University Library); von Schlegel, "De l'origine des Hindous," 137–214; "Prichard on the Celtic Languages"; Kuhn, Review of *Eastern Origin*; Meyer, "Celtische sprachen."
81. Van Hal, "From Jones to Pictet," 6–8; Augstein, *James Cowles Prichard's Anthropology*, 157–70.
82. Dillon, *Celts and Aryans*, 8–10; Turley, *Politics of Language*, 131–36; Griffith, "History of Welsh Scholarship," 219; Winning, *Manual of Comparative Philology*; [Brown], "Celtae," 273–77; Welsford, *On the Origin and Ramifications*, v–vi; Donaldson, *New Cratylus*, 46–47; Garnett, *Philological Essays*,

78-111; Mackinnon, *University of Edinburgh*, 17-18; C. Bunsen, *Outlines of the Philosophy*, 47-49; Ian Stewart, email, 2021. For his analysis of Prichard's book and its place in the history of linguistics, see Stewart, "James Cowles Prichard"; Stewart, "After Sir William Jones."

83. Prichard to Traherne, August 26, 1834, and September 5, 1834, Traherne Collection, NLW, 6598D 70, 105 and 105A, 106. He continued to press Traherne to professionalize the Welsh Antiquarian Society, July 30, [1840], March 24, [1841], Traherne Collection, 109, 110.

84. Benjamin Hall (1802-67); Augusta Hall (1802-67). Prichard to Du Ponceau, October 26, 1838, William S. Gilbert Collection, College of Physicians of Philadelphia Library. See also Gurden-Williams, "Lady Llanover."

85. Théodore Claude Henri, vicomte Hersart de la Villemarqué (1815-95). Christian Charles Josias von Bunsen (1791-1860). Prichard to Bunsen, November 10, 1838, Geheimes Staatsarchiv Preußischer Kulturbesitz; Hersart de la Villemarqué, *La villemarqué*, 52, 54; Bunsen to Prichard, October 19, 1839, Birthday Book, 76.

86. Rees, *Liber Landavensis*, iii, vii; Prichard, *Ethnography of the Celtic Race*; John Davies, "Cymreigyddion y Fenni and Its Work," Papers of or from the library of John Davies, NLW, MS.11415B. For influence on the translator Lady Charlotte Guest, see Obey, *Wunderkammer of Lady Charlotte Guest*, 119-20, 200.

87. Prichard to Bunsen, September 28, [1842], ff. 215-16, October 7, [1842], ff. 223-24, October 12, 1842, ff. 225-26, Geheimes Staatsarchiv Preußischer Kulturbesitz; Prichard, "Adjudication of the Great Prize," NLW, 13,961E, 73.

88. "South Wales: The Abergavenny Cymreigyddion," *Bristol Mirror*, October 22, 1842, 3; *Monmouthshire Merlin*, October 22, 1842, 4; *Bristol Mercury*, October 22, 1842, 2; Abergavenny Cymreigyddion Society, *Hereford Times* (Supplement), October 22, 1842, 1, where Prichard's adjudication is in cols. 2-3, preceded by an apology for his absence owing to being on duty in his new government commission; James Cowles Prichard, Adjudication of Abergavenny Cymreigyddion Prize, 1842, NLW, 13,961E, 73; Prichard to Bunsen, October 20, [1842], ff. 241-42, Geheimes Staatsarchiv Preußischer Kulturbesitz.

89. Prichard to Bunsen, October 7, [1842], ff. 223-24, Geheimes Staatsarchiv Preußischer Kulturbesitz; Prichard to Buschmann, April 10, 1845, Darmstaedter Collection 3 l, State Library of Prussian Cultural Heritage.

90. "Twelfth Anniversary of the Abergavenny Cymreigyddion Society," *Hereford Times* (Supplement), October 25, 1845, 1, Prichard's adjudication in cols. 7-9; "Abergavenny Cymreigddion," *Monmouthshire Merlin and South Wales Advertiser*, October 25, 1845, 3; and *Cambrian Journal* 1 (March 1854): 5-11.

91. Prichard to Traherne, September 10, 1846, Traherne Collection, 108.

92. Prichard, *Eastern Origin* (1857); [Stokes], "Dr. Latham's Celtic Philology"; Ewald, Review of *The Eastern Origin*; Review of *The Eastern Origin*, *Archaeologia Cambrensis*; Cull and Williams, Review of *The Eastern Origin*. Latham earned £30, while the Prichard family was paid £23, 12 shillings.

Personal communication, letter from E. M. Dring, Bernard Quaritch, Ltd, May 23, 1974.
93. See also Prichard's speech on comparative philology: "On the Various Methods of Research."
94. Prichard, "Memoir, Part 2," 247–48.
95. Prichard, "Memoir, Part 2," 246, 255–56.
96. Prichard, "Memoir, Part 2," 269.
97. Prichard, "Memoir, Part 2," 278–79.
98. Orange, "Origins of the British Association," 152–61.
99. William Vernon Harcourt (1789–1871). Prichard to Phillips, August 25, 1831, Correspondence of John Phillips, Archive of the British Association for the Advancement of Science, Bodleian Libraries, UO, 1; Prichard to Harcourt, September 22, [1831], Correspondence and Papers of William Vernon Harcourt, 1817–71, Papers of the Harcourt Family, Bodleian Libraries, UO, MS. Eng. d. 3873; List of Members' Signatures, Archive of the British Association for the Advancement of Science, 2.
100. Prichard, "Memoir, Part 2," 249, 252. Prichard and Gilby are signatures nos. 157 and 158 for the year 1831 in the BAAS List of Members' Signatures, Archive of the British Association for the Advancement of Science, 2.
101. Conybeare to William Vernon Harcourt, September 8, 1831, Correspondence of William Vernon Harcourt, 1822–73, Papers of the Harcourt Family, Bodleian Libraries, UO, MS. Eng. d. 3876; Morrell, "Individualism and the Structure," 184–87; Harcourt to Whewell, postmarked October 17, 1831, Whewell Papers, Trinity College, Cambridge, Add.MS. a. 205; Notebook of John Phillips, Oxford Meeting, [32], and Notebook of John Phillips Cambridge [and Edinburgh], 21, Archive of the British Association for the Advancement of Science. For the role of the BAAS in the development of anthropology, see chapter 12. Prichard served on the subcommittee in 1832 and 1833.
102. Prichard to [Yates], May 27, 1833, John Rylands Library, University of Manchester, Rylands English MS. 382/1646/1.
103. Orange, "Idols of the Theatre," 277–94.
104. Poole, "To Be a Bristolian," 76–95; M. Harrison, "'To Raise and Dare Resentment,'" 557–85.
105. Atkinson, "Early Example of the Decline," 74–75.
106. Conybeare to Harcourt, November 13, 1831, Phillips, Smith, Conybeare, 1821–1873, letter 124, Correspondence of William Vernon Harcourt, 1822–73, MS. Eng. d. 3876. Funding compensation for the 1831 Bristol riots crippled the city's finances for years.
107. See chapter 5.
108. "Cholera Morbus," *FFBJ*, November 19, 1831, 3; [Appointment of James Cowles Prichard to the Bristol Board of Health, March 22, 1832, and copy of correspondence March 22 to July 20, 1832], 59, 214, 253, Central Board of Health, Letter Books February 21, 1832–April 28, 1832, April 30, 1832–July 20, 1832, NA, MSS, PC1/94, PC1/95, pp. 564–66.

109. "Board of Health in This City," *Bristol Mirror*, November 19, 1831, 3; "Subscriptions for the Relief of the Poor and the Prevention of Cholera," FFBJ, December 31, 1831, 2.
110. "Bristol Election. [Requisition to Sir Rich. Rawlinson Vyvyan, Bart, October 11, 1832]," *Bristol Mirror*, October 13, 1832, 3.
111. Butcher, *Bristol Corporation of the Poor*, 164–65.
112. Hardcastle, *Life of John, Lord Campbell*, 74–75.
113. Matthews to J. R. Hay, August 1832, John Rylands University Library, Manchester, Rylands English MSS., 1196, nos. 41, 42, quoted in Neve, "Natural Philosophy, Medicine," 275–76.
114. Hardcastle, *Life of John, Lord Campbell*, 74–75.
115. George Cumberland, Diary for 1832, Department of Manuscripts, BL, Add. MS. 36,521G.
116. St. Peter's Hospital, Report of a Meeting of Court, undated news clipping, in BIBM, 11:540; Central Board of Health Privy Council, Orders in Council for Boards of Health July 25, 1832–October 9, 1832, 88, NA, MSS, PC1/98. St. Peter's Hospital and its records were destroyed by enemy action on November 24, 1940. Prichard, "Memoir, Part 2," 266. See also De la Beche and Playfair, "Report on the Sanatory Condition of Bristol," 241–64.
117. Prichard, "Memoir, Part 2," 267, 279.
118. This first of four Victorian cholera epidemics had a British death toll of about thirty-one thousand. See also McLean, *Public Health and Politics*; Hardiman, *1832 Cholera Epidemic*.

11. Life and Reputation at the Red Lodge

1. Prichard, "Memoir, Part 2," 290–91.
2. Mary Prichard, Journal of a Tour to Paris, Pocock Papers, BA, 46875/J/1. For Prichard's reference to French psychiatrists, see chapter 8.
3. Prichard, "Memoir, Part 2," 282–84.
4. Munro Smith, *History of the Bristol Royal Infirmary*, 378–81; A. Prichard, *Bristol Medical School*; [Parker], *Schola Medicinae Bristol*. The exact date and degree of amalgamation are unclear.
5. List of Officers, Members.
6. Munro Smith, "Notes on Some Bristol Medical Societies," 277–78. See also "Bristol Meeting of the British Medical Association"; McMenemey, *Life and Times of Sir Charles Hastings*, 98–101.
7. Bristol Medical and Surgical Association, Inaugural Meeting Held at the Medical Library, FFBJ, June 20, 1840, 2; Munro Smith, "Notes on Some Bristol Medical Societies," 278.
8. Prichard, "Address Delivered at the Opening of the Bristol Branch of the Provincial Medical Association, by Dr. Prichard," *Bristol Mirror*, July 4, 1840, 4.
9. Provincial Medical and Surgical Association, Minutes of Proceedings of the Bath District Branch, November 18, 1836–June 27, 1842, and the Bath and Bristol Branch, June 30, 1842–July 15, 1854, ff. 29v–34r, Clinical Society of

Bath Archives, Bath Record Office, 1265. Prichard attended this meeting and dinner on June 3, 1841.
10. "Bath and Bristol Branch."
11. B. Harrison, "Drink and Sobriety," 218, 244; seven temperance tracts in BA, 13063(1); Bristol Auxiliary Temperance Society, *First Report*, 5. Prichard attended its third anniversary meeting on July 29, 1833, BIBM, 11:623.
12. Ram Mohan Roy (1772-1833). Bayly, "Rammohan Roy."
13. Martin, *Memories of Seventy Years*, 170-71. See also Barot, *Bristol and the Indian Independence Movement*.
14. M. Carpenter, *Last Days in England*, 138-47. See also "Ram Mohun Roy"; Banerji, "Sutherland's Reminiscences of Rammohun Roy." Roy's portrait, statue, and mausoleum are in Bristol, where his life is commemorated annually.
15. Daniel to Hare, Sunday morning, addressed to Richard Smith, BIBM, 11:682.
16. Prichard to Daniel, December 23, 1833, BIBM, 11:684.
17. Prichard, "Memoir, Part 2," 300-309, 314-15, 318-20, 329; Journal Book of the Royal Society, vol. 47, May 9, 1833-June 16, 1836, 524, Royal Society of London Archives.
18. Prichard to Clark, [1834], Letters to G. T. Clark, letter 5; Bristol Institution, *Three Lectures*; Prichard, *Lectures on the Mummies*, a reprint from *Bristol Mirror*, April 5, 1834; Bristol Institution, Advertisement for a Course of Lectures on Egypt, Egyptian Antiquities and the Rosetta Stone, FFBJ, March 22, 1834, 3; Bristol Institution, *Proceedings of the Twelfth Annual Meeting*, 17. The well-connected London surgeon Thomas Joseph Pettigrew (1791-1865) was an entertaining mummy-unwrapper at this time. Prichard subscribed to his illustrated book on the subject and wrote to him in 1833 about the copper color of Egyptian skin, Prichard to Pettigrew, July 2, 1833, WC, Autograph Letter File. Prichard's wax seal depicts the Egyptian image of reared serpent and priest.
19. Dr. Prichard's First of Three Lectures on Egyptian Mummies, Egyptian Antiquities, and the Rosetta Stone, *Bristol Gazette*, April 3, 1834, 3; "Bristol Institution: Dr. Prichard's Lectures on Egyptian Mummies and Antiquities," *Bristol Mercury*, April 5, 1834, 3, and April 12, 1834, 4.
20. "Lectures on Egyptian Mummies, Egyptian Antiquities, and the Rosetta Stone," abstract and report, FFBJ, April 5, 1834, 2. Prichard sent the manuscript of his lectures to FFBJ, but much of it was printed in long articles in the *Bristol Gazette*, April 10, 1834, 4, and April 17, 1834, 4, and in the *Bristol Mirror*, April 5, 1834, 3-4, and April 12, 1834, 4.
21. "Lecture III, Lectures on the Mummies and Antiquities of Egypt," report, *Bristol Mirror*, April 19, 1834, 4.
22. Report of Annual General Meeting of the Bristol Institution, FFBJ, February 14, 1835, 3.
23. Sanders to Clark, April 7, 1834, and Conybeare to Clark, October 7, 1834, Letters to G. T. Clark, letters 30 and 37.
24. *Bristol Institution*, vol. 1, *Its Origin and Progress* (1896), 264, BA, 32079/BI/H/4.

25. Conybeare to Clark, received December 1834, and Conybeare to Clark, received 1835?, Letters to G. T. Clark, letters 45 and 49; "Ethnographical Memoir on the Nations of Slavonian Race, Part 1"; "Ethnographical Memoir on the Nations of Slavonian Race, Part 2". He had lectured the Phil & Lit on "An Ethnographical Memoir of the Slavonic Nations, with Remarks on Their Mythology," January 10, 1833, List of Papers Read before the Public Meetings of the Philosophical and Literary Society, from its Commencement to 26th May 1836, No. 128, BA, 32079.
26. Conybeare to Clark, November 9, 1835, Letters to G. T. Clark, letter 71. For the BAAS, see chapter 12.
27. Bristol Philosophical and Literary Society, Annual General Meeting for the year 1838–39, *FFBJ*, June 8, 1839, 4.
28. William Herapath (1796–1868), lecturer at the Bristol Medical School, sometime Radical local politician. Wetherell, *Trial of Mary Ann Burdock*; Munro Smith, *History of the Bristol Royal Infirmary*, 270–71; Report of a Trial at Bristol Quarter Sessions, January 11, 1830, *Bristol Mirror*, January 16, 1830, 3; "Poisoning at the Bristol Infirmary," 109; "Inquest [on the Body of Mary Mabbett, December 3, 1839]," *Bristol Mercury*, December 7, 1839, 8.
29. Prichard, "Memoir, Part 2," 320–21, 330–33, 343–44, 350, 355, 360, 361, 368, 372, 377, 378; Mary Jane Moline to Edith Pocock, October 4, NY, Records of Rev. Theodore Innes Pocock, BA, 46875/Co/3. "Rigors" could also refer to a recurrent fever, as from malaria. A "remittance man" was a person who had become an embarrassment to his family and was sent a regular remittance on promising not to return to Britain.
30. Prichard to [Carrington?], December 4, 1845, Album, Special Collections, University of Iowa Libraries.
31. Neve, "Natural Philosophy, Medicine," 309–16.
32. Neve, "Natural Philosophy, Medicine," 323–30.
33. John Kidd (1775–1851); Charles Giles Bridle Daubeny (1795–1867); Rev. Dr. William Buckland (1784–1856). Prichard to Daubeny, June 22, 1835, Magdalen College Library, UO, MS. 400/36; "Provincial Medical and Surgical Association," 551. Dr. Buckland proposed a geological theory that reconciled geological evidence with scriptural history. The Radcliffe Library is now known as the Radcliffe Camera.
34. Buxton and Gibson, *Oxford University Ceremonies*, 84–91; Symonds, *Some Account*, 10.
35. Sir Charles Bell (1774–1842). Report of the Third Anniversary Meeting of the Provincial Medical and Surgical Association, *Bristol Gazette*, August 6, 1835, 4; "Provincial Medical and Surgical Association"; "Provincial Medical & Surgical Association," *Oxford University, City, and County Herald*, July 25, 1835, 2; Prichard, *Address Delivered at the Third Anniversary Meeting*; Review of James Cowles Prichard's Retrospective Address, *British and Foreign Medical Review*; Siemers, Review of James Cowles Prichard's Retrospective Address, *Zeitschrift fur die gesammte medicin*; Certificate of the Honorary Degree of Doctor of Medicine from the University of Oxford, granted to James Cowles Prichard on July 3, 1835, BA, 16082 (2).

36. "Provincial Medical and Surgical Association."
37. William Ley (1815-87); Dionysius Lardner (1793-1859); William West (1803-37); William Wilde (1815-76). Ticknor, *Life, Letters*, 418-25; *Proceedings of the Fifth Meeting*.
38. Charles Babbage (1791-1871). Notebook of John Phillips, Arrangements, etc. for Dublin, 1835, 130-33, Archive of the British Association for the Advancement of Science.
39. William Rowan Hamilton (1805-65). Ticknor, *Life, Letters*, 423; Prichard, "Memoir, Part 2," 323-24. Prichard was elected honorary member of the Royal Irish Academy; James Cowles Prichard, Certificate of election to Honorary Membership of the Royal Irish Academy, January 25, 1836, BA, 16082(3); Minutes of the Academy, vol. 2, January 1827-March 1849, Archives, Royal Irish Academy, Dublin. Prichard was elected honorary fellow of the College of Physicians of Ireland; College of Physicians of Ireland, *Register of the King and Queen's College*, 114; Widdess, *History of the Royal College*.
40. Robert James Graves (1797-1853). Williams, *Memoirs*, 113.
41. Prichard to Harcourt, November 3, 1835, Correspondence and Papers of William Vernon Harcourt, 1817-71, MS. Eng. d. 3873, ff. 21-27.
42. Susanna Estlin to Mary Anne Estlin, July 28, 1836, Estlin Papers, BA.
43. Greenough to Clark, August 21, 1836, "James Burton's letters," Greenough Papers, UCL; Harcourt to Conybeare, August 22, 1835, on which is continued Conybeare to Clark, postmarked August 25, 1835, Letters to G. T. Clark, letter 66.
44. Phillips to Harcourt, August 5 and August 3, 1836, Correspondence and papers of William Vernon Harcourt, 1817-71, MS. Eng. d. 3876.
45. Report of the Meeting of the British Association for the Advancement of Science, *FFBJ*, August 27, 1836, 2; Prichard, "On the Treatment of Some Diseases."
46. Report of the Meeting.
47. Thomas Moore (1779-1852); Baron Charles Dupin (1784-1873), mathematician and pioneer of thematic mapping, and Prichard's London friend James Yates stayed at the Red Lodge. *List of Members of the British Association*, 9, 32; Moore, *Journal of Thomas Moore*, 1814-1821.
48. R. P. Graves, *Life of Sir William Rowan Hamilton*, 185.
49. Alexander von Humboldt (1769-1859); William Whewell (1794-1866). Wulf, *Invention of Nature*; Bristol Library Register, BCL, B7485-500; Goldman, "Origins of British 'Social Science,'" 602.
50. Bristol Statistical Society, *Proceedings of the First Annual Meeting*, and reports for 1838-1841, BCL, B4592-96, 4597; "Bristol Statistical Society," editorial, *FFBJ*, November 12, 1836, 3; Bristol Statistical Society, Report of the Annual Meeting, November 21, 1840, *FFBJ*, December 12, 1840, 2; Mayhew, *London Labour*, 175-76.
51. Goldman, "Origins of British 'Social Science,'" 590. See also Cullen, *Statistical Movement*; and Westergaard, *Contributions to the History*.
52. Neve, "Natural Philosophy, Medicine," 307.
53. Carpenter to Acland, October 21, 1839, Acland Papers, Box 11 (ii)/34, Devon Heritage Centre.

54. Carpenter, *Nature and Man*, 1888, in Neve, "Natural Philosophy, Medicine," 308.
55. Desmond and Moore, *Darwin's Sacred Cause*, 184–92; Gibson, *Lecture, Introductory to a Course*, 11–15.
56. W. Carpenter, *Principles of General and Comparative Physiology*, vii, 141; Carpenter, Comments Made Following the Presidential Address to Section D, BAAS, *Bristol Mercury*, August 28, 1875, 4, and *Saturday Bristol Times and Mirror*, August 28, 1875, 5.
57. Ashmolean Society, *Rules*, 9.
58. Benjamin Parsons Symons (1785–1878); Harriet Marineau (1802–76); Lucy Aikin (1781–1864). Prichard, "Memoir, Part 2," 358. See chapter 10 for the Sanskrit professorship.
59. Desmond and Moore, *Darwin's Sacred Cause*, 254.
60. Kenyon, *History Men*, 144–48.
61. Prichard to Daubeny, June 22, 1835, Magdalen College Library, UO, MS. 400/36.
62. Prichard to Whewell, July 15, 1842, Whewell Papers, Add.MS. a. 210-181.
63. Prichard to Whewell, July 28, [1842], Whewell Papers, Add.MS. a. 210-182.
64. Bell, *University Reform in Nineteenth-Century Oxford*, 61–62.
65. Olgivie to Howley, July 26, 1842, Peel Papers, vol. 332, BL, MS. 40,512, ff. 97–98.
66. Buckland to Whewell, July 22, 1842, Whewell Papers, Add.MS. a. 55-35.
67. William Ewart Gladstone (1809–98). Gladstone to Whewell, July 23, 1842, Whewell Papers, Add.MS. c. 88-100; Todhunter, *William Whewell*, 431, where when writing to Charles Lyell about the evolution of languages, he refers to Prichard as one of his masters in the science of language.
68. Prichard to Peel, July 23, 1842, Peel Papers, ff. 93–94.
69. John Anthony Cranmer (1793–1848). Howley to Peel, July 26, 1842, Peel to Cramer, July 21, 1842, and Cranmer to Peel, July 30, 1842, Peel Papers, ff. 57–58, 55–56, 59–60; Kenyon, *History Men*, 148.
70. Prichard to William Buckland, March 8, 1845, Buckland Correspondence, Royal Society of London Archives, MS.251/111.
71. "Bristol Institution [Lecture on Philology and Baron Cuvier's Division of Nations into Three Distinct Races]," *Bristol Mirror*, April 28, 1832, 3.
72. Prichard to Clark, June 23, 1837, Letters to G. T. Clark, letter 86.
73. Prichard, "A Specimen of the Oldest Language of Europe, viz. The Cantabrian," Charlotte Wilkins' Album, Special Collections, University Library, UB, DM931; Wilkins, "Goebel's Journey in Southern Russia"; Prichard to Washington, February 18, June 4, [1840], and June 10, 1840, Correspondence Collection, RGS-IBG Collections; Prichard to Blackwood, August 19, 1848, Blackwood Correspondence 1848 N-Z, NLS, MS. 4085, ff. 24–25.
74. Prichard, [Poem], April 3, 1832, and other entries in Mary Prichard's Album, Special Collections, University Library, UB, DM. 931; Farmayan, "Forces of Modernization," 121–24; Avery, "Printing, the Press and Literature," 815–17; P. Jones, *Life and Journals of Kah-ke-wa-quo-ma-by*, 303. It is likely that Jones was introduced to Prichard by their mutual friend Thomas Hodgkin, for which see Laidlaw, *Protecting the Empire's Humanity*, 258.

75. Dupin, Inscription to Mary Prichard, August 28, 1831, Mary Prichard's Album.
76. "Report of a Conversazione," 604; Carpenter, "Record of the First Year at Red Lodge," Red Lodge Journal, 1855–57, BA, 12693 (1); [M. Carpenter], *Red Lodge Girls' Reformatory School*. Mary complained of the rubbish left behind by Augustin Prichard and his apprentices, including a human foot found in the outhouse; Prichard to Schlegel, June 30, 1842, Manuscripts, Sächsische State Library, Dresden, Mscr. Dresd.e90.XIX, Bd.17, nr.50.
77. John Thelwall (1764–1834) had lectured at the Bristol Institution, and Prichard's poem in praise of his oratorical magic, January 28, 1829, is in Mary Prichard's Album.
78. F. Bunsen, *Memoir of Baron Bunsen*, 1:476.
79. Prichard, "Memoir, Part 2," 380.
80. William Budd (1811–80). A. Prichard, *A Few Medical & Surgical Reminiscences*, 28, 87; Prichard Jr. to Muncke, n.d., and Prichard to Muncke, November 16, c. 1837, Bibliotheca Walleriana, Collection of Axel Erik Waller, Uppsala University Library.
81. Prichard Jr., "Patri dilectissimus," flyleaf of a booklet in Birthday Book.
82. In 1948 two Prichard descendants remembered being told about the volumes of the *Red Lodge Intelligencer* but could not locate them. Script of a drama performed at the Red Lodge, Birthday Book.
83. A. Prichard, *Some Incidents*, 51–53.
84. Symonds, *Some Account*, 51.
85. American Philosophical Society, letter from the secretary of the APS, Philadelphia, informing Prichard of his election as a member, April 21, 1837, BA, 16082(4); Institut de France, Académie des Sciences Morales et Politiques, *Notices biographiques*, 371, where Prichard's election date is January 4, 1834; F. A. M. A. Mignet, two letters from the secretary of the Academy of Moral and Political Sciences, Institut de France, Paris, informing Prichard of his election as a member, July 19, 1837, and concerning his work as a corresponding member, November 11, 1837, BA, 16082(5)a and b; François Arago, Letter from the secretary of the Royal Academy of Science, Institut de France, Paris to Prichard, acknowledging receipt of the second volume of *Natural History of Man*, February 28, 1842, BA, 16082(7).
86. Symonds, *Some Account*, 9, 47.
87. Broadside Advertisement for the Sale of the Red Lodge, BIBM, 11:554; Bennett to Prichard, Monday night, and Prichard to J. Levitt, n.d., BA, 5535 (50)e. Mary Carpenter's school was shut at the end of World War I, then renovated and held in cooperation with a club in a contiguous building, leaving the Red Lodge itself restored and part of the city's museum and art gallery. Bristol Museum and Art Gallery files 703 and 2631.
88. Prichard Jr., *Sermons*, xii–xiii, xviii.
89. "Literary and Scientific Intelligence"; Church, *Life and Letters*, 18–22, 40.
90. Pattison, *Memoirs*, 163; Richard William Church was in competition with James Jr. They were both awarded fellowships; Prichard, "Memoir, Part 2," 374.

91. Prichard, "Memoir, Part 2," 415; 1841 Census, Enumeration District no. 7, NA, H.O.107/371, f. 29. During that summer three members of the Ley family and Charlotte Wilkins were staying at the Red Lodge, making a heavy workload for the Prichards' two domestic servants. Prichard to Bunsen, October 20, [1842], Deutsches Zentrales Staatsarchiv, ff. 241–42; Letters and documents by Richard and William Simpson, James Cowles Prichard Jr., and Nicholas Pocock, 1841–48, Simpson Papers, Merton Heritage Service; Prichard Jr. and Simpson in the right of his wife, Emily, Deed of Covenant, October 19, 1841, Papers of the Diocese of Winchester, Greater London Record Office, DW OP 1841/12.

92. Obituary of James Cowles Prichard Jr., *FFBJ*, September 16, 1848, 5; Obituary of Anna Maria Sarah Prichard, *Bristol Times and Mirror*, October 4, 1888, 7; Prichard Jr., *Sermons*, xiv–xvii; Prichard Jr., *Life and Times of Hincmar*. Jem's widow and daughter became Roman Catholics.

93. Prichard, "Memoir, Part 2," 421–22.

94. Barrington, *Life of Walter Bagehot*, 95.

95. Prichard, "Memoir, Part 2," 350.

96. Prichard's published and unpublished correspondence concern at least sixty-two of his patients, mostly on the subject of continuing consultations and asylum committals but also on high-profile legal cases.

12. New Scientists, New Organizations

1. A Countryman, "On the Tendency of Doctrines," 483. See chapter 6 for Lawrence.

2. Robert Grant (1793–1874). Desmond, "Robert E. Grant"; Chambers, *Vestiges of the Natural History*.

3. Schwebber, "Scientists as Intellectuals," 1–3, 18.

4. Bynum, "Time's Noblest Offspring," 230–33; Gurney, "An Autobiography," 109, Manuscript Volume s.357, Archives and Manuscripts, Society of Friends Library.

5. For natural theologians' domination of scientific thought, see chapter 2.

6. Étienne Geoffroy Saint-Hilaire (1772–1844). Conlin, *Evolution and the Victorians*, 56–57; Douglas, "'Novus Orbis Australis,'" 101–5.

7. "Oneness of the Human Race"; "Mosaic Account of the Unity"; Burnett, "Common Origin of Mankind"; [Craik], "The Unity of Mankind"; "Types of Mankind"; Société Ethnologique de Paris, "Liste des membres," xx.

8. Burnett, *Power, Wisdom, and Goodness*; Tullidge, *Triumphs of the Bible*; Spring, *First Things*. A later monogenist heavily influenced by Prichard is J. W. Dawson, *Archaia* and *Origin of the World*.

9. William Buckland, DD, later dean of Westminster, presided over the first meeting of the BAAS, giving a lecture indicating nature as evidence of the Almighty's design. One of several BAAS organizers whose science was based on scriptural truth, he wrote the Bridgewater Treatise *Geology and Mineralogy Considered with Reference to Natural Theology* in 1836.

10. Rupke, *Richard Owen: Victorian Naturalist*, 58–60, 68, 107–9, 179, 220–23.

11. Pierre Jean Georges Cabanis (1757–1808), physiologist. Prichard, *Natural History*, 1843, 132.
12. Gottfried Wilhelm Leibniz (1646–1716); Adam Kollar (1718–83), Slovak jurist; Adrien Balbi (1782–1848), Italian geographer. Staum, *Labeling People*, 125.
13. For the history of early Continental anthropology and its nomenclature, see Vermeulen, *Before Boas* and "Origins and Institutionalization," in which he explains how social/cultural anthropology is rooted in the ethnology and ethnography of eighteenth-century German speakers associated with the Russian Academy of Sciences, the University of Göttingen, and the Imperial Library in Vienna. Prichard, however, seems to have conceived of his science of humankind unaware of these earlier German efforts. Di Brizio, *Histoire du concept de couvade*, thoroughly explores early nineteenth-century Prichardian anthropology.
14. Christoph Meiners (1747–1810). For Prichard's influence on later race theorists like Gobineau, see Vermeulen, *Before Boas*, 383–85. The considerable shift in the meaning of certain of Prichard's own terms and even the titles of his books led later generations to misapprehend his views. A case in point is his description of "miserable savages," the adjective being an expression of sympathy for their harsh living conditions and the noun a rather neutral term for a stage in cultural development. "Culture" and "ethnic" had not yet acquired their modern anthropological meaning. He used the terms "race," "species," "type," "variety," "group," "genus," "stock," "family," and "nation" neutrally and somewhat interchangeably, allowing him, for instance, to write about a race of plants and to define a species as that which is characterized by a "distinctness of race." "Race" seems not to have acquired its stricter human biological connotation in Britain until the third decade of the nineteenth century and its negative connotations only from midcentury, so Prichard's use of the term is not derogatory. The titles of Prichard's books are now misleading; "natural history" and "physical" imply biology, to the detriment of their considerable linguistic, historical, and cultural content. Prichard was a stickler for what he considered correct (non-Continental) terminology, and his choice of nomenclature is a factor of time, culture, and nationality. For Prichard's views on race and for post-Prichardian race science and anthropology, see chapter 13.
15. For the BAAS and Prichard's involvement in it, see also chapter 10.
16. Prichard, *Abstract of a Comparative Review*, [1832], offprint at BCL 572/1983; and "Abstract of a Comparative Review," in *Edinburgh New Philosophical Journal* and BAAS *Report*; abstracted in *Gentleman's Magazine*; translated and with an introduction as "Des essais de classification," translated as "Philologische und physische." Prichard had previously rehearsed this speech as a lecture combined with a criticism of Cuvier's "three race" theory at the Bristol Phil & Lit on April 26, 1832, List of Papers Read before the Public Meetings. John Phillips, an organizer of the BAAS, considered Prichard's paper "a very elegant dissertation" but was sorely challenged by Prichard's insistence that it could not be intelligently conveyed in an abstract, Phillips to Vernon Harcourt, July

29, 1832, and August 1, 1832, Correspondence of William Vernon Harcourt, 1822–73, MS. Eng. d. 3876.
17. Thomas Hodgkin (1798–1866). In his "On the Importance of Studying and Preserving the Languages Spoken by Uncivilised Nations" Hodgkin stressed the historical linguistic approach to tracing human origin. He published on cholera, anatomy, morbid anatomy, medical education, public health, medical reform, antislavery, colonization for emancipated slaves, preservation of native languages, civilizing Indigenous peoples, and ethnology. See also Kass and Kass, *Perfecting the World*; and Rosenfeld, *Thomas Hodgkin*.
18. Gibson, *Lecture, Introductory to a Course*, 25–28.
19. Prichard to Hodgkin, February 28, 1838, Hodgkin Family, WC, PP/HO/D/A995-2300.
20. Heartfield, *Aborigines' Protection Society*, 3–6.
21. Thomas Fowell Buxton (1786–1845), ex-Quaker. Heartfield, *Aborigines' Protection Society*, 9–18; *House of Commons Report*.
22. Heartfield, *Aborigines' Protection Society*, 19–20.
23. Richard King (1810–76). [Fox Bourne], *Aborigines Protection Society*, 3, 14.
24. Prichard to Thomas Hodgkin, June 23, 1838, Rhodes House Library, UO, MS. Brit. Emp. s18, c122/51.
25. Eleventh Anniversary Meeting of the Aborigines Protection Society, May 2, 1848, *Colonial Intelligencer; or, Aborigines' Friend* 2 (May and June 1848): 5–20, 19.
26. Heartfield, *Aborigines' Protection Society*, 24–28; *First Annual Report of the Aborigines Protection Society*, [3].
27. Antoine Thomson d'Abbadie d'Arrast (1810–97). Hodgkin copy to Prichard, May 17, 1839, Hodgkin Family, WC, PP/HO/D/A/2301-2412a.
28. Prichard, "Letter from Dr. Prichard to Dr. Hodgkin," 56–58.
29. Hodgkin copy to Prichard, August 10, 1839, and October 8, 1839, Hodgkin Family, WC, PP/HO/D/A/2301-2412a.
30. Prichard to Hodgkin, February 28, 1838, and June 23, 1838, and Hodgkin copy to Prichard, January 1, 1841, Hodgkin Family, WC, PP/HO/D/A995-2300 and PP/HO/D/A/2301-2412a.
31. Hodgkin had previously proposed a questionnaire, concentrating on languages but also benefiting ethnologists and humanitarian efforts, under the auspices of the Philological Society of London, Hodgkin, *On the Importance of Studying*; Hodgkin copy to Prichard, August 10, 1839, Hodgkin Family, WC, PP/HO/D/A/2301-2412a.
32. Prichard to Du Ponceau, August 23, 1839, Simon Gratz Collection, Box 225, Case 12, Box 12, Historical Society of Pennsylvania.
33. [Hannah Mary Rathbone Jr.] to Richard Reynolds Rathbone, September 1, [1839], Rathbone Papers, VII. 1. 20, University of Liverpool; Prichard, "On the Extinction of Human Races," 1–3, reprinted in the *Literary Gazette*, *Monthly Chronicle*, *Edinburgh New Philosophical Journal*, BAAS Report, *Edinburgh Journal of Natural History*, abstracted in *Calcutta Journal of Natural History*,

offprinted as Prichard, *Letter from Dr. Prichard to Dr. Hodgkin*, and Aborigines Protection Society, *Second Annual Report*, 3, and translated as "Ueber das aussterben von menschenracen." For Prichard's article on the extermination of the Guanches, see chapter 10.

34. Gibson, *Rambles in Europe*, 274–76; [Watson], "Phrenology and the British Association."
35. Albrecht Meier (1528?–1603). Staum, *Labeling People*, 98, 132; Vermeulen, *Before Boas*, 422–23; Sera-Shriar, *Making of British Anthropology*, 54–56, 66–71; Hodgen, "Anthropology in the BAAS," 805–6; Martineau, *How to Observe*.
36. A total of £75 and 11 shillings was granted to it between 1839 and 1852 for producing and reprinting the initial questionnaire and later editions, including the *Races of Man*. In the 1850s it involved members of the ESL. BAAS Minute Book of the Committee of Recommendations, 1834–1852, 32, Archives of the British Association for the Advancement of Science.
37. The committee members were Prichard, Hodgkin, the Rev. James Yates, Mr. Gray, Charles Darwin, Mr. R. Taylor, Dr. Wiseman, and Mr. Yarrell. Hodgkin copies to Prichard, October 8, 1839, and December 21, 1839, and Prichard to Hodgkin, August 17, 1840, and September 7, 1840, Hodgkin Family, WC, PP/HO/D/A/2301-2412a and PP/HO/D/A995-2300; Darwin, *Descent of Man*, xxvi–xxvii.
38. Hodgkin to Phillips, December 21, 1840, Phillips Correspondence, Geological Collections, University Museum, Oxford, 1840/41; *Queries respecting the Human Race*.
39. *Queries respecting the Human Race*.
40. Report on the Queries, 690; Report of the Committee for Queries, 828.
41. "Report of Section D," 628.
42. Prichard to Traherne, November 11, [1844], Traherne Collection, 107. Prichard attended the 1844 BAAS meeting: British Association for the Advancement of Science, *List of Resident & Non-resident Members*, 21.
43. King, *Address to the Ethnological Society of London, 25th May, 1844*, 15; Laidlaw, *Protecting the Empire's Humanity*, 96–97. For the relationship among the Select Committee, APS, and ESL, see Rainger, "Philanthropy and Science."
44. *Prospectus of the Society*.
45. Hodgkin to Jerdan, November 3, 1843, Letters to William Jerdan, 1817–50, vol. 1, Bodleian Libraries, UO, MS. Eng. lett. D. 113, ff. 249–50.
46. [King], *Ethnological Society Prospectus*; Hodgkin to John Scouler, December 22, 1843, Papers of Dr. John Scouler, Mitchell Library, Glasgow, SR189.
47. [King], *Ethnological Society Prospectus*; Dieffenbach, *On the Study of Ethnology*; King, "Address to the Ethnological Society of London," 20.
48. Société Ethnologique de Paris, "Liste des membres," xvi–xxi. See page xviii for Prichard's being the first name on this undated list of corresponding members. Reviews of *Researches*, 3rd ed., vols. 1 and 2, are in *Mémoires de la Société Ethnologique* 1 (1841): 109–28; and review of *Histoire naturelle* is in *Mémoires de la Société Ethnologique* 2 (1845): xxviii–xxxix.

49. Vermeulen, *Before Boas*, 422–23; Sera-Shriar, *Making of British Anthropology*, 54–56. The first ethnographical museum was established in Saint Petersburg in 1836, and an academic chair in ethnography was established at the Academy of Sciences in 1837.
50. George Bellas Greenough (1778–1855). Greenough draft to [Richard King, 1844], Greenough Papers, UCL, GREENOUGH/B/4/K/7.
51. King lived in straitened circumstances, gained some public recognition as a wronged man, and died in 1876, leaving his family the object of charity, according to the Royal Literary Fund Archives, London. Review of *Narrative of a Journey*; Wallace, "Arctic Profiles"; Wallace, *The Navy*, 20–48; *Arctic Expedition*.
52. Reports of Sub-section E.
53. Hodgkin copy to Prichard, January 4, 1844, Hodgkin Family, WC, PP/HO/D/A/2301-2412a; Prichard to Hodgkin, February 15, [1844], Durham County Record Office, D/HO/C38/34, containing the rarely used term "anthropology." In Prichard to Morton, February 17, 1840, American Philosophical Society, Philadelphia, SR189, Prichard describes Hodgkin's interest in ethnography as instrumental to his philanthropic goals.
54. Extract of a letter from Prichard to Pickering, October 27, 1845, in Pickering, *Life*, 511. Prichard had expressed the same sentiments in Prichard to Hodgson, November 13, 1844, Telfair Family Papers, Dep Ms. 793, Box 19, Folder 173, item 655, Georgia Historical Society.
55. Asad, "Afterword," 315.
56. For discussion of phrenology's impact on Victorian science, see Poskett, *Materials of the Mind*; see also chapter 8.
57. William Frédéric Edwards (1777–1842); François-Joseph-Victor Broussais (1772–1838). Staum, *Labeling People*, 58–59.
58. Prideaux, "British Association and Cerebral Physiology," 473–77; Minute Book, vol. 3, September 10, 1841–December 12, 1870, 120–26, Papers of the Phrenological Society, EUL, Gen.608/2. Combe to Channing, April 23, 1839, Letter Copy Book, America, December 27, 1838–August 23, 1839, Papers of George Combe, NLS, MS. 7396, ff. 52–54. For anti-Prichard comments, see Papers of George Combe, NLS. See also Jenkins, "Phrenology, Heredity and Progress"; Desmond and Moore, *Darwin's Sacred Cause*, 161–66; and Poskett, *Materials of the Mind*.
59. Isaac La Peyrère (1596–1676); J. B. Bory de Saint Vincent (1778–1846); Julien-Joseph Virey (1775–1846).
60. Staum, *Labeling People*, 11–13, 98, 100, 121–22.
61. Staum, *Labeling People*, 132; Stewart, "William Edwards."
62. Williams, *Physical and the Moral*, 224–31; Staum, *Labeling People*, 136–49, 151. Like the Société Phrénologique, the organization was undone by the 1848 revolution; its archives and finances were absorbed into the notoriously biological Anthropological Society in 1873.
63. Staum, *Labeling People*, 6, 117–19. See also chapter 13.
64. Stoddart, "RGS and the 'New Geography,'" 190–91.

65. Twenty-eight letters from Prichard to Washington, 1838–40, and from Constantine Estlin Prichard, 1850, to the Geographical Society of London in Correspondence Collection, RGS-IBG Collections. Prichard, draft articles: "On the Ethnography of High Asia," "Dr. S. G. Morton. Crania Americana," and "Analyses of Japan, Nippon, Documents for the description of, by von Siebold. Published Leden 1832–39," in Correspondence, [Autograph manuscripts of articles for publication in the *Journal of the Royal Geographical Society*]. Articles, partial articles, and book reviews written by Prichard in *Journal of the Royal Geographical Society of London* are referred to in Washington, "Sketch of the Progress," 261–66; Prichard, "Dr. Mueller on the Ural"; Prichard, "A. Th. D'Abbadie"; Prichard, "On the Ethnography of High Asia"; Prichard, *On the Ethnography of High Asia*, reprinted in Royal Geographical Society, *The Country of the Turkomans*, offprint from the *Journal of the Geographical Society of London* available at Thane Library, University College, London, Anth.42.(A).1; Prichard, "Von Siebold on Japan"; Prichard, Obituary Notice of Johann Friedrich Blumenbach; Prichard, "Dr. Morton's 'Crania Americana.'" Captain John Washington, RN (1800–1863) was also a committee member of the APS during this period. Hodgkin was involved in the Geographical Society and corresponded with its officers, especially to get access to visiting Indigenous peoples, for which see Laidlaw, *Protecting the Empire's Humanity*, 94, 150f.
66. Julian Jackson (1790–1853). Five letters from Prichard to Jackson, 1841, in Correspondence Collection, RGS-IBG Collections; Nomination form of James Cowles Prichard, October 12, 1842, Membership Records, RGS; Prichard to the Secretary of the Royal Geographical Society, October 29, 1847, RGS Correspondence, RGS-IBG Collections. Prichard resigned October 29, 1847, but continued borrowing books.
67. *Statement of Facts*; Committee of Zoology and Animal Physiology, Minutes (November 23, 1838–November 21, 1849), Royal Society of London Archives, CMB/289; Certificates of Election and Candidature, vol. 8, 1830–1840, f. 241, and vol. 9, 1840–1860, ff. 122, 132, 164, 217, Royal Society of London Archives.
68. John Pickering (1777–1846); Peter Stephen Du Ponceau (1760–1844). Ticknor to Pickering, August 10, 1835, Prichard to Pickering, March 29, 1836, Pickering copy to Prichard, May 26, 1837, Prichard to Pickering, September 25, 1837, Papers of John Pickering VI, Pickering Family Papers, MSS 400, Phillips Library, Peabody Essex Museum.
69. Prichard to Pickering, March 20, 1844, and October 27, 1845, in Pickering, *Life*, 495–96, 511–12.
70. Albert Gallatin (1761–1849). Prichard to Du Ponceau, October 26, 1838, William S. Gilbert Collection; Du Ponceau to Gallatin, February 13, 1837, and March 16, 1837, Gallatin Papers, New York Historical Society.
71. Prichard to Du Ponceau, October 26, 1838, William S. Gilbert Collection.
72. William Brown Hodgson (1801–71). Prichard to Hodgson, November 13, 1844, Telfair Family Papers; Hodgson, extract of a letter to Pickering, May 17, 1844, and George R. Gliddon (1809–57), extract of a letter to John Pickering, November 14, 1845, in Pickering, *Life*, 499–500, 509.

73. "Report of the Anniversary Meeting," 659; Ethnological Society, Council Minute Book (January 2, 1844–January 26, 1869), A1, Royal Anthropological Institute of Great Britain and Ireland; Abstract of Prichard's "Brief Survey," 165.
74. Prichard, *On the Relations of Ethnology*, 1847; Prichard, "On the Relations of Ethnology," *Journal of the Ethnological Society of London*, 302, 304, 312, 329; *Dr. Prichard on the Progress of Ethnology*, University of Edinburgh Library, P.441/9; Prichard, "On the Relations of Ethnology," *Edinburgh New Philosophical Journal*; Prichard, "Anniversary Address for 1848," *Journal of the Ethnological Society of London*; Prichard, "Anniversary Address, for 1848," *Edinburgh New Philosophical Journal*; Prichard, "Mixture of Human Races."
75. Prichard, "On the Various Methods of Research," 231, 237, in which he complained that ethnology had had to struggle for recognition at the BAAS; Prichard, *Report on the Various Methods*; "Meeting of Sub-section D," 773.
76. Friedrich Max Müller (1823–1900). Müller, "Comparative Philology," 306–9, where he evaluates Prichard's philology; Müller, *My Autobiography*, 212. An appreciative review by French geographer Louis Vivien de St.-Martin (1802–96) is Review of Seventeenth Meeting, 316–24; further reviews were published in France and the United States.
77. Prichard to Owen, May 29, [1840 or 1841], Scientific Correspondence of Sir Richard Owen, vol. 22 (Pri-Rut), ff. 12–13, British Museum (Natural History) Library.
78. Prichard to Hodgkin, December 7, 1830, Hodgkin Family, WC, PP/HO/D/A/995-2300.
79. Prichard to Washington, April 3, [1840], Correspondence Collection, RGS-IBG Collections; "Dr. Prichard on Insanity," *Boston Medical and Surgical Journal*, 417.
80. Prichard, *Researches into the Physical History of Mankind*, 3rd ed., 3:vii–viii, xvii–xxii; "On Sepulchral Remains," translated as "Sur les tombeaux des anciens peuples."
81. Carl Gustaf Santesson (1819–86); Anders Adolf Retzius (1796–1860). Prichard to Santesson, November 28, [1847], Karolinska Institutets Bibliotek. Prichard to Retzius, May 2, 1847, March 15, 1848, and Saturday, [n.d.], Kungliga Vetenskapsakademien Biblioteket, Si. Fol. Kat, 5 Brev till A. A. Retzius.
82. Prichard to John Phillips, March 28, [1848], and March 14, [1848], Correspondence of John Phillips, Phillips Correspondence, Geological Collections, Museum of Natural History, UO.
83. Prichard to Retzius, February 20, 1848, and October 21, 1848, Kungliga Vetenskapsakademien Biblioteket, Si. Fol. Kat, 5 Brev till A. A. Retzius; Retzius, "Cranier ur gamla grafvar"; Retzius, "Present State of Ethnology," 253, reports that Prichard sent him two skulls to identify their ethnic type.
84. Robert James Graves (1796–1853). R. J. Graves, "Letter from Dr. Prichard," reprinted in R. J. Graves, *Studies in Physiology and Medicine*, 346.
85. Morton, *Crania Americana*; Pichard to Morton, October 3, 1839, Samuel George Morton Microfilm (Film 1413), American Philosophical Society, letter

16, 143053 Series IV; Morton to Prichard, November 25, 1838, Documents Relating to James Cowles Prichard and Augustin Prichard, BA, 16082(6).
86. Prichard to Morton, August 23, 1839, and February 17, 1840, American Philosophical Society, Mss.B.M843.
87. Prichard to Morton, March 24, 1841, Samuel George Morton Microfilm, letter 18; Prichard to Morton, February 17, 1840, American Philosophical Society, Mss.B.M843.
88. Combe to Morton, January 13, 1840, American Philosophical Society, SR189.
89. Morton to Combe, May 24, 1840, NLS, MS. 7256, ff. 50, 51.
90. Prichard to Morton, February 17, 1840, American Philosophical Society, SR189.
91. Prichard, extract from a letter to Pickering, in Pickering, *Life*, 468.
92. Prichard to Morton, March 24, 1841, Samuel George Morton Microfilm, letter 18. See Poskett, *Materials of the Mind*, 89–96, 106–7, for the struggle between ethnology and phrenology over *Crania Americana*; and 113, for images in promoting science; see Daston and Galison, *Image of Objectivity*, for images in promoting science.
93. Hack Tuke, *Prichard and Symonds*, 26.
94. Caldwell to Combe, August 14, 1841, Papers of George Combe, NLS, MS. 7258, ff. 110, 111.
95. Caldwell to Combe, August 30, 1839, Papers of George Combe, NLS, MS. 7242, ff. 145, 146.
96. Caldwell to Combe, August 12, 1837, Papers of George Combe, NLS, MS. 7242, ff. 46, 47.
97. Gliddon and Nott, *Types of Mankind*; Quine, "Destiny of Races."
98. Davis, "Catalogue of Crania," Royal College of Surgeons of England, London, MS0562/5/2/1-4; Davis to Combe, January 27, 1857, Papers of George Combe, NLS, MS. 7362, ff. 7–9.
99. Laidlaw, *Protecting the Empire's Humanity*. For later anthropology, see chapter 13.

13. Christian Humanitarian Anthropology

1. Prichard, "Memoir, Part 2," 308.
2. Newman to John Rickards Mozley, May 22, 1889, Paleography Room, Special Collections, University of London Library, AL 342/23.
3. Benoît de Maillet (1656–1738).
4. Prichard to [James Yates?], c. 1845–48, and October 16, 1839, Letters of Scientists: 1766–1886, American Philosophical Society, Philadelphia, 509/L56.23D.
5. Prichard to Johnes, November 22, [1843], Llanidloes Deposit (Miscellaneous), NLW, GB 0210, GLAERN; Prichard to Johnes, November 22, [1843], Glansevern Estate Records, Correspondence, Letters to Arthur James Johnes, NLW, 3837.
6. Prichard to Morton, February 17, 1840, American Philosophical Society, SR189; Prichard, "Dr. Morton's 'Crania Americana.'"
7. Prichard, *Researches into the Physical History of Mankind*, 3rd ed., 1:vi.

8. Prichard, "Instances of Longevity," reprinted as "Instances of Longevity," *Bristol Mercury*, December 30, 1837, 4; An Essay on the Native Races of America, "Philosophical and Literary Society," undated news clipping, BIBM, 11:647. For his correspondence with linguists, see chapter 12.
9. Prichard, *Researches into the Physical History of Mankind*, 3rd ed., vol. 2. In the volume's subtitle, *Containing Researches into the Physical Ethnography of the African Races*, "physical ethnography" is an example of how the second word is just coming into use in English, and "races," in the plural, means "cultures" as opposed to the later biological concept.
10. Prichard to Morton, February 17, 1840, American Philosophical Society, SR189; Prichard, *Researches into the Physical History of Mankind*, 3rd ed., vol. 3.
11. For Prichard's struggle against phreno-anthropology and his noting the importance of archaeology, see chapter 12.
12. Prichard to Pickering, March 23, [1843], in Pickering, *Life*, 490.
13. Prichard, *Researches into the Physical History of Mankind*, 3rd ed., vol. 4.
14. Johann Karl Eduoard Buschmann (1805–80); Wilhelm von Humboldt (1767–1835); Robert Hermann Schomburgk (1804–65). Prichard to Gallatin, February 19, 1847, Gallatin Papers; Prichard to Buschmann, April 10, 1845, Darmstaedter Collection 3 l, 1830, State Library of Prussian Cultural Heritage; Prichard, extracts of letters to Pickering, March 23, [1843], March 20, 1844, and October 27, 1845, in Pickering, *Life*, 489–90, 495–96, 511.
15. Prichard, *Researches into the Physical History of Mankind*, 3rd ed., vol. 5; Douglas, "'Novus Orbis Australis,'" 131–33.
16. Prichard to Yates, October 16, 1839, American Philosophical Society, Philadelphia, 509/L56.23D; Prichard, *Researches into the Physical History of Mankind*, 3rd ed., 3:[xvii]. The many images of Ram Mohan Roy produced after his death, having been derived from an original monochrome engraving, depict his skin in a great range of colors from pinkish to dark brown. Prichard was exacting in requiring adjustment to the hues of his books' maps, so he was likely satisfied with the color of the skin in Ram Mohan Roy's portrait; however, the exact darkness of tone might have been a factory painter's uncorrected lack of subtlety. Given Prichard's statement that his patient had been of very dark complexion and as this illustration is not known to have been criticized as darker than reality, the claim in Simpson, "Historicizing Humans in Colonial India," 113–37, that Prichard distorted the image to support his theory seems incorrect.
17. Prichard to Hodgkin, February 28, 1838, and June 23, 1838, Hodgkin Family, WC, PP/HO/D/A.
18. For an exposition of Prichard's creation of taxonomic terminology in this edition in an effort to limit the concept of race and establish his science of humankind, see Henze, "Scientific Definition in Rhetorical Formations."
19. Carl Ritter (1779–1859) visited Prichard for some days in August 1841; see chapter 15. For Prichard's use of Ritter, see Augstein, *James Cowles Prichard's Anthropology*, 139–40; for a discussion of the correlation between environmentalism, liberalism, and monogenism, see Schiebinger, *Nature's Body*, 138; Prichard, *Researches into the Physical History of Mankind*, 3rd ed., 3:4.

20. See also Gardner, "'Faculty of Faith.'" For the attribution of the formulation of "psychic unity" in the 1860s to the "father of German anthropology" Adolf Bastian (1826–1905), and later "appropriated" by E. B. Tylor, see Eriksen and Nielsen, *History of Anthropology*, 28–29. These authors also consider Tylor influenced by Bastian and German anthropology and overlook Prichard (31).
21. Prichard, *Researches into the Physical History of Mankind*, 3rd ed., 4:611. See also Di Brizio, *Histoire du concept de couvade*, 265–319, for the history of degeneration theory.
22. Prichard, *Researches into the Physical History of Mankind*, 3rd ed., 2:225. For an exposition of Friedrich Schlegel's (1772–1829) influence on Prichard's linguistics and for Prichard's views on language and monotheism and the search for language links, see Augstein, *James Cowles Prichard's Anthropology*, 159–62.
23. Prichard, *Researches into the Physical History of Mankind*, 3rd ed., vol. 5; Prichard, *Researches into the Physical History of Mankind*, 2nd ed., 2:595. In turn, theologian Cardinal Wiseman considered Prichardian anthropology's single origin of humankind as confirmatory of the scriptural account, for which see Wiseman, *Twelve Lectures* (1836), vol. 1, 9–10, in Di Brizio, *Histoire du concept de couvade*, 234–36.
24. Alexander Burns (1805–41), military officer, explorer, and author of the popular *Travels into Bokhara*, 1835. Prichard to Du Ponceau, August 23, 1839, Simon Gratz Collection, Case 12, Box 12, Historical Society of Pennsylvania.
25. Prichard to Retzius, October 21, 1848, Kungliga Vetenskapsakademien Biblioteket, Stockholm; Prichard to Bunsen, March 9, 1848, Deutsches Zentrales Staatsarchiv, ff. 36a–36b; for Blumenbach's original choice of "Caucasian" to denote a race, an idea later called the "Caucasian mystery," see Schiebinger, *Nature's Body*, 126–33.
26. Prichard, *Naturgeschichte des menschengeschlechts*; Wagner, *Prospectus*; L. A., Review of *Naturgeschichte des menschengeschlechts*, *Gazette médicale de Paris*; Review of *Naturgeschichte des menschengeschlechts*, *Blätter für literarische Unterhaltung*; Wagner, *Naturgeschichte des menschen*; Prichard to Rudolph Wagner, April 30, 1841, Cod. Ms. R. Wagner VI: Prichard, Manuscripts and Scientific Collections, Niedersächsische State and University Library.
27. The Society for the Diffusion of Useful Knowledge was a Whig organization dedicated to providing "improving" scientific and technical literature to autodidacts. Hodgkin offered to edit a series on the races of man with moral and political considerations, promising Prichard's help. Together they submitted a detailed proposal explaining the series' aim to demonstrate the affinities among races physically, linguistically, and culturally, stressing the evils inflicted on Indigenous populations by the civilized; this would convince the government to stem such destruction. The series would also suggest ways of bringing the benefits of commerce to the uncivilized and preparing colonists for contact with them. For good measure, the proposal quoted Prichard's appeal to preserve endangered populations so that scientists might fathom the universal human mind, the nature of language, and human physiology. The project stalled and

was finally shelved in June 1841, just as the *Ethnological Queries* was being launched. This Society for the Diffusion of Useful Knowledge project is one strand of Prichard and Hodgkin's ethnological humanitarian and scientific program. "On the Races and Varieties of Man," [1840], Papers of the Society for the Diffusion of Useful Knowledge 27, UCL; Hodgkin, copy of a letter to Prichard, December 21, 1839, Hodgkin Family, WC, PP/HO/D/A2301-2412a.

28. Lightman, *Victorian Popularizers of Science*, 220–22; Prichard, extract of a letter to Pickering, March 23, [1843], in Pickering, *Life*, 489–90; Prichard, *Natural History of Man* (1843). The first of ten monthly numbers of *Natural History* was actually published on January 1, 1842; Ghosh, *Annals of English Literature*, 189, lists it as one of the significant publications of 1843.
29. Prichard to Bunsen, August 26, 1842, Geheimes Staatsarchiv Preußischer Kulturbesitz, ff. 187–88; Prichard, *Histoire naturelle de l'homme*.
30. Prichard to Bunsen, September 28, [1842], and August 26, 1842, Geheimes Staatsarchiv Preußischer Kulturbesitz, ff. 215–16, 187–88.
31. George Catlin (1796–1872). Prichard, *Illustrations to the Researches*; Qureshi, *Peoples on Parade*, 84–86. For an example of convincing imagery of the time, in this case contrasting images of the same person undergoing Europeanization, see Richards, *Darwin and the Making*, 43, 44. In *Physical History* and later *Natural History* there is a sameness in the gray-brown skin color of many illustrations and some instances of extremely red Native Americans.
32. Prichard, *Six Ethnographical Maps*; Prichard to Hippolyte Baillière, January 6, [1843], Manuscripts and Archives, New York Academy of Medicine, MS.1308; Prichard, *Six Ethnographical Maps*.
33. Poskett, *Materials of the Mind*, 84.
34. Prichard, *Natural History of Man* (1843), vii–viii, 1–8.
35. Prichard, *Natural History of Man* (1843), 5.
36. For an exploration of past and continuing European views of the Other, see Athreya and Ackemann, "Colonialism and Narratives."
37. Poskett, *Materials of the Mind*, 80.
38. Prichard, *Natural History of Man*, 2nd ed., 1845; 3rd ed., 1848; 4th ed., 1855.
39. Examples: [Hope], "On the Diversity of Origin"; "Dr. Prichard on the Physical History of Mankind"; [Wagner], Review of *Researches into the Physical History*. An abstract "On the Artificially Distorted Skulls of a Peruvian Race" from *Natural History* was printed in the *Phrenological Journal*. *Natural History* and its later editions and translations were reviewed in a much broader range of periodicals, as would be expected of a book for general readers. An example of this is his friend Sir William Robert Grove's (1811–96) review in *Blackwood's Edinburgh Magazine* 56 (September 1844): 312–30, and reviews in *Baptist Record, and Biblical Repository* 1 (January 1844): 16–27; *Dublin Review* 19 (September 1845): 67–98; *Calcutta Review* 26 (June 1856): 474–548; and Advertisement of the First Number, *Athenaeum* (January 1842): 22. The second edition was reviewed in *Massachusetts Quarterly Review* 2 (September 1849): 428–37; and *London Quarterly Review* 1 (December 1853): 328–53.

The third edition was reviewed in *British and Foreign Medico-Chirurgical Review* 3 (January 1849): 222–24; and *Methodist Quarterly Review* 33 (July 1851): 345–77. The fourth edition, edited and enlarged by Edwin Norris in 1855, was reviewed in *American Journal of Science and Arts*, 2nd ser., 20 (September 1855): 302. The French translation was reviewed by François Jules Pictet in *Bibliothèque universelle de Genève* 45 (June 1843): 358–77; by Gustave d'Eichthal in *Mémoires de la Société Ethnologique* 2 (1845): xxx–xlvii; and in *Gazette médicale de Paris*, 2nd ser., 11 (July 1843): 473–78. Zoologist William C. L. Martin's popular *A General Introduction to the Natural History of Mammiferous Animals*, 1841, approved of Prichard's criterion for species unity as the capability to be civilized.

40. "Physical History of Man," 338; "Prichard's Physical History of Mankind," *New Quarterly Review*, 132–33.
41. "Natural History of the Varieties of Man," *Athenaeum* 1226 (1851): 447, cited in Sera-Shriar, *Making of British Anthropology*, 23; [Holland], "Natural History of Man"; Prichard, *Appendix to First Edition*; [W. Carpenter], "Dr. Prichard on the Physical," 51, 481.
42. John Beddoe (1826–1911). Beddoe, *Races of Britain*, cited in Augstein, *James Cowles Prichard's Anthropology*, 236. The Society for the Diffusion of Useful Knowledge Library of Entertaining Knowledge received prospectuses for "Natural History of Man" by William Rhind in 1830 and H. W. Dewhurst in 1840, Papers of the Society for the Diffusion of Useful Knowledge 27, UCL. See Di Brizio, *Histoire du concept de couvade*, 89, 235–38, 297, for Prichard's influence on Wiseman, Taylor, Chambers, and Tylor. For his influence on a physiologist, see Herbert Mayo's *Outlines of Human Physiology*, 2nd ed. (1829), in which particularly pages 517–71 are based on or extracted from *Physical History*. For anthropology, see also Victor Courtet de l'Isle, *Tableau ethnographique du genre humain* (1849); Eusèbe François de Salles, *Histoire générale des races humaies ou philosophie ethnographique* (1849); Dominique Alexandre Godron, *De l'espèce et des races dans les êtres organisés: Et spécialement de l'unité de l'espèce humaine* (1859); Jean Louis Armand de Quatrefages de Bréau, *Rapport sur les progress de l'anthropologie* (1867).
43. Robert Gordon Latham (1812–88). Prichard to Latham, December 23, [1848], Newport Correspondence, Linnean Society of London, Archives, MS.236.
44. "Dr. Latham's Ethnological Works"; Latham and Forbes, *Natural History Department*; Quirk, *Study of the Mother-Tongue*; "Dr. R. G. Latham [Obituary]"; Qureshi, *Peoples on Parade*, 216–17. See Sera-Shriar, *Making of British Anthropology*, for a discussion of Latham's place in the development of British Anthropology and Hake, *Memoirs of Eighty Years*, 205–12, for a hilarious portrayal of Latham as he transmogrified from a professor who dressed like a respectable clergyman into a Dickensian character, unable to manage his financial affairs: "No one could help liking and disliking him. He was logical in mind, illogical in action," unpredictable and forever on the scrounge "with an outward display of poverty, almost amounting to boastfulness."

45. Edward Forbes (1815-54). Rupke, *Richard Owen: Victorian Naturalist*, 179, 224-25. For an account of several pre-Darwinian evolutionary theorists, see Stott, *Darwin's Ghosts*.
46. Prichard's books owned by Darwin at CUL-DAR.LIB.511 and CUL-DAR.LIB.512, Library of Charles Darwin, Special Collections, Cambridge University Library (darwin-online.org.uk); Darwin, Descent Portfolios 1st ed., Scraps (including Man), 80, 85, Correspondence, 98, manuscript notes, notebooks, lists, vols. 575-80; and for Darwin's notes from *Physical History* and *Natural History*, on sexual selection, sterility, hybridism, transmutation, and use of analogy, see Abstracts of Scientific Books and abstracts of scientific books, journals, and pamphlets, 71: 1-5, 139-45, 119, 120, 122, 128, Darwin Papers, Special Collections, Cambridge University Library.
47. Desmond and Moore, *Darwin's Sacred Cause*, 158. For these issues and a historical overview of aesthetic evaluation in racial classification from Winckelmann, 1755 onward, see Richards, *Darwin and the Making*, 126-59 (Prichard on 142-46). Blyth, "Attempt to Classify the Variety," and Blyth, "On the Psychological Distinction," quoted in Wells, "Sir William Lawrence (1783-1867)," 344-47, 355-59. Both of Blyth's articles rehearse Prichard's views, and Blyth discussed Prichard's *Natural History*, 1843, extensively in his letters to Darwin, 1855, in vol. 98, a25-a55, Darwin Papers.
48. Richards, *Darwin and the Making*, 146, points out this annotation but notes that Darwin did not own the earlier and more evolutionary editions of *Physical History*; Darwin, *Descent of Man*, xiv, xxv-xxvi, xxix, xxxi, xxxvii.
49. See chapter 12.
50. John Frederick William Herschel (1792-1871). Prichard, "Ethnology," postprinted as Prichard, *Ethnology*, [1849]; *Manual of Scientific Enquiry*, 2nd ed., 1851; 3rd ed., 1859; and its offprint *Manual of Ethnology*, [1859]; and *Manual of Scientific Enquiry*, 4th ed., revised by Edward Burnett Tylor, 1871. The first edition was reviewed in *Athenaeum* and *Literary Gazette*; James Cowles Prichard and Constantine Estlin Prichard, Letters to Sir John Frederick William Herschel, March 16, 1848-January 9, 1849, Herschel Papers, HS.14.61-65, 187, Royal Society of London Archives. Prichard's five letters and his son's single letter to Herschel concern Prichard's contribution to the *Manual of Scientific Enquiry*, especially the phonetic alphabet he had devised for it. It appears that the Admiralty's *Manual of Scientific Enquiry* had been in the planning stages for several months before Prichard was asked to contribute to it. Rather than payment for the task, authors were given free copies of the book, a supply of offprints of their article, and the prestige of involvement. For this, see Behrisch, "En Route with the British Admiralty's *Manual*."
51. Prichard, "Ethnology," 253-54. For the significance of Prichard's "Ethnology" in the development of anthropology, see Sera-Shriar, *Making of British Anthropology*, 71-73; Stocking, "From Chronology to Ethnology," xcix-c.
52. Prichard's 1849 "Ethnology" appeared in the Admiralty's *Manual of Scientific Enquiry*, 1859 edition, with the addition of only one sentence, the deletion of Prichard's appendix on vocabulary collection, and the misleading claim of

having been edited on behalf of the ESL. Tylor completely rewrote the 1849/1871 version, renaming the chapter "Anthropology" for the Admiralty's *Manual of Scientific Enquiry*, 1889 edition. As for Prichard's conception of what would only later be termed "culture," in his *Researches into the Physical History of Mankind*, 3rd ed., vol. 3, the phrase "moral characteristics" often appears in the heading of sections concerning culture. Where he does use "culture," it is most often collocated with "mental" and other words indicating development or sophistication. The three examples of his use of "culture," still implying sophistication, are "eastern culture," "culture of the Finnish race," and "social and national culture." See especially Leopold, *Culture in Comparative*, for an exposition of the development of the anthropological concept of culture from the eighteenth century through earlier German writers to Tylor's contemporaries during the later nineteenth century. The author suggests Tylor may have been influenced by Johann Christoph Adelung and Johann Severin Vater but more likely the Humboldts and several later German ethnographers.

53. For discussion of Prichardian anthropology carried on by his immediate successors contrasted with rival developments in polygeny, including Tylor's adopting unacknowledged several of Prichard's ideas such as the relevance of cultural artifacts, see especially Di Brizio, *Histoire du concept de couvade*, 238–40, 244–57, 263, and 476. Some years before Tylor's involvement in Prichard's *Manual of Scientific Enquiry* chapter, he took notes on Prichard's *Physical History* (Tylor, Reading Notebook II, c. 1862–63, 168–81, Pitt Rivers Museum, UO) but did not often cite Prichard. Tylor's 1880 speech outlining the history of British anthropology represents him as the embodiment of the early discipline, nevertheless; here Tylor particularly notes Prichard's recognition of the role of archaeology in the science of humankind (Tylor, President's Annual Address). Five years later, Tylor's *Encyclopaedia Britannica* article describes Prichard as the "founder of ethnology or anthropology in England," reflecting the discipline's name in transition, and he notes Prichard's innovative integration of the study of bodily form, language, and state of civilization (culture). In other words, Prichard had pulled together the elements of anthropology, as he had expressed it in the *Manual of Scientific Enquiry*. Tylor felt that Prichard's *Natural History* "remains a standard work of the anthropologist's library," presumably including his own (Tylor, "James Cowles Prichard," 722, 723). In 1910 he still considered Prichard the "founder of modern anthropology" (Tylor, "Anthropology," 108).

54. Johnes had expanded his essay into a book following Prichard's recommendation. Prichard to Johnes, July 24, 1843, Glansevern Collection, NLW, GB 0210, GLAERN, 3837. This letter is quoted in advertisements for Johnes's book and in Jones, "Letters of Arthur James Johnes," 264.

55. Arnold, "Inaugural Lecture," 28; Binns, "Prodromus towards a Philosophical Inquiry"; Smith, *Natural History*; Burke, *Ethnological Journal*, 7–8, in Di Brizio, *Histoire du concept de couvade*, 247. This trend in Britain continued with Robert Knox's earlier views of race being stripped of its humanitarian content and turned into a manifesto for growing racialism as expressed by

later members of the ASL, for which see Richards, "'Moral Anatomy' of Robert Knox."

56. Caldwell, *Phrenology Vindicated*, 75–87; Caldwell, *Thoughts on the Original Unity*.
57. Van Amringe, *Investigation of the Theories*; Cartwright, "Diseases and Physical"; Ely, "On the Common Origin."
58. Jean Louis Agassiz (1807–73). See also Brantlinger, *Dark Vanishings*; and Bynum, "Time's Noblest Offspring," 397–435.
59. Lester, "Settler Colonialism, George Grey." See also Lester and Dussart, *Colonization and the Origins*.
60. Knox, *Races of Men*; Campbell, *Negro-mania*, 50–77; "Hair of Different Races of Men"; Browne, *Classification of Mankind*; Van Evrie, *Negroes and Negro "Slavery."* George Stocking considers Knox as having established the modern, biological concept of race.
61. Arthur Joseph de Gobineau (1816–62), *Essai sur l'inégalité*; Gobineau, *Moral and Intellectual Diversity*, 315; Nott and Gliddon, *Types of Mankind*. An excerpt from *Physical History* is in Count, *This Is Race*, 60–67. See also Bernasconi, "Introduction."
62. For a discussion of the rise of the term "race" in its biological sense, see Hudson, "From Nation to 'Race'"; and Douglas, "Climate to Crania," 33–96.
63. After several years of skirmishes between the Ethnologicals and Anthropologicals, the ESL and ASL merged awkwardly. A new generation of anthropologists continued for a time their preoccupation with race.
64. Desmond and Moore, *Darwin's Sacred Cause*, 332–33; Richards, *Ideology and Evolution*, 120. For the classic account of the fortunes of institutional anthropology in nineteenth-century Britain, see Stocking, "What's in a Name."
65. A. E. R. A. Serres (1786–1868); Pierre Paul Broca (1824–80); Alphonse Bertillon (1853–1914). Turda and Quine, *Historicizing Race*, 91–93.
66. Daniel Wilson (1816–92); Giustiniano Nicolucci (1819–1904). Kidd, *Forging of Races*, 132–34; Quine, "Destiny of Races," 83.
67. Williams, *Physical and the Moral*, 233–38; Turda and Quine, *Historicizing Race*, 93. For a discussion of craniometry, racial knowledge, and European exceptionalism, see Perrin and Anderson, "Reframing Craniometry." For the late nineteenth-century French scientific debate on specific unity represented by de Quatrefages v. Broca, see Livingstone, *Adam's Ancestors*, 122; Laidlaw, *Protecting the Empire's Humanity*; Stepan, *Idea of Race in Science*.
68. Athreya and Ackemann, "Colonialism and Narratives."
69. Conlin, *Evolution and the Victorians*, 146; Darwin, *Descent of Man*, xxvii.
70. Sera-Shriar's *Making of British Anthropology* makes a case for the continuity of Prichard, Lawrence, and later nineteenth-century anthropologists' observational practice with modern methodology, while Rosa and Vermeulen's *Ethnographers before Malinowski* describes some of the ethnographic resources of the period.
71. "Natural History of the Varieties of Man," 447, cited in Sera-Shriar, *Making of British Anthropology*, 23.

72. C. Bunsen, "On the Results of the Recent Egyptian," 265.
73. Max Müller, *My Autobiography*, 212–13.

14. From the Red Lodge to Asylumdom

1. "Asylum Life Office," *Bristol Mercury*, January 12, 1833; "Britannia Life Assurance Company," *FFBJ*, November 25, 1837, 1; "National Loan Fund Life Assurance Society," *Bristol Mercury*, June 30, 1838, 1.
2. Gibson, *Rambles in Europe*, 276–78.
3. Carlyle, *Life of John Sterling*, 245–46; Griffin to Hitch, postmarked March 5, 1840, Letters to Dr. Samuel Hitch, Gloucestershire Archives, D3848 1/1 (bundle 4). Prichard was George Griffin's physician.
4. Kramer, *Carl Ritter*, 272–73.
5. Susanna (Bishop) Estlin to Parkes, February 15, 1840, Estlin Papers, BA.
6. Mary Prichard Ley, 13 letters to Edith Prichard, Records of Rev. Theodore Innes Pocock, BA, 46875/Co/7. Mary wrote that she was proud whenever someone recognized her as Prichard's daughter. Nicholas Pocock (1814–97), grandson of the famous marine painter of the same name, gave up his Oxford career as an excellent lecturer in mathematics at about the time of his marriage to Edith on January 13, 1852. They settled in Bristol, where, though ordained, he devoted his time to writing history books. Their fourth son, Reginald Innes (1863–1947), preserved his mother's biography of Prichard and other family papers. Obituary of Nicholas Pocock, *Times*, March 11, 1897, 10; *Boase's Modern English Biography*, col. 408.
7. Prichard, "Memoir, Part 2," 405–6.
8. Prichard, "Memoir, Part 2," 402–3; A. Prichard, *Some Incidents*, 33–34. Fearing being buried alive, Eden made Prichard promise to certify his death; Augustin performed the service.
9. A. Prichard, *A Few Medical & Surgical Reminiscences*, 10–14.
10. Obituary of John Bishop Estlin, *Bristol Gazette*, June 10, 1855, 8.
11. Frederick Douglass (c. 1817–95). [James], "Memoir of John Bishop Estlin"; Taylor, "Some American Reformers," 32–34; Quarles, *Frederick Douglass*, 48, 53; Rice, "Scottish Factor in the Fight," 397–431; Clark to John Bishop Estlin, December 4, 1838, Estlin Papers, BA; Mary Carpenter to Mary Anne Estlin, December 25, [1846], Estlin Papers, BA; Bristoliensis, "The Easterlings," 659. Estlin forged links with American antislavery activists and tackled sectarianism among British ones. His will directed that the £40 that would normally be wasted on funeral pomp should be divided among the poor of nearby parishes.
12. William Wilde (1815–76), father of Oscar. Wilson, *Victorian Doctor*, 86–87, 133–39; "Remarkable Discovery of Skulls," 219–20, references frequent correspondence between Prichard and Wilde; "Dr. Wilde's Madeira," 470; "Sir William Wilde."
13. "Bristol. Institution for the Deaf and Dumb," *FFBJ*, August 22, 1840, 2, 4; Bristol Institution for the Deaf and Dumb, Financial Records, BA, 40861/F/1.
14. "Bristol Established Church Society and Book Association," *FFBJ*, December 11, 1841, 3; Bristol Established Church and Book Association, *First Annual*

Report; First Anniversary Meeting of the Bristol Established Church and Book Association, *Bristol Mirror*, December 11, 1841, 2; Bristol Established Church and Book Association, *Third Annual Report*.

15. Certificate of James Cowles Prichard's Honourary Membership of the Royal Medical Society of Edinburgh, April 2, 1841, BA, 16082(8).
16. Cohen, Bristol College [Annual General Meeting, February 20, 1841], in BIBM, 11:678–80.
17. Metropolitan Commissioners in Lunacy, "Account of All Monies," 457–58; Prichard, Invoices and receipts for visiting Gloucestershire Lunatic Asylums for October 12, 1824, to March 4, 1845, Quarter Sessions Archives, Gloucestershire Archives, Q/AL 42/1-3. For the duties of a Medical Visitor to madhouses, see Parry-Jones, *Trade in Lunacy*, appendix C; Latcham to Bloxham notifying the resignation of James Cowles Prichard as visiting physician to Gloucestershire Private Asylums, October 13, 1845, and Prichard's reports and invoices for visiting Gloucestershire private asylums as visiting physician and commissioner in lunacy, 1828–1848, Quarter Sessions Archives, Gloucestershire Archives, Q/AL 40/27 and Q/AL40/39, 40, 42.jk.
18. William Budd to Richard Budd, September 5, 1842, Budd Family of N. Tawton, Devon, WC, MS.5153/A/24.
19. "Bristol Infirmary," news clipping annotated February 1842, in BIBM, 11:540.
20. Announcement of the Appointment of the Metropolitan Commissioners in Lunacy, *London Gazette*, August 26, 1842; F. Bunsen, *Memoir of Baron Bunsen*, 2:32–33; Prichard to Bunsen, August 26, 1842, Geheimes Staatsarchiv Preußischer Kulturbesitz, ff. 187–88. The need to demonstrate Tory party affiliation was also apparent in his 1842 application for an Oxford professorship (see page 355 of the current volume).
21. "Bristol Infirmary," *Bristol Gazette*, March 31, 1842, 4; Bristol Infirmary Weekly Committee Book, 1840–1848, 50–55, BA, 35983/2 h.
22. Prichard did not acknowledge his honorary appointment as consulting physician until prompted. On March 17, 1848, he asked for his name to be removed from the Infirmary Annual Reports as it was absurd, considering his residence in London. Bristol Infirmary Weekly Committee Book, 1840–1848, 181, 219–20, 451; Munro Smith, *History of the Bristol Royal Infirmary*, 290–94.
23. A. Prichard, *Some Incidents*, 19–20.
24. A. Prichard, *A Few Medical & Surgical Reminiscences*, 32–87; Ritter, Permit and Introduction for Mr. Prichard, M.D., August 17, 1841, Birthday Book.
25. A. Prichard, *A Few Medical & Surgical Reminiscences*; "Report of the Conversazione."
26. *Plarr's Lives of the Fellows*, 1:199–200; Wood, *American Encyclopedia and Dictionary*, 10370–71; Weller, "To Sleep, Perchance"; Munro Smith, *History of the Bristol Royal Infirmary*, 471–72; [Swayne], "In Memoriam."
27. Augustin Prichard, Lecture on National Peculiarities in the Form of the Cranium, Philosophical and Literary Society, *Bristol Mirror and General Advertiser*,

April 4, 1846, 8; A. Prichard, "On the Crania." Humboldt disliked Augustin's pirated translation of *Kosmos*, 2 vols., 1845–1848. Collection of Human Skulls and Casts, Bristol Museum and Art Gallery, Bristol, file 1642.

28. Strachey to Elphinstone, December 14, [1844], Mountstuart Elphinstone Papers, BL, MSS.Eur.F.88, Box 4C, Bundle 17; Prichard, The Parent's or Guardian's Certificate for Illtudus Thomas Prichard upon his Application for Cadetship for the Bengal Infantry of the East India Company, dated May 6, 1845, East India Company, BL, Cadet Papers 331–444, 1844–45, /MIL/9/210, ff. 126r–128v; Hanifi, "Mountstuart Elphinstone." Elphinstone conducted ethnographic research in Afghanistan and took extensive notes on Prichard's books.

29. "Called to the Bar" refers to becoming a barrister, an elite form of lawyer. Boase, "Iltudus Thomas Prichard"; "Notices of Works by Iltudus Prichard"; Obituary of Illtudus Thomas Prichard, *Saturday Bristol Times and Mirror*, January 9, 1875, 2.

30. See also chapter 8.

31. Prichard to Johnes, November 22, [1843], Llanidloes Deposit (Miscellaneous), NLW.

32. Bynum, "Psychiatry in Its Historical Context"; Prichard to Rathbone, March 24, [1848], Manuscript Collection, Menninger Foundation, O D Misc Box #2, Prichard, 1.

33. Fox, Return for Northwoods Private Lunatic Asylum, June 6, 1843, Quarter Sessions Archives, Gloucestershire, Private Asylums: copy reports, applications for licenses, etc., Gloucestershire Archives, Q/AL 40/24. Prichard seemed to work particularly well with his Infirmary colleague Dr. Fox, signing the committal certificates of five of the twenty-one patients in his asylum in 1843.

34. Prichard to Johnes, November 22, [1843], NLW, Llanidloes Deposit (Miscellaneous).

35. Eghigian, *From Madness to Mental Health*, 116–23.

36. Hervey, "Lunacy Commission," 31; Commissioners in Lunacy, *Further Report*, 144, for statement that most victims of mistreatment were paupers; 267–68, for the opinion that two-thirds of lunatics in workhouses had congenital defects and were unlikely to benefit from asylum treatment; 177–220, for experts' opinions on therapeutics frequently differing.

37. Tourney, "History of Therapeutic Fashions," 785–87.

38. Prichard to Robertson?, December 25, [c. 1843], fastened to Charles Alexander Lockhart Robertson's copy of Prichard, *Treatise on Insanity*, Royal College of Psychiatrists, London. In this letter to an asylum owner, Prichard clarifies his definition of monomania and encloses the commissioners' questionnaire.

39. Metropolitan Commissioners in Lunacy, *Report of the Metropolitan Commissioners*; *An Act (8 & 9 Vict. c. 100) for the Regulation of the Care and Treatment of Lunatics* (1845). For the history of public asylums and the Lunacy Commission, see Smith, *"Comfort and Safe Custody"*; Hervey, "The Lunacy Commission 1845–60"; Watkin, *Documents on Health*; Scull, *Museums of Madness*, and others of his publications.

40. Reports on nine of Prichard's visits during this period are located mostly in quarter sessions archives in the county record offices of Gloucestershire, Oxfordshire, Herefordshire, Dorsetshire, Kent, and East Sussex.
41. Court of Chancery Commission on George King, third Earl of Kingston, *Times*, July 23, 1833, 6; "Commission in Lunacy. Extraordinary Loss of Memory," *Times*, January 25, 1844, 8; Prichard to Yates, [1830], Darmstaedter Collection 3 l, 1830, State Library of Prussian Cultural Heritage; *Sir Herbert Jenner Fust*.
42. Walk and Walker, "Gloucester and the Beginnings," 628; Walk, "Royal College of Psychiatrists," 135–36. Prichard referred several patients to Hitch, Samuel Hitch Papers, Gloucestershire Archives, D3848 1/1, bundle 4.
43. Examination Papers Royal College of Physicians 1838–1854, March 1845, Library of the Royal College of Physicians of London Archives, c.06.067.1.
44. Royal College of Physicians of London, License of James Cowles Prichard, March 17, 1845, sealed, BA, 16082 (9).
45. Commissioners in Lunacy, Minute Book, vol. 1, August 14, 1845–December 3, 1846, 14–22, NA, M.H. 50/1; Shaftesbury, August 9, 1845, in Diary, June 9, 1845–August 17, 1847, Diaries, Miscellaneous Papers and Correspondence, 1825–1885, Special Collections, University of Southampton Library, SHA/PD/4; Lutwidge to the Lords Commissioners of Her Majesty's Treasury, October 8, 1845, NA, T1 5121 X/LO7400.
46. Prichard, "Memoir, Part 2," 425–29.
47. Prichard, "Memoir, Part 2," 434–39.
48. W. Ley, "Memoir of Thomas Prichard extracted from the *Red Lodge Intelligencer*," in Birthday Book; Prichard, "Memoir, Part 2," 230–32.
49. Death of Thomas Prichard Esq., extracted from the *Journal of the Royal Agricultural British School*, Ross, August 28, 1843, property of the Prichard family.
50. [T. Prichard], "Britannia's New Vow," property of the Prichard family; T. Prichard, *Remarks Suggested by the Perusal*.
51. Prichard, "Memoir, Part 2."
52. Prichard to Hodgkin, February 15, [1844], Durham County Record Office, D/HO/C38/34.
53. "Bristol Medical School [Report of Prize Giving]," *FFBJ*, April 26, 1845, 6; "Monument to Southey," *FFBJ*, July 20, 1844, 3. At least sixty-two items of Prichard's published and unpublished correspondence concern his patients, mostly on the subject of continuing consultations and asylum committals. A letter from Southey to Prichard was exhibited in 1912, reported in "Bristoliana. Notable Exhibition at the University," *Bristol Times and Mirror*, February 7, 1912, 5.

15. Public Service and Private Misery

1. Summerson, *Georgian London*, 153, 154; British Museum Register of Admission to the Reading Room, 1836–1848, British Museum Administration. Prichard's friend James Yates recommended his admission on April 17, 1837, and he changed his address to 1 Woburn Place on April 27, 1846.
2. Eight letters from Anna Maria Prichard to Emily (Cranmer) Simpson, 1845–46, Box 27, Simpson Papers.

3. Bagehot copy of a letter to Thomas Watson Bagehot, September 7, 1845, and copy of a letter to Edith Stuckey Estlin Bagehot, September 9, 1846, St. John-Stevas family private collection.
4. William Lloyd Garrison (1805–79). Bagehot copy of a letter to Thomas Watson Bagehot, September 1846, St. John-Stevas family private collection; Quarles, "Ministers without Portfolio," 31; Prichard to John Bishop Estlin, December 31, [1847], Department of Rare Books and Manuscripts, Boston Public Library, MS.962.
5. F. Bunsen, *Memoir of Baron Bunsen*, 2:117–18. For a description of the exacting etiquette at Bunsen's breakfasts at the magnificent Prussian legation, a source of scientific and social contacts, see Max Müller, *My Autobiography*, 205–7.
6. Sir Alexander Morison (1779–1866). Diaries, 1807–1862, Collection of Sir Alexander Morison, Royal College of Physicians of Edinburgh, DEP/MOR. See especially volumes 18 and 19 for his relationship with Prichard.
7. Ward, *History of the Athenaeum*, 119; Athenaeum Club, *Catalogue of the Library*, 251; Athenaeum Club, *Supplement*, 132. Prichard was one of the nine men eminent "in arts, science or literature" the committee was allowed to elect for the year 1832
8. American Ethnological Society (founded 1842), "Honorary Members," vii–viii; American Oriental Society (founded 1842), "Officers of the American Oriental Society," xii (Prichard is sixth on this list, so presumably an early honorary member of the society); "Extracts from the Proceedings of the Society," 449; Cambridge Philosophical Society, entry for the meeting of March 4, 1844, in General Meetings Minute Book, vol. 2, April 26, 1830–February 24, 1851, Cambridge Philosophical Society Papers, GBR/0279/CPS 3/1/2. Prichard was also an honorary member of the Cambridge Antiquarian Society, according to the title pages of his books.
9. Shaftesbury, August 28, 1845, in Diary, June 9, 1845–August 17, 1847. Prichard's reports of his visits to Hanwell where he would have met Dr. Conolly are in the asylum's *Annual Reports*. *First Report of the Committee*, 28–29. See Prichard and William George Campbell's report of a visit to Stafford County Asylum, October 14, 1847, Stafford County Asylum, Minutes, Staffordshire County Record Office, D550/1. Forty-eight of Prichard's commissioner in lunacy inspection reports were examined in asylum and quarter sessions records in many county archives offices. For an administrative history of the Commissioners in Lunacy, see Mellett, "Bureaucracy and Mental Illness."
10. Prichard to Hodgson, November 13, 1844, no. 655, Telfair Academy of Arts and Sciences; Prichard to Herschel, March 18, 1843, Royal Society of London Archives, II.S.14.62; Commissioners in Lunacy, *Copy of Report*, 407; Hervey, "Lunacy Commission."
11. Hervey, "Lunacy Commission," 32–33, 116–27, 134.
12. MacKenzie, "Family Asylum," 145; Bristol Guardians of the Poor Meeting, FFBJ, October 13, 1847, 8; Commissioners in Lunacy, *Further Report*, 95–96.
13. John Robert Hume (1781–1857); Brian Waller Procter (1787–1874); R. W. S. Lutwidge (1802–73). Procter, *Literary Recollections of Barry Cornwall*, 9–13; Renton, "Chapters in the English Law," 493.

14. Jansson, *From Melancholia to Depression*, 74–75.
15. Phillips, "Old Private Lunatic Asylum," 42. Prichard's seven positive reports on Northwoods, 1842–48, were eventually printed in Extracts of Reports to Northwoods Asylum, *Bristol Mirror and General Advertiser*, July 19, 1851, 4, and July 26, 1851, 4.
16. Hervey, "Lunacy Commission," 142; MacKenzie, "Family Asylum," 172–76.
17. McCandless, "Dangerous to Themselves," 84–85.
18. Commissioners in Lunacy, *Haydock Lodge Lunatic Asylum*; Roberts, "England's Poor Law Commissioners."
19. James William Mylne (1800–1855); William George Campbell (d. 1881, aged seventy). Commissioners in Lunacy, *Further Report*, 137–43; Crowther, *Observations on the Management*, 50.
20. Suzuki, *Madness at Home*, 154–58. See also chapter 8.
21. Hervey, "Advocacy or Folly"; Commissioners in Lunacy, *Further Report*; Crowther, *Observations on the Management*. The Alleged Lunatics' Friend Society can be seen as ancestral to both the modern antipsychiatry movement and the charity Mind. See also chapter 8.
22. Prichard to [Amariah Brigham], n.d. [1848], extracted in Brigham, Obituary of James Cowles Prichard, 384.
23. Caroline Susanna Estlin to Anna Maria Prichard, June 15, 1846, Birthday Book, 162.
24. Seymour, *Letter to the Right Honourable*, 6–8.
25. Bloxam, *Register of the Presidents*, 7:349.
26. Robert Simpson to William Simpson, June 25, 1844, Simpson Papers; The's Egyptian artwork and several letters from Egypt mostly to his mother are in Records of Rev. Theodore Innes Pocock in Bristol Archives. In Prichard, "Memoir, Part 2," 431–34, Thomas Prichard tells his grandson Roger in 1842 to accept and prepare his soul for impending death, as his case was hopeless.
27. Anna Maria Prichard to Emily (Cranmer) Simpson, n.d., but after March 2, 1846, Simpson Papers, Merton Heritage Service.
28. Theodore Innes Pocock (Edith's son) to Edward Cowles Prichard, November 21, 1953, Prichard family private collection. Pocock labeled The's letters in BA similarly.
29. Constantine Estlin Prichard to Augustin Prichard, January 3, 1860, Woods family private collection.
30. Constantine Estlin Prichard to Augustin Prichard, January 18, 1860.
31. Augustin Prichard, "A Family Chronicle," Prichard family private collection.
32. Strahan, *Suicide and Insanity*, 197–201.
33. Obituary of T. J. Prichard; Certified Copy of an Entry of Death, Theodore James, February 25, 1846, Case Book, Male, Private Pauper, D. December 18, 1841–August 7, 1845, entry 1763; Undertaking to Pay [for T. J. Richards], June 16, 1845, and Medical Certificate for [T. J. Richards]; Gloucester Lunatic Asylum Day Book, January 1, 1844–February 7, 1859, all in Archives of the Gloucester Lunatic Asylum, Gloucestershire Archives, HO 22 70/4, HO 22 83/2/23, HO 22 32/45.

34. Concerning Dr. Hitch and the Gloucester Lunatic Asylum, see Smith, "'A Worthy Feeling Gentleman'"; Gloucester Lunatic Asylum House Committee Journal, February 6, 1835–February 22, 1848, entry for c. February 20, 1845, Archives of the Gloucester Lunatic Asylum, Gloucestershire Archives, HO 22 3/2.
35. Gloucester Lunatic Asylum, Minute Book of the Committee, January 29, 1813–October 24, 1851, 526, 528–30, 535–36, 537–38, Archives of the Gloucester Lunatic Asylum, Gloucestershire Archives, HO 22 1/1; Commissioners in Lunacy, Minute Book, vol. 1, 137. See Waller Family Pedigree, GRO, D4183 2/1, for a description of Hitch as a man who could out-charm any man in England, married well three times, and spent his wives' £60,000 on medical experiments, agricultural equipment, and other ladies.
36. Suzuki, *Madness at Home*, 137–39.
37. Bagehot copy to Edith Stuckey Estlin Bagehot, February 6, 1847, St. John-Stevas family private collection.
38. Prichard, "Memoir, Part 2," 324, 327; Prichard, copy to Charles Balston, January 26, 1841, Correspondence of Henry Balston (1816–40) and associated material, Bodleian Libraries, UO, MS. Eng. lett. D. 346, f. 242.
39. "Constantine Estlin Prichard," 536.
40. Prichard to Constantine Prichard, February 11, [1847], in Birthday Book, bound between 216 and 217.
41. "Constantine Estlin Prichard," 536; Birmingham Oratory, *Correspondence of John Henry Newman*, 222.
42. Obituary of Constantine Estlin Prichard, *Guardian*, October 13, 1869, 1126; Prichard, Selected Poems, 1851–1869, Woods family private collection.
43. John Duke Coleridge (1820–94). Coleridge, *Life and Correspondence*, 165; Shairp, *Glen Desseray*, 212–14.
44. Michael Faraday (1791–1867). Certificate of Election of James Cowles Prichard to Correspondent Membership in the Russian Geographical Society, Documents relating to James Cowles Prichard and Augustin Prichard, BA, 16082(10); "Meeting of the British Association [at Oxford, July 26–30, 1847]," *Jackson's Oxford Journal*, July 3, 1847, 3.
45. Prichard, "On the Various Methods of Research"; Barrington, *Life of Walter Bagehot*, 178–79.
46. Bagehot copy to Edith Stuckey Estlin, received February 10, 1848, St. John-Stevas family private collection.
47. Personal communication, the Rev. Edward Cowles Prichard, 1974; Albert Hermann Prichard, Index to the Catalogue of the [Bristol] Library, Manuscripts, BCL, 26789; Bristol Library Society, General Meeting Minutes, December 2, 1772–March 28, 1870, BA, 32079/LS/M/7; Constantine Estlin Prichard to Augustin Prichard, [1858–60], Woods family private collection; Register of Deaths England and Wales, NA, 2 Q1912, Probate.
48. Edith Mary Pocock, Sketch of the Life of Dr. Prichard, 5, Prichard family private collection. According to Symonds, "his opinions, during the greater part of his life, were in strict conformity with the doctrines embodied in the book

of Common Prayer." The phrase "greater part of his life" corroborates Edith's statement.
49. Bagehot copy to Thomas Watson Bagehot, December 1848, St. John-Stevas family private collection.
50. Constantine Prichard to Mary Anne Estlin London, December 27, 1848, Records of Rev. Theodore Innes Pocock, BA, 46875/Co/3; A. Prichard, *A Few Medical & Surgical Reminiscences*, 53; Pocock, Sketch of the Life of Dr. Prichard, 3; Hodgkin, "Obituary," 205. Edith Pocock considered Hodgkin's assessment of Prichard's character to be fair and accurate, and she described him as "eagerly addicted to studying." On page 207 of "Obituary" Hodgkin directly states Prichard's death was caused by his arduous job.
51. Newman to James Martineau, February 26, 1849, and Newman to James Martineau, January 17, 1849, Letters from F. W. Newman to James Martineau, 1846–1893, Special Collections, Tate Library, Harris Manchester College, GB133 UCC/2/21/2.
52. Scores of obituary notices and memoirs appeared in periodicals in Britain, the United States, France, and Germany. Some of Prichard's possessions owned by the Rev. Edward Cowles Prichard were donated to the Royal Anthropological Institute, London. Others are still scattered among his descendants.

Conclusion

1. W. Osler (1849–1919). Hodgkin, "Obituary," 206; Osler to Cunningham, February 11, 1908, Papers of Cunningham, UE, Gen. 2003 c.12.
2. Sanders, *Celebrities of the Century*, 842; Traill, *Encyclopaedia Britannica*, 512; Tylor, "James Cowles Prichard," 722–23; Allibone, "James Cowles Prichard"; Odom, "James Cowles Prichard," 136–38; [W. Carpenter], "Ethnology."
3. Keith, *Autobiography*, 551.
4. Rolleston, "Address to the Department," 153.

Bibliography

Archives and Manuscript Materials
American Philosophical Society, Philadelphia. Letters of Scientists, 1766–1886; Samuel George Morton Papers.
BA. Bristol Archives, Bristol, UK. Records of Bristol Royal Infirmary, 1735–1980; Bristol Apprentice Register, 1802–1819; Bristol Diocesan Registry; Records of the Bristol Institution for the Advancement of Science, Literature and the Arts, the Bristol Library Society, the Bristol Museum and Library, and the Philosophical and Literary Society, 1700s–1950s; Documents relating to James Cowles Prichard and Augustin Prichard; Estlin Papers; Mary Carpenter, Red Lodge Journal; Records of Rev. Theodore Innes Pocock—papers relating to the Pocock, Prichard and extended families; Bristol Institution for the Deaf and Dumb; Society of Friends, Bristol, Men's Monthly Meeting Minutes, 1801–1809, 1810–1818.
Bath Record Office. Clinical Society of Bath Archives.
BCL. Bristol Central Library, Bristol. Library Society Records; Bristol Commercial Rooms Records.
Berkshire Record Office, Reading. Justices Roll, 1801–1895, Q/JL1.
BL. British Library, London. Department of Manuscripts. Broughton Papers; Peel Papers.
Boston Public Library. Department of Rare Books and Manuscripts.
Bristol Museum and Art Gallery, Bristol. Correspondence and Catalogue of Collection of Human Skulls and Casts, file 1642.
Cambridge Philosophical Society, Cambridge. Archives.
College of Physicians of Philadelphia Library. William S. Gilbert Collection.
Deutsches Zentrales Staatsarchiv. Historische Abteilung II, Merseburg. Rep. 92, Dep. K.J.V. Bunsen. B. No. 36.
Devon Heritage Centre, Exeter. Acland Papers.
Geheimes Staatsarchiv Preußischer Kulturbesitz, Berlin. GStA PK, VI. HA, FA Bunsen, v., Karl Josias, B. No. 36.
Georgia Historical Society, Savannah. Manuscripts. Telfair Family Papers.
Gloucestershire Archives, Gloucester. Samuel Hitch Papers; Quarter Sessions Archives; Archives of the Gloucester Lunatic Asylum.
Greater London Record Office. Papers of the Diocese of Winchester, DW OP 1841/12.
Harvard University Library, Cambridge MA. Houghton Rare Book Library, Autograph File.
Historical Society of Pennsylvania, Philadelphia. Simon Gratz Collection.
Karolinska Institutets Bibliotek, Stockholm.

Kungliga Vetenskapsakademien Biblioteket, Stockholm.
Linnean Society of London. Archives.
Medical Reading Society, Bristol. Archives.
Menninger Foundation, Topeka, Kansas. Manuscript Collection.
Merton Heritage Service, London Borough of Merton. Simpson Papers.
NA. National Archives, UK. Census; Records of the Lunacy Commission, Board of Control and Special Hospitals; Records of the General Register Office; Registered Copy Wills.
New York Academy of Medicine, New York. Archives and Manuscripts.
New York Historical Society, New York. Manuscript Collections, Gallatin Papers.
New York Hospital–Cornell Medical Center, Cornell, New York. Oskar Diethelm Historical Library, Department of Psychiatry Library.
Niedersächsische State and University Library, Göttingen. Manuscripts and Scientific Collections.
NLS. National Library of Scotland, Edinburgh. Archives and Manuscript Collections. Papers of George Combe; Sir Henry Holland Letters to His Father; Blackwood Correspondence.
NLW. National Library of Wales, Aberystwyth. Archives and Manuscripts. Glansevern Estate Records; Iolo Morganwg Manuscripts; G. T. Clark Manuscripts; Taliesin ab Iolo Manuscripts; Papers of or from the library of John Davies; Llanidloes Deposit (Miscellaneous); Traherne Collection.
NMW. Amgueddfa Cymru, National Museum of Wales, Cardiff. De la Beche Papers.
Peabody Essex Museum, Rowley, Massachusetts. Phillips Library. Pickering Family Papers.
RGS. Royal Geographical Society of London. Manuscript Archives. Membership Records; Correspondence Collection, including manuscripts of articles for publication in the *Journal of the Royal Geographical Society*.
RMSE. Royal Medical Society of Edinburgh. Archives (uncataloged).
Royal Anthropological Institute of Great Britain and Ireland, London. Ethnological Society Records.
Royal College of Physicians of Edinburgh. Archives. Collection of Sir Alexander Morison.
Royal College of Physicians of London. Archives. Presidential Addresses; Examination Papers.
Royal College of Psychiatrists, London. Library.
Royal College of Surgeons of England, London. Archives.
Royal Irish Academy, Dublin. Archives. Minutes of the Academy.
Royal Society of London. Archives. Committee of Zoology and Animal Physiology, Minutes; Herschel Papers; Journal Book of the Royal Society; Buckland Correspondence; Certificates of Election and Candidature for Fellowship of the Royal Society, 1731–.
Sächsische State Library, Dresden. Manuscripts. August Wilhelm von Schlegel, Mscr. Dresd.e90.XIX, Bd. 17, No. 50.
Society of Friends Library, London. Archives and Manuscripts.
Staffordshire County Record Office. Stafford County Asylum, Minutes.

St. Andrews University, St. Andrews. University Muniments.
State Library of Prussian Cultural Heritage (Staatsbibliothek Preußischer Kulturbesitz), Berlin. Darmstaedter Collection 3 l.
UB. University of Bristol. University Library. Special Collections.
UCL. University College, London. Special Collections, Archives. Brougham Papers; Papers of the Society for the Diffusion of Useful Knowledge; College Correspondence; Greenough Papers.
UE. University of Edinburgh. Centre for Research Collections. University Archives; Library Archives; Papers of Cunningham; Notes on Lectures.
University of Cambridge, Cambridge. Matriculations; Trinity College Library, Whewell Papers.
University of Iowa, Iowa City. Libraries. Special Collections.
University of Liverpool, Liverpool. Sydney Jones Library. Special Collections Department. Rathbone Papers.
University of London Library, London, Paleography Room.
University of Manchester. John Rylands Library. Special Collections.
University of Reading. Special Collections. Longman Group Archive.
University of Southampton. Library. Special Collections. Anthony Ashley-Cooper, Seventh Earl Shaftesbury, Diaries, Miscellaneous Papers and Correspondence, 1825–1885.
UO. University of Oxford.
  Bodleian Libraries. Special Collections. Archive of the British Association for the Advancement of Science; Papers of the Harcourt Family; Archive of the Anti-Slavery Society; Correspondence of Henry Balston (1816–1840).
  Harris Manchester College. Tate Library.
  Hope Department of Zoology (Ent), University Museum. Papers of Sir Edward Bagnall Poulton.
  Magdalen College Library. Archives. Papers of Charles Daubeny.
  Museum of Natural History. Geological Collections. Phillips Correspondence.
  Pitt Rivers Museum. Manuscript Collections. E. B. Tylor Papers.
Uppsala University, Uppsala, Sweden. University Library. Bibliotheca Walleriana.
WC. Wellcome Collection, London. Budd Family of N. Tawton, Devon; Hodgkin Family; Autograph Letter File; Medical Society of London Archives.
Westminster Public Library, London. Burial Register, St Anne, Westminster.

Published Works

Abstract of Prichard's "Brief Survey of the Actual State of Ethnology" at a Meeting of the Ethnological Society on November 11, 1846. *Medical Times* 15 (November 1846): 165.
Advertisement of the First Number of *The Natural History of Man. Athenaeum* (January 1842): 22.
Aigner, B. Robert, and Donald W. Mulder. "Myoclonus." *AMA Archives of Neurology* 2 (January–June 1960): 600–615.
Alford, Henry. "The Bristol Infirmary in My Student Days, 1822–1828." *Bristol Medico-Chirurgical Journal* 8 (September 1890): 165–91.

Alison, W. P. "Reflections on the Results of Experience as to the Symptoms of Internal Inflammations, and the Effects of Blood-Letting, during the Last Forty Years." *Edinburgh Medical Journal* 1 (March 1856): 769–88.

Allibone, Samuel Austin. "James Cowles Prichard [with citations of reviews of his works]." In *A Critical Dictionary of English Literature, and British and American Authors, Living and Deceased, from the Earliest Accounts to the Middle of the Nineteenth Century. Containing Thirty Thousand Biographies and Literary Notices, with Forty Indexes of Subjects*, vol. 2, 1680–81. Philadelphia: J. B. Lippincott, 1870.

American Ethnological Society. "Honorary Members." *Transactions of the American Ethnological Society* 1 (1845): vii–viii.

"An Analysis of the Egyptian Mythology." *Antijacobin Review, and Protestant Advocate: or, Monthly, Political, and Literary Censor* 57 (January 1820): 401–12.

Anderson, Nancy Fix. "Cousin Marriage in Victorian England." *Journal of Family History* 11 (July 1986): 285–301.

Andrews, Jonathan. "'Of the Termination of Insanity in Death,' by James Cowles Prichard (1835)." *History of Psychiatry* 23, no. 1 (2012): 129–36.

Annual Report of the National Society for Promoting the Education of the Poor in the Principles of the Established Church. London: Printed at the Free-School, Gower's Walk, Whitechapel, 1812.

Arctic Expedition. Copies of Letters to Sir John Franklin, R.N. London: House of Commons, 1848. Parliamentary Papers, Accounts and Papers, Session (November 18, 1847–September 5, 1848), vol. 41, no. 264.

Armstrong, John. *Facts and Observations, Relative to the Fever Commonly Called Puerperal*. London: Longman, Hurst, Rees, Orme & Brown, 1814.

Arnold, Thomas. "An Inaugural Lecture on the Study of Modern History: Delivered in the Theatre, Oxford, Dec. 2, 1841." In *Race Relations*, by Michael Banton. London: Tavistock, 1967.

———. *Observations on the Nature, Kinds, Causes, and Prevention of Insanity, Lunacy, or Madness*. London: Printed by G. Ireland, 1782, 1786.

Arrowsmith's Dictionary of Bristol. 2nd ed. Bristol: J. W. Arrowsmith, 1906.

Asad, Talal. "Afterword: From the History of Colonial Anthropology to the Anthropology of Western Hegemony." In *Colonial Situations: Essays on the Contextualization of Ethnographic Knowledge*, edited by George W. Stocking, 314–24. Madison: University of Wisconsin Press, 1992.

Ashmolean Society. *Rules*. Oxford: Bagster Printer, [1841].

Ashworth, J. H. "Charles Darwin as a Student in Edinburgh, 1825–1827." *Proceedings of the Royal Society of Edinburgh* 55 (1935): 97–113.

Aspinall, A., ed. *King George IV: The Correspondence of George, Prince of Wales, 1770–1812*. Vol. 6. London: Cassell, 1963–71.

Athenaeum Club. *A Catalogue of the Library of the Athenaeum*. London: Printed for the Members by T. C. Savill, 1845.

———. *Supplement to the Catalogue of the Library of the Athenæum, Printed in 1845*. London: Printed for the Members, 1851.

Athreya, Sheela, and Rebecca Rogers Ackemann. "Colonialism and Narratives of Human Origins in Asia and Africa." In *Interrogating Human Origins: Decolonisation and the Deep Human Past*, edited by Martin Porr and Jacqueline M. Matthews, 72–95. London: Routledge, 2020.

Atkinson, B. J. "An Early Example of the Decline of the Industrial Spirit? Bristol 'Enterprise' in the First Half of the Nineteenth Century." *Southern History: A Review of the History of Southern England* 9 (1987): 71–89.

Augstein, Hannah F. *James Cowles Prichard's Anthropology: Remaking the Science of Man in Early Nineteenth-Century Britain*. Amsterdam: Editions Rodolpi, 1999.

Avery, Peter. "Printing, the Press and Literature in Modern Iran." In *The Cambridge History of Iran*, vol. 7, edited by P. Avery, G. R. G. Hambly, and C. Melville, 815–69. Cambridge: Cambridge University Press, 1991.

Babbington, William, and James Curry. *Outlines of a Course of Lectures on the Practice of Medicine, as Delivered in the Medical School of Guy's Hospital*. London: J. M'Creery, 1811.

Bachman, Maria K. "'Furious Passions of the Celtic Race': Ireland, Madness and Wilkie Collins's 'Blind Love.'" In *Victorian Crime, Madness and Sensation*, edited by Andrew Maunder and Grace Moore, 179–94. Aldershot: Ashgate, 2004.

Baker Brown, Isaac. *On the Curability of Certain Forms of Insanity, Epilepsy, Catalepsy, and Hysteria in Females*. London: Robert Hardwicke, 1866.

Ball, W. W. R., and J. A. Venn, eds. *Admissions to Trinity College, Cambridge*. Vol. 4. London: Macmillan, 1911.

Banerji, Brajendranath. "Sutherland's Reminiscences of Rammohun Roy." *Calcutta Review: An Illustrated Monthly*, 3rd ser., 57 (October 1935): 58–70.

[Barbauld, Anna Letitia]. "Memoir of the Late Rev. John Prior Estlin, LL.D." *Monthly Repository of Theology and General Literature* 12 (October 1817): 573–75.

"Barclay and Prichard on the Principle of Life; S.T. Coleridge on the Theory of Life." *Edinburgh Medical and Surgical Journal* 72 (October 1849): 396–436.

Barfoot, James. "James Gregory (1753–1821) and Scottish Scientific Metaphysics, 1750–1800." PhD dissertation, University of Edinburgh, 1983.

Barot, Rohit. *Bristol and the Indian Independence Movement*. Bristol Branch of the Historical Association Local History Pamphlets no. 70. Bristol: Alan Sutton, 1988.

Barrington, Emilie Isabel. *Life of Walter Bagehot*. London: Longmans, Green, 1914.

Barry, Jonathan. "Bristol Pride: Civic Identity in Bristol c. 1640–1775." In *The Making of Modern Bristol*, edited by Madge Dresser and Philip Ollerenshaw, 25–47. Tiverton: Redcliffe Press, 1996.

"Bath and Bristol Branch of the Provincial Medical and Surgical Association Annual Meeting." *Provincial Medical and Surgical Journal* 9 (July 23, 1845): 475–76.

Bayly, C. A. "Rammohan Roy and the Advent of Constitutional Liberalism in India, 1800–1830." *Modern Intellectual History* 4, no. 1 (2007).

Beddoes, Thomas. *Hygeia: Or, Essays Moral and Medical, on the Causes Affecting the Personal State of Our Middling and Affluent Classes*. 3 vols. Bristol: J. Mills, 1802.

Beeson, Anthony. *Bristol in 1807: Impressions of the City at the Time of Abolition*. Bristol: Redcliffe Press and Bristol Libraries, 2009.
Behrisch, Erika. "En Route with the British Admiralty's 'Manual of Scientific Enquiry' (1849)." In *Discovery, Innovation, and the Victorian Admiralty: Paper Navigators*, 111–48. Cham, Switzerland: Palgrave Macmillan, 2022. https://doi.org/10.1007/978-3-031-06749-5_4.
Bell, E. G. W. *University Reform in Nineteenth-Century Oxford: A Study of Henry Halford Vaughan, 1811–1885*. Oxford: Clarendon Press, 1973.
"Beobachtungen uber die Beziehung des Gedächtnisses zum Gehirn." Translation of *Treatise*, 14–22. *Zeitschrift für anthropologie* 1 (1824): 243–51.
Bernasconi, Robert. "Introduction." In *Crania Americana; or, A Comparative View of the Skulls of Various Aboriginal National of North and South America; Crania Ægyptiaca*, by Samuel George Morton, v–xiii. American Theories of Polygenesis 1. Bristol: Thoemmes, 2002.
Berrios, German E. *The History of Mental Symptoms: Descriptive Psychopathology since the Nineteenth Century*. Cambridge: Cambridge University Press, 1996.
——— . "Hypochondriasis: History of the Concept." In *Hypochondriasis: Modern Perspectives on an Ancient Malady*, edited by Vladen Starcevic and Don R. Lipsitt, 3–20. Cary: Oxford University Press, 2001.
Bettany, George Thomas. *Eminent Doctors: Their Lives and Work*. 2 vols. London: John Hogg, 1885.
——— . "John Haighton (1755–1823)." In *Dictionary of National Biography*, vol. 23, edited by Leslie Stephen and Sidney Lee, 441–42. London: Elder Smith, 1890.
——— . "Sir Astley Paston Cooper (1768–1841)." In *Dictionary of National Biography*, vol. 12, edited by Leslie Stephen and Sidney Lee, 137–39. London: Elder Smith, 1887.
Bettey, Joseph. *St. James's Fair, Bristol, 1137–1837*. ALHA Booklet no. 16. Bristol: Bristol Branch of the Historical Association, 2014.
Beveridge, Allan. "Reading about . . . the History of Psychiatry." *British Journal of Psychiatry* 200, no. 5 (2012): 431–33. https://doi.org/10.1192/bjp.bp.111.107565.
Binns, Edward. "Prodromus towards a Philosophical Inquiry into the Intellectual Powers of the Negro." *Simmonds's Colonial Magazine and Foreign Miscellany* 1 (April 1844): 464–70; 2 (May/June 44): 48–59, 154–84.
"Biographical: Dr. Thomas Charles Hope, Professor of Chemistry." *Cheilead, or University Coterie* 1 (1827): 157–59.
"Biographical Notice of the Late Dr. Gregory of Edinburgh." *London Medical Repository, Monthly Journal, and Review* 15 (1821): 423–29.
Biographical Sketch of Renn Hamden. In *Who's Who of British Members of Parliament: A Biographical Dictionary of the House of Commons based on Annual Volumes of "Dod's Parliamentary Companion" and Other Sources*, vol. 1, *1832–1885*. Hassocks, Sussex: Harvester Press, 1976.
"Biographical Sketch of the Late Dr. Chisholm." *Edinburgh Medical and Surgical Journal* 23 (April 1825): 428.
"Biography of the Late Professor Jameson." *Monthly Journal of Medical Science* 18 (1854): 572–75.

Birmingham Oratory, ed. *Correspondence of John Henry Newman with John Kebel and Others 1839–1845*. London: Longmans, Green, 1917.

Blakey, Robert. *History of the Philosophy of Mind: Embracing the Opinions of All Writers on Mental Science from the Earliest Period to the Present Time*. 4 vols. London: Trelawney Wm. Saunders, 1848.

Blandford, G. Fielding. *Insanity and Its Treatment: Lectures on the Treatment, Medical and Legal, of Insane Patients*. Edinburgh: Oliver and Boyd, 1871.

Bloxam, John Rouse. *A Register of the Presidents, Fellows, Demies, Instructors in Grammar and in Music, Chaplains, Clerks, Choristers, and Other Members of Saint Mary Magdalen College in the University of Oxford, from the Foundation of the College to the Present Time*. 8 vols. Oxford: William Graham, 1853–85.

Blyth, Edward. "An Attempt to Classify the Variety of Animals." *Magazine of Natural History* 8 (1835): 40–53.

Boase's Modern English Biography. Vol. 6. Truro: Netherton and Worth, 1921.

Bonfigli, Clodomiro. "Ulteriore considerazione sull'argomento della cosiddetta pazzia morale. Ulterior Considerations on the Discussion of the So-Called Moral Insanity." *American Journal of Insanity* 36 (October 1879; April 1880): 224–29; 476–96.

Bostock, John. *An Elementary System of Physiology*. London: Baldwin and Cradock, 1836.

[———]. "Prichard's Researches into the Physical History of Man." *Monthly Review; or Literary Journal*, ser. 2, 75 (October 1814): 127–34.

Bower, Alexander. *The Edinburgh Student's Guide: or, an Account of the Classes of the University, Arranged under the Four Faculties; with a Detail of What Is Taught in Each*. Edinburgh: Waugh and Innes, 1822.

Bowles, [Francis Cheyne], and [Richard] Smith Jr. Announcement of a Course of Seven or Eight Lectures to a Female Audience, Chiefly concerning the Senses of Vision, Hearing at the Red Lodge, December 1797. Bristol: n.p., 1797.

Boyer, Jodie. "Religion, 'Moral Insanity,' and Psychology in Nineteenth-Century America." *Religion and American Culture: A Journal of Interpretation* 24 (2014): 70–99.

Braid, James. *Neurypnology; or, the Rationale of Nervous Sleep Considered in relation with Animal Magnetism*. London: John Churchill, 1843.

Braithwaite, Joseph Bevan, ed. *Memoirs of Joseph John Gurney, with Selections from his Journal and Correspondence*. Vol. 1. Norwich: Fletcher and Alexander, 1854.

Brantlinger, Patrick. *Dark Vanishings: Discourse on the Extinction of Primitive Races, 1800–1930*. Ithaca: Cornell University Press, 2014.

[Brigham, Amariah]. Obituary of James Cowles Prichard. *American Journal of Insanity* 5, no. 4 (April 1849): 383–84.

Bristol Auxiliary Temperance Society. *The First Report, June 14th [1832]*. Bristol: Wright & Bagnall, 1832.

Bristol College. *Proceedings of the Fourth Annual Meeting, Held February 27, 1834*. Bristol: Printed by J. Chilcott, 1834.

Bristol College Theological Lecture Fund. Bristol: n.p., 1829.

Bristol Corporation of the Poor. *Bye-Laws, Rules, and Regulations, for the Conduct and Government of all and Every the Members of the Corporation, of the Governor, Deputy-Governor, Assistants, and Guardians of the Poor*. Bristol: Printed by A. Brown, Mirror Office, [1825].

Bristol Established Church Society and Book Association. *The First Annual Report of the Bristol Established Church Society and Book Association*. Bristol: Printed by A. and H. Hill, 1842.

———. *The Third Annual Report of the Bristol Established Church Society and Book Association Feb. 14, 1844*. Bristol: Printed by D. Vickery, 1844.

Bristoliensis. "The Easterlings." *Gloucestershire Notes and Queries* 2 (1882–84): 657–59.

Bristol Infirmary. *Proceedings in Relation to a Proposed Extension of the Number of Pupils Admissible to Witness the Medical and Surgical Practice of the Infirmary*. Bristol: J. G. Fuller, 1838.

———. *Proposed Rules for the Government of the Bristol Infirmary, for Consideration and Adoption at a Special General Board of The Trustees, June 1, 1824*. Bristol: Printed by T. J. Manchee, 1824.

———. *Report by the Committee of Enquiry to a General Board of Trustees*. Bristol: Evans & Grabham, 1811.

———. *Report of the Special Committee to the General Board, Held the 29th of October, 1824*. Bristol: Printed at the Bristol Observer Office by John Evans, 1824.

———. *Rules Confirmed by the Subscribers to the Bristol Infirmary At their several General Boards, From the first Institution of the Society in the Year 1727, to the 15th of April, 1806*. Bristol: Printed by W. Pine, 1806.

———. *Rules for the Government of the Bristol Infirmary, for Consideration and Adoption at a Special General Board of The Trustees, June 1, 1824*. Bristol: Printed by T. J. Manchee, 1824.

———. *State of the Infirmary, 1816*. Bristol: Printed by Browne and Manchee, 1816.

Bristol Institution. *Proceedings of the Annual Meeting, Held February 10, 1825, and of the General Meeting, Held March 10, 1825*. Bristol: A. Brown, [1825].

———. *Proceedings of the Twelfth Annual Meeting [February 12, 1835]*. Bristol: Printed for the Bristol Institution, [1835].

———. *Proceedings of the Twenty-Third Annual Meeting . . . for the Years 1836 to 1845*. Bristol: Printed at the Journal Office by James Martin, [1846].

———. *Report of the Proceedings of the Institution, from the Year 1846 to the Close of the Year 1860*. Bristol: T. D. Taylor, Printer, Mirror Office, [1861].

———. *Three Lectures on Egyptian Mummies, Egyptian Antiquities, and the Rosetta Stone*. Bristol: Printed at the Mirror Office by John Taylor, 1834.

"The Bristol Meeting of the British Medical Association, 1894." *Bristol Medico-Chirurgical Journal* 12 (September 1894): 161–224.

Bristol Refuge Society. *The First Report of the Bristol Refuge Society, for the Restoration of Females, 6 Month 30, 1815*. Bristol: Philip Rose, [1815].

Bristol Statistical Society. *Proceedings of the First Annual Meeting, Held November 10th, 1837, with the Report of the Council*. Bristol: Printed at the Mirror Office by John Taylor, [1837].

British Association for the Advancement of Science. *List of Resident & Non-resident Members, Fourteenth Meeting.* York: n.p., 1844.

———. *Queries respecting the Human Race, to Be Addressed to Travellers and Others.* Drawn up by a committee appointed in 1839. London: Printed by Richard and John E. Taylor, 1840.

[Bronson, Henry]. Review of *Thoughts on the Original Unity of the Human Race. Quarterly Christian Spectator* 3, no. 3 (March 1831): 56–75.

[Brown, Andrew]. *Notice of the Life and Character of Alexander Christison, A.M., Late Professor of Humanity in the University of Edinburgh.* Edinburgh: Printed by Abernethy & Walker, 1820.

[Brown, James]. "Celtae." In *Encyclopaedia Britannica*, 7th ed., vol. 7, 273–77. Edinburgh: Adam and Charles Black, 1842.

Browne, P[eter]. A[rrell]. *The Classification of Mankind by the Hair and Wool of Their Heads: With an Answer to Dr. Prichard's Assertion, that "the Covering of the Head of the Negro Is Hair, Properly So Termed, and Not Wool": Read before the American Ethnological Society, November 3, 1849.* Philadelphia: A. Hart, 1850.

Bruce, James. *Travels to Discover the Source of the Nile, in the Years 1768, 1769, 1770, 1771, 1772 and 1773.* Edited by Alexander Murray. 3rd ed. Edinburgh: Printed by George Ramsay for Archibald Constable, 1813.

Buchanan, Francis. *A Journey from Madras through the Countries of Mysore, Canara, and Malabar.* London: T. Cadell and W. Davies, 1807.

Buchwald, Jed Z., and Diane Greco Josefowicz. *The Zodiac of Paris: How an Improbable Controversy over an Ancient Egyptian Artifact Provoked a Modern Debate between Religion and Science.* Princeton NJ: Princeton University Press, 2010.

Buckland, William. *Geology and Mineralogy Considered with Reference to Natural Theology.* 2 vols. Bridgewater Treatise 6. London: William Pickering, 1836.

Bucknill, John Charles, and Daniel Hack Tuke. *A Manual of Psychological Medicine: Containing the History, Nosology, Description, Statistics, Diagnosis, Pathology, and Treatment of Insanity.* London: John Churchill, 1858.

[Budd, Henry]. *A Memoir of the Rev. Henry Budd: Comprising an Autobiography; Letters, Papers, & Remains.* London: Seeley, Jackson and Halliday, 1855.

Bunsen, Christian Charles Josias von. "On the Results of the Recent Egyptian Researches in Reference to Asiatic and African Ethnology, and the Classification of Languages." In *Three Linguistic Dissertations Read at the Meeting of The British Association in Oxford*, 254–99. London: Printed by Richard and John E. Taylor, 1848.

———. *Outlines of the Philosophy of Universal History, Applied to Language and Religion.* Vol. 1. London: Longman, Brown, Green, and Longmans, 1854.

Bunsen, Frances. *A Memoir of Baron Bunsen Late Minister, Late Minister Plenipotentiary and Envoy Extraordinary of his Majesty Frederic William IV at the Court of St. James.* 2 vols. London: Longmans, Green, 1868.

Bureaud Riofrey, A. M. "Retrospective Review of the Therapeutical Progress of Medicine and Surgery during the Year 1837." *Continental and British Medical Review, or Monthly Therapeutical Journal* 2 (January 1838): 1–11.

Burke, John G. "Kirk and Causality in Edinburgh, 1805." *ISIS: An International Review Devoted to the History of Science and Its Cultural Influences* 61 (1970): 340–54.
Burnett, Charles. "The Common Origin of Mankind." *Church of England Magazine* 11 and 12 (1841–42).
Burnett, C. M. *The Power, Wisdom, and Goodness of God, as Displayed in the Animal Creation: Shewing the Remarkable Agreement between This Department of Nature and Revelation; in a Series of Letters*. London: James Burns, 1838.
Butcher, E. E. *Bristol Corporation of the Poor: Selected Records, 1696–1834*. Bristol: Printed for the Bristol Record Society by J. W. Arrowsmith, 1932.
Buxton, L. H. Dudley, and Strickland Gibson. *Oxford University Ceremonies*. Oxford: Clarendon, 1935.
Bynum, W. F. "Theory and Practice in British Psychiatry from J. C. Prichard (1785–1848) to Henry Maudsley (1835–1918)." *Nihon Ishigaku Zasshi: Journal of the Japan Society of Medical History* 27 (January 1981): 73–94.
Bynum, William F. "Psychiatry in Its Historical Context." In *Handbook of Psychiatry*, vol. 1, *General Psychopathology*, edited by M. Shepherd and O. L. Zangwill, 6–38. Cambridge: Cambridge University Press, 1983.
Bynum, William Frederick. "Time's Noblest Offspring: The Problem of Man in the British Natural Historical Sciences, 1800–1863." PhD dissertation, University of Cambridge, 1974.
Caldwell, Charles. *Phrenology Vindicated, and Antiphrenology Unmasked*. Lexington KY: J. Clarke, 1835.
———. *Thoughts on the Original Unity of the Human Race*. New York: E. Bliss, 1830; 2nd ed., 1852.
"Caldwell on the Unity of the Human Race." *North American Medical and Surgical Journal* 12 (October 1831): 363–91.
Cameron, H. C. "Richard Bright at Guy's." *Guy's Hospital Reports* 107, special issue (1958): 263–93.
Campbell, John. *Negro-mania: Being an Examination of the Falsely Assumed Equality of the Various Races of Men; Demonstrated by the Investigations of Champollion [and Others]*. Philadelphia: Campbell & Power, 1851.
Camper, Petrus. *Verhandeling van Petrus Camper, over het natuurlijk verschil der wezenstrekken in menschen van onderscheiden landaart en ouderdom*. Utrecht: B. Wild en J. Altheer, 1791.
Carlyle, Thomas. *The Life of John Sterling*. London: Chapman and Hall, 1851.
Carpenter, J. Estlin. *James Martineau, Theologian and Teacher: A Study of His Life and Thought*. London: Philip Green, 1905.
Carpenter, Mary. *The Last Days in England of the Rajah Rammohun Roy*. London: Truebner, 1866.
[———]. *Red Lodge Girls' Reformatory School, Bristol: Certified under the Act 17 and 18 Vict. cap. 86*. Bristol: Arrowsmith, 1875.
[Carpenter, William Benjamin]. "Ethnology, or the Science of Races." *Edinburgh Review* 88 (October 1848): 429–87. Reprinted in the *Eclectic Magazine of Foreign Literature, Science, and Art* 16 (January 1849): 55–87.

[———]. "Dr. Prichard on the Physical and Natural History of Mankind." *British and Foreign Medical Review* 24 (July/October 1847): 49–81, 441–82.
[———]. "[Oration at the] Centenary of the Royal Medical Society of Edinburgh." *London Medical Gazette* 20 (1837): 85–86.
———. *Principles of General and Comparative Physiology: Intended as an Introduction to the Study of Human Physiology: and as a Guide to the Philosophical Pursuit of Natural History*. London: John Churchill, 1839.
Carrick, A. *Observations Submitted to the Trustees of the Bristol Infirmary, on the Exclusion of the Medical Officers from the House Committee; and Other Subjects Connected with the General Management of the Charity*. Bristol: Printed by J. M. Gutch, 1825.
Carrick, Andrew. *Address on the Opening of the Bristol College, the 17th January, 1831*. Bristol: Gutch and Martin, [1831].
Cartwright, Samuel A. "The Diseases and Physical Peculiarities of the Negro Race." *Charleston Medical Journal and Review* 6 (September 1851): 643–52.
[Chambers, Robert]. *Vestiges of the Natural History of Creation*. London: John Churchill, 1844.
Childe-Pemberton, William S. *The Romance of Princess Amelia, Daughter of George III (1783–1810)*. London: Eveleigh Nash, 1910.
Chisholm, C[olin]. "On the Statistical Pathology of Bristol and of Clifton, Gloucestershire." *Edinburgh Medical and Surgical Journal* 13 (July 1817): 265–300.
Chisholm, Colin. "Extract of a Letter from Colin Chisholm, M.D. F.R.S. &c. Addressed to Dr. Hosack: Dated Clifton, August 21, 1811." *American Medical and Philosophical Register* 2 (April 1812): 456–61.
Chitnis, Anand Chidamber. "The Edinburgh Professoriate, 1790–1826, and the University's Contribution to Nineteenth Century British Life." PhD dissertation, University of Edinburgh, 1968.
Christison, Alex[ander]. *The General Diffusion of Knowledge: One Great Cause of the Prosperity of North Britain*. Edinburgh: Printed for Peter Hill, 1802.
Church, Mary C., ed. *Life and Letters of Dean Church*. 2nd ed. London: Macmillan, 1897.
Clark, John Willis. "The Foundation and Early Years of the Society." *Proceedings of the Cambridge Philosophical Society* 7 (1891): ii.
Coleridge, Ernest Hartley, ed. *Life and Correspondence of John Duke Lord Coleridge, Lord Chief Justice of England*. Vol. 2. London: Hilliam Heinemann, 1904.
College of Physicians of Ireland. *Register of the King and Queen's College of Physicians in Ireland, to Which Is Appended a Roll of the Presidents and Fellows, from 1654 to 1865*. Dublin: Hodges and Smith, 1866.
Colley, Linda. "The Apotheosis of George III: Loyalty, Royalty and the British Nation, 1760–1820." *Past & Present* 102 (February 1984): 94–129.
Colley, Noel G. "Medical Chemistry at Guy's Hospital (1770–1850)." *Ambix* 35 (1988): 155–68.
Colquhoun, John Campbell. *Hints on Animal Magnetism*. Edinburgh: Maclachlan & Stewart, 1838.

[Combe, Andrew]. "Cyclopaedia of Practical Medicine—Dr. Prichard and Phrenology." *Phrenological Journal and Miscellany* 8 (June 1834): 649–57.

———. "Dr. Prichard and Phrenology." In *On the Functions of the Cerebellum, by Drs Gall, Vimont, and Broussais, translated by George Combe; Also Answers to the Objections Urged Against Phrenology by Drs Roget, Rudolphi, Prichard, and Tiedemann, by George Combe and Dr. A. Combe*, edited by George and Andrew Combe, 248–90. Edinburgh: Maclachlan & Stewart, 1838.

[———]. "Dr Pritchard and Phrenology." *Phrenological Journal and Miscellany* 2 (August 1824): 47–55.

Combe, George. *Essay on the Constitution of Man, and Its Relations to External Objects*. Edinburgh: Printed by P. Neill, 1827.

"Comedies of Aristophanes, viz. The Clouds, Plutus, the Frogs, the Birds. Translated into English, with Notes. London. 1812." *British Review, and London Critical Journal* 4 (May 1813): 384–402.

Commissioners in Lunacy. *Copy of Report to the Lord Chancellor of the Number of Visits Made, the Number of Patients Seen, and the Number of Miles Travelled by the Several Commissioners in Lunacy, during the Six Months ending the 4th of February 1846*. In House of Commons, *Accounts and Papers*, vol. 33, 407–8. [London]: Ordered by the House of Commons to Be Printed, 1846.

———. *Further Report of the Commissioners in Lunacy, to the Lord Chancellor Presented to Both Houses of Parliament by Command of Her Majesty*. London: Shaw and Sons, 1847.

———. *Haydock Lodge Lunatic Asylum. A Copy of a further Report of the Commissioners in Lunacy to the Secretary of State for the Home Department relative to the Haydock Lodge Lunatic Asylum*. London: Ordered by the House of Commons to Be Printed, 1847.

———. *Report of the Metropolitan Commissioners in Lunacy to the Lord Chancellor: Presented to Both Houses of Parliament by Command of Her Majesty*. London: Bradbury and Evans, 1844.

Conlin, Jonathan. *Evolution and the Victorians: Science, Culture and Politics in Darwin's Britain*. London: Bloomsbury, 2014.

Conolly, John. *Enquiry concerning Indications of Insanity*. 1830. In *Madness at Home: The Psychiatrist, the Patient, and the Family in England, 1820–1860*, by Akihito Suzuki. Berkeley: University of California Press, 2006.

[———]. *Familiar Views of Lunacy and Lunatic Life: with Hints on the Personal Care and Management of those who are Afflicted with Temporary or Permanent Derangement*. London: John W. Parker, 1850.

[——— ?]. "Prichard, Esquirol, Allen, Ellis, Ferrarese, Greco, Farr, Crowther, &c. on Insanity." *British and Foreign Medical Review or Quarterly Journal of Practical Medicine and Surgery* 7 (January 1839): 1–55.

"Constantine Estlin Prichard." In *Crockford's Clerical Directory for 1868: Biographical and Statistical Book of Reference for Facts Relating to the Clergy and the Church*, 536. London: Horace Cox, 1868.

Conybeare, William Daniel. *An Elementary Course of Theological Lectures*. London: John Murray, 1834.

———. *Inaugural Address on the Application of Classical and Scientific Education to Theology; and on the Evidences of Natural and Revealed Religion. Delivered as Introductory to a Course of Theological Lectures for the Use of the Pupils of Bristol College, Being Members of the Established Church.* London: John Murray, 1831.

Conybeare, William Daniel, and William Phillips. *Outlines of the Geology of England and Wales: with an Introductory Compendium of the General Principles of that Science, and Comparative Views of the Structure of Foreign Countries.* Part 1. London: William Phillips, 1822.

Cooke, John. *History and Method of Cure of the Various Species of Epilepsy: Being the Second Part of the Second Volume of a Treatise on Nervous Diseases.* London: Longman, Hurst, Rees, Orme and Brown, 1823.

Cooter, Roger James. "The Cultural Meaning of Popular Science: Phrenology and the Organisation of Consent in Nineteenth Century Britain." PhD dissertation, University of Cambridge, 1978.

Cottle, Basil. *Robert Southey and Bristol.* [Bristol]: Bristol Branch of the Historical Association, 1980.

Count, Earl Wendel. *This Is Race: An Anthology Selected from the International Literature on the Races of Man.* New York: Henry Schuman, 1950.

A Countryman. "On the Tendency of Doctrines Maintained by Some Modern Physiologists." *Evangelical and Literary Magazine* 5 (September 1822): 480–84.

[Craik, James]. "The Unity of Mankind." *Church Review and Ecclesiastical Register* 9 (January 1857): 530–46.

"Cranier ur gamla grafvar i England." *Öfversigt af Kongl: Vetenskaps-Akademiens Förhandlingar* 5 (April 1848): 71–72.

Creuzer, [Georg Friedrich]. *Religions de l'antiquité, considérées principalement dans leurs formes symboliques et mythologiques.* Translated and expanded by J. D. Guigniaut. Vol. 1, part 2. Paris: Treuttel et Wurtz, 1825.

Critical Analysis of James Cowles Prichard's "Cases of Typhus Fever." *London Medical and Physical Journal* 38 (November 1817): 406–11.

Critical Analysis of the Review of Dr. Prichard's *A History of the Epidemic Fever* Published in the London Medical Repository. *Medical Intelligencer* 1, no. 9 (July 1820): 219–20.

Cross, F. Richardson. "Early Medical Teaching in Bristol: The Bristol Medical School and Its Association with the University College." *Bristol Medico-Chirurgical Journal* 44 (Summer 1927): 73–112.

Crossley Evans, M. J. *Hannah More.* Bristol Branch of the Historical Association no. 99. Bristol: Printed by the Malago Press, 1999.

Crowther, Caleb. *Observations on the Management of Madhouses.* Part 3. London: Simpkin, Marshall, 1849.

Cull, Richard, and J. H. Williams. Review of *The Eastern Origin of the Celtic Nations,* New Edition. *Traethodydd* 14 (May 1858): 131–32.

Cullen, M. J. *The Statistical Movement in Early Victorian Britain: The Foundations of Empirical Social Research.* Hassocks, Sussex: Harvester Press, 1975.

[Cullimore, Isaac]. "The Trinity of the Gentiles: Egyptian Mythology." *Frazer's Magazine* 20 (July–September 1839): 1–10, 200–211, 326–32.

Curry, James. *Examination of the Prejudices Commonly Entertained against Mercury, as Beneficially Applicable to the Greater Number of Liver Complaints, and to Various Other Forms of Disease, as well as to Syphilis.* London: J. M'Creery, 1809.

Curtis, Lewis Perry, Jr. *Apes and Angels: The Irishman in Victorian Caricature.* Washington DC: Smithsonian Institution Press, 1971.

Cuvier, Georges. *Essay on the Theory of the Earth.* Edinburgh: William Blackwell, 1813.

"The Cyclopaedia of Practical Medicine." *London Medical and Surgical Journal* 3 (February 1833): 27–28.

The Cyclopaedia of Practical Medicine. Revised by Robley Dunglison. Philadelphia: Lea & Blanchard, 1845.

Dain, Norman. *Concepts of Insanity in the United States, 1789–1865.* New Brunswick NJ: Rutgers University Press, 1964.

Darnell, Regna. "A Critical Paradigm for the Histories of Anthropology: The Generalization of Transportable Knowledge." *Bérose-Encyclopédie internationale des histoires de l'anthropologie.* https://www.berose.fr/article2718.html.

Darwin, Charles. *The Descent of Man, and Selection in Relation to Sex.* 1871. Repr., London: Penguin, 2004.

———. *More Letters of Charles Darwin.* Edited by Francis Darwin. Vol. 1. London: John Murray, 1903.

Darwin, Erasmus. *Zoonomia; or, the Laws of Organic Life.* London: J. Johnson, 1796.

Daston, Lorraine, and Peter Galison. *The Image of Objectivity.* New York: Zone, 2007.

Davies, David. *Letters on Medical Consultation, to and from Dr. Prichard, M.D. with Some Observations on Medical Usage, and the Inseparability of Medical Surgery & Medicine.* Bristol: Printed by T. J. Manchee, [1826].

Davies, Edward. *Celtic Researches, on the Origin, Traditions & Language of the Ancient Britons: With Some Introductory Sketches, on Primitive Society.* London: Printed for the Author, 1804.

Dawson, J. W. *Archaia: or, Studies of the Cosmogony and Natural History of the Hebrew Scriptures.* Montreal: B. Dawson and Son, 1860.

———. *The Origin of the World according to Revelation and Science.* London: Hodder & Stoughton, 1877.

Dawson, Warren Royal, and Eric P. Uphill. *Who Was Who in Egyptology: A Biographical Index of Egyptologists: of Travellers, of Explorers, and Excavators in Egypt.* 2nd ed. London: Egypt Exploration Society, 1972.

De La Beche, H. T., and Lyon Playfair. "Report on the Sanatory Condition of Bristol." In *Second Report of the Commissioners for Inquiring into the State of Large Towns and Populous Districts,* 241–64. 2 vols. London: Printed by William Clowes and Sons, for Her Majesty's Stationery Office, 1845.

Desmond, Adrian. "Robert E. Grant: The Social Predicament of a Pre-Darwinian Transmutationist." *Journal of the History of Biology* 17 (Summer 1984): 189–223.

Desmond, Adrian, and James Moore. *Darwin's Sacred Cause: Race, Slavery and the Quest for Human Origins*. London: Allen Lane, 2009.

Di Brizio, Maria Beatrice. *Histoire du concept de couvade: Edward B. Tylor et l'ethnologie victorienne*. Paris: L'Harmattan, 2021. https://doi.org/10.7340/anuac2239-625X-5269.

Dieffenbach, Ernest. *On the Study of Ethnology*. Read at a Meeting Preliminary to the Formation of the Ethnological Society, Held at Dr. Hodgkin's, 9 Lower Brook Street, Grosvenor Square, January 31, 1843. London: Printed by Richard Watts, [1843].

Digby, Ann. *Making a Medical Living: Doctors and Patients in the English Market for Medicine, 1720–1911*. Cambridge: Cambridge University Press, 1994.

Dillon, Myles. *Celts and Aryans: Survivals of Indo-European Speech and Society*. Simla: Registrar, Indian Institute of Advanced Study, 1975.

Donaldson, John William. *The New Cratylus: Or, Contributions towards a More Accurate Knowledge of the Greek Language*. London: John W. Parker, 1850.

Douglas, Bronwen. "Climate to Crania: Science and the Racialization of Human Difference." In *Foreign Bodies: Oceania and the Science of Race, 1750–1940*, edited by Bronwen Douglas and Chris Ballard, 33–96. Canberra: ANU Press, 2008.

——— . "'Novus Orbis Australis': Oceania in the Science of Race, 1750–1850." In *Foreign Bodies: Oceania and the Science of Race, 1750–1940*, edited by Bronwen Douglas and Chris Ballard, 99–155. Canberra: ANU Press, 2008.

Dresser, Madge. *Bristol: Ethnic Minorities and the City, 1000–2001*. Chichester, UK: Phillimore, 2007.

——— . "Protestants, Catholics, and Jews." In *The Making of Modern Bristol*, edited by Madge Dresser and Philip Ollerenshaw, 96–123. Tiverton: Redcliffe Press, 1996.

"Dr. Latham's Ethnological Works." *British and Foreign Medico-Chirurgical Review or Quarterly Journal of Practical Medicine and Surgery* 10 (October 1852): 520–22.

"Dr. Pope and the Highwayman." *Journal of the Friends' Historical Society* 5, no. 4 (October 1908): 200.

"Dr. Prichard on Diseases of the Nervous System." *London Medical and Physical Journal* 47 (February 1822): 129–40.

"Dr. Prichard on Diseases of the Nervous System." *Medico-Chirurgical Review, and Journal of Medical Science* 3 (June 1822): 122–51.

"Dr. Prichard on Epidemic Fever." *London Medical and Physical Journal* 44 (August 1820): 132–42.

"Dr. Prichard on Fever." *Medico-Chirurgical Review, and Journal of Medical Science* 1 (December 1820): 381–87.

"Dr. Prichard on Insanity." *Boston Medical and Surgical Journal* 22 (August 5, 1840): 417.

"Dr. Prichard on Insanity." *Medical Quarterly Review* 4 (April 1835): 1–32.

"Dr. Prichard on Insanity." *Medico-Chirurgical Review, and Journal of Practical Medicine*, n.s., 22 (April 1835): 442–48 and (July 1835): 106–22.

"Dr. Prichard on the Physical History of Mankind." *Dublin Journal of Medical Science* 10 (November 1837): 331–32.

"Dr Prichard on the Vital Principle." *Medico-Chirurgical Review, and Journal of Practical Medicine*, n.s., 12 (January 1830): 316–21.

"Dr. Prichard—Physical History of Mankind." *British Critic: Quarterly Theological Review and Ecclesiastical Record* 4 (July 1828): 33–61.

"Dr. Prichard's Pathology of Paralysis, Epilepsy, and Chorea." *Anderson's Quarterly Journal of the Medical Sciences* 1 (April 1824): 300.

"Dr. Prichard's Pathology of Paralysis, Epilepsy, and Chorea." *Journal of Foreign Medical Science and Literature* 4 (July 1824): 377.

"Dr. Pritchard on the 'Physical History of Man.'" *Annals of Philosophy* 5 (May 1815): 379–82.

"Dr. R. G. Latham [Obituary]." *The Athenaeum* 1 (January–June 1888): 340–41.

Drummond, James, and Charles Barnes Upton. *The Life and Letters of James Martineau*. Vols. 1 and 2. New York: Dodd, Mead, 1902.

"Dr. Wilde's Madeira and the Mediterranean." *Dublin University Magazine* 15 (April 1840): 451–70.

Duncan, Andrew, Jr. *Additional Testimonials in Favour of Dr. Duncan, Jun.* Edinburgh: Printed by George Ramsay, 1821.

———. *Reports of the Practice in the Clinical Wards of the Royal Infirmary of Edinburgh, during the Months of November and December 1817, and January 1818, and May, June and July, 1818*. Edinburgh: Archibald Constable, 1818.

Duncan, P. Martin. "On Insanity." *Quarterly Journal of Science* 7 (April 1870): 165–86.

Duppa, Richard. *Travels on the Continent, Sicily, and the Lipari Islands*. 2nd ed. London: Longman, Rees, Orme, 1829.

Earle, Pliny. "Psychologic Medicine: Its Importance as a Part of the Medical Curriculum." *American Journal of Insanity* 24 (January 1868): 257–80.

Ebel, Hermann Wilhelm. *Celtic Studies*. Translated by William K Sullivan. London: Williams and Norgate, 1863.

Eden, John. *The Book of Psalms, in Blank Verse*. London: Hamilton, Adams, 1841.

"Edward Bird, Esq. R. A." *Gentleman's Magazine and Historical Chronicle* 89, pt. 2 (November 1819): 470–71.

Eghigian, Greg, ed. *From Madness to Mental Health: Psychiatric Disorder and Its Treatment in Western Civilization*. New Brunswick: Rutgers University Press, 2009.

Eigen, Joel Peter. *Unconscious Crime: Mental Absence and Criminal Responsibility in Victorian London*. Baltimore: Johns Hopkins University Press, 2003.

Elliott-Binns, L. E. *The Early Evangelicals: A Religious and Social Study*. London: Lutterworth, 1953.

Ely, H. E. "On the Common Origin of the Human Races." *DeBow's Review, Agricultural, Commercial, Industrial Progress and Resources* 17 (July 1854): 25–39.

"The Epidemic Fever." *Edinburgh Medical and Surgical Journal* 17 (October 1821): 602–34.

Eriksen, Thomas Hylland, and Finn Sivert Nielsen. *A History of Anthropology*. London: Pluto, 2013.

Esquirol, E. *Des maladies mentales considérées sous les rapports médical, hygiénique et médico-légal.* Vol. 2. Paris: J. B. Baillière, 1838.

Ewald, Heinrich. Review of *The Eastern Origin of the Celtic Nations*, New Edition. *Göttingische gelehrte Anzeigen* 1 (March 1858): 433–38.

"Exposition of the Present State of the Profession of Physic in England, and of the Laws Enacted for Its Government." *Edinburgh Medical and Surgical Journal* 16 (1820): 481–509.

"Extracts from the Proceedings of the Society." *Journal of the Bombay Branch of the Royal Asiatic Society* 2 (July 1847): 442–79.

Farmayan, Hafez Farman. "The Forces of Modernization in Nineteenth Century Iran: A Historical Survey." In *Beginnings of Modernization in the Middle East: The Nineteenth Century*, edited by William R. Polk and Richard L. Chambers, 119–51. Chicago: University of Chicago Press, 1968.

The First Annual Report of the Aborigines Protection Society. Presented at the Meeting at Exeter Hall, with List of Officers, Subscribers, and Benefactors, May 16, 1838. London: Printed for the Society by P. White and Son, 1838.

The First Report of the Committee of Visitors of the County Lunatic Asylum, at Hanwell, April Quarter Session. London: John Thomas Norris, 1846.

Fischer-Homberger, Esther. "Hypochondriasis of the Eighteenth Century—Neurosis of the Present Century." *Bulletin of the History of Medicine* 46 (July–August 1972): 391–401.

Fissell, Mary Elizabeth. "The Physic of Charity: Health and Welfare in the West Country, 1690–1834." PhD dissertation, University of Pennsylvania, 1988.

Flinn, Derek. "James Hutton and Robert Jameson." *Scottish Journal of Geology* 16 (1980): 251–58.

Foster, John. *Letters from John Foster to Thomas Coles, M.A. Now First Published.* Edited by Henry Coles. London: H. G. Bohn, 1864.

———. *The Life and Correspondence of John Foster.* Edited by Jonathan Edwards Ryland and John Sheppard. London: Jackson and Walford, 1848.

Foster, Joseph, comp. *Alumni Oxonienses: The Members of the University of Oxford, 1715–1886.* Oxford: Parker, 1888.

Foster, W. D. "William Charles Wells Physician St. Thomas' Hospital (1795–1817)." *St. Thomas's Hospital Gazette* 57 (1959): 75–78.

Foucault, Michel. *Histoire de la folie à l'âge classique—Folie et déraison.* Paris: Plon, 1960.

[Fox Bourne, Henry Richard]. *The Aborigines Protection Society: Chapters in Its History.* London: P. S. King & Son, 1899.

Frampton, Sally. "Science in the Nineteenth-Century Periodical: Reading the Magazine of Nature." In *Science Periodicals in Nineteenth-Century Britain: Constructing Scientific Communities*, edited by Gowan Dawson, Bernard Lightman, Sally Shuttleworth, and Jonathan R. Topham, 309–69. Chicago: University of Chicago Press, 2020.

Galt, J. G. "The Letters Testimonial of the English Bishops and the Lambeth M.C." *History of Medicine* 6 (1975): 10–17.

Galt, John Minson. *The Treatment of Insanity.* New York: Harper & Brothers, 1846.

Ganz, Melissa J. "Carrying On like a Madman: Insanity and Responsibility in 'Strange Case of Dr. Jekyll and Mr. Hyde.'" *Nineteenth-Century Literature* 70, no. 3 (2015): 363–97.

Gardner, Helen. "The 'Faculty of Faith': Evangelical Missionaries, Social Anthropologists, and the Claim for Human Unity in the 19th Century." In *Foreign Bodies: Oceania and the Science of Race, 1750–1940*, edited by Bronwen Douglas and Chris Ballard, 259–82. Canberra: ANU Press, 2008.

Garnett, Richard. *The Philological Essays of the Late Rev. Richard Garnett of the British Museum*. London: Williams and Norgate, 1859.

[———]. "Prichard on the Celtic Nations." *Quarterly Review* 57 (September 1836): 80–110.

Georgii, Ludwig. "Prichard, 'Darstellung der Ägyptischen Mythologie.'" *Jahrbücher für wissenschaftliche Kritik* 2 (November 1839): cols. 665–72, 673–77, 681–88.

Ghosh, J. C. *Annals of English Literature, 1475–1950*. 2nd ed. Oxford: Clarendon, 1961.

Gibson, William. *Lecture, Introductory to a Course on the Principles and Practice of Surgery: in the University of Pennsylvania, delivered November 1, 1841*. Philadelphia: J. G. Auner, 1847.

———. *Rambles in Europe, in 1839: With Sketches of Prominent Surgeons, Physicians, Medical Schools, Hospitals, Literary Personages, Scenery, Etc.* Philadelphia: Lea and Blanchard, 1841.

Gilby, W. H. "A Geological Description of the Neighbourhood of Bristol." *Philosophical Magazine and Journal* 44 (October 1814): 241–48.

———. "Geological Observations." *Philosophical Magazine and Journal* 46 (September 1815): 182–91.

Gliddon, George, and Josiah Nott. *Types of Mankind: or, Ethnological Researches Based upon the Ancient Monuments, Paintings, Sculptures, and Crania of Races, and upon Their Natural, Geographical, Philological and Biblical History*. Philadelphia: Lippincott, 1854.

Gobineau, Arthur Joseph de. *Essai sur l'inégalité des races humaines*. 4 vols. Paris: Librairie de Firmin Didot frères, 1853, 1855; 2nd ed., 2 vols., Paris: Librairie de Firmin Didot, 1884.

———. *The Moral and Intellectual Diversity of Races: With Particular Reference to Their Respective Influence in the Civil and Political History of Mankind*. Translated by H. Hotz. Philadelphia: J. B. Lippincott, 1856.

Goldman. Lawrence. "The Origins of British 'Social Science': Political Economy, Natural Science and Statistics, 1830–1835." *Historical Journal* 26, no. 3 (1983): 587–616.

Goldstein, Jan. *Console and Classify: The French Psychiatric Profession in the Nineteenth Century*. Chicago: University of Chicago Press, 2001.

Good, John Mason. *The Study of Medicine*. 2nd ed., 5 vols. London: Baldwin, Cradock, and Jay, 1825.

Goodfield-Toulmin, June. "Blasphemy and Biology." *Rockefeller University Review* 4 (September–October 1966): 9–18.

———. "Some Aspects of English Physiology: 1780–1840." *Journal of the History of Biology* 2 (Fall 1969): 283–320.

Gordon, John. "The Doctrines of Gall and Spurzheim." *Edinburgh Review* 25 (June 1815): 227–68.
Goshen, Charles Ernest, ed. *Documentary History of Psychiatry: A Source Book on Historical Principles*. London: Vision, 1967.
Gowers, W. R. *Epilepsy and Other Chronic Convulsive Diseases: Their Causes, Symptoms, & Treatment*. London: J. & A. Churchill, 1881.
"Graduations at Edinburgh in 1808." *Edinburgh Medical and Surgical Journal* 4 (1808): 507–8.
Graham, Thomas J. *Modern Domestic Medicine: A Popular Treatise Illustrating the Character, Symptoms, Causes, Distinction, and Correct Treatment of All Diseases Incident to the Human Frame*. 6th ed. London: Simpkin and Marshall, 1835.
Grant, Alexander. *The Story of the University of Edinburgh during Its First Three Hundred Years*. 2 vols. London: Longmans, Green, 1884.
Graves, Robert James. "Letter from Dr. Prichard on the Subject of Mr. Wallace's Opinion concerning the Want of Sagittal Suture in Certain Tribes of Negroes [Addressed to Robert James Graves, July 20, 1836]." *Dublin Journal of Medical Science* 10 (September 1836): 138–39.
——. *Studies in Physiology and Medicine*. London: John Churchill & Sons, 1863.
Graves, Robert Perceval. *Life of Sir William Rowan Hamilton, Andrews Professor of Astronomy in the University of Dublin and Royal Astronomer of Ireland*. Vol. 2. Dublin: Hodges, Figgis, 1882–89.
Greene, John C. *The Death of Adam: Evolution and Its Impact on Western Thought*. Ames: Iowa State University Press, 1959.
[Gregory, James]. "Notes of the Lectures of the Late Professor Gregory, of Edinburgh [on Treatment of Diseases of the Nervous System]." *London Medical Gazette* 35 (April 1845): 855–59, 917–23, 954–58.
Gregory, Olinthus Gilbert. *A Brief Memoir of the Life of Robert Hall*. London: Holdsworth and Ball, 1833.
Gregory, Philip Spencer. *Records of the Family of Gregory*. London: Privately printed [by Veale, Chifferiel], 1886.
Griffiths, L. M. *The Medical Reading Society, Bristol*. Bristol: Reprinted from the *Bristol Medico-Chirurgical Journal* by J. W. Arrowsmith, 1907.
Griffiths, O. M. "Side Lights on the History of Presbyterian-Unitarianism from the Records of Lewin's Mead Chapel, Bristol." *Transactions of the Unitarian Historical Society* 6 (1936): 116–29.
Grimm, Jacob Ludwig Karl. *Kleinere Schriften*. Hildesheim: Georg Olms Verlagsbuchhandlung, 1965.
Griscom, John. *A Year in Europe: Comprising a Journal of Observations in England, Scotland, Ireland, France, Switzerland, the North of Italy, and Holland in 1818 and 1819*. Vol. 1. New York: Collins and E. Bliss & E. White, 1823.
Griscom, John H. *Memoir of John Griscom, LL.D. Late Professor of Chemistry and Natural Philosophy; with an Account of the New York High School; Society for the Prevention of Pauperism; the House of Refuge; and other Institutions*. New York: Robert Carter and Brothers, 1859.

Gruetter, Thomas. *Johannes von Müllers Begegnung mit England. Ein Beitrag zur Geschichte der Anglophilie im späten 18. Jahrhundert*. Basel: Verlag von Helbing & Lichtenhahn, 1967.

Gruppe, [Paullus] Otto. *Geschichte der klassischen Mythologie und Religionsgeschichte während des Mittelalters im Abendland und während der Neuzeit*. Leipzig: Verlag und druck von B. G. Teubner, 1921.

Guardian Society for the Preservation of Public Morals. *Eighth Report of the Committee*. London: Printed for the Society by A. D. White, 1827.

Gurden-Williams. Celyn. "Lady Llanover and the Creation of a Welsh Cultural Utopia." PhD dissertation, Cardiff University, 2008.

Hack Tuke, Daniel. *Chapters in the History of the Insane in the British Isles*. London: Kegan Paul, Trench, 1882.

———. *A Dictionary of Psychological Medicine*. 2 vols. London: J. & A. Churchill, 1892.

———. *Prichard and Symonds in Especial Relation to Mental Science with Chapters on Moral Insanity*. London: J. & A. Churchill, 1891.

"Hair of Different Races of Men." *Transactions of the American Medical Association* 3 (1850): 61–62.

Hake, Gordon. *Memoirs of Eighty Years*. London: Richard Bentley and Son, 1892.

Hall, Robert. *The Works of Robert Hall, A.M.* Edited and with a memoir by Olinthus Gilbert Gregory. 6 vols. London: Holdsworth and Ball, 1832.

Hall, Thomas Steele. *Ideas of Life and Matter: Studies in the History of General Physiology, 600 B.C.–1900 A.D.* 2 vols. Chicago: University of Chicago Press, 1969.

Hancock, Thomas. *Essay on Instinct, and Its Physical and Moral Relations*. London: William Phillips, 1824.

———. *The Laws and Progress of the Epidemic Cholera, Illustrated by Facts and Observations*. London: Hamilton, Adams, 1832.

———. *Researches into the Laws and Phenomena of Pestilence; Including a Medical Sketch and Review of the Plague of London, in 1665; and Remarks on Quarantine*. London: William Phillips, 1821.

Hanifi, M. Jamil. "Mountstuart Elphinstone: An Anthropologist before Anthropology." In *Mountstuart Elphinstone in South Asia: Pioneer of British Colonial Rule*, edited by Shah Mahmoud Hanifi. Oxford: Oxford University Press, 2019. https://doi.org/10.1093/oso/9780190914400.003.0003.

Hapgood, Kathleen. *The Friends to Literature: Bristol Library Society, 1772–1894*. Bristol: Printed by David Harrison for ALHA, 2011.

Hardcastle, Mary Scarlett Campbell. *Life of John, Lord Campbell Lord High Chancellor of Great Britain; Consisting of a Selection from His Autobiography, Diary, and Letters*. Jersey City: Frederick D. Linn, 1881.

Hardiman, Sue. *The 1832 Cholera Epidemic and Its Impact on the City of Bristol*. Bristol: Malago Press, 2005.

Hare, Augustus J. C. *The Life and Letters of Maria Edgeworth*. Vol. 1. New York: Houghton, Mifflin, 1895.

[Harris, George?]. "The Plea of Insanity in Criminal Cases. The Criminality of the Insane." *British and Foreign Review; or, European Quarterly Journal* 15, no. 29 (1843): 152–69.

Harrison, Brian. "Drink and Sobriety in England, 1815–1872: A Critical Bibliography." *International Review of Social History* 12, no. 2 (1967): 204–76.

Harrison, Mark. "'To Raise and Dare Resentment': The Bristol Bridge Riot of 1793 Re-examined." *Historical Journal* 26, no. 3 (September 1983): 557–85.

Hawson, G. "Robert Pope, M.D." *Baptist Magazine* 20, no. 4 (April 1828): 172–73.

Hayward, Arthur Ralph. "Murder and Madness: A Social History of the Insanity Defence in Mid-Victorian England." PhD dissertation, University of Oxford, 1982.

Heartfield, James. *The Aborigines' Protection Society: Humanitarian Imperialism in Australia, New Zealand, Fiji, Canada, South Africa, and the Congo, 1836–1909*. London: Hurst, 2011.

Heinrich, C. B. "Kritische Abhandlung über die von Prichard als moral insanity geschilderte Krankheitsform." *Allgemeine zeitschrift für psychiatrie und psychisch-gerichtliche medicin* 5 (1848): 501–39.

Henderson, A. S. "Epidemiology of Alzheimer's Disease." *British Medical Bulletin* 42, no. 1 (1986): 3–10.

Henze, Brent. "Scientific Definition in Rhetorical Formations: Race as 'Permanent Variety' in James Cowles Prichard's Ethnology." *Rhetoric Review* 23, no. 4 (2004): 311–31.

Hersart de la Villemarqué, Théodore Claude Henri. *La villemarqué: Sa vie et ses oeuvres*. Paris: Librairie ancienne, 1926.

Hervey, Nicholas Bethell. "Advocacy or Folly: The Alleged Lunatics' Friend Society, 1845–1863." *Medical History* 30 (July 1986): 245–75.

———. "The Lunacy Commission 1845–60, with Special Reference to the Implementation of Policy in Kent and Surrey." Vol. 1. PhD dissertation, University of Bristol, 1987.

Heusinger, [Karl Friedrich]. "Anthropologie, London: *Researches into the Physical History of Mankind*, by James Cowles Prichard." *Allgemeine literatur-zeitung*. Ergänzungsblätter 4 (March 1830): col. 228–32, 233–36.

Hickey, John Edward. *History of the Old Chapel Sunday School, Dukinfield, 1800–1950*. Dukinfield: Sydney H. Cliffe, 1950. https://www.unitarian.org.uk/pages/history.

"History of the Firm John and Arthur Arch, of Cornhill." *Bookseller: A Newspaper of the British and Foreign Literature* (June 1873): 455.

Hobhouse, John Cam. *Recollections of a Long Life with Additional Extracts from His Private Diaries*. Edited by Charlotte (Hobhouse) Carleton, Lady Dorchester. Vol. 1. London: John Murray, 1909–11.

Hodgen, Margaret Trabue. "Anthropology in the BAAS, Its Inception." *Scientia: Rivista di Scienza* 108 (September–December 1973): 803–11.

Hodgkin, [Thomas]. "Obituary of Dr. Prichard: Read before the Ethnological Society, 28 February 1849." *Journal of the Ethnological Society of London* 2 (1850): 182–207.

Hodgkin, Thomas. "On the Importance of Studying and Preserving the Languages Spoken by Uncivilised Nations, with the View of Elucidating the Physical History of Man." *London and Edinburgh Philosophical Magazine and Journal of Science*, 3rd ser., 7 (July–August 1835): 27–36, 94–106.

———. *On the Importance of Studying and Preserving the Languages Spoken by Uncivilized Nations, with the View of Elucidating the Physical History of Man*. London: Richard Taylor, 1835.

Hodgson, William. *The Society of Friends in the Nineteenth Century: A Historical View of the Successive Convulsions and Schisms Therein during That Period*. Vol. 1. Philadelphia: Smith, English & Co.; the Author, 1876.

Hoffbauer, Johann Christoph. *Die psychologie in ihren hauptanwendungen auf die rechtspflege nach den allgemeinen gesichtspunkten der gesetzgebung*. Halle: Schimmelpfennig, 1808.

Hole, Charles. *The Early History of the Church Missionary Society for Africa and the East*. London: Church Missionary Society, 1896.

[Holland, Henry]. "Natural History of Man." *Quarterly Review* 86 (December 1849): 1–40.

———. *Recollections of Past Life*. 4th ed. London: Longmans, Green, 1873.

Homo. "XL. On Jameson's *Preface* to Cuvier's *Theory of the Earth*." *Philosophical Magazine and Journal* 46, no. 209 (September 1815): 225–29. https://doi.org/10.1080/14786441508638526.

Hooper, Robert. *Lexicon Medicum; or Medical Dictionary: Containing an Explanation of the Terms in anatomy, botany, chemistry, materia medica, midwifery, mineralogy, pharmacy, physiology, practice of physic, surgery, and the various branches of natural philosophy connected with medicine*. 7th ed. London: Longmans, Orme, and Col, 1839.

[Hope, Matthew Boyd]. "On the Diversity of Origin of the Human Races." *Biblical Repertory and Princeton Review* 22 (October 1850): 603–42.

Horn, D. B. *A Short History of the University of Edinburgh, 1556–1889*. Edinburgh: Edinburgh University Press, 1967.

Horsman, Reginald. "Origins of Racial Anglo-Saxonism in Great Britain before 1850." *Journal of the History of Ideas* 37 (July–September 1976): 387–410.

Hosack, [David]. "Memoir of the Life and Writings of the Late Colin Chisholm M.D., F.R.S. & Formerly Inspector General of Ordnance Hospitals in the West Indies." *American Journal of the Medical Sciences* 4 (August 1829): 394–402.

House of Commons Report from the Select Committee on Aborigines (British Settlements); Together with the Minutes of Evidence, Appendix and Index. London: Ordered by the House of Commons to Be Printed, 1836, 1837.

Hudson, Nicholas. "From Nation to 'Race': The Origin of Racial Classification in Eighteenth-Century Thought." *Eighteenth-Century Studies* 29, no. 3 (1996).

Hughes, C. H. "Moral (Affective) Insanity-Psycho-Sensory Insanity." *Alienist and Neurologist* 5 (April 1884): 297–314.

Huie, Richard. *Harveian Oration for MDCCCXXIX; Being a Tribute of Respect for the Memory of the Late Andrew Duncan Sen. M.D. Professor of the Institutions of Medicine in the University of Edinburgh*. Edinburgh: Printed for the Society by P. Neill, 1829.

Humboldt, Friedrich Alex Wilhelm Heinrich von. *Kosmos: A General Survey of the Physical Phenomena of the Universe*. Translated by J. P. T. and Augustin Prichard. 2 vols. London: Hippolyte Baillière, 1845–48.

Hunter, Richard, and Ida Macalpine. *Three Hundred Years of Psychiatry, 1535–1860: A History Presented in Selected English Texts*. London: Oxford University Press, 1963.

Hunter, Richard A. "Status Epilepticus: History, Incidence and Problems." *Epilepsia: Journal of the International League Against Epilepsy* 4 (December 1959): 162–88.

Hy., W. Review of Prichard's Vital Principle. *Göttingische gelehrte Anzeigen* 3 (December 1831): 1985–96.

Inkster, Ian. "The Public Lecture as an Instrument of Science Education for Adults: The Case of Great Britain, c. 1750–1850." *Paedagogica Historica: International Journal of the History of Education* 20 (1980): 80–107.

Institut de France, Académie des Sciences Morales et Politiques. *Notices biographiques et bibliographiques*. Paris: Distribué par la Librairie d'Argences, 1960.

"Interlineal Translations." *Gentleman's Magazine* 97, pt. 1 (May 1827): 445.

Irvine, William. *Walter Bagehot*. London: Longmans, Green, 1939.

J. Review and Notice of Twenty-Four Works on Fever. *Magazin der ausländischen literatur der gesammten heilkunde und arbeiten des ärztlichen vereins zu Hamburg* 1 (January–February 1821): 189; 3 (January–June 1822): 377–96.

Jablonski, Paul Ernst. *Pantheon Aegyptiorum, sive De Diis eorum commentarius, cum prolegomenis de religione et theologia Aegyptiorum*. Francofurti: Scumptibul Ioan. Christ. Kleyb, 1750.

James, William. "Memoir of John Bishop Estlin, Esq., F.L.S., F.R.C.S." *Christian Reformer*, n.s., 11 (August 1855): 461–81.

Jansson, Åsa. *From Melancholia to Depression: Disordered Mood in Nineteenth-Century Psychiatry*. Cham: Springer International, 2020.

"J. C. Prichard's *Treatise on Diseases of the Nervous System*." *Magazin der ausländischen literatur der gesammten heilkunde* 3 (May and June 1823): 524.

Jenkins, Bill. "Phrenology, Heredity and Progress in George Combe's Constitution of Man." *British Journal of the History of Science* 48 (September 2015): 455–73.

Jenkinson, Jacqueline. "Medical Societies and the Scottish Enlightenment." In *Association and Enlightenment: Scottish Clubs and Societies, 1700–1830*, edited by Mark C. Wallace and Jane Rendall, 69–84. New York: Bucknell University Press, 2020.

———. "The Role of Medical Societies in the Rise of the Scottish Medical Profession, 1730–1939." *Social History of Medicine* 4 (1991): 253–75.

Jewson, N. D. "Medical Knowledge and the Patronage System in 18th Century England." *Sociology: Journal of the British Sociological Association* 8 (September 1974): 369–85.

John Birch (1745?–1815). *Gentleman's Magazine and Historical Chronicle* 86 (1816): 189.
John Hudson (1773–1843). *Gentleman's Magazine*, n.s., 20 (December 1843): 662.
"John Playfair." MacTutor. 2018. https://mathshistory.st-andrews.ac.uk/Biographies/Playfair/.
Johnson, J. *A Guide for Gentlemen Studying Medicine at the University of Edinburgh*. London: Printed for G. G. J. and J. Robinson, 1792.
Johnson, James. *An Address to the Inhabitants of Bristol, on the Subject of the Poor-Rates, with a View to their Reduction, and the Ameliorating the Present Condition of our Poor*. Bristol: Printed and Sold by Browne & Manchee, 1820.
——— . *Transactions of the Corporation of the Poor, in the City of Bristol, during a Period of 126 Years*. Bristol: Printed and Sold by P. Rose, 1826.
Jones, D. W. "Moral Insanity and Psychological Disorder: The Hybrid Roots of Psychiatry." *History of Psychiatry* 28, no. 3 (2017): 263–79.
Jones, Marian Henry. "The Letters of Arthur James Johnes, 1809–71." *National Library of Wales Journal* 10, no. 3 (1958): 233–64.
Jones, Mary Jeanne A., and Chalmers L. Gemmill. "The Notebook of Robley Dunglison, Student of Clinical Medicine in Edinburgh, 1815–1816." *Journal of the History of Medicine and Allied Sciences* 22 (1967): 261–73.
Jones, M. G. *Hannah More*. Cambridge: Cambridge University Press, 1952.
Jones, Peter. *Life and Journals of Kah-ke-wa-quo-ma-by (Rev. Peter Jones), Wesleyan Missionary*. Toronto: Anson Green, 1860.
Jones, Philip D. "The Bristol Bridge Riot and Its Antecedents: Eighteenth-Century Perception of the Crowd." *Journal of British Studies* 19, no. 2 (1980): 74–92.
Kames, Henry Home. *Sketches of the History of Man*. Edinburgh: W. Creech; W. Strahan and T. Cadell, 1774.
Kass, Amalie M., and Edward H. Kass. *Perfecting the World: The Life and Times of Dr. Thomas Hodgkin, 1798–1866*. Boston: Harcourt Brace Jovanovich, 1988.
Kaufman, Matthew H. *Edinburgh Phrenological Society: A History*. Edinburgh: William Ramsay Henderson Trust, 2005.
——— . *Medical Teaching in Edinburgh during the 18th and 19th Centuries*. Edinburgh: Royal College of Surgeons of Edinburgh, 2003.
Kaufman, Paul. "John Peace to William Wordsworth: Four Unpublished Letters." *English Language Notes* 11, Supplement (1974): 193–99.
Keel, Terence. "Blumenbach's Race Science in the Light of Christian Supersessionism." In *Johann Friedrich Blumenbach: Race and Natural History, 1750–1850*, edited by Nicolaas Rupke and Gerhard Lauer, 123–41. Milton: Taylor & Francis, 2018.
Keith, Arthur. *An Autobiography*. London: Watts, 1950.
Kendler, Kenneth S. "Philippe Pinel and the Foundations of Modern Psychiatric Nosology." *Psychological Medicine* 50, no. 16 (2020): 2667–72.
Kenyon, John. *The History Men: The Historical Profession in England since the Renaissance*. London: Weidenfeld and Nicolson, 1983.
Kerslake, Thomas. *T. Kerslake's Catalogue of Books Including a Portion of the Library of the Learned James Cowles Prichard Esq. M.D. &c Author of the Physical*

History of Man . . . and also that of Dr. Edward Jenner. Bristol: Printed and published by Thomas Kerslake, [November 1854].

Kidd, Colin. *The Forging of Races: Race and Scripture in the Protestant Atlantic World, 1600-2000*. Cambridge: Cambridge University Press, 2006.

King, Richard. *Address to the Ethnological Society of London, Delivered at the Anniversary Meeting on the 25th May, 1844*. London: Printed by W. Watts, 1844.

———. "Address to the Ethnological Society of London, Delivered at the Anniversary, 25 May 1844." *Journal of the Ethnological Society of London* 1 (1848).

[———]. *Ethnological Society Prospectus*. [London]: R. Watts, Printer, [1842].

Knight, D. M. "The Vital Flame." *Ambix* 23 (March 1976).

Knox, Robert. *The Races of Men: A Fragment*. London: Henry Renshaw, 1850.

Kofoid, Charles A. "An American Pioneer in Science: Dr. William Charles Wells, 1757-1817." *Scientific Monthly* 57 (1943): 77-80.

Kramer, Gustav. *Carl Ritter: Ein Lebensbild nach seinem handschriftlichen Nachlass*. Vol. 2. Halle: Verlag der Buchhandlung des Waisenhauses, 1864-70.

Kuhn, Franz Felix Adalbert. Review of *The Eastern Origin of the Celtic Nations*. *Jahrbücher für wissenschaftliche Kritik* 1 (April 1840): cols. 581-98.

L. A. Review of *Naturgeschichte des menschengeschlechts*. *Gazette médicale de Paris*, 2nd ser., 9 (January 1841): 62-64.

Laidlaw, Zoë. *Protecting the Empire's Humanity: Thomas Hodgkin and British Colonial Activism, 1830-1870*. Cambridge: Cambridge University Press, 2021.

Lamarck, Jean Baptiste Pierre Antoine de Monet de. *La philosophie zoologique exposition des considerations relative a l'histoire naturelle des animaux*. Vol. 1. Paris: Denty et L'Auteur, 1809.

Lamoine, G. *Literature and Politics in Bristol (1789-1800)*. Extrait des Actes du congrès de Nantes (1974). Études Anglaises no. 66. Paris: Didier, 1977.

Lanska, D. J., and J. T. Lanska. "Franz Anton Mesmer and the Rise and Fall of Animal Magnetism: Dramatic Cures, Controversy, and Ultimately a Triumph for the Scientific Method." In *Brain, Mind and Medicine: Essays in Eighteenth-Century Neuroscience*, edited by H. Whitaker, C. U. M. Smith, and S. Finger, 301-20. Boston: Springer, 2007.

Large, David. *Radicalism in Bristol in the Nineteenth Century*. Bristol: Bristol Record Society, 1981.

"The Late Professor Christison." *Edinburgh Magazine, and Literary Miscellany* 7 (August 1820): 186-87.

Latham, R. G., and Edward Forbes. *The Natural History Department of the Crystal Palace Described*. London: Crystal Palace Library and Bradbury & Evans, 1854.

Latimer, John. *The Annals of Bristol in the Nineteenth Century*. Bristol: W. and F. Morgan, 1887.

Lawrence, Christopher. "The Edinburgh Medical School and the End of the 'Old Thing,' 1790-1830." In *History of Universities*, vol. 7, 259-86. Oxford: Oxford University Press, 1988.

Lawrence, S. C. "Entrepreneurs and Private Enterprise: The Development of Medical Lecturing in London, 1775-1820." *Bulletin of the History of Medicine* 62, no. 2 (Summer 1988): 171-92.

Lawrence, Susan C. "'Desirous of Improvements in Medicine': Pupils and Practitioners in the Medical Societies at Guy's and St. Bartholomew's Hospitals, 1795–1815." *Bulletin of the History of Medicine* 59 (1985): 89–104.
Lawrence, William. *Lectures on Physiology, Zoology, and the Natural History of Man: Delivered at the Royal College of Surgeons.* London: J. Callow, 1819.
Lefmann, Salomon. *Franz Bopp, sein Leben und seine Wissenschaft.* Vol. 2. Berlin: Druck und Verlag von Georg Reimer, 1891–97.
Leidesdorf, Max. "Sandon und die folie affective, morale der Franzosen oder die moral insanity Prichard's." *Wiener Medizinische Wochenschrift* 15 (August 1865): 1185–89.
[Lennox, William Pitt]. *Three Years with the Duke of Wellington in Private Life.* London: Saunders and Otley, 1853.
Leopold, Joan. *Culture in Comparative and Evolutionary Perspective: E. B. Tylor and the Making of Primitive Culture.* Berlin: Dietrich Reimer, 1980.
Lester, Alan. "Settler Colonialism, George Grey and the Politics of Ethnography." *Environment and Planning D: Society and Space* 34, no. 3 (2016): 492–507.
Lester, Alan, and Fae Dussart. *Colonization and the Origins of Humanitarian Governance: Protecting Aborigines across the Nineteenth-Century British Empire.* Cambridge: Cambridge University Press, 2014.
Leupoldt, Johann Michael. *Lehrbuch der psychiatrie.* Leipzig: Verlag von Leopold Voss, 1837.
Lewinstein, Stephen R. "The Historical Development of Insanity as a Defense in Criminal Actions." *Journal of Forensic Sciences* 14, no. 3 (July 1969): 275–93, 469–500.
"The Library of the Bristol Medico-Chirurgical Society Fortieth List of Books." *Bristol Medico-Chirurgical Journal* 19, no. 72 (June 1901): 183–87.
"The Library of the Bristol Medico-Chirurgical Society Twenty-Eighth List of Books." *Bristol Medico-Chirurgical Journal* 16, no. 60 (June 1898): 186–93.
Lightman, Bernard. "Introduction." In *A Companion to the History of Science,* edited by Bernard Lightman, 30–35. Hoboken: John Wiley & Sons, 2016.
———. *Victorian Popularizers of Science: Designing Nature for New Audiences.* Chicago: University of Chicago Press, 2007.
"Liste des membres de la Société." *Mémoires de la Société Ethnologique de Paris* 1 (1841): xx–xxi.
[Lister, William]. Obituary of William Charles Wells. *Gentleman's Magazine and Historical Chronicle* 87 (1817): 467–71.
List of Members of the British Association for the Advancement of Science, Not Residing in Bristol; Enrolled at Bristol, August, 1836. Bristol: Printed by J. Chilcott, 1836.
List of Officers, Members of the Provincial Medical and Surgical Association. *Transactions of the Provincial Medical and Surgical Association* 1 (1833): [iv–xviii].
"Literary and Scientific Intelligence." *Gentleman's Magazine,* n.s., 4 (July 1835): 74.
Living, Edward. *Bristol's Gas Supply, 1811–1923.* Bristol: Bristol Gas Company, 1923.

"Living Authors, Natives of Bristol, or Residing in That City and Its Vicinity [Continued]." *Bristol Memorialist*, issues published 1816–23, compiled in a single volume. Bristol: William Tyson, 1823.

Livingstone, David N. *Adam's Ancestors: Race, Religion, and the Politics of Human Origins*. Baltimore: Johns Hopkins University Press, 2008.

———. *The Preadamite Theory and the Marriage of Science and Religion*. Transactions of the American Philosophical Society 82. Philadelphia: American Philosophical Society, 1992.

"Lodging Houses." *Cheilead, or University Coterie* 1 (1826): 70.

London Friends' Institute. *Biographical Catalogue: Being an Account of the Lives of Friends*. London: Friends' Institute, 1888.

Long, Edward. *The History of Jamaica; or, General Survey of the Antient and Modern State of that Island: with Reflections on its Situation, Settlements, Inhabitants, Climate, Products, Commerce, Laws, and Government*. London: T. Lowndes, 1774.

"Lord Grenville." *Literary Panorama and Annual Register* 8 (August 1810): 708–12.

Loudon, Irvine. *Medical Care and the General Practitioner, 1750–1850*. Oxford: Clarendon Press, 1986.

Loudon, I. S. L. "The Origins and Growth of the Dispensary Movement in England." *Bulletin of the History of Medicine* 55 (September 1982): 322–42.

Mackenzie, Charles. "Analysis of Compact Feldspar from Pentland Hills." *Memoirs of the Wernerian Natural History Society* 1 (1808–10): 616–19.

———. *Notes on Haiti, Made during a Residence in That Republic*. Vol. 1. London: Henry Colburn and Richard Bentley, 1830.

MacKenzie, Charlotte. "A Family Asylum: A History of the Private Madhouse at Ticehurst in Sussex, 1792–1917." PhD dissertation, University College, London, 1986.

Mackenzie, Patrick. *Practical Observations on the Medical Powers of the Most Celebrated Mineral Waters and of the Various Modes of Bathing, Intended for the Use of Invalids*. London: Printed for Burgess and Hill, 1819; 2nd ed., enlarged, 1820.

Mackinnon, Donald. *University of Edinburgh, Celtic Chair: Inaugural Address*. Edinburgh: Maclachlan & Stewart, 1883.

Malpass, Peter. *The Bristol Dock Company*. [Bristol]: Printed for Avon Local History & Archaeology, 2010.

Mann, Edward C. A. *Manual of Psychological Medicine and Allied Nervous Diseases*. London: J. & A. Churchill, 1883.

Marino, Mario. "At the Roots of Racial Classification: Theory and Iconography in the Work and Legacy of Johann Friedrich Blumenbach." *Bérose—Encyclopédie internationale des histoires de l'anthropologie*. https://www.bcrose.fr/.

Markham, W. O. *Bleeding and Change in Type of Diseases: Being the Gulstonian Lectures for 1864*. London: John Churchill & Sons, 1866.

Marmion, V. J. *The Bristol Eye Hospital: A Monograph*. Bristol: JCL Graphics, 1986.

Marshall, Peter. *The Anti-Slave Trade Movement in Bristol*. Bristol Branch of the Historical Association. Dursley, Gloucestershire: Printed by F. Bailey and Son, 1968.

Martin, Mary E. *Memories of Seventy Years, by One of a Literary Family.* London: Griffith & Farran, 1884.
Martineau, Harriet. *How to Observe: Morals and Manners.* New York: Harper and Brothers, 1838.
Mason, Tom. *The Story of Southgate and Other Local Essays.* 2nd ed. Enfield: Meyers Brooks, 1948.
Mathews's Annual Bristol Directory. Bristol: Printed and Sold by M. Mathew and Son, 1832.
Matthews's New Bristol Directory, for the Year 1793-4. Bristol: Printed and Sold by William Matthews, [1793].
May, Samuel Joseph. *Memoir of Samuel Joseph May.* Boston: Roberts Brothers, 1873.
Mayhew, Henry. *London Labour and the London Poor: A Cyclopaedia of the Condition and Earnings of Those That Will Work, Those That Cannot Work, and Those That Will Not Work.* Vol. 1. London: Office, 1851.
McCallum, David. *Personality and Dangerousness: Genealogies of Antisocial Personality Disorder.* Cambridge: Cambridge University Press, 2001.
McCandless, Peter. "Dangerous to Themselves and Others: The Victorian Debate over the Prevention of Wrongful Confinement." *Journal of British Studies* 23 (Fall 1983): 84-104.
McCartney, Paul. "Facts, Opinions, and Possibilities: Melville's Treatment of Insanity through 'White-Jacket.'" *Studies in the Novel* 16 (Summer 1984): 167-81.
McDade, Katie. "'A Particular Spirit of Enterprise': Bristol and Liverpool Slave Trade Merchants as Entrepreneurs in the Eighteenth Century." PhD dissertation, University of Nottingham, 2011.
McIntyre, Silvia. "The Mineral Water Trade in the Eighteenth Century." *Journal of Transport History* 2, no. 1 (February 1973): 1-19.
McKenzie, Isabel. "Social Activities of the English Friends in the First Half of the Nineteenth Century." PhD dissertation, Columbia University, 1935.
McLean, David. *Public Health and Politics in the Age of Reform: Cholera, the State and the Royal Navy in Victorian Britain.* London: I. B. Tauris, 2005.
McMenemey, William Henry. *The Life and Times of Sir Charles Hastings, Founder of the British Medical Association.* Edinburgh: E. & S. Livingstone, 1959.
"Medical Education in 18th Century Hospitals." *Scottish Society of the History of Medicine: Report of the Proceedings* (Session 1969-70): 27-46.
Medical Reading Society. *Rules of the Medical Reading Society, 1820.* Bristol: Printed by J. Norton, 1820.
"Meeting of Sub-section D—Ethnology at the British Association at Oxford, July 26-30, 1847." *Athenaeum Journal of Literature, Science, and the Fine Arts* (July 17, 1847): 773.
Mellett, D. J. "Bureaucracy and Mental Illness: The Commissioners in Lunacy 1845-1890." *Medical History* 25 (1981): 221-50.
Mellor, Penny, and Mary Wright. *Kingsdown: Bristol's Vertical Suburb.* Chichester, UK: Phillimore, 2009.
A Member of the Royal College of Surgeons. *An Address to the Shareholders of the Intended New College.* Bristol: Printed by John Wansbrough, 1829.

Metropolitan Commissioners in Lunacy. "An Account of All Monies received for Licenses, and of all Monies received and paid out . . . the Metropolitan Commissioners in Lunacy, from the 1st August 1844 to the 4th August 1845." In House of Commons, *Accounts and Papers*, vol. 33, 457–58. [London]: Ordered by the House of Commons to Be Printed, 1846.

———. *Report of the Metropolitan Commissioners in Lunacy to the Lord Chancellor.* Presented to both Houses of Parliament by command of Her Majesty. London: Bradbury and Evans, Printers, 1844.

Meyer, Karl. "Celtische sprachen." Review of *Eastern Origin of the Celtic Nations* and Other Works. *Jahrbücher der Literatur* 104 (October–December 1843): 28–69.

Michael, John S. "Nuance Lost in Translation: Interpretations of J. F. Blumenbach's Anthropology in the English Speaking World." *NTM International Journal of History & Ethics of Natural Sciences Technology & Medicine* 25, no. 3 (July 2017): 281–309.

Michie, Archibald. *A Challenge to Phrenologists; or, Phrenology Tested by Reason and Facts.* London: James S. Hodson, 1839.

[Millard, Simeon Warner]. "T. W. Dyer, M.D." *Gentleman's Magazine* 103, pt. 2, no. 3 (September 1833): 278.

Minchinton, W. E. "Bristol—Metropolis of the West in the Eighteenth Century." *Transactions of the Royal Historical Society* 4 (1954): 69–89.

———. *The British Tinplate Industry: A History.* Oxford: Clarendon, 1957.

M'Lauchlan, Thomas. *Celtic Gleanings; or, Notices of the History and Literature of the Scottish Gael, in Four Lectures.* Edinburgh: Maclachlan and Stewart, 1857.

Monboddo, Lord James Burnett. *Of the Origin and Progress of Language.* Edinburgh: J. Balfour, 1774.

Moore, James, and Adrian Desmond. "Introduction." In Charles Darwin, *The Descent of Man, and Selection in Relation to Sex*, xi–lviii. London: Penguin, 2004.

Moore, Thomas. *The Journal of Thomas Moore.* Vol. 5, *1836–42.* Newark: University of Delaware Press, 1988.

Moorhead, Robert. "William Budd and Typhoid Fever." *Journal of the Royal Society of Medicine* 95 (2002): 561–64.

Mora, George. "History of Psychiatry." In *Comprehensive Textbook of Psychiatry*, edited by Alfred M. Freedman, Harold I. Kaplan, and Benjamin J. Sadock, 2–34. Baltimore: Williams & Wilkins, 1967.

Morgan, Bayard Quincy. *A Critical Bibliography of German Literature in English Translation, 1481–1927.* 2nd ed. Stanford: Stanford University Press, 1938.

Morgan, Kenneth. "The Economic Development of Bristol, 1700–1850." In *The Making of Modern Bristol*, edited by Madge Dresser and Philip Ollerenshaw. Tiverton: Redcliffe Press, 1996.

[Morgan, Susanna]. *An Appeal to the Good Sense and Humanity of the Inhabitants of Bristol & Clifton, on the Expediency of Forming an Institution for the Cure and Prevention of Contagious Fever.* Bristol: Printed by Browne and Manchee, 1819.

———. *Hints towards the Formation of a Society, for Promoting a Spirit of Independence among the Poor.* 2nd ed. Bristol: Printed by E. Bryan, [1812].

Morrell, J. B. "Individualism and the Structure of British Science in 1830." *Historical Studies in the Physical Sciences* 3 (1971): 183–204.

———. "Medicine and Science in the Eighteenth Century." In *Four Centuries: Edinburgh University Life, 1583–1983*, edited by Gordon Donaldson, 38–52. Edinburgh: Edinburgh University Press, 1983.

———. "Practical Chemistry in the University of Edinburgh, 1799–1843." *Ambix* 16 (1969): 66–80.

———. "The University of Edinburgh and Academic Structure." *Isis: An International Review Devoted to the History of Science and its Cultural Influences* 62 (1971): 158–71.

Morris, R. J. *Class, Sect and Party: The Making of the British Middle Class, Leeds, 1820–1850*. Manchester: Manchester University Press, 1990.

Mortimer, Russell S. "Quaker Printers, 1750–1850: Presidential Address to the Friends' Historical Society." *Journal of the Friends; Historical Society* 50 (1963): 100–133.

Morton, Samuel George. *Crania Americana; or, A Comparative View of the Skulls of Various Aboriginal Nations of North and South America: To Which Is Prefixed an Essay on the Varieties of the Human Species*. Philadelphia: J. Dobson; London: Simpkin, Marshall, 1839.

"The Mosaic Account of the Unity of the Human Race, Confirmed by the Natural History of the American Aborigines." *American Biblical Repository*, 2nd ser., 10 (July 1843): 29–80.

"Mr. John Peace [1785–1861], of Bristol." *Gentleman's Magazine and Historical Review* 210 (1861): 577–78.

Mueller, Johannes von. *An Universal History, in Twenty-Four Books*. Translated from the German [by James Cowles Prichard and William Tothill]. 3 vols. London: Printed for Longman, Hurst, Rees, Orme, and Brown, 1818.

Müller, Friedrich Max. "Comparative Philology." *Edinburgh Review* 94 (October 1851): 297–339.

———. *My Autobiography: A Fragment*. New York: Charles Scribner's Sons, 1901.

Munby, A. N. L. *The Formation of the Phillipps Library from 1841 to 1872*. Cambridge: University Press, 1956.

Munk, William. *The Roll of the Royal College of Physicians of London: Comprising Biographical Sketches of all the eminent physicians whose names are recorded in the Annals, from the foundation of the college in 1518 to its removal in 1825*. Vol. 2. London: Published by the College, 1878.

Munro Smith, G. *A History of the Bristol Royal Infirmary*. Bristol: J. W. Arrowsmith, 1917.

———. "Notes on Some Bristol Medical Societies." *Bristol Medico-Chirurgical Journal* 32 (December 1913): 268–86.

Neale, A. V. *Medical Progress in Bristol: The Long Fox Memorial Lecture, 1963*. Bristol: John Wright & Sons, 1964.

Neve, Michael. "Science in a Commercial City: Bristol, 1820–60." In *Metropolis and Province: Science in British Culture, 1780–1850*, edited by Jack Morrell and Ian Inkster, 179–204. London: Taylor & Francis, 2007.

Neve, Michael Raymond. "Natural Philosophy, Medicine and the Culture of Science in Provincial England: The Case of Bristol, 1790–1850." PhD dissertation, University of London, 1985.
Niebyl, Peter H. "The English Bloodletting Revolution, or Modern Medicine before 1850." *Bulletin of the History of Medicine* 51 (Fall 1977): 464–83.
Niekerk, Carl. "Buffon, Blumenbach, Lichtenberg, and the Origins of Modern Anthropology." In *Johann Friedrich Blumenbach: Race and Natural History, 1750–1850*, edited by Nicolaas Rupke and Gerhard Lauer, 27–52. Milton: Taylor & Francis, 2018.
Notice of the Second Edition of *Researches into the Physical History of Mankind. Summarium des Neuesten aus der gesammten Medicin* 3, nos. 3 and 4 (1830): 554–55.
Notice of *Treatise on Diseases of the Nervous System. London Medical Repository* 17 (January 1822): 87.
"Notices of Works by Iltudus Prichard, Esq., Barrister-at-Law." *Journal of the East India Association* 7 (1873): 192–94.
Nott, Josiah C., and George R. Gliddon. *Types of Mankind: or, Ethnological Researches Based upon the Ancient Monuments, Paintings, Sculptures, and Crania of Races, and upon Their Natural, Geographical, Philological and Biblical History.* 7th ed. Philadelphia: J. B. Lippincott, Grambo, 1855.
Obey, Erica. *The Wunderkammer of Lady Charlotte Guest.* Bethlehem PA: Lehigh University Press, 2007.
"Obituary: John Addington Symonds, M.D., F.R.C.P., F.R.S.E., Vice-President of the British Medical Association." *British Medical Journal*, no. 1 (March 1871): 268.
Obituary of Colin Chisholm. *Gentleman's Magazine and Historical Chronicle* 95, pt. 1 (January–June 1825): 647–48.
Obituary of Dr. Alexander Tweedie. *Lancet* 1, no. 3172 (June 1884): 1101.
Obituary of Edward Rochemont Estlin. *Monthly Repository of Theology and General Literature* 20 (October 1825): 626–28.
Obituary of James Hamilton. *Gentleman's Magazine*, n.s., 5 (1836): 102.
Obituary of James Yates. *Proceedings of the Royal Society of London* 20 (November 1871–June 1872): i–iii.
Obituary of Richard Smith. *Gentleman's Magazine*, n.s., 19, no. 3 (March 1843): 323–25.
Obituary of Thomas Stock. *Gentleman's Magazine*, n.s., 10, no. 2 (August 1838): 215.
Obituary of T. J. Prichard. *Gentleman's Magazine*, n.s., 25 (April 1846): 444.
Odom, Herbert H. "James Cowles Prichard." In *Dictionary of Scientific Biography*, vol. 11, 136–38. New York: Charles Scribner's Sons, 1975.
"Officers of the American Oriental Society . . . Honorary Members of the Society to January, 1847." *Journal of the American Oriental Society* 1 (1851): x–xii.
Oldroyd, David Roger. *Darwinian Impacts: An Introduction to the Darwinian Revolution.* Milton Keynes: Open University Press, 1980.
"Oneness of the Human Race." *The Church*, n.s., 2 (May 1848): 125–26.
"On Sepulchral Remains of Ancient Nations Dispersed through the North of Europe." *Edinburgh New Philosophical Journal* 31 (October 1841): 378–82.

"On the Artificially Distorted Skulls of a Peruvian Race." *Phrenological Journal, and Magazine of Moral Science* 17 (October 1844): 342–45.

"On the Physical History of Mankind." *London Medical Repository*, 3rd ser., 4 (February 1827): 112–44.

Orange, Arthur Derek. "Idols of the Theatre: The British Association and its Early Critics." *Annals of Science* 32 (1975): 277–94.

———. "The Origins of the British Association for the Advancement of Science." *British Journal for the History of Science* 6 (1972): 152–76.

"Origin and Affinity of the Languages of Asia and Europe." *Asiatic Journal* 7 (January 1832).

"Origin and Antiquity of the Zodiac[, a review of three volumes by C.G.S., 1813]." *British Review, and London Critical Journal* 8 (November 1816): 359–87.

"Osservazione sulla paralisia; del sig. Prichard." *Annali universali di medicina* 33 (March 1825): 442–44.

Outline of the Plan of Education to Be Pursued in the Bristol College. Bristol: Printed for the Council by John Taylor, 1830.

Owen, Robert. *The Life of Robert Owen, Written by Himself: With Selections from His Writings and Correspondence.* Vol. 1. London: Effingham Wilson, 1857.

Oxonian. *Observations on Medical Reform by a Member of the University of Oxford.* Reprinted from *The Pamphleteer*, London, 1814.

Paley, William. *Natural Theology; or, Evidences of the Existence and Attributes of the Deity, Collected from the Appearances of Nature.* London: R. Faulder, 1802.

Palfreman, John. "Mesmerism and the English Medical Profession: A Study of a Conflict." *Ethics in Science & Medicine* 4 (1977): 51–66.

"Paralysis." *Medico-Chirurgical Review, and Journal of Medical Science* 4 (March 1824): 926–27.

[Parker, George]. *Schola Medicinae Bristol: Its History, Lecturers, and Alumni, 1833–1933.* Bristol: John Wright & Sons, 1933.

Parkinson, James. *The Hospital Pupil: or An Essay Intended to Facilitate the Study of Medicine and Surgery.* London: Printed for H. D. Symonds; Cox, Murray and Highley, Callow, and Boosey; Bell and Bradfute, 1800.

Parry-Jones, William Ll. *The Trade in Lunacy: A Study of Private Madhouses in England in the Eighteenth and Nineteenth Centuries.* Abingdon: Routledge, 2007.

Parsons, F. G. *The History of St. Thomas's Hospital.* Vol. 2. London: Methuen, 1932.

Parssinen, T. M. "Popular Science and Society: The Phrenology Movement in Early Victorian Britain." *Journal of Social History* 8 (Fall 1974): 1–20.

Part of the Evidence Given by J.H. Jerrard, D.C.L., before the House of Commons on the 28th and 29th of March 1836. 1842?

Pattison, Mark. *Memoirs.* London: Macmillan, 1885.

Payne, Joseph Frank. "John Birch (1745–1815)." In *Dictionary of National Biography*, vol. 5, edited by Leslie Stephen and Sidney Lee, 64–65. London: Elder Smith, 1886.

———. "William Babbington (1756–1833)." In *Dictionary of National Biography*, vol. 2, edited by Leslie Stephen and Sidney Lee, 314–15. London: Elder Smith, 1885.

[Peace, John]. *Axiomata Pacis*. With a preface containing a biographical sketch of the author. London: Longman, Green, Longman, and Roberts, 1862.

Peacock, Thomas Love. "Memoirs of Percy Bysshe Shelley." In *The Works of Thomas Love Peacock*, vol. 8. London: Constable, 1834.

Pellegrino, Edmund D. "The Sociocultural Impact of Twentieth-Century Therapeutics." In *The Therapeutic Revolution: Essays in the Social History of American Medicine*, edited by Morris J. Vogel and Charles E. Rosenberg, 245–66. Philadelphia: University of Pennsylvania Press, 1979.

Penn, Granville. *A Comparative Estimate of the Mineral and Mosaical Geologies*. 2nd ed. London: Printed for James Duncan, 1825.

Penn, Virginia. "Philhellenism in England (1821–1827)." *Slavonic (and East European) Review* 14 (January and April 1936): 363–71; 647–60.

Penny, John. *Up, Up and Away! An Account of Ballooning in and around Bristol and Bath, 1784–1999*. Bristol: Bristol Branch of the Historical Association, 1999.

Percival, Edward. *Practical Observations on the Treatment, Pathology, and Prevention of Typhous Fever*. Bath: Printed by Richard Cruttwell, 1819.

Perrin, Colin, and Kay Anderson. "Reframing Craniometry: Human Exceptionalism and the Production of Racial Knowledge." *Social Identities* 19, no. 1 (February 2013): 90–103.

Perry, C. Bruce. *The Bristol Royal Infirmary, 1904–1974*. Bristol: Portishead, 1981.

———. "British Hospitals, Their Early History and Development: The Bristol Royal Infirmary." *Medical Press and Circular* 203 (April 1940): 278–82.

———. *The Voluntary Medical Institutions of Bristol*. [Bristol]: Alan Sutton for the Bristol Branch of the Historical Association, 1984.

Perry, Henry. "Observations on Blood-Letting." *London Medical Repository, Monthly Journal, and Review* 17 (February 1822): 112–15.

Phillips, Howard Temple. "The Old Private Lunatic Asylum at Fishponds." *Bristol Medico-Chirurgical Journal* 85 (April 1970): 41–44.

"Physical History of Man." *British Quarterly Review* 1 (May 1845): 337–68.

Pickering, Mary Orne. *Life of John Pickering*. Boston: Printed for Private Distribution, 1887.

Pitschaft, J. A. "Miscellanen, rhapsodien und erfahrungen im gebiete der medicin." *Journal der practischen heilkunde* 77 (September 1833): 3–24.

Plarr's Lives of the Fellows of the Royal College of Surgeons of England. 2 vols. Bristol: John Wright & Sons, 1930.

"Poisoning at the Bristol Infirmary from Prussic Acid!!!" Reprinted from the *Bristol Mercury*. *Medical Times* 1 (December 1839): 109.

Pole, Thomas. *Prospectus of a Course of Lectures, including the General Oeconomy of Nature; to Be Delivered in the City of Bristol*. Bristol: J. Mills, 1802.

Pollok, Robert. *The Course of Time: A Poem, in Ten Books*. Edinburgh: William Blackwood, 1827.

Poole, Steve. "Documents in Focus: The Stogursey Rising of 1801." *Regional Historian: The Newsletter of the Regional History Centre at the University of the West of England, Bristol*, no. 9 (Summer 2002): 2–6.

———. "To Be a Bristolian: Civic Identity and the Social Order, 1750–1850." In *The Making of Modern Bristol*, edited by Madge Dresser and Philip Ollerenshaw, 76–95. Bristol: Redcliffe, 1996.
Poskett, James. *Horizons: A Global History of Science*. London: Viking, 2022.
———. *Materials of the Mind: Phrenology, Race, and the Global History of Science, 1815-1920*. Chicago: University of Chicago Press, 2019.
Post-Office Annual Directory, from Whitsunday 1807, to Whitsunday 1808. Edinburgh: Printed by Abernethy & Walker, 1807.
Pott, August Friedrich. *Etymologische forschungen auf dem Gebiete der Indo-Germanischen sprachen*. Vol. 2. Lengo: Verlage der Meyerschen Hofbuchhandlung, 1833–36.
Poulton, E. B. "A Remarkable Anticipation of Modern Views on Evolution." *Science Progress* 1 (1897): 278–96.
Powell, A. G. *Bristol Commercial Rooms*. Bristol: Printed by J. W. Arrowsmith, 1951.
Prichard, Arthur W. "Reminiscences of the Bristol Royal Infirmary." *Bristol Medico-Chirurgical Journal* 18 (September 1900): 193–203.
Prichard, Augustin. *Bristol Medical School*. Reprinted with additions from the *Bristol Medico-Chirurgical Journal*, 1892. Bristol: J. Arrowsmith, [1894].
———. "The Early History of the Bristol Medical School." *Bristol Medico-Chirurgical Journal* 10 (December 1892): 264–91.
———. *A Few Medical & Surgical Reminiscences*. Bristol: J. W. Arrowsmith, 1896.
[———]. Obituary of Crosby Leonard. *Bristol Royal Infirmary Reports* 1 (1878–79): 342–60.
———. "On the Crania of the Laplanders and Finlanders, with Observations on the Differences They Present from Other European Races." *Proceedings of the Zoological Society of London* 12 (1844): 129–35.
———. *Some Incidents in General Practice: Being a Second Series of Reminiscences*. Bristol: J. W. Arrowsmith, 1898.
Prichard, Edward. *Marriage with a Deceased Wife's Sister: A Reply to the Article upon the Subject in the 'Quarterly Review' for June, 1849: Together with a Short Statement of the Facts Bearing upon the Question*. London: E. Newman, 1849.
———. *Observations on the Changes in the Currency*. Ross: B. Powle, [1830].
———. *A Reply to the Chapter of Dr. Chalmers' Bridgewater Essay upon the "Affections which Conduce to the Economic Well-Being of Society"; Being upon the Subjects of Tithe, Poor-Law, and Political Economy*. London: W. Dinmore, 1834.
Prichard, [James Cowles]. "A Short Description of a Collection of Engraved Stones, Deposited by B. H. Bright, Esq. in the Museum of the Bristol Institution." *Friends' Monthly Magazine* 1 (October 1830): 687–91.
P[richard], J[ames] C[owles]. "Horae Africanae." *Friends' Monthly Magazine* 1 (August 1830): 477–82.
———. "Horae Africanae, No. 2.—History of the Guanches." *Friends' Monthly Magazine* 1 (November 1830): 737–43.
Prichard, James Cowles. "Abstract of a Comparative Review of Philological and Physical Researches, as Applied to the History of the Human Species." *Edinburgh New Philosophical Journal* 15, no. 30 (October 1833): 308–26.

———. "Abstract of a Comparative Review of Philological and Physical Researches as Applied to the History of the Human Species." *Report of the First and Second Meetings of the British Association for the Advancement of Science; at York in 1831, and at Oxford in 1832* 2 (1832): 529–44.

———. *The Address Delivered at the Third Anniversary Meeting of the Provincial Medical and Surgical Association, Held at Oxford, on Thursday, July 23rd, 1835*. London: Sherwood, Gilbert, and Piper; Worcester: Deighton, 1835.

———. "An Address Delivered at the Third Anniversary Meeting of the Provincial Medical and Surgical Association, July 23, 1835." *Transactions of the Provincial Medical and Surgical Association* 4 (1836): 1–54.

———. *An Analysis of the Egyptian Mythology, in which the Philosophy and the Superstitions of the Ancient Egyptians Are Compared with Those of the Indians and Other Nations of Antiquity; To Which Is Added a Translation of the Preliminary Essay Prefixed by A. W. von Schlegel to the German Edition of the Same Work by James Yates*. London: Sherwood, Gilbert, and Piper, 1838.

[———]. "An Analysis of the Egyptian Mythology, to Which Is Added, a Critical Examination of the Remains of Egyptian Chronology." *Classical Journal* 26 (September 1822): 89–100.

———. *An Analysis of the Egyptian Mythology: To Which Is Subjoined, a Critical Examination of the Remains of Egyptian Chronology*. London: Printed for John and Arthur Arch, 1819.

———. "Anniversary Address, for 1848, to the Ethnological Society of London, on the Recent Progress of Ethnology." *Edinburgh New Philosophical Journal* 45, no. 90 (October 1848): 336–46; and 46, no. 91 (January 1849): 53–72.

———. "Anniversary Address for 1848, to the Ethnological Society of London on the Recent Progress of Ethnology by the President." *Journal of the Ethnological Society of London* 2 (1850): 119–49.

———. *Appendix to First Edition of the Natural History of Man*. London: Hippolyte Baillière; Paris: J. B. Baillière; Leipsic: T. O. Weigel, 1845.

———. "A. Th. D'Abbadie and Aug. Chaho on the Euskarian Language." *Journal of the Geographical Society of London* 8 (1838): 397–400.

———. "Cases of Typhus Fever, with Observations on the Nature and Treatment of That Disease." *Edinburgh Medical and Surgical Journal* 13 (October 1817): 413–27.

[———]. "*The Character of Moses Established for Veracity as an Historian, recording Events subsequent to the Deluge*. By the Rev. Joseph Townsend, 1815, [and] *Mithridates oder allgemeine sprachenkunde. Mithradates; or a General History of Languages, with the Lord's Prayer as a specimen, in nearly five hundred Languages and Dialects*. By Johann Christoph Adelung, 1813." *British Review, and London Critical Journal* 6 (November 1815): 476–523.

[———]. "Chronology." *Westminster Review* 16 (April 1832): 327–41.

———. "A Clinical Lecture Delivered to the Pupils of the Bristol Infirmary." *London Medical Gazette; Being a Weekly Journal of Medicine and the Collateral Sciences* 27 (September 1840): 8–13.

———. *Darstellung der Ägyptischen Mythologie: verbunden mit einer kritischen Untersuchung der Überbleibsel der Ägyptischen Chronologie*. Übersetzt und mit Anmerkungen begleitet von L. Haymann; nebst einer vorrede von A. W. von Schlegel. Bonn: E. Weber, 1837.

———. "Delirium." In *The Cyclopaedia of Practical Medicine*, vol. 1, edited by Sir John Forbes, Alexander Tweedie, and John Conolly, 506–10. London: Sherwood, Gilbert, and Piper, 1833–35.

———. *Della Pazzia*. Extracted from the *Cyclopaedia of Practical Medicine* and translated from the English. Livorno: Fratelli Vignozzi e Nipote, 1839.

———. "Des essais de classification de en l'epèce humaine." *Revue l'encyclopédique* 58, no. 173 (June 1833): 383–405.

———. *Disputatio inauguralis de generis humani varietate . . . Eruditorum examini subjicit*. Edinburgh: Abernethy & Walker, 1808.

———. "Dr. Morton's 'Crania Americana.'" *Journal of the Royal Geographical Society of London* 10 (1841 [sic, 1840]): 552–61.

———. "Dr. Mueller on the Ural and Caucasus." *Journal of the Geographical Society of London* 8 (1838): 389–90.

———. "Dr. Prichard on the Use of Issues in Disorders of the Nervous System." *Monthly Journal of Medicine* 3 (March 1824): 176–78.

———. *The Eastern Origin of the Celtic Nations Proved by a Comparison of Their Dialects with the Sanskrit, Greek, Latin, and Teutonic Languages. Forming a Supplement to Researches into the Physical History of Mankind*. Oxford: Printed by S. Collingwood, Printer to the University; London: Sherwood, Gilbert, and Piper; J. and A. Arch, London, 1831. New edition with a supplementary chapter edited by Robert Gordon Latham, London: Houlston and Wright; Bernard Quaritch, 1857.

———. "Ethnographical Memoir on the Nations of Slavonian Race, Part 1." *West of England Journal of Science and Literature* 1, no. 1 (January 1835): 11–29.

———. "Ethnographical Memoir on the Nations of Slavonian Race, Part 2." *West of England Journal of Science and Literature* 1, no. 2 (April 1835): 48–62.

———. *Ethnography of the Celtic Race*. [Oxford]: n.p., [1840].

———. "Ethnology." In *A Manual of Scientific Enquiry Prepared for the Use of Her Majesty's Navy and Adapted for Travellers in General*, edited by John F. W. Herschel, 423–40. London: John Murray, 1849; 2nd ed., 1851; 3rd ed., revised by Thomas Wright and Marie Armand Pascal d'Avezac, 1859; 4th ed., revised by Edward Burnett Tylor, 1871.

———. *Ethnology*. Postprinted from *A Manual of Scientific Enquiry Prepared for the Use of Her Majesty's Navy and Adapted for Travellers in General*, edited by John F. W. Herschel, 1849. London: Printed by William Clowes and Sons, [1849].

———. "Evacuation of Fluid from the Thorax by Means of the Common Grooved Needle." *London Medical Gazette* 30 (March 1842): 19.

———. "Geography of Palestine: The Substance of a Paper Read before the Literary and Scientific Institution at Bristol." *Bath and Bristol Magazine; or, Western Miscellany* 3 (1834): 14–26.

———. "Geological Observations on North Wales." *Annals of Philosophy* 6 (November 1815): 363–66.

———. *Histoire naturelle de l'homme, comprenant des recherches sur l'influence des agens physiques et moraux considérés comme causes des variétés qui distinguent entre elles les différentes races humaines*. Translated from English by Dr. F[rançois Désiré] Roulin. 2 vols. Paris: J.-B. Baillière; London: H. Baillière, 1843.

———. *A History of the Epidemic Fever which Prevailed in Bristol, During the Years 1817, 1818, and 1819; Founded on Reports of St. Peter's Hospital and the Bristol Infirmary*. London: Printed for John and Arthur Arch, 1820.

———. "Hypochondriasis." In *The Cyclopaedia of Practical Medicine; Comprising Treatises on the Nature and Treatment of Disease, Materia Medica and Therapeutics, Medical Jurisprudence, Etc., Etc.*, vol. 2, edited by John Forbes, Alexander Tweedie, and John Conolly, 548–57. London: Sherwood, Gilbert, and Piper and Cradock and Baldwin, 1833.

———. *Illustrations to the Researches into the Physical History of Mankind: Atlas, of Forty-Four Coloured and Five Plain Plates, Engraved on Steel*. London: Hippolyte Baillière, Publisher and Foreign Bookseller to the Royal College of Surgeons, 1844.

———. "Insanity." In *The Cyclopaedia of Practical Medicine; Comprising Treatises on the Nature and Treatment of Disease, Materia Medica and Therapeutics, Medical Jurisprudence, Etc., Etc.*, vol. 2, edited by John Forbes, Alexander Tweedie, and John Conolly, [824]–75. London: Sherwood, Gilbert, and Piper and Cradock and Baldwin, 1833.

———. "Instances of Longevity (from 'Researches in the Physical History of Mankind,' Third Edition, 1836, Vol. 1)." *Edinburgh Medical and Surgical Journal* 48 (October 1837): 550–52.

———. *Lectures on the Mummies and Antiquities of Egypt. Lecture I*. Bristol: Mirror Office, 1834.

———. "Letter from Dr. Prichard to Dr. Hodgkin, [May 20, 1839]." *Extracts from the Papers and Proceedings of the Aborigines' Protection Society* 1, no. 2 (June 1839): 56–58.

———. *Letter from Dr. Prichard to Dr. Hodgkin*. [Bristol, 1839].

———. "[Letter to Alexander Tilloch] On the Cosmogony of Moses." *Philosophical Magazine and Journal* 48 (December 1816): 300.

———. "[Letter to Alexander Tilloch] On the Cosmogony of Moses; in Reply to F. E——s." *Philosophical Magazine and Journal* 48 (August 1816): 111–17.

———. "[Letter to Alexander Tilloch] On the Cosmogony of Moses; with Some Preliminary Observations on Dr. Gilby's Communication in Number 209." *Philosophical Magazine and Journal* 46 (October 1815): 285–90.

———. *Manual of Ethnology*. Postprinted from *A Manual of Scientific Enquiry*, 1859. Revised by Thomas Wright and Marie Armand Pascal d'Avezac on the part of the Ethnological Society. London: Printed by W. Clowes and Sons, [1859].

———. "The Mixture of Human Races [Extracted from Anniversary Address for 1848, to the Ethnological Society of London]." *Journal of the Indian Archipelago and Eastern Asia* 4 (January 1850): 54.

———. *The Natural History of Man; Comprising Inquiries into the Modifying Influence of Physical and Moral Agencies on the Different Tribes of the Human Family.* London: H. Baillière; Paris: J. B. Baillière; Leipsic: T. O. Weigel, 1843; 2nd ed., London: Hippolyte Baillière; Paris: J. B. Baillière; Leipsic: T. O. Weigel, 1845; 3rd ed., London: Hippolyte Baillière; Paris: J. B. Baillière; Leipsic: T. O. Weigel, 1848; 4th ed., edited and enlarged by Edwin Norris, London: H. Baillière; New York: H. Baillière; Paris: H. B. Baillière; Madrid: Bailly Baillière, 1855.

———. *Naturgeschichte des menschengeschlechts.* Translated by Rudolf Wagner. 5 vols. Leipzig: Verlag von Leopold Voss, 1840, 1840, 1842, 1845, 1848.

———. "Observations on the Connexions of Insanity with Diseases of the Organs of Physical Life." *Phrenological Journal, and Magazine of Moral Science* 17 (April 1844): 168–72.

———. "Observations on the Connexions of Insanity with Diseases of the Organs of Physical Life." *Provincial Medical and Surgical Journal, and Retrospect of the Medical Sciences* 7, no. 174 (January 27, 1844): 323–24.

———. "Observations sur les altérations du système nerveux dans la chorée." *Archives générales de médecine* 8 (June 1825): 273–74.

———. "Observations sur les altérations du système nerveux dans la chorée." *Journal complémentaire du Dictionnaire des Sciences Médicales* 22 (September 1825): 283.

———. *Om Sindssygdommene og andre sygelige Sjælstilstande.* Translated and annotated by Harald Selmer. Kobenhavn: C. A. Reitzel, 1842.

[———]. "On Oneirophantia & Daemonology." *Collegian* 1 (1831): 49–53.

———. *On the Different Forms of Insanity, in Relation to Jurisprudence, Designed for the Use of Persons Concerned in Legal Questions Regarding Unsoundness of Mind.* London: Hippolyte Baillière, 1842.

———. *On the Different Forms of Insanity, in Relation to Jurisprudence, Designed for the Use of Persons Concerned in Legal Questions Regarding Unsoundness of Mind.* 2nd ed. London: Hippolyte Baillière; Paris: J. B. Baillière, 1847.

———. "On the Ethnography of High Asia." *Journal of the Geographical Society of London* 9 (1839): 192–215.

———. "On the Extinction of Human Races." In *Ethnological Extracts [from the Monthly Chronicle],* 1–3. London: Printed by A. Spottiswoode, [1840].

[———]. "On the Genealogies of Matt. i and Luke iii." *Christian Observer* 25 (June 1825): 338–43.

———. "On the Relations of Ethnology to Other Branches of Knowledge." *Edinburgh New Philosophical Journal* 43 (October 1847): 307–35.

———. "On the Relations of Ethnology to Other Branches of Knowledge." *Journal of the Ethnological Society of London* 1 (1848): 301–29.

———. *On the Relations of Ethnology to Other Branches of Knowledge, Delivered at the Anniversary Meeting of the Ethnological Society, 22d June 1847.* Edinburgh: Printed by Neill, 1847.

———. "On the Treatment of Hemiplegia, and Particularly on an Important Remedy in Some Diseases of the Brain." *London Medical Gazette* 7 (January 1831): 425–28.

———. "On the Treatment of Some Diseases of the Brain." *Report of the Sixth Meeting of the British Association for the Advancement of Science, Held at Bristol in August 1836*. Vol. 5. London: John Murray, 1837.

———. "On the Various Methods of Research which Contribute to the Advancement of Ethnology, and of the Relations of That Science to Other Branches of Knowledge." *Report of the Seventeenth Meeting of the British Association for the Advancement of Science; Held at Oxford in June 1847* 17 (1847): 230–53.

[———]. "Origin of Pagan Idolatry, ascertained from Historical Testimony and Circumstantial Evidence. By G. S. Faber, 1816, [and] Ueber die Sprache und Weisheit der Indier, 1808." *British Review, and London Critical Journal* 8 (November 1816): 359–87.

———. "Paralysis." *Medico-Chirurgical Review, and Journal of Medical Science* 4 (March 1824): 926–27.

———. "Philologische und physische Untersuchungen ruckaichtlich der Geschichte der Menschenarten." *Notizen aus dem Gebiete der Natur-und Heilkunde* 38, nos. 834–35 (December 1833): cols. 305–12, 321–29.

———. "Remarks on the Older Floetz Strata of England." *Annals of Philosophy* 6 (July 1815): 20–26.

[———]. "Remarks on the Poetry of the Hebrews, As Distinguished from That of Other Nations; with a New Translation of the Song of Deborah, in Judges, Chap. 5." *Friends' Monthly Magazine* 1 (Fifth Month, 1830): 311–18.

———. "Remarks on the Treatment of Epilepsy, and Some Other Nervous Diseases." *Edinburgh Medical and Surgical Journal* 11 (October 1815): 458–66.

———. "Remarks on the Treatment of Paralysis, and Some Other Diseases, by Issues and Blisters." *London Medical Repository*, n.s., 1 (January 1824): 1–15.

———. *Report on the Various Methods of Research which Contribute to the Advancement of Ethnology, and of the Relations of That Science to Other Branches of Knowledge*. London: Printed by Richard and John Taylor, 1848. Available at BL 572/1982.

———. *Researches into the Physical History of Man*. London: Printed for John and Arthur Arch, Cornhill, and B. and H. Barry, Bristol, 1813.

———. *Researches into the Physical History of Mankind*. 2nd ed., 2 vols. London: John and Arthur Arch, 1826.

———. *Researches into the Physical History of Mankind*. 3rd ed., vol. 1. London: Sherwood, Gilbert, and Piper; J. and A. Arch, 1836.

———. *Researches into the Physical History of Mankind: Containing Researches into the History of the Asiatic Nations*. 3rd ed., vol. 4. London: Sherwood, Gilbert, and Piper, 1844.

———. *Researches into the Physical History of Mankind: Containing Researches into the History of the European Nations*. 3rd ed., vol. 3. London: Sherwood, Gilbert, and Piper, 1841.

———. *Researches into the Physical History of Mankind: Containing Researches into the History of the Oceanic and of the American Nations.* 3rd ed., vol. 5. London: Sherwood, Gilbert, and Piper, 1847.

———. *Researches into the Physical History of Mankind: Containing Researches into the Physical Ethnography of the African Races.* 3rd ed., vol. 2. London: Sherwood, Gilbert, and Piper; J. and A. Arch, 1837.

———. *A Review of the Doctrine of a Vital Principle, as Maintained by Some Writers on Physiology, with Observations on the Causes of Physical and Animal Life.* London: Sherwood, Gilbert, and Piper; J. and A. Arch, 1829.

———. *Six Ethnographical Maps with a Sheet of Letterpress: In Illustration of His Works:—"The Natural History of Man," and "Researches into the Physical History of Mankind."* London: Hippolyte Baillière, Moyes and Barclay, 1843; 2nd ed., London and New York: Hippolyte Baillière; London: Moyes and Barclay, Printers, 1851, 1861.

———. "Somnambulism and Animal Magnetism." In *Cyclopaedia of Practical Medicine*, vol. 4, edited by John Forbes, Alexander Tweedie, and John Conolly, 21–39. London: Sherwood, Gilbert, and Piper, 1835.

———. "Soundness and Unsoundness of Mind." In *Cyclopaedia of Practical Medicine*, vol. 4, edited by John Forbes, Alexander Tweedie, and John Conolly, 39–55. London: Sherwood, Gilbert, and Piper, 1835. Also preprinted by London: Marchant, 1834.

———. "Successful Case of Transfusion of Blood." *Provincial Medical Journal, and Retrospect of the Medical Sciences* 6 (July 1843): 345.

———. "Temperament." In *The Cyclopaedia of Practical Medicine*, vol. 4, edited by John Forbes, Alexander Tweedie, and John Conolly, 159–74. London: Sherwood, Gilbert, and Piper, 1835. Preprinted by London: Marchant, 1834.

[———]. "Townsend's Character of Moses Established for Veracity as an Historian, Recording Events from the Creation to the Deluge, 1813." *British Review, and London Critical Journal* 6 (August 1815): 26–50.

———. *A Treatise on Diseases of the Nervous System: Part the First: Comprising Convulsive and Maniacal Affections.* London: Printed for Thomas and George Underwood, 1822.

———. *A Treatise on Hypochondriasis.* In *The Cyclopaedia of Practical Medicine*. London: Marchant, 1832.

———. *A Treatise on Insanity.* Philadelphia: E. L. Carey and A. Hart, 1837.

———. *Treatise on Insanity.* In *The Cyclopaedia of Practical Medicine.* London: Marchant, Printer, 1833.

———. *A Treatise on Insanity and Other Disorders Affecting the Mind.* London: Sherwood, Gilbert, and Piper, 1835.

———. "Ueber das aussterben von menschenracen." *Neue notizen aus dem gebiete der natur-und heilkunde*, 2nd ser., 13 (March 1840): cols. 273–77.

———. "Von Siebold on Japan, and the Adjacent Countries." *Journal of the Royal Geographical Society of London* 9 (1839): 477–81.

Prichard, J[ames] C[owles], and A[aron] Hartnell. *Circular Announcing the Concluding Part of J. C. Prichard's Lecture on Pestilences.* Bristol: For the Bristol Institution, 1828.

Prichard, James Cowles, Lamuel Seyer, and Charles Abraham Elton. *Cause of the Greeks.* Bristol: J. M. Gutch, 1824.

Prichard, James Cowles, [Jr.] *The Life and Times of Hincmar, Archbishop of Rheims.* Littlemore: Masson; London: J. H. Parker, 1848.

——. *Sermons. With a Memoir of the Author.* London: Joseph Masters, 1849.

Prichard, Thomas. *Remarks Suggested by the Perusal of a Portraiture of Primitive Quakerism, &c.* London: William Phillips, 1813.

"Prichard, Winslow, Crichton, Rumball &c. on the Pleas of Insanity in Criminal Cases." *British and Foreign Medical Review or Quarterly Journal of Practical Medicine and Surgery* 16 (July 1843): 81–110.

"Prichard and Georget on the Nervous System." *London Medical Repository* 17 (February 1822): 115–56.

"Prichard on a Vital Principle." *Eclectic Review,* 3rd ser., 3 (May 1830): 460–66.

"Prichard on Diseases of the Nervous System." *American Medical Recorder of Original Papers and Intelligence in Medicine and Surgery* 5 (October 1822): 726–60.

"Prichard on Epidemic Fever." *London Medical Repository* 14 (July 1820): 36–40.

"Prichard on Insanity." *Boston Medical and Surgical Journal* 17, no. 18 (December 1837): 288.

"Prichard on Insanity." *Lancet,* no. 2 (August 1835): 703–5.

"Prichard on the Celtic Languages." *Eclectic Review* 8 (July 1840): 26–41.

"Prichard on the Celtic Nations." *Eclectic Review,* 3rd ser., 7 (February 1832): 145–57.

"Prichard on the Diseases of the Nervous System." *Quarterly Journal of Foreign and British Medicine and Surgery* 4 (January 1822): 130–42. Reprinted in *Journal of Foreign Medical Science and Literature* 2 (July 1822): 487–98 and *Monthly Journal of Medicine* 1 (April 1823): 214–25.

"Prichard on the Egyptian Mythology." *Monthly Review* 92 (July 1820): 225–42.

"Prichard's Analysis of Egyptian Mythology." *British Critic* 14 (July 1820): 55–69.

"Prichard's Physical History of Mankind." *New Quarterly Review; or, Home, Foreign, and Colonial Journal* 8 (October 1846): 95–134.

"Prichard's Researches." *Critical Review, or, Annals of Literature,* ser. 5, 1 (February–March 1815): 89–106, 266–75.

Prideaux, T. S. "The British Association and Cerebral Physiology." *Zoist: A Journal of Cerebral Physiology & Mesmerism, and Their Applications to Human Welfare* 4 (January 1847): 473–80.

Priestly, Joseph. *Disquisitions Relating to Matter and Spirit.* London: J. Johnson, 1777.

Pritchard, John E. "Bristol Archaeological Notes, 1913–1919." *Transactions of the Bristol and Gloucestershire Archaeological Society for 1920* 40 (1920): 125–48.

"Pritchard's 'Physical History of Man.'" *Literary and Statistical Magazine for Scotland* 1 (February/May 1817): 179–88; 288–97.

Proceedings of the Fifth Meeting of the British Association for the Advancement of Science, Held in Dublin, during the Week from the 10th to the 15th of August, 1835, Inclusive. Dublin: Printed by Philip Dixon Hardy, 1835.

Procter, Bryan Waller. *The Literary Recollections of Barry Cornwall.* Boston: Meador, 1936.

Prospectus of a College for Classical and Scientific Education, to Be Established in or near the City of Bristol. Bristol: Wright & Bagnall, [1829].

Prospectus of the Society for the Extinction of the Slave Trade and the Civilization of Africa: Instituted June, 1839. London: n.p., 1840.

"Provincial Medical and Surgical Association: Third Anniversary Meeting, Held at Oxford, July 23, 1835." *Lancet* 2 (July 25, 1835): 551–59.

Quarles, Benjamin. *Frederick Douglass.* New York: Athenaeum, 1968.

———. "Ministers without Portfolio." *Journal of Negro History* 39, no. 1 (January 1954): 27–42.

"Questions Proposed to a Candidate for the Degree of M.D. at Edinburgh." *Lancet* 278, no. 276 (December 13, 1828): 340–42.

Quine, Maria Sophia. "The Destiny of Races 'Not Yet Called to Civilization': Giustiniano Nicolucci's Critique of American Polygenism and Defense of Liberal Racism." In *National Races: Transnational Power Struggles in the Sciences and Politics of Human Diversity, 1840–1945*, edited by Richard McMahon, 69–104. Lincoln: University of Nebraska Press, 2019.

Quirk, Randolph Charles. *The Study of the Mother-Tongue: An Inaugural Lecture Delivered at University College London, 21 February 1961.* London: For the College by H. K. Lewis, 1961.

Qureshi, Sadiah. *Peoples on Parade: Exhibitions, Empire, and Anthropology in Nineteenth Century Britain.* Chicago: University of Chicago Press, 2011.

Rainger, Ronald. "Philanthropy and Science in the 1830s: The British and Foreign Aborigines' Protection Society." *Man: The Journal of the Royal Anthropological Institute,* n.s., 15, no. 4 (December 1980): 702–17.

Raison, Jennifer, and Michael Goldie. *The Servant Girl Princess Caraboo: The Real Story of the Grand Hoax.* Moreton-in-Marsh, Gloucestershire: Windrush, 1994.

Raistrick, Arthur. *Quakers in Science and Industry: Being an Account of the Quaker Contributions to Science and Industry during the 17th and 18th Centuries.* New ed. Newton Abbot: David & Charles, 1968.

"Ram Mohun Roy." *Asiatic Journal* 12, pt. 1 (November 1833): 195–213; (December 1833): 287–90.

The Red Lodge. 4th ed. Bristol: Printed for the City Art Gallery, 1965.

Rees, William, ed. *The Liber Landavensis, Llyfr Teilo, or the Ancient Register of the Cathedral Church of Llandaff.* Llandovery: William Rees, 1840.

"Remarkable Discovery of Skulls near Jerusalem." *Phrenological Journal, and Magazine of Moral Science* 14, no. 68 (1841): 217–27.

"Remarks on the Review of Dr. Prichard's Work." *Asiatic Journal* 22 (February/March 1837): 105–14, 221–31.

Renton, A. Wood. "Chapters in the English Law of Lunacy, III: Moral Insanity." *Green Bag: An Entertaining Magazine for Lawyers* 9 (November 1897): 481–93.

"Report of a Conversazione Held at the Red Lodge August 25, 1836." *Literary Gazette; and Journal of Belles Lettres, Arts, Sciences, &c.* (September 17, 1836): 604.

"Report of Section D of the British Association for the Advancement of Science, 1841." *Athenaeum Journal of Literature, Science, and the Fine Arts* (August 28, 1841): 627–28.

"Report of the Anniversary Meeting of the Ethnological Society of London, Held on May 29, 1846." *Athenaeum* (June 27, 1846): 659.

Report of the Committee for Queries to Section D of the BAAS, Thirteenth Meeting of the British Association of Science. *Athenaeum Journal of Literature, Science, and the Fine Arts* (September 9, 1843): 823–31.

Report of the Conversazione, or First Quarterly Meeting of the Bath and Bristol Branch of the Provincial Medical and Surgical Association, September 27, 1849. *Provincial Medical and Surgical Journal* 13 (October 3, 1849): 551.

Report of the Council on the General State of the Leeds Philosophical and Literary Society, 1822–1823. Leeds: Edward Baines, 1823.

Report of the Provisional Committee of the Bristol Institution for the Advancement of Science and Literature and the Arts. [Bristol: J. M. Gutch, 1823].

Report on the Queries to Section D of the BAAS Meeting of 1842. *Athenaeum Journal of Literature, Science, and the Fine Arts* (July 30, 1842): 690.

Reports of Sub-section E.—Ethnology Meetings of the British Association for the Advancement of Science 1846, Southampton. *Athenaeum Journal of Literature, Science, and the Fine Arts* (1846): 971, 1005, 1050.

Retzius, Anders Adolf. "Present State of Ethnology in relation to the Form of the Human Skull." *Annual Report of the Board of Regents of the Smithsonian Institution, Showing the Operations, Expenditures, and Condition of the Institution for the Year 1859* (1860): 251–70.

Review of *A Treatise on Diseases of the Nervous System*. *Annali universali di medicina* 30, nos. 88–89 (April–May 1824): 191–250.

Review of *A Treatise on Diseases of the Nervous System*. *Göttingische gelehrte Anzeigen* (June 1823): 1033–36.

Review of *A Treatise on Insanity, 1835*. *Göttingische gelehrte Anzeigen*, no. 8 (January 1838): 78–80.

Review of James Cowles Prichard, *Remarks on the Treatment of Epilepsy*. *London Medical and Physical Journal, Containing the Earliest Information on Subjects of Medicine, Surgery, Pharmacy, Chemistry, and Natural History* 34 (December 1815): 517–19.

Review of James Cowles Prichard's Retrospective Address, Oxford, 1835. *British and Foreign Medical Review or Quarterly Journal of Practical Medicine and Surgery* 3 (January 1837): 106–61.

Review of *Narrative of a Journey to the Shores of the Arctic Ocean in 1833-4-5, under the Command of Captain Back, RN*. By Richard King. *Athenaeum*, no. 473 (November 19, 1836): 812–14.

Review of *Naturgeschichte des menschengeschlechts*. *Blätter für literarische Unterhaltung* 1 (June 1842): 653–56, 657–59, 661–64, 665–57.

Review of *Om Sindssygdommene*. *Bibliothek for Læger*, 2nd ser., 9 (1843): 401–26.

Review of *Om Sindssygdommene*. *Journal for litteratur og Kunst* 1 (1843): 236–37.
Review of *On the Different Forms of Insanity, in Relation to Jurisprudence*. *Athenaeum* (December 3, 1842): 1037–38.
Review of *On the Different Forms of Insanity, in Relation to Jurisprudence*. *London Medical Gazette; Being a Weekly Journal of Medicine and the Collateral Sciences* 31 (January 1843): 557–59.
Review of *The Eastern Origin of the Celtic Nations*, New Edition. *Archaeologia Cambrensis: The Journal of the Cambrian Archaeological Association* 3 (October 1857): 404–8.
Review of the English Translation of Johannes von Muller's *An Universal History, in Twenty-Four Books*. *Gentleman's Magazine and Historical Chronicle* 88 (August 1818): 150.
"Rev. Samuel Seyer, M.A." *Gentleman's Magazine and Historical Chronicle* 101, pt. 2, no. 5 (November 1831): 471–72.
Reynolds, John Russell. *Epilepsy: Its Symptoms, Treatment, and Relation to Other Chronic Convulsive Diseases*. London: John Churchill, 1861.
Rhodes, Philip. "Mr. Cline's Surgical Lectures at St. Thomas's in 1805 and 1806." *St. Thomas's Hospital Gazette* 68, no. 3 (1970): 6–9.
Rice, Charles Duncan. "The Scottish Factor in the Fight against American Slavery, 1830–1870." PhD dissertation, Edinburgh, 1969.
Richards, Evelleen. *Darwin and the Making of Sexual Selection*. Chicago: University of Chicago Press, 2017.
———. *Ideology and Evolution in Nineteenth Century Britain: Embryos, Monsters, and Racial and Gendered Others in the Making of Evolutionary Theory and Culture*. Milton: Taylor & Francis, 2020.
———. "The 'Moral Anatomy' of Robert Knox: The Interplay between Biological and Social Thought in Victorian Scientific Naturalism." *Journal of the History of Biology* 22, no. 3 (Autumn 1989): 373–436.
Risse, Guenter B. "The Renaissance of Bloodletting: A Chapter in Modern Therapeutic." *Journal of the History of Medicine and Allied Sciences* 34 (January 1979): 3–22.
Ritchie, James. "A Double Centenary—Two Notable Naturalists, Robert Jameson and Edward Forbes." *Proceedings of the Royal Society of Edinburgh. Section B (Biology)* 66 (1955–56): 29–58.
Ritter, Sabine. "Natural Equality and Racial Semantics." In *Racism and Modernity*, edited by Iris Wigger and Sabine Ritter. Festschrift for Wulf D. Hund. Munster: Lit-verlag, 2012.
Roach, J. P. C. "Victorian Universities and the National Intelligentsia." *Victorian Studies* 3 (1959): 131–50.
Roberts, Andrew. "England's Poor Law Commissioners and the Trade in Pauper Lunacy, 1834–1847." http://www.studymore.org.uk/.
Roget, Peter Mark. *Treatises on Physiology and Phrenology: From the Seventh Edition of the Encyclopaedia*. Edinburgh: Adam and Charles Black, 1838.
Rolleston, George. "Address to the Department of Anthropology by the President of the Department." *Nature* 12 (September 1875): 382–86.

Rollin, Charles. *Histoire ancienne des egyptiens*. 6 vols. Paris: Veuve Estienne, 1740.

——— . *Histoire Romaine depuis la fondation de Rome jusqu'a la bataille d'Actium, c'est-a-dire jusqu'à la fin de la République*. 16 vols. Paris: Veuve Estienne, 1738–81.

Romberg, Moritz Heinrich. *A Manual of the Nervous Diseases of Man*. Translated from the German in 2 vols. London: Printed for the Sydenham Society, 1853.

Romeyn, Theodric, and John B. Beck. *Elements of Medical Jurisprudence*. 6th ed. London: Longman, Orme, Brown, Green, and Longmans, 1938.

Rosa, Frederico Delgado, and Han F. Vermeulen, eds. *Ethnographers before Malinowski: Pioneers of Anthropological Fieldwork, 1870-1922*. New York: Berghahn, 2022.

Rosen, George. *Madness in Society: Chapters in the Historical Sociology of Mental Illness*. London: Routledge & Kegan Paul, 1968.

Rosenberg, Charles E. "The Therapeutic Revolution: Medicine, Meaning, and Social Change in Nineteenth-Century America." *Perspectives in Biology and Medicine* 20 (Summer 1977): 485–506.

Rosenfeld, Louis. *Thomas Hodgkin: Morbid Anatomist and Social Activist*. Lanham MD: Madison, 1993.

Rosner, Lisa M. *Medical Education in the Age of Improvement: Edinburgh Students and Apprentices*. Edinburgh: Edinburgh University Press, 1991.

Rowntree, J. Wilhelm, and Henry Bryan Binns. *A History of the Adult School Movement*. London: Headley Brothers, 1903.

Royal Geographical Society. *The Country of the Turkomans: An Anthology of Exploration from the Royal Geographical Society*. Introduction by Duncan Cumming. London: Oguz Press and the Royal Geographical Society, 1977.

Royal Medical Society of Edinburgh. *Dissertations by Eminent Members of the Royal Medical Society*. Edinburgh: David Douglas, 1892.

——— . *General List of Members of the Medical Society of Edinburgh*. Edinburgh: Printed for the Society, 1823.

——— . *General List of Members of the Medical Society of Edinburgh*. Edinburgh: Printed for the Society, 1850.

——— . *The Record of the Royal Society of London*. 3rd ed. London: Printed for the Society by Oxford University Press, 1912.

Rubinstein, W. D. "The End of 'Old Corruption' in Britain 1780-1860." *Past & Present* 101 (November 1983): 55–86.

Rupke, Nicolaas. "The Origins of Racism and Huxley's Rule." In *Johann Friedrich Blumenbach: Race and Natural History, 1750-1850*, edited by Nicolaas Rupke and Gerhard Lauer, 233–47. Milton: Taylor & Francis, 2018.

——— . *Richard Owen: Victorian Naturalist*. New Haven: Yale University Press, 1994.

Rush, Benjamin. *Medical Inquiries and Observations, upon the Diseases of the Mind*. Philadelphia: Kimber & Richardson, 1812.

Russell, Michael. *A Connection of Sacred and Profane History, from the Death of Joshua to the Decline of the Kingdoms of Israel and Judah (Intended to Complete the Works of Shuckford and Prideau)*. London: Printed for C. & J. Rivington, 1827.

Ryland, John. *Pastoral Memorials: Selected from the Manuscripts of the Late Revd. John Ryland, D. D. of Bristol.* Edited and with a memoir of the author by Jonathan Edwards Ryland. Vol. 2. London: B. J. Holdsworth, 1826–28.

Sanders, Lloyd C., ed. *Celebrities of the Century: Being a Dictionary of Men and Women of the Nineteenth Century.* London: Cassell, 1887.

Saunders, Charles J. G. *A History of the United Bristol Hospitals.* Bristol: Printed by J. W. Arrowsmith, for the Board of Governors of the United Bristol Hospitals, 1965.

Schaeffer, Karl. Review of Prichard's *A Treatise*. *Jahrbücher der in-und ausländischen gesammten Medicin* 10 (1836): 137–43.

Schiebinger, Londa L. *Nature's Body: Gender in the Making of Modern Science.* New Brunswick NJ: Rutgers University Press, 2013.

Schlegel, August Wilhelm von. "De l'origine des Hindous." *Nouvelles annales des voyages et des sciences géographiques* 80 (October–December 1838): 137–214.

Schwebber, S. S. "Scientists as Intellectuals: The Early Victorians." In *Victorian Science and Victorian Values: Literary Perspectives*, edited by James Paradis and Thomas Postlewait, 1–37. New York: New York Academy of Sciences, 1981.

Scott, Walter. *The Lady of the Lake: A Poem.* Edinburgh: John Ballantyne, 1810.

Scull, Andrew T. *Museums of Madness: The Social Organization of Insanity in 19th Century England.* New York: St. Martin's Press, 1979.

Second Annual Report of the Bristol Infant School. Bristol: Printed by D. G. Goyder, 1824.

Sera-Shriar, Efram. *The Making of British Anthropology, 1813–1871.* Pittsburgh: University of Pittsburgh Press, 2016.

Seyer, Samuel. *Outline of Proposals concerning Expansion of the Library into New Premises.* Bristol: Printed by J. M. Gutch, 1814.

Seymour, Edward J. *A Letter to the Right Honourable the Earl of Shaftesbury Etc. Etc. on the Laws which Regulate Private Lunatic Asylums: with a Comparative View of the Process "de lunatico inquirendo" in England and the Law of "Interdiction" in France.* London: Longman, Brown, Green, Longmans, & Roberts, 1859.

Shairp, John Campbell. *Glen Desseray and Other Poems Lyrical and Elegiac.* London: Macmillan, 1888.

Shryock, Richard Harrison. "The Strange Case of Wells' Theory of Natural Selection (1813)." In *Studies and Essays in the History of Science and Learning Offered in Homage to George Sarton on the Occasion of His Sixtieth Birthday, 31 August 1944*, edited by M. F. Ashley Montagu, 195–207. New York: Henry Schuman, 1946.

Siemers, [J. F.] Review of James Cowles Prichard's Retrospective Address, Oxford, 1835. *Zeitschrift fur die gesammte medicin* 2, no. 1 (September 1836): 36–48.

Sieveking, Henry Edward. *On Epilepsy and Epileptiform Seizures, Their Causes, Pathology, and Treatment.* London: John Churchill, 1858.

[Silliman, Benjamin]. *A Journal of Travels in England, Holland and Scotland, and of Two Passages over the Atlantic, in the Years 1805 and 1806.* 3rd ed., 3 vols. New Haven: S. Converse, 1820.

Simmons, Samuel Foart, comp. *The Medical Register for the Year 1779.* London: Printed for J. Murray, 1779.

Simond, Louis. *Journal of a Tour and Residence in Great Britain, during the Years 1810 and 1811.* Vol. 1. Edinburgh: Archibald Constable, 1817.

Simpson, A. R. "History of the Chair of Midwifery and the Diseases of Women and Children in the University of Edinburgh. An Introductory Lecture." *Edinburgh Medical Journal* 28 (1882): 481–98.

Simpson, Thomas. "Historicizing Humans in Colonial India." In *Historicizing Humans: Deep Time, Evolution, and Race in Nineteenth-Century British Sciences*, edited by Eftam Sera-Shriar, 113–37. Pittsburgh: University of Pittsburgh Press, 2018.

Singer, Charles, and S. W. F. Holloway. "Early Medical Education in England in Relation to the Pre-history of London University." *Medical History* 4 (1960): 1–17.

Sir Herbert Jenner Fust, A Medical Man, Dr. S. Ashwell, Obtains a Will from a Sick Lady during the Absence of her Husband, whom he Deprives of 25,000l. Judgment of Sir H. Jenner-Fust. London: n.p., 1850.

"Sir William Wilde, 1815–1876." *Journal of the Irish Colleges of Physicians and Surgeons* 5 (April 1976): 147–48; 150–52.

Slee, Peter. "The Oxford Idea of a Liberal Education, 1800–1860: The Invention of Tradition and the Manufacture of Practice." *History of Universities* 7 (1988): 61–87.

Sloan, Phillip. "Evolutionary Thought before Darwin." In *The Stanford Encyclopedia of Philosophy*, winter 2019, edited by Edward N. Zalta. https://plato.stanford.edu/archives/win2019/entries/evolution-before-darwin/.

Smith, Charles Hamilton. *The Natural History of the Human Species, Its Typical Forms, Primaeval Distribution, Filiations, and Migrations.* Edinburgh: W. H. Lizars, 1848.

Smith, Henry Nash. "The Madness of Ahab." *Yale Review* 66 (October 1976): 14–32.

Smith, Leonard. "Lunatic Asylum in the Workhouse: St Peter's Hospital, Bristol, 1698–1861." *Medical History* 61, no. 2 (April 2017): 225–45.

Smith, Leonard D. *"Comfort and Safe Custody": Public Lunatic Asylums in Early Nineteenth Century England.* London: Leicester University Press, 1999.

———. "'A Worthy Feeling Gentleman': Samuel Hitch at Gloucester Asylum, 1828–1847." In *150 Years of British Psychiatry*, vol. 2, *The Aftermath*, edited by Hugh L. Freeman and German E. Berrios, 479–99. London: Athlone Press, 1996.

Smith, Richard. *An Address, Delivered on Opening the Bristol Medical School, in the Old-Park, on Tuesday, the 14th of October, 1834.* Bristol: Mirror Office, 1834.

Smith, Samuel Stanhope. *An Essay on the Causes of the Variety of Complexion and Figure in the Human Species.* Philadelphia: Robert Aitken, 1787.

Smith, W. D. A. "A History of Nitrous Oxide and Oxygen Anaesthesia Part IVa: Further Light on Hickman and His Times." *British Journal of Anaesthesia* 42 (1970): 347–53.

Soemmerring, Samuel Thomas von. *Vom Baue des menschlichen Körpers.* Frankfurt am Main: L. Voss, 1791–96.

"Some Famous Bristol Doctors." *Bristol Medico-Chirurgical Journal* 98, no. 365 (January/April 1983): 4–17.
Southey, Robert. *The Doctor, &c.* London: Longman, Rees, Orme, Brown, Green and Longman, 1834.
Spring, Gardiner. *First Things: A Series of Lectures on the Great Facts and Moral Lessons First Revealed to Mankind.* New York: M. W. Dodd, 1855.
Stafford, William. "Religion and the Doctrine of Nationalism in England at the Time of the French Revolution and Napoleonic Wars." In *Religion and National Identity: Papers Read at the Nineteenth Summer Meeting and the Twentieth Winter Meeting of the Ecclesiastical History Society,* edited by Stuart Mews, 381–96. Oxford: Basil Blackwell, 1982.
Stanley, Arthur Penrhyn. *The Life and Correspondence of Thomas Arnold, D.D.: Late Head-Master of Rugby School, and Regius Professor of Modern History in the University of Oxford.* Vol. 2. Boston: Ticknor and Fields, 1868.
Statement of Facts concerning the Proposed Election of Officers and Council of the Royal Society for the Ensuing Year. N.p.: n.p., [1848].
State of the Bristol Dispensaries, in North-Street and Bath-Street, for the Year 1814. [Bristol]: Printed by J. M. Gutch, [1814].
Staum, Martin S. *Labeling People: French Scholars on Society, Race, and Empire, 1815–1848.* Montreal: McGill-Queen's University Press, 2003.
Stepan, Nancy. *The Idea of Race in Science: Great Britain, 1800–1960.* London: Macmillan, 1982.
Stephens, Michael D., and Gordon W. Roderick. "Nineteenth Century Educational Finance: The Literary and Philosophical Societies." *Annals of Science: An International Review of the History of Science and Technology Since the Renaissance* 31, no. 4 (1974): 335–49.
Steven, William. *The History of the High School of Edinburgh.* Edinburgh: Maclachlan & Stewart, 1849.
Stewart, Dugald. *Elements of the Philosophy of the Human Mind.* Edinburgh: A. Strahan and T. Cadell, 1792.
Stewart, Ian. "After Sir William Jones: British Linguistic Scholarship and European Intellectual History." *Journal of Modern History* 95 (2023).
———. "James Cowles Prichard and the Linguistic Foundations of Ethnology." *Berichte Zur Wissenschaftsgeschichte/History of Science and Humanities* 46 (2023): 76–91.
Stewart, Ian B. "William Edwards and the Study of Human Races in France, from the Restoration to the July Monarchy." *History of Science* 58, no. 3 (September 2020): 275–300.
Stinson, Daniel T. *The Role of Sir William Lawrence in 19th Century English Surgery.* Zurich: Juris Druck, 1969.
Stock, Paul. "'Almost a Separate Race': Racial Thought and the Idea of Europe in British Encyclopedias and Histories, 1771–1830." *Modern Intellectual History* 8, no. 1 (2011): 3–29.
Stocking, George W., Jr. "From Chronology to Ethnology: James Cowles Prichard and British Anthropology 1800–1850." In *Researches into the Physical History*

of Man, by James Cowles Prichard, reprint edition, edited by George W. Stocking Jr., ix–cx. Chicago: University of Chicago Press, 1973.

———. "What's in a Name: The Origins of the Royal Anthropological Institute (1837–71)." *Man*, n.s., 6 (September 1971).

Stoddart, D. R. "The RGS and the 'New Geography': Changing Aims and Changing Roles in Nineteenth Century Science." *Geographical Journal* 146 (July 1980): 190–202.

[Stokes, Whitley]. "Dr. Latham's Celtic Philology." *Saturday Review of Politics, Literature, Science, and Art* 6 (August 1858): 139–41.

Stott, Anne. *Hannah More: The First Victorian*. New York: Oxford University Press, 2004.

Stott, Rebecca. *Darwin's Ghosts: In Search of the First Evolutionists*. London: Bloomsbury, 2012.

Strahan, Samuel Alexander Kenny. *Suicide and Insanity: A Physiological and Sociological Study*. London: Swan Sonnenschein, 1893.

Sturge, Elizabeth. *Reminiscences of My Life and Some Account of the Children of William and Charlotte Sturge and of the Sturge Family of Bristol*. Bristol: J. W. Arrowsmith, 1928.

Sturge, William. *Some Recollections of a Long Life*. [Bristol]: J. W. Arrowsmith for private circulation, 1893.

Summerson, John. *Georgian London*. London: Pleiades, 1945.

"Sur les tombeaux des anciens peuples qui habitaient le Nord de l'Europe." *Bibliothèque universelle de Genève*, n.s., 38 (March 1842): 99–102.

Suzuki, Akihito. *Madness at Home: The Psychiatrist, the Patient, and the Family in England, 1820–1860*. Berkeley: University of California Press, 2006.

[Swayne, Joseph Griffiths]. "In Memoriam: Augustin Prichard." *Bristol Medico-Chirurgical Journal* 16 (March 1898): 1–15.

Sweet, Jessie M., and Charles D. Waterston. "Robert Jameson's Approach to the Wernerian Theory of the Earth, 1796." *Annals of Science* 23 (1967): 81–95.

Symonds, John Addington. *Our Institution and Its Studies: An Introductory Lecture, Delivered at the Bristol Institution for the Advancement of Science, Literature and the Arts, on Monday, September 23, 1850*. London: J. Churchill; Bristol: Evans & Abbott, 1850.

[———]. Review of "Insanity." *Cyclopaedia of Practical Medicine. Bath and Bristol Magazine; or, Western Miscellany* 2, no. 6 (1833): 231–34.

———. Review of Prichard's Vital Principle. *Bath and Bristol Magazine; or, Western Miscellany* 2 (1833): 498–507.

———. *Some Account of the Life, Writings, and Character of the Late James Cowles Prichard, M.D., F.R.S, M.R.I.A., Corresponding Member of the National Institute of France; Etc., Etc*. [Bristol: Evans and Abbott, Printers], 1849.

Taylor, [Gloria] Clare. "Some American Reformers and Their Influence on Reform Movements in Great Britain from 1830 to 1860." PhD dissertation, University of Edinburgh, 1960.

[Taylor, John Pitt]. "On MacNaughten's Trial, and the Plea of Insanity in Criminal Cases: Review of James Cowles Prichard's 'On the Different Forms of Insanity' [and Three Other Publications]." *Legal Observer, or Journal of Jurisprudence* 26 (May 1843): 81–89.

Taylor, Michael A., and Hugh S. Torrens. "Saleswoman to a New Science: Mary Anning and the Fossil Fish Squaloraja from the Lias of Lyme Regis." *Proceedings of the Dorset Natural History and Archaeological Society* 108 (1986): 135–48.

[Taylor, William]. "Muller's *Universal History*." *Monthly Review; or Literary Journal*, 2nd ser., 88 (March 1819): 225–34.

T. B. H. "William Lister, M.D." *Gentleman's Magazine and Historical Chronicle* 100, pt. 1 (1830): 563–64.

Temkin, Owsei. *"The Falling Sickness": A History of Epilepsy from the Greeks to the Beginnings of Modern Neurology*. Baltimore: Johns Hopkins University Press, 1945.

"Thomas Stock, Esq." *Gentleman's Magazine*, n.s., 10 (August 1838): 215.

Ticknor, George. *Life, Letters, and Journals of George Ticknor*. Vol. 1. London: Sampson Low, 1876.

Todhunter, Isaac. *William Whewell, D.D., Master of Trinity College, Cambridge: An Account of his Writings; with Selections from his Literary and Scientific Correspondence*. Vol. 2. London: Macmillan, 1876.

Toogood, Jonathan. "On the Advantages of Counter-Irritation." *Provincial Medical and Surgical Journal* 2 (September 1841): 518–19.

———. *Reminiscences of a Medical Life, with Cases and Practical Illustrations*. Taunton: Frederick May, 1853.

Tourney, Garfield. "A History of Therapeutic Fashions in Psychiatry, 1800–1966." *American Journal of Psychiatry* 124 (December 1967): 784–96.

Traill, Thomas Stuart, ed. *Encyclopaedia Britannica*. Vol. 18. Edinburgh: Adam and Charles Black, 1859.

"Traitement de l'hémiplégie." *Gazette médicale de Paris* 2 (August 1831): 300.

"Trattamento dell'emiplegia." *Bullettino delle scienze mediche pubblicata per cura della Società Medico-Chirurgica di Bologna* 4 (1831): 198.

"A Treatise on Diseases of the Nervous System." *Medicinische-chriurgische Zeitung* 3 (July 18 and 22, 1822): 81–95, 97–105.

"A Treatise on Diseases of the Nervous System." *Medico-Chirurgical Review, and Journal of Medical Science* 3 (September 1822): 277–306.

"Treatment of Hemiplegia." *North American Medical and Surgical Journal* 12 (July 1831): 240.

Trotter, David. *Paranoid Modernism: Literary Experiment, Psychosis, and the Professionalization of English Society*. Oxford: Oxford University Press, 2001.

A Trustee to the Infirmary. *The House-Committee of the Bristol Infirmary Vindicated, and the Late Proceedings of the Trustees Examined, in a Letter to Dr. Carrick, being a Reply to the Observations of that Gentleman Recently Published*. Bristol: Printed by T. J. Manchee, [1825].

Tuke, Samuel. *Description of The Retreat, An Institution near York, for Insane Persons of the Society of Friends*. York: Printed for W. Alexander, 1813.

Tullidge, Henry. *Triumphs of the Bible, with the Testimony of Science to Its Truth*. New York: Charles Scribner, 1863.

Turda, Marius, and Maria Sophia Quine. *Historicizing Race*. London: Bloomsbury, 2018.
Turley, Richard Marggraf. *The Politics of Language in Romantic Literature*. Basingstoke: Palgrave Macmillan, 2002.
Tweedie, Alexander, ed. *A System of Practical Medicine*. 5 vols. Philadelphia: Lea & Blanchard, 1840-41; 2nd American ed. in 3 vols., 1842.
Tylor, Edward Burnett. "Anthropology." In *Encyclopaedia Britannica*, vol. 2, 108-19. Cambridge: University Press, 1910.
[————]. "James Cowles Prichard." In *Encyclopaedia Britannica*, vol. 19, 722-23. Edinburgh: Adam and Charles Black, 1885.
[————]. President's Annual Address. *Journal of the Anthropological Institute of Great Britain and Northern Ireland* 9 (1879-80): 443-58.
"Types of Mankind—Ethnology and Revelation." *British Quarterly Review* 22 (July 1855): 1-45.
Tyson, Blake. "A Cumbrian Medical Student at Edinburgh University in 1806-7." *Transactions of the Cumberland & Westmorland Antiquarian & Archaeological Society* 91 (1991): 199-211.
"Ueber die Arten, Natur, Ursachen und Behandlung der Geistesstörungen." *Allgemeines Repertorium der medizinisch-chirurgischen Journalistik des Auslandes* 20 (July 1835): 273-80.
"University of Edinburgh (List of Medical Classes for 1806-7)." *Edinburgh Medical and Surgical Journal* 2 (1806): 506.
"University of Edinburgh (List of Medical Classes for 1807-8)." *Edinburgh Medical and Surgical Journal* 3 (1807): 498-99.
V. "Prichard—'Diseases of the Nervous System.'" *New-England Journal of Medicine and Surgery* 13 (January 1824): 58-73.
Van Amringe, W. F. *An Investigation of the Theories of the Natural History of Man by Lawrence, Prichard, and Others: Founded upon Animal Analogies: and an Outline of a New Natural History of Man: Founded upon History, Anatomy, Physiology and Human Analogies*. New York: Baker & Scribner, 1848.
Van Evrie, J. H. *Negroes and Negro "Slavery": The First an Inferior Race, the Latter Its Normal Condition*. New York: Van Evrie, Horton, 1861.
Van Hal, Toon. "From Jones to Pictet: Some Notes on the Early History of Celtic Linguistics." *Beiträge zur Geschichte der Sprachwissenschaft* 15, no. 2 (2005): 219-43.
Venn, J. A., comp. *Alumni Cantabrigienses*. Part 2, vol. 1. Cambridge: Cambridge University Press, 1940.
Vermeulen, Han F. *Before Boas: The Genesis of Ethnography and Ethnology in the German Enlightenment*. Lincoln: University of Nebraska Press, 2015.
——— . "Origins and Institutionalization of Ethnography and Ethnology in Europe and the USA, 1771-1845." In *Fieldwork and Footnotes: Studies in the History of European Anthropology*, edited by Arturo Alvarez Roldan and Han Vermeulen, 39-59. London: Taylor & Francis, 1995.
Vivien de St.-Martin, Louis. Review of Seventeenth Meeting of the BAAS, June 1847. *Nouvelles annales des voyages et des sciences géographiques* 123 (September 1849): 312-24.

[Wagner, Andreas Johann]. Review of *Researches into the Physical History of Mankind*, vol. 1, 1836. *Gelehrte Anzeigen* 4 (June 1837): cols. 925–30, 933–47.

Wagner, F. J. H. R. *Naturgeschichte des menschen: Handbuch der populären anthropologie für vorlesungen und zum selbstunterricht*. 2 vols. Kempten: Druck und Verlag von Tob. Dannheimer, 1831.

Wagner, Rudolph. *Prospectus: James Cowles Prichard, "Researches into the Physical History of Mankind," Vol. I and II*. In *Lehrbuch der Physiologie für Vorlesungen und zum Selbstunterricht und mit vorzüglicher Rücksicht auf das Bedürfnis der Ärzte*. Leipzig: Leopold Boss, 1839.

Walk, Alexander. "The Royal College of Psychiatrists." *St. Bartholomew's Hospital Journal* 77 (May 1973): 135–39.

Walk, Alexander, and D. Lindsay Walker. "Gloucester and the Beginnings of the R.M.P.A." *Journal of Mental Science* 107 (July 1961): 603–32.

Wallace, Edwin R., and John Gach, eds. *History of Psychiatry and Medical Psychology: With an Epilogue on Psychiatry and the Mind-Body Relation*. New York: Springer, 2008.

Wallace, Hugh N. "Arctic Profiles: Richard King (1810–1876)." *Journal of the Arctic Institute of North America* 40 (December 1987): 350–51.

———. *The Navy, the Company, and Richard King*. Montreal: McGill, 1980.

Ward, [Thomas] Humphry. *History of the Athenaeum, 1824–1925*. London: Printed for the Club, by William Clowes and Sons, 1926.

Warner, John Harley. "Therapeutic Explanation and the Edinburgh Bloodletting Controversy: Two Perspectives on the Medical Meaning of Science in the Mid-Nineteenth Century." *Medical History* 24 (July 1980): 241–58.

Washington, John. "A Sketch of the Progress of Geography." *Journal of the Geographical Society of London* 8 (1838): 235–66.

Watkin, Brian, ed. *Documents on Health and Social Services, 1834 to the Present Day*. London: Methuen, 1975.

Watkin, David. *The Life and Work of C. R. Cockrell*. London: A. Zuemmer, 1974.

[Watson, Hewett C.] "Phrenology and the British Association." *Phrenological Journal, and Magazine of Moral Science* 12 (October 1839): 412–14.

Wedmore, Edmund Tolson. *Thomas Pole, M.D., with notes by Norman Penney. Friends' Historical Society Journal*, supplement, no. 7. London: Headley Brothers; Philadelphia: Herman Newman; New York: David S. Faber, 1908.

Weeks, Mary Elvira. "Daniel Rutherford and the Discovery of Nitrogen." *Journal of Chemical Education* 11 (1934): 101–7.

Weiss, Kenneth J. "American Forensic Psychiatry Begins: Setting Standards." In *The Evolution of Forensic Psychiatry: History, Current Developments, Future Directions*, edited by Robert Sadoff, 3–19. Cary: Oxford University Press, 2015.

Weller, R. M. "To Sleep, Perchance? A Surgeon's Eye View of Anaesthesia, Bristol, 1850–1860." *Anaesthesia Points West* 9 (Spring 1976): 13–18.

Wells, Kentwood D. "Sir William Lawrence (1783–1867): A Study of Pre-Darwinian Ideas on Heredity and Variation." *Journal of the History of Biology* 4 (Fall 1971): 319–61.

Welsford, Henry. *On the Origin and Ramifications of the English Language: Preceded by an Inquiry into the Primitive Seats, Early Migrations, and Final Settlements of the Principal European Nations*. London: Longman, Brown, Green, and Longmans, 1845.
Westergaard, Harald. *Contributions to the History of Statistics*. London: P. S. King & Son, 1932.
Wetherell, Charles. *Trial of Mary Ann Burdock for the Willful Murder of Mrs. Clara Ann Smith, by Administering Arsenic, Before the Recorder, Sir Charles Wetherell, April 10, 11, and 13, 1835*. London: Printed by P. Rose and Son, 1835.
Whalley, Lawson. "A Vindication of the University of Edinburgh (as a School of Medicine), from the Aspersions of 'A Member of the University of Oxford,' with Remarks on Medical Reform." *Pamphleteer* 13 (1818–19): 429–52.
Wharton, Francis. *A Treatise on Mental Unsoundness, Embracing a General View of Psychological Law*. 3rd ed. Philadelphia: Kay & Brother, 1873.
[Wheaton, Henry]. "Egyptian Antiquities." *North American Review* 29 (October 1829): 361–88.
White, Charles. *An Account of the Regular Gradation in Man, and in Different Animals and Vegetables*. London: C. Dilly, 1799; Verhandeling van Petrus Camper, Utrecht: B. Wild en J. Altheer, 1791.
Whitfield, Michael. *The Dispensaries: Healthcare for the Poor before the NHS; Britain's Forgotten Health-Care System*. Milton Keynes: Printed for AuthorHouse and Michael Whitfield, 2016.
Whitlock, F. A. "Prichard and the Concept of Moral Insanity." *Australian & New Zealand Journal of Psychiatry* 1 (June 1967): 72–79.
Widdess, J. D. H. *A History of the Royal College of Physicians of Ireland 1654–1963*. Edinburgh: E. & S. Livingstone, 1963.
Wilkins, [Charlotte]. "Goebel's Journey in Southern Russia." *Journal of the Royal Geographical Society* 10 (1840): 537–43.
Wilkinson, Ethel M. "French Emigres in England, 1789–1802: Their Reception and Impact on English Life." Dissertation, University of Oxford, 1952.
Wilkinson, J. Gardner. *The Manners and Customs of the Ancient Egyptians*. New ed. London: John Murray, 1878.
Wilkinson, Nathaniel Spire Mender. "Nelson in Ross." *Ross-on-Wye and District Civil Society Newsletter* 78 (Autumn 2002). http://www.rosscivic.org.uk/index.php?page=civic_510-Nelson_in_Ross.
Williams, Elizabeth A. *The Physical and the Moral: Anthropology, Physiology, and Philosophical Medicine in France, 1750–1850*. Cambridge: Cambridge University Press, 1994.
Williams, Griffith John. "The History of Welsh Scholarship." *Studia Celtica* 8 9 (1973–74): 195–219.
Williams, Jeanie. "Bristol in the General Elections of 1818 and 1820." *Transactions of the Bristol and Gloucestershire Archaeological Society* (1968): 173–201.
Williams, W. R. *The Parliamentary History of the County of Gloucester, including the Cities of Bristol and Gloucester, and the Boroughs of Cheltenham, Cirencester,*

Stroud, and Tewkesbury, from the Earliest Times to the Present Day, 1213–1898. Hereford: Privately printed for the author by Jakeman and Carver, 1898.

Wilson, T. G. *Victorian Doctor: Being the Life of Sir William Wilde*. New York: L. B. Fischer, 1846.

Winning, William Balfour. *A Manual of Comparative Philology, in Which the Affinity of the Indo-European Languages Is Illustrated*. London: Printed for J. G. & F. Rivington, 1838.

Winter, Alison. *Mesmerized: Powers of Mind in Victorian Britain*. Chicago: University of Chicago Press, 1998.

Wiseman, Nicholas Patrick. *Twelve Lectures on the Connexion between Science and Revealed Religion. Delivered in Rome*. Vol. 1. London: J. Booker, 1836.

Wofinden, R. C. "Public Health in Bristol: Some Historical Aspects." *Public Health: The Journal of the Society of Medical Officers of Health* 69 (1956): 124–29.

Wood, Casey A. *The American Encyclopedia and Dictionary of Ophthalmology*. Vol. 13. Chicago: Cleveland Press, 1918.

Wood, Jane. *Passion and Pathology in Victorian Fiction*. Oxford: Oxford University Press, 2001.

Woolrich, A. "An American in Gloucestershire and Bristol: The Diary of Joshua Gilpin, 1796–97." *Transactions of the Bristol and Gloucestershire Archaeological Society for 1973* 92 (1974): 169–89.

Wrobel, Arthur. "Orthodoxy and Respectability in Nineteenth-Century Phrenology." *Journal of Popular Culture* 9 (Summer 1975): 38–50.

Wulf, Andrea. *The Invention of Nature: The Adventures of Alexander von Humboldt, the Lost Hero of Science*. London: John Murray, 2015.

Y. "Account of Medical Education in Edinburgh, with Remarks." *Medical and Physical Journal* 6 (1801): 301–8.

Yates, S. A. T., ed. *Memorials of the Family of the Rev. John Yates*. London: Privately printed, 1890–91.

Young, J. H. "James Hamilton (1767–1839), Obstetrician and Controversialist." *Medical History* 7 (1963): 62–73.

Youngson, Alexander John. *The Scientific Revolution in Victorian Medicine*. London: Croom Helm, 1979.

Zegger, Robert E. "Greek Independence and the London Committee, Revolution in the 1820s." *History Today* 20 (April 1970): 236–45; 297–98.

Zirkle, Conway. "Natural Selection before the 'Origin of Species.'" *Proceedings of the American Philosophical Society* 84 (April 1941): 71–123, 104–6.

Index

Page numbers in italics refer to illustrations.

Abergavenny Eisteddfod, 317; prize adjudication at (1838), 317, 318; prize adjudication at (1842), 318, 319, 320; prize adjudication at (1845), 320
Abernethy, John, 294
Aborigines' Protection Society, 377, 378, 379, 380, 381, 383–84, 389, 407
Acland, Maria, 467
Admiralty Manual of Scientific Enquiry, 432, 433, 552n50, 552n52, 553n53
African achievements, Prichard on, 309
Albert, Prince, 476
Alleged Lunatics' Friend Society, 250, 457, 468–69
Allen, William, 48, 375
American Colonization Society, 379
American Ethnological Society, 386
analogy and analogical reasoning, 160, 169, 171–72, 187, 430, 552
An Analysis of the Egyptian Mythology (1819), 202, 203–5
An Analysis of the Egyptian Mythology (1838), preface in, 205
Anatomy Act (1832), 326
Anchor Society, 113
Anglicans. *See* Church of England
animal magnetism, 216, 227, 228, 333
anthropological fieldwork, 383, 386, 388, 441. See also *Ethnological Queries*
anthropological societies, 386
Anthropological Society of London, 437, 438
anthropology: contributions to, 480; definition of (1847), 398; as history, 354, 355; history of, 155–56, 157, 158, 439, 440, 441, 442; Prichard's reputation as founder of, 479, 480; as race science, 372–73; rare use of term of, 544n53; Russian, 386; varieties of, 371–72, 484n2
anthropology, British institutional. *See* Aborigines' Protection Society; Ethnological Society of London; Ethnology Subsection (BAAS); Geographical Society of London
anthropology, Prichardian: influence of, 428, 429, 430, 431, 433–34; later Christian defense of, 439–40; later nineteenth-century, 439–40, 553n53; legacy of, 440, 441, 442; and observational practice, 441
antislavery cause, 330–31, 447. *See also* Bristol: and anti-slave trade; Bristol: and Triangular Trade
anti-slave trade letter, 110, 500n65
archaeology, 153, 260, 398, 399, 400, 553n53
Armstrong, John, 192, 278
Arnold, Thomas (asylum physician), 213, 230
Arnold, Thomas (headmaster of Rugby), 315–16, 356, 434–35
Arnould, Joseph, 79–80, 476
Ashley, Lord, 450, 458, 459, 464, 465, 470
asylum inspections, 456, 464, 559n9; at Fishponds House Private Lunatic Asylum, 467; at Gate Hemsley Retreat, 468; at Haydock Lodge Private Asylum, 467–68; at Northwoods Asylum, 467; at Warwick Workhouse, 468

617

asylum legislation: County Asylums Act (1808), 455–56; Lunacy Act (Shaftesbury's Act) (1845), 456–57, 458; Madhouse Act (1828), 456. *See also* Commissioners in Lunacy
asylums, 453–54, 455, 465; and the ALFS, 468–69; complaints about, 467, 468, 469; John Conolly's non-restraint in, 454; moral management in, 455; moral treatment in, 222, 230, 454, 455; reform of American, 455; tour of French, 333. *See also* insanity; psychiatry
Athenaeum Club, 463
attitudes, Scottish and English: on Edinburgh medical education, 39; on progress, status, and education, 54, 55; on Scotland, 54; on universities, 54–55, 59

Babbage, Charles, 347, 349, 354
Babbington, William, 48
Baconian observationism, 215
Bagehot, Walter, 288–90, 305, 474, 477
balloon flights, 88, 98, 349
Barclay, John, 74
Barnard, Hannah, 23–24, 87
Bear's Cub Club, 210–11
Beddoes, Thomas, 35, 42–43, 213, 256
Beddoes's Medical Institution, 119, 144
Bellingham, John, 235
Bertillon, Alphonse, 439
biblical chronology in *Physical History of Mankind* (3rd ed.), 418–19
biblical genealogy, 271
Biddulph, Thomas, 86, 107, 304
biogeographical evidence, 182, 429
biographies and eulogies, 479
Birch, John, 50
Bird, Edward, 134, 200
The Birds (Aristophanes), 110
Black, Joseph, 58, 60
Black to white skin theory, 172–73, 181, 182
bloodletting, 141, 142–43, 277, 278, 279;

decline of, 282, 518n29; publications on, 277–78; self-, 278; for typhus, 193, 195
blood transfusions, 278
Blumenbach, Johann Friedrich, 160, 161, 164, 175, 179, 371; on beauty, 510n46; dedication of *Physical History of Man* (1813) to, 180; five races of, 183; mistranslation of, 509n16; visit to, 298
Blyth, Edward, 431, 552n47
body snatching, 139–40, 326
books, 96; borrowed, 42, 95, 163, 200, 269, 277, 394, 489n20, 490n31, 490n36, 491n48, 494n69, 501n83, 512n79, 515n44, 515n46, 524n24; owned, x, 96, 498n24; as resources, 164, 165, 167, 168, 169; in reviews, 96
Bopp, Franz, 183, 185, 314, 316
Bory de Saint-Vincent, Jean-Baptiste, 392
Bostock, John, 177, 297, 428
Bridgewater Treatises, 370
Brigham, Amariah, 240, 244, 470
Bristol, 4, 5, 7, 8, 11–12, 13–14, 20, 91; and anti-slave trade, 8, 9; charities in, 100, 106, 107, 255–56; Corporation, 18, 91–92, 102, 198, 205, 206, 255, 363–64; docks and Floating Harbour of, 20–21, *310*; in 1810s, 90, 91, 92, 93, 94; elections, politics, and economics of, 16, 17, 18, 19, 20, 21, 91, 92, 93, 102, 105, 106, 198, 199, 205, 364, 486n55; gas lighting, water, and sanitation in, 102–3, 269; Hannah More in, 16, 17; Jews and Catholics in, 299, 300; manufacturing in, 9–11; medical education in, 333–34, 335; poverty in, 19–20, 328; press gang in, 487n60; riots in, 18–19, 91, 92, 325; science in, 97, 256; sectarianism in, 299, 300; socializing, tourism, and leisure in, 11, 12, 13, 14–15, 97, 210–11, 364, 448; transport in and around, 97–98,

198; and Triangular Trade, 8, 9, 485n20. *See also* Bristol religion; cholera epidemic
Bristol Auxiliary Temperance Society, 335–36
Bristol Baptist College, 100, 299
Bristol Board of Health, 197, 326, 327, 328
Bristol College, 299, 300, 302–3, 304, 305, 306–7, 529n43; and Bristol Baptist College, 299; and Bristol Medical School, 334; and *Collegian*, 305; Establishment opposition to, 300, 301, 302, 303, 304, 307; and London University, 300, 301
Bristol Commercial Rooms, 92–93
Bristol Deaf and Dumb Institution, 448
Bristol Dispensaries, 129, 191
Bristol Established Church Society and Book Association, 448–49
Bristol Eye Dispensary, 149–50, 507n94
Bristol General Hospital, 324–25
Bristol Infirmary, 125–26, 130, 135, 136, *136*; accommodation at, 135; bloodletting at, 141, 142–43; career enhancement from, 118–19; disputes at, 147, 148, 149, 271, 451; dissection at, 139; expectant therapeutics at, 143; faculty and duties at, 136, 140–41, 143–44; fever at, 193, 194; heroic therapeutics at, 141, 142; medical lectures at, 135, 137–38; organization and management of, 130–31, 141, 148; paid staff of, 136; physician colleagues at, 144, 145, 146; poisoning at, 342; pupils of, 136–37, 143, 505n55; resignation from, 152, 450, 451; surgeon colleagues at, 146, 147
Bristol Infirmary physicians' elections, 119; of 1810, 131; of 1811, 131, 132; of 1816, 132, 133, 134, 135
Bristol Institution, 257, 258, *258*, 264; building, 257, 523n6; Egyptology lectures at, *261*, 262, 339, 340; founding of, 257; geology at, 259–60; lectures

at, 258–59, 260, 262, 263, 264; parlous state of, 263–64, 340, 341; Philosophical and Literary Society of, 259, 260; professorships at, 263; religion, politics, and class at, 258; running of, 257, 258; and *West of England Journal*, 340, 341
Bristol Institution Philosophical and Literary Society lectures, 180, 260, 262, 264; "Abraxean Stones," 260, 262; on Africans, 262; "Application of Philological Researches to the History of Mankind," 307; "Distribution of Plants and Animals," 260; on Egyptian antiquities, *261*, 262, 339, 340; on interlinear translations, 263; on native races of America, 262–63; "Palestinian Geography," 307; on pestilences, 263; on phrenology and mesmerism, 263; on vital principle, 263
Bristol Library Society, 42, 94, 95, 96, 497n17, 498n23. *See also* books
Bristol Medical and Surgical Association, 151
Bristol medical charities, 119. *See also* Beddoes's Medical Institution; Bristol Dispensaries; Bristol Eye Dispensary; Bristol General Hospital; Bristol Infirmary; Castle Green Dispensary; Clifton Dispensary
Bristol Medical Library Society, 334
Bristol Medical School, 138, 333–34
Bristol medical societies. *See* Bristol Medical and Surgical Association; Bristol Medical Library Society; Medical Book Society; Medical Reading Society
Bristol Memorialist, 209–10
Bristol Refuge Society, 150
Bristol religion, 98–99, 100; and Baptists, 100; and Dissenters, 99–100; and evangelicalism, 99; and High Church, 99; and Low Church, 99; and Unitarians, 100, 101–2. *See also*

Index · 619

Bristol religion (*continued*)
  Church of England; Friends, Society of; Unitarianism
Bristol Riot (1831), 325. *See also* Bristol: riots in
Bristol Statistical Society, 350, 351
Bristol Zoological Society and Zoo, 344
Britain: Chartism in, 332, 381, 427; elections in, 198, 205, 321; postwar hardship in, 112; science progress in, 256–57; social and political unrest in, 273, 309, 310, 332, 368, 427, 477
British Association for the Advancement of Science (BAAS), 322, 323, 324, 373; Bristol meeting of (1836), 348, 349, 350; "A Comparative Review of Philological and Physical Researches" at, 373–74; Dublin meeting of (1835), 346, 347; "On the Extinction of Human Races" at, 380–81; and Oxford speech (1847), 398; Statistical Section of, 349, 350. *See also Ethnological Queries*; Ethnology Subsection (BAAS)
British Museum Reading Room, 558n1
Broca, Pierre Paul, 439
Bronte, Charlotte, 250
Broussais, François-Joseph-Victor, 391
Bruce, James, 201
Buckland, William, 345, 355–56, 369, 540n9
Budd, William, 360, 514n14
Buffon, Georges-Louis Leclerc, 157, 158, 164
Bunsen, Christian Charles Josias von, 316, 318, 319, 360, 395, 398, 419, 422, 450, 476
burgess of Bristol, 105
Burke, Luke, 435
Burns, Alexander, 419
Burrows, George Man, 225
Buschmann, J. K. E., 413
Buxton, Thomas Fowell, 376, 377

Caldwell, Charles, 185–86, 383, 404–5, 406, 513n85
Cambridge, University of, 84–85. *See also* Oxbridge (Oxford and Cambridge)
Camper, Petrus, 158, 392
capital punishment, abolition of, 236–37
Carpenter, Mary, 359
Carpenter, William Benjamin, 305, 351–52, 353, 396, 428
Carpenter family, 290, 351
Carrick, Andrew, 142, 144, 334
case histories. *See* medical statistics
"Cases of Typhus Fever" (1817), 192–93
Castle Green Dispensary, 119–20
Catholic emancipation and civil rights, 299–300, 486n48
Catholicism, 477
Catlin, George, 423
Cause of the Greeks, 269–70
Celtic, 73–74, 115–16, 161, 163, 175, 185, 320. *See also* Abergavenny Eisteddfod; *The Eastern Origin of the Celtic Nations* (1831)
Chambers, Robert, 368
Champollion, Jean-François, 205, 262, 339, 340
charities. *See* Bristol: charities in
Charrúas, 333, *424*
Chartism. *See* Britain: Chartism in
child factory labor, 331–32
Chisholm, Colin, 122, 127, 192, 503n21
cholera epidemic, 197, 326, 327, 328. *See also* typhus and typhus epidemic
Christian thought and human unity, 153, 154, 155
Christison, Alexander, 66, 165
Church Missionary Society, 107
Church of England: conversion to, 86; corruption and apathy in, 206; and education, 449; pluralism in, 206; preferment in, 206; reform in, 206. *See also* Bristol College
civilization, detriments of, 233, 235, 309
Clark, George Thomas, 339, 340, 341

Clifton Dispensary, 125, 126–27, 128, 135
climate. *See* environmentalism
Cline, Henry, 50
Clutterbuck, Henry, 277–78
coat of arms and social status, 284
Coleridge, Samuel Taylor, 16, 101
colonialism, 308, 376, 384, 389–90, 407, 432, 434, 436–37
Combe, Andrew, 222–23
Combe, George, 242, 243, 244, 245, 402, 403
Commissioners in Lunacy, 458, 465; asylum inspection reports of, 559n9; colleagues in, 466, 468; duties and powers of, 465, 466, 467; *The Further Report of the Commissioners in Lunacy* (1847), 469; *General Report* (1846), 466; and legal profession, 468; special investigations by, 468; suspicion of, 467; *Treatise on Insanity*'s nosology for, 466. *See also* Alleged Lunatics' Friend Society; asylum legislation; asylums; Metropolitan Commissioners in Lunacy
commission in lunacy (de lunatico inquirendo), 213, 225, 235–36, 457
communication revolution, 410
comparative psychology, 237, 417
"A Comparative Review of Philological and Physical Researches" (1832), 373–74
"connection" and biblical history, 312
Conolly, John, 225, 226, 240, 244, 246, 454, 559n9
contagion, theory of, 196, 281, 514n14
Conybeare, William Daniel, 185, 259, 260, 303–4, 323, 340, 341; accident of, 298; and professorship application, 354, 355
Cooper, Astley, 50, 71
counterirritation, 280, 348. *See also* heroic therapeutics
Cowles, James (great uncle), 27

Cowles, Joseph (relative), 28, 207, 516n58
Cowles, William (great uncle), 26–27
Crania Americana, 401, 402, 403, 404
crania and craniology, 399, 400, 401, 402, 403, 404; Anders Adolph Retzius and, 400, 401; atlas of British, 404; classifying and describing, 170–71, 183–84, 262–63, 404; collecting, 399–400, 483n3; and criminology, 439; and human unity, 170; lectures on, 262–63; in *Physical History*, 400, 401; Robert James Graves and, 401; Samuel George Morton and, 401, 402, 403, 404; terminology for, 183. *See also* phreno-anthropology; phrenology; race and race science
Crania Britannica, 406
creation: and catastrophic destruction, 369; multiple centers of, 182, 410; post-diluvian, 260, 429–30; successive, 183
criminology and degeneration theory, 252
Cross, John, 24
Cross, John Brent, 24, 84, 120
Cross, Margaretta, 24, 487n80
cross-cultural research, 173–74, 203
Cullen, William, 58
cultural relativism, 171, 414, 416
culture, 185–86, 373, 398, 408, 433, 552n52
cupping. *See* bloodletting
Curry, James, 49
Cuvier, Georges, 369, 392
Cyclopaedia of Practical Medicine (1833, 1835), 225–26; "Delerium," 226; "Hypochondriasis," 228–29; "Insanity," 229; moral insanity in, 229; "Somnambulism and Animal Magnetism," 227, 228; "Soundness and Unsoundness of Mind," 227; "Temperament," 226, 227

d'Abbadie, Antoine Thomson, 378

Index · 621

Daniel, Henry, 147, 337–38
Darstellung der Ägyptischen Mythologie (1837), 205, 515n53
Darwin, Charles, 171, 187, 382, 430, 431–32
Darwin, Erasmus, 159
Daubeny, Charles, 344, 357
Davies, Davies, 273–74
Davies, Edward, 41, 313, 489n17
Davis, Joseph Barnard, 406
degeneration theory, 156, 160, 251–52, 372, 393, 418, 439
De generis humani varietate (1808), 165, 495n92
de Gobineau, Arthur, 437
de lunatico inquirendo. *See* commission in lunacy (de lunatico inquirendo)
dementia, 232–33
Dendera Zodiac, 116
descendants, x–xi
diffusion, 182, 183. *See also* migration theory
dissection, 139, 140; for cerebral pathology, 224–25, 230; in Edinburgh, 65, 74; in insanity, 221; of John Horwood, 208. *See also* body snatching
dissent and Dissenters, 15, 16, 299, 322; civil rights of, 198, 299; and exceptions to discrimination, 486n48, 498n31; at Oxbridge, 324; at Scottish universities, 36
Dolphin Society, 112–13, 149
Douglass, Frederick, 447, 463
dualism, mind-body, 178, 214, 216
Duncan, Andrew, 75
Dupin, Charles, 349, 359
Du Ponceau, Peter Stephen, 396, 419
Dyer, Samuel, 22, 487n70
Dyer, Thomas Webb, 131–32, 133, 135

Earl, Pliny, 240
The Eastern Origin of the Celtic Nations (1831), 312, 314; achievement of, 321; and Celtic migration from southwest Asia, 315; citations of Franz Bopp in, 314; comparative linguistic methodology in, 314; dedication of, to Jacob Grimm, 314; as inspiration to Celtic linguists, 316–17; proof of Celtic as Indo-European language in, 314; reviews and opinions of, 315, 316, 317
The Eastern Origin of the Celtic Nations (1857), 320–21
ecstatic affections. *See* animal magnetism; somnambulism
Eden, John, 210, 259, 260, 271–72, 304, 446
Edgeworth, Maria, 95
Edinburgh, journey to, 51–52
Edinburgh, public health resources in, 63
Edinburgh, University of, 57; Celtic studies at, 64, 65, 66, 76; curriculum at, 63–64; education at, 38, 39; fees at, 64, 65; freedom of discussion at, 63; geology at, 58–59, 76–77; graduates of, 56; graduation from, 82–83; science at, 58, 59; student life at, 61–63
Edinburgh, University of, Medical School, 56, 57, 58; advice about, 65; choice of, 36; and the city, 57; courses at, 65, 66, 71, 72, 74, 75; curriculum of, 492n36; examinations at, 81, 82, 83; medical theory at, 74–75; method of education at, 56–57; professors' benefits and detriments at, 59–60; and the Royal Infirmary, 56–57, 64–65. *See also* Royal Medical Society (RMS) of Edinburgh
Edinburgh Phrenological Society, 242
Edinburgh Royal Infirmary, 56–57, 64–65
education, homelife, and leisure (early, of Prichard), 3, 4, 5, 6–7, 23, 25
Edwards, William Frédéric, 391, 393
Egypt, lectures on, *261*, 262, 339, 340
Egypt and India, comparison of, 167, 203

Egyptian chronology, 203, 204, 420
Egyptian mythology. See *An Analysis of the Egyptian Mythology* (1819)
environmentalism, 162–63, 164, 416, 420, 425–26. *See also* evolution and evolutionary theory
epidemics. *See* cholera epidemic; typhus and typhus epidemic
epilepsy, 113, 220, 222, 224
Esquirol, Jean-Étienne Dominique, 229, 230, 239, 249, 333
Established Church. *See* Church of England
the Establishment, 485n16
Estlin, Edward Rochemont, 140, 273
Estlin, John Bishop, 70, 101, 134, 149–50, 310, 446–47, 502n5; and anti-slavery, 330–31, 447, 463. *See also* Bristol Eye Dispensary
Estlin, John Prior, 104, 189, 190
Estlin, Mary Anne, 330, 447
Estlin, Susanna (Bishop; mother-in-law), 446
Estlin family, 104
ethnographic data, 180–81, 184, 412, 475
Ethnological Queries, 381, 382, 383, 389, 542n31. *See also* Ethnology Subsection (BAAS)
Ethnological Society of London, 385, 386, 387, 397, 398, 554n63; administration of, 386; aims of, 385–86; foundation of, 385; later history of, 389; membership of, 387, 397; presidential address to, 398
"Ethnology" (1849), 432, 433
ethnology, terminology of, 371–72. *See also* anthropology
Ethnology Subsection (BAAS), 374, 380, 383, 391, 398. *See also* British Association for the Advancement of Science (BAAS); *Ethnological Queries*
European exceptionalism, xvii, 157, 390, 437
evolution and evolutionary theory, 158, 159, 162, 430, 431–32; and British

society, 368; and Darwinism, 186–87; F. W. Newman discussion about, 409, 410; transcendental anatomy and, 343–44; of varieties, 170, 171, 172. *See also* natural theologians and natural theology
expectant therapeutics, 143, 274, 277. *See also* heroic therapeutics
extra-Europeans and "the Other," 190, 251, 252, 393

Faber, G. S., 116
Factories Act, 331–32
family life. *See* education, homelife, and leisure (early, of Prichard); Red Lodge
Faraday, Michael, 476
fever hospital, 191, 192, 193–94, 281. *See also* Morgan, Susanna
fieldwork, anthropological, 383, 386, 388, 432, 441, 444. See also *Admiralty Manual of Scientific Enquiry*; *Ethnological Queries*
First Cause, 159, 295, 368. *See also* natural theologians and natural theology; science and religion
Fisher, Francis (uncle), 21, 131
Fisher, George, Jr., 113, 120
Fisher, Sarah (Prichard; aunt), 21
Fishponds House Private Lunatic Asylum, 467
Fodéré, François-Emmanuel, 238
Forbes, Edward, 429
Forbes, John, 225
Forster, Georg, 157
Forster, Johann Reinhold, 157
Foville, Achille-Louis, 332
Fox, Edward Long, 19, 124, 132–33, 467
Fox, Henry Hawes: at Bristol Infirmary, 132, 135, 145, 328; at St. Peter's Hospital, 122, 123–24, 125
France, 264–68, 332, 333
Friends, Society of, 5–6; ancestors' membership of, 25–26; and anti-slave trade, 8, 154, 308; in Bristol,

Index · 623

Friends, Society of (*continued*) 485n17; and doctrinal issues, 87–88; erosion in faith in, 23; poor opinion of, 86–87; resignation from, 86
Friends Monthly Magazine, 308
The Further Report of the Commissioners in Lunacy (1847), 469

"Gagging Acts," 205
Gall, Franz Joseph, 216, 226–27, 242, 244
Gallatin, Albert, 395, 396, 397, 413
Garrison, William Lloyd, 463
Gate Helmsley Retreat, York, 468
Gayton (near Ross), 27–28
general paralysis of the insane (GPI), 232, 234
General Report (1846), 466
Geoffroy Saint-Hilaire, Étienne, 296, 369
Geographical Society of London, 393, 394, 395
geologizing, 109, 113
geology, 58, 59, 158, 183, 259, 260
geology articles, 113–14. *See also* science and religion
George III, 102, 205, 213
Georget, Étienne-Jean, 233, 238
German: ethnology, 541n13; historians, 354; learning of, 111, 199; linguists, 316, 320, 396, 397; resources in *Physical History*, 183, 510n40; sentiment against, 398; translation of *Physical History of Mankind* (3rd ed.), 420
Germany, visit to, 298
germ theory of disease, 196–97
Gibson, William, 443
Gilby, William Hall, 109, 114, 127
Gliddon, George, 397, 405–6, 437
Gloucestershire Madhouses, Medical Visitor to, 449–50, 467
Grant, Robert, 368
Graves, Robert James, 401, 411
Great Chain of Being, 156, 160, 390

Greeks, 269–70
Greenough, George Bellas, 387, 395
Gregorian physic, 71–72
Gregory, James, 60, 71–72, 277
Griscom, John, 202, 515n40
Guanches, 308–9
Guide for Gentlemen Studying Medicine (J. Johnson), 65
Guislain, Joseph, 238
Guy's Hospital, London, 47, 48, 49

Haighton, John, 47, 48–49
Hall, Benjamin. *See* Llanover, Baron
Hamden, Renn, 80
Hamilton, James, 72
Hamilton, William Rowan, 347, 349, 395
Hancock, Thomas, 69–70, 79, 88, 292
Harcourt, William Vernon, 323, 348, 352
Harford, John Scandrett, 257–58, 293
Harfords, 2–3
Haydock Lodge Asylum, 467–68
Hebrew poetry, 308
Heinroth, J. C. A., 238
Herapath, William, 342
heroic therapeutics, 71–72, 113, 141, 142–43, 222, 274, 277, 278, 282. *See also* bloodletting; counterirritation; medical philosophy
Herschel, John, 432, 552n50
Hetling, William, 146
A History of the Epidemic Fever (1820), 194–97. *See also* typhus and typhus epidemic
Hodgkin, Thomas, 374, 375; anthropological network of, 375–76, 378, 379–80, 389, 545n65; and the Ethnological Society of London, 371, 385, 386; humanitarian anthropology of, 375–76, 411, 421; publications of, 542n17; and Select Committee on Aborigines, 376. *See also* Aborigines' Protection Society; *Ethnological Queries*; Ethnological Society

of London; Ethnology Subsection
(BAAS)
Hodgson, William Brown, 397
Hoffbauer, Johann Christoph, 236
holidays in France and Switzerland,
  264–68, 332, 333
Holland, Henry, 81–82, 83, 274, 428
Home, James, 75
homes (of Prichard): 1 Woburn Place,
  London, 462; 12 Berkeley Square,
  105, 208; 39 College Green, 107, 108,
  499n57; 47 Park Street, 4–5, 487n73;
  Ross, 1, 21; Somerset Street, 1–2
honorary MD, Oxford, 344, 345, 346
Hope, Thomas Charles, 58, 65–66
Horwood, John, 207, 208
The Hospital Pupil (Parkinson), 35, 36
Hotwells, 11, 12, 91, 503n25. *See also*
  Clifton Dispensary
Howell, John, 145–46
Hudson, John, 85
human species. *See* polygenism and
  monogenism; unity of human
  species
"human zoo," 421
Humboldt, Alexander von, 175, 350,
  419, 420
Humboldt, Wilhelm von, 413
Hume, John Robert, 466
humoral medicine, 276–77. *See also*
  medical philosophy
Hunt, Henry "Orator," 91, 105
hypnotism. *See* Mesmer, Anton, and
  mesmerism
hypochondriasis, 228–29, 518n39

idiots, congenital, 454–55
illness, final, 177, 178
illustrations, 392, 400, 408, 422–23,
  548n16
"improvement," 35, 92, 197, 206, 213,
  242
incoherence. *See* dementia
India and Egypt, comparison of, 167,
  203

Indigenous peoples, extermination of,
  309, 377, 378, 425, 436
inheritance of acquired characteristics. *See* Lamarck, Jean Baptist, and
  Lamarckism
insanity: causes of, 217, 221–22, 230,
  233, 234, 235, 249; and civilization,
  217, 230, 233–34, 250; and criminal
  responsibility, 225, 230; curability
  of, 218; definition of, 220–21, 231;
  in family and society, 225, 235, 236;
  among friends and family, 24, 25;
  inspiration to study, 212; jurisprudence of, 235, 236, 246–47, 248;
  moral treatment of, 215, 222, 230,
  234, 250, 454, 455, 469, 517n9; and
  pessimism, 249, 250; prognosis in,
  233; psychicist or mentalist theory
  of, 237, 238; somatist theory of, 237,
  238; statistical evidence of, 233–34,
  235; stigma of, 470–71; suicide and,
  237; visceral origin of, 218, 221–22,
  238, 249. *See also* moral insanity;
  On the Different Forms of Insanity
  (1842); *A Treatise on Diseases of the
  Nervous System* (1822); *A Treatise
  on Insanity* (1835)
"instinctive hereditary propensities,"
  426
interbreeding theory in *Natural History*, 426
Iolo Morganwg, 115–16
irresistible impulse, 227, 236, 247

Jablonski, Paul Ernst, 202
Jacobi, K. W. M., 238, 249
Jameson, Robert, 59, 76–77, 162,
  492n18
Jews, civil rights of, 486n48
Jews and Catholics in Bristol, 299, 300
Jones, William, 165, 168, 174, 315
*Journal of the Ethnological Society of
  London*, 387
*Journal of the Geographical Society of
  London*, 394, 395

Index · 625

Kames, Lord, 161
Kant, Immanuel, 156
Keith, Arthur, 479
Kentish, Edward, 122, 129
Kidd, John, 344, 345, 346
King, Richard, 377, 387–88, 544n51; and Ethnological Society of London, 385, 386, 387
Kingston, Earl of, 225
Klaproth, Julius, 184–85, 425
Knox, Robert, 437, 553n55
Koreans in *Natural History*, 424

Lamarck, Jean Baptist, and Lamarckism, 166, 170, 416. See also evolution and evolutionary theory
language: as anthropological tool, 165, 312, 314–15; as evidence of monogenism, 165; Indo-European, 312, 314, 315; learning French, 3, 23; love of Welsh, 312–13. See also *The Eastern Origin of the Celtic Nations* (1831); linguistics
La Peyrère, Isaac, 156, 392
Laromiguière, Pierre, 238
Latham, Robert Gordon, 320–21, 397, 429, 551n44
laughing gas, 42–43, 362
Lavater, Johan Caspar, 242
Lawrence, William, 178, 179, 294, 430–31, 511n65
leeching. See bloodletting
legal profession and Lunacy Commission, 468
Leibniz, Gottfried Wilhelm, 165, 510n40
Lepsius, D. R., 318, 319
Leslie, John, 55–56
Lewis, John (maternal grandfather), 29, 30
Lewis, Mary (Morgan; maternal grandmother), 29, 30
Ley, Mary (Prichard; daughter), 189, 343, 358–59, 360, 470
linguistics: comparative, 168; contributions to, 317, 321, 480–81; in *Eastern Origin*, 314; Indo-European, 315; in MD dissertation, 165; in *Physical History of Man* (1813), 167, 173; in *Physical History of Mankind* (1826), 184–85; in *Physical History of Mankind* (3rd ed.), 419
linguists, American, 396, 397
Linnean Society of London, election to, 179–80, 512n66
Llanover, Baron, 317, 318. See also Abergavenny Eisteddfod
Llanover, Lady, 317
London: homelife in, 462, 463; move to, 462; scientific societies in, 463; social life in, 463
London Labour and the London Poor, 351
Long, Edward, 158
Lowe, Richard, 146, 507n85
lunacy. See insanity
Lunacy Act (1845), 456–57. See also Commissioners in Lunacy
Lunacy Commissioners. See Commissioners in Lunacy; Metropolitan Commissioners in Lunacy
Lutwidge, R. W. S., 466
Lyell, Charles, 341, 354, 431, 538n67

Mackenzie, Charles, 80–81
Mackenzie, Kenneth Francis, 80
Mackenzie, Patrick, 81
mad-doctors. See insanity; psychiatry
madhouses. See insanity; psychiatry
madness. See insanity
mania, 230, 231, 233
manie sans délire. See moral insanity
manuscripts and family documents, x, 446
Martineau, Harriet, 353–54, 381
Martineau, James, 290
materialism, 154, 159, 179, 295, 297, 352, 366–67. See also evolution and evolutionary theory; science and religion
Maupertuis, Pierre Louis, 158
Max Muller, Friedrich, 398, 442
MD dissertation, 165, 495n92

Medical Book Society, 150
medical charities. *See* Bristol medical charities
medical degrees, testimonial versus university, 37-38, 133, 134
medical education, 36, 333, 334, 335, 488n6; history of, 38-39; at Oxbridge, 39; with Robert Pope, 45, 46; at St. Thomas and Guy's Hospitals, 47, 48, 49, 50; with Thomas Pole, 42, 43, 44; with William Tothill, 46-47. *See also* Edinburgh, University of, Medical School
medical etiquette, 37, 273-74
medical lectures, 110, 132
Medical Officers of Asylums and Hospitals for the Insane, 457
medical philosophy, 275, 276, 277. *See also* humoral medicine
medical profession, 34, 35, 36, 37, 38, 274-75, 334, 335
medical progress, 139, 197, 276, 280-81, 282, 481
Medical Reading Society, 150-51
Medical Reform Bill, 335
medical statistics, 191, 192, 193, 194; at Clifton Dispensary, 127; on insanity, 233, 235
medical therapeutics. *See* bloodletting; expectant therapeutics; heroic therapeutics
Melville, Herman, 250
memberships, honorary: Académie des Sciences Morales et Politiques, Institut de France, 362; Académie Nationale de Médecine, 362; Academy of Science of Siena, 259; American Oriental Society, 396; American Philosophical Society, 362; Bombay Branch of the Royal Asiatic Society, 463-64; Royal College of Physicians of Ireland, 537n39; Royal Irish Academy, 537n39; Royal Medical Society, 449
Mesmer, Anton, and mesmerism, 216, 227-28

Metropolitan Commissioners in Lunacy, 422, 450, 456, 457, 556n17. *See also* asylum legislation; Commissioners in Lunacy
Meyer, Karl, 319, 320
migration theory, 165, 172, 176, 312
Miller, J. S., 257
Mithridates (Adelung), 115
M'Naghten Rules, 248
Moline, Mary (Prichard; sister), 111, 254
Monboddo, James Burnet, Lord, 161-62
monogenism and monogenists. *See* unity of human species
monomania (partial insanity), 231
monotheism, original, 116, 168, 336, 384, 417-18
Monro, Alexander, 60, 74
Montesquieu, 156
Moore, Thomas, 349
moral insanity: American views on, 240; definition of (1822), 221; definition of (1833), 229; definition of (1835), 231-32; goals in gaining acceptance of, 232; and irresistible impulse, 236; in later psychiatric nosology, 252; legal profession's criticisms of, 247-48; objections to, 239, 252; research on, 230, 231; variations in, 232. *See also* insanity
moral management, 455
moral treatment, 222, 230, 234, 454, 455
More, Hannah, 16, 17
Morgan, Kitty, 4, 44-45
Morgan, Susanna, 106, 193
Morgan family, 29-30
Morison, Alexander, 214, 463
Morton, Samuel George, 391, 401, 402, 403, 404, 411. *See also Crania Americana*
Mosaic Records, 508n2
moxas, 280. *See also* counterirritation
Müller, Johannes von. *See An Universal History, in Twenty-Four Books* (1818)
Muller, W. J., 523n15

Murray, Alexander, 201
Mylne, William James, 468

Napoleon, abdication of, 109
Nasse, C. F., 238
National Society for the Education of the Poor in the Principles of the Established Church, 111
Native peoples, extermination of, 309, 377, 378, 425, 436
natural historical methodology, 159
The Natural History of Man (1843), 421–22, *424*; dedication of, to Baron von Bunsen, 422; environmentalism in, 425–26; ethnographic maps in, 423, 425; illustrations in, 422–23, *424*; influence of, 428–29; "instinctive hereditary propensities" in, 426; interbreeding theory in, 426; later editions of, 427; motivation to publish, 425; racialist expressions in, 426–27; reviews of, 427–28
natural philosophy. *See* science
natural theologians and natural theology, 158, 159, 369. *See also* science and religion
necroscopical researches, 234
Nelson, Lord, 41
neologisms. *See* terminology and neologisms
neurosis. *See* hypochondriasis
New Harmony IN, opinion of, 272
Newman, Elizabeth (aunt), 284, 290–91
Newman, Francis William, 305, 409, 410, 478
Newman, Josiah (uncle), 291
newspapers, 97
Nicolucci, Giustiniano, 440
non-restraint, 454
Northwoods Asylum, 467
Nott, Josiah, 405–6, 437

On the Different Forms of Insanity (1842), 246, 247–49

"On the Extinction of Human Races" (1840), 380–81
"On the Relations of Ethnology to Other Branches of Knowledge" (1847), 398
Origin of Pagan Idolatry (Faber), 116
"the Other," 251, 252, 393, 421
Owen, Richard, 399, 429–30
Oxbridge (Oxford and Cambridge), 85, 86, 88. *See also* Cambridge, University of; Oxford, University of
Oxford, University of, 86, 88, 354. *See also* Oxbridge (Oxford and Cambridge)
Oxford honorary MD, 344, 345, 346
Oxford Movement, 365
Oxford professorships, 353, 354; of modern history, 354, 355, 356–57; of philology, 357; of Sanskrit, 353

paleontology and archaeology, 398, 399, 400
Paley, William, 158, 159
Parkinson, James, 35–36
patients, 282–84, 498n32
Peace, John, 96
Peel, Robert, 355
"permanent varieties" in *Physical History of Mankind* (3rd ed.), 416, 431
pessimism and insanity, 249, 250
Pettigrew, Thomas Joseph, 535n18
Phil & Lit. *See* Bristol Institution: Philosophical and Literary Society of; Bristol Institution Philosophical and Literary Society lectures
philology. *See* linguistics
phreno-anthropology, 390, 391, 392. *See also* phrenology
phrenologists, 243, 244–45
phrenology, 216, 242, 243; alienists and, 244; attack on, 237; criticisms of, 244, 245; *Cyclopaedia* attack on, 227; decline of, 246; French, 245; lecture against, 245; legacy of, 245;

thriving state of, 243–44. *See also* phreno-anthropology

Physical History of Man (1813), 166, 167, 177, 178; anti-polygenism in, 171; biogeography and geology in, 172; biological argument in, 167, 169, 170, 171, 172, 173; Black to white skin theory in, 172–73; civilization (domestication) and human variation in, 171–72; craniometry in, 170–71; credibility of data in, 174; culture in, 166, 167, 173, 174; environmentalism in, 169–70, 172; ethnology in, 173, 174, 175, 176; evolution of varieties in, 170, 171, 172; linguistics in, 166, 167, 168; migration in, 176; publication of, 108–9; resources for, 167, 168, 169; reviews of, 177; Scripture in, 168–69; sexual selection in, 171; single human origin in, 174–76; spontaneous congenital variation in, 170; unity of human species in, 166–67

Physical History of Mankind (1826), 180, 181, 182; biological adaptation in, 181; catastrophism (successive creations) in, 183; Celtic in, 185; civilization in, 181, 182; craniometry in, 183; culture in, 185; diffusion in, 182; environmentalism in, 181, 182; ethnographic data in, 180–81, 184; five human varieties in, 183; German citations in, 183; the "germ" in, 181; linguistic data in, 184–85; multiple centers of creation in, 182, 183; race in, 183–84; reviews of, 185–86; Scripture references in, 183; sexual selection in, 181; skin color in, 181–82, 183; spontaneous connate variation in, 181, 182; unity of human species in, 184

Physical History of Mankind (3rd ed.), 408–9, 411, 412; adjustments to arguments in, 420; cultural relativism in, 414, 416; futility of racial boundaries in, 414; illustrations in, 414; influence of, 428–29; migration and origin in biblical lands in, 416–17; motivation to publish, 420–21; "permanent varieties" in, 416; psychic unity in, 414, 417; Scripture as evidence in, 418–19, 420; seven human varieties in, 416; social evolution in, 414, 415, 417–18; translation of, 420; varieties through congenital change in, 416; volume 1 of, 411–12; volume 2 of, 412; volume 3 of, 412–13; volume 4 of, 413; volume 5 of, 413

Physical Society of Guy's Hospital, 49

Pickering, John, 395, 396, 399, 435, 463

Pinel, Philippe, 221, 229, 230, 454, 517n9

Pinkerton, John, 313, 315

Playfair, John, 59, 73

plumping, 105, 499n52

pluralism, 206. *See also* Church of England

plurality, human. *See* polygenism and monogenism; unity of human species

Pocock, Edith (Prichard; daughter), 298, 446, 555n6

Pocock, Theodore (descendant), xi–xii

Pole, John, 44, 47

Pole, Thomas, 42, 43, 44

polygenism and monogenism, 163, 185–86, 435–36, 437, 508n5. *See also* race and race science; unity of human species

Poor Law, 341

Pope, Robert, 46, 490n33

portrait by Nathan Branwhite, *xv*, 272

postal service, 98

pre-Adamism and non-Adamism, 156. *See also* race and race science

preferment, 206. *See also* Church of England

Index · 629

Price, Thomas "Carnhuanawc," 320
Prichard, Albert Hermann (son), 312, 447
Prichard, Ann (Cowles; paternal grandmother), 26–27
Prichard, Anna Maria (daughter), 105
Prichard, Anna Maria (Estlin; wife), 103, *104*, 499n60
Prichard, Augustin (son), 206, 358, 451–53
Prichard, Constantine Estlin (son), 206, 366, 475, 476
Prichard, Edward (brother), 84, 101, 105, 108, 112, 208, 310, 311, 500n71
Prichard, Edward (great grandfather), 26
Prichard, Edward Cowles (descendant), xi
Prichard, Francis (son), 189
Prichard, Illtudus Thomas ("Illty," "Hillty"; son), 273, 453
Prichard, James Cowles, Jr. ("Jem"; son), 109, 321–22, 357, 364, 365, 366
Prichard, James Cowles, works of: *Admiralty Manual of Scientific Enquiry*, 432–33, 552n50, 552n52, 553n53; *An Analysis of the Egyptian Mythology* (1819), 202–5; *An Analysis of the Egyptian Mythology* (1838), 205; "Cases of Typhus Fever" (1817), 192–93; "A Comparative Review of Philological and Physical Researches" (1832), 373–74; *Cyclopaedia of Practical Medicine* articles (1833, 1835), 225–29; *Darstellung der Ägyptischen Mythologie* (1837), 205, 515n53; *De generis humani varietate* (1808), 165, 495n92; *The Eastern Origin of the Celtic Nations* (1831), 312–21; *The Eastern Origin of the Celtic Nations* (1857), 320–21; *Ethnological Queries*, 381–83, 389, 542n31; "Ethnology" (1849), 432–34; *A History of the Epidemic Fever* (1820), 194–97; *The Natural History of Man* (1843), 421–48; *On the Different Forms of Insanity* (1842), 246–49; "On the Extinction of Human Races" (1840), 380–81; "On the Relations of Ethnology to Other Branches of Knowledge" (1847), 398; "Remarks on the Treatment of Paralysis" (1824), 224, 269; "Retrospective Address" (PMSA) (1835), 345–46; *Review of the Doctrine of a Vital Principle* (1829), 292–97; *Six Ethnographical Maps* (1843), 423, 425; *A Treatise on Diseases of the Nervous System* (1822), 216–24; *A Treatise on Insanity* (1835), 229–41; "Treatment of Some Diseases of the Brain" (1831), 348; *An Universal History, in Twenty-Four Books* (1818), 199–201. See also *Physical History of Man* (1813); *Physical History of Mankind* (1826); *Physical History of Mankind* (3rd ed.)
Prichard, Mary "Polly" (Lewis; mother), 28–29
Prichard, Roger (ancestor), 26
Prichard, Samuel (relative), 207, 496n101
Prichard, Theodore Joseph ("The"; son), 208, 471–74
Prichard, Thomas (father), 4, 5, 6, 22, 28, 52–54, 82, 84, 103, 228, 229, 254, 269, 285, 286, 291, 292, 328, 331, 332, 487n65; advice from, 69, 70, 71, 73, 209, 270, 322, 323; business interests of, 2, 9, 11, 21, 22, 83–84, 273; character and death of, 459–60; on Church of England corruption, 201; memoir of, xi, xii, *xxiv*, 1, 475; on Peace Society, 292; politics of, 73, 270–71, 285, 310; proposed baptism of, 459; and sacred poetry, 291; and theology, 68–69, 70, 104, 201, 209, 254–55, 270, 271, 285, 333

Prichard, Thomas I (grandfather), 26
Prichard, Tom (brother), 41–42, 84, 101, 108, 112, 190, 254, 284, 297–98, 321, 342–43
Prichard children, education of, 298, 357–58. *See also* Bristol College
Prichard children's names, 207
"Prichard issue" or "tomahawk," 280. *See also* counterirritation
Priestly, Joseph, 100, 293
Princess Caraboo, 190
Procter, Brian Waller, 466
professorships. *See* Oxford professorships
Provincial Medical and Surgical Association (PMSA), 334–35, 344
Provincial Medical and Surgical Journal, 249
Prudent Man's Friend Society, 106
psychiatric profession. *See* Medical Officers of Asylums and Hospitals for the Insane
psychiatry, 212–13, 214, 215, 216; contributions to, 481; County Asylums Act (1828) and, 215; dualism and materialism and, 214, 216–17, 218; early history of, 214, 215; German theories and, 216; House of Commons Select Committee Report (1815) and, 213; humoral terminology in, 519n45; influence on later, 251; later biological determinism in, 251; later degeneration theory in, 251–52; mad-doctors and madhouses and, 213–14; medical statistics in, 215–16; mesmerism and phrenology in, 216; psychicist or mentalist theory in, 237–38; reformism and, 213; science and, 215, 216, 251–52; in society, 213, 470–71; somatist theory in, 238; use of terminology of, anachronistically, 516n2. *See also* Commissioners in Lunacy; insanity; phrenology; *A Treatise on Insanity* (1835)

psychicist or mentalist theory, 237–38
psychic unity in *Physical History of Mankind* (3rd ed.), 414, 416, 417, 549n20
publishing, promotion and rewards of, 410–11

race and race science, xvi–xvii, 156, 157, 160, 161, 183–84, 434, 435; adapted to psychiatry, 439; American, 185, 186, 435, 436, 438; and Anthropological Society of London, 437–38; ascendancy of, in Britain, 434, 435, 436–37, 438; "biologizing," 438, 439; and degenerationist anthropometry, 439; and "extinction discourse," 438; in France, 392, 393, 437, 439; invalidity of anthropometry in, 439; in later nineteenth century, 437, 438, 439, 440; in *Physical History of Mankind* (3rd ed.), 414. *See also* Caldwell, Charles; *Crania Americana*; crania and craniology; Gliddon, George; Morton, Samuel George; polygenism and monogenism
radicals and radicalism, 91, 92, 206, 368
railways, 325, 364
Rask, Rasmus, 204–5
Ray, Isaac, 240
Red Lodge, 112, 358–59, 360, 363; BAAS at, 349; building, 287–88, 289, 361, 363, 539n87; Carl Ritter at, 445, 446; family life at, 358, 361–62, 446; social life at, 288, 330, 349, 359, 360; Walter Bagehot at, 288, 289–90
reform and reformism, 310, 311, 332; of asylums, 213; Bristol Auxiliary Temperance Society and, 335–36; and child factory labor and Factories Act, 331–32; and Church of England, 206; Electoral Reform Bill and Act (1832) and, 325, 327, 332; and insanity in society, 225;

reform and reformism (*continued*)
of Oxbridge education, 354; statistics and, 350, 351
religion: and biblical evidence in *Natural History*, 426; and biblical evidence in *Physical History*, 418, 420; and personal belief in Revelation, 200–201; as social evolutionary process, 417, 418. *See also* Bristol religion; science and religion
"Remarks on the Treatment of Paralysis" (1824), 224, 269
remittance man, 536n29
Report of the Metropolitan Commissioners in Lunacy (1844), 456
"Retrospective Address" (PMSA) (1835), 345, 346
Retzius, Anders Adolph, 400, 401, 438
Review of the Doctrine of a Vital Principle (1829), 292–93, 294, 295, 296, 297
Reynolds, Richard, 3, 27, 106, 499n54, 505n45
Riley, Henry, 140, 146, 343, 344
riots. *See* Bristol: riots in
Ritter, Carl, x, 183, 354, 445–46
Roget, Peter Mark, 244
Rolleston, George, 479–80
Rosetta Stone, 339, 340
Rotch, Benjamin, 21
Roy, Ram Mohan, 336–37, 338, 414, 415, 548n16
Royal College of Physicians license examination, 458
Royal Medical Society (RMS) of Edinburgh, 66–68, 78–79; Azygotic friendships in, 79, 80, 81; case histories of, 77, 78; committee involvement with, 78; dissertation for, 77, 78, 162, 163
Royal Society, 284, 395–96
Rutherford, Daniel, 75

salvage ethnology, 437
Sanders, Thomas, 135

Schlegel, August Wilhelm von, 205, 316, 359, 513n84
Schlegel, Friedrich, 116
Schomburgk, R. H., 379, 413
science: in Bristol, 42, 43; in British society, 370; early interest in, 32–33; of humankind, 156–57, 178, 323; introduction of modern term of, 489n25; medicine as, 34; professionalization of, 369; Scottish Enlightenment and, 55, 56, 157. *See also* First Cause; natural theologians and natural theology; *Review of the Doctrine of a Vital Principle* (1829); science and religion
science and religion, 33, 157, 158, 159, 177, 178, 341–42, 352, 367–68, 369, 370, 409–10, 508n3; at the BAAS, 323–24; in geology, 58–59; Thomas Prichard's views on, 69. *See also* dualism, mind-body; First Cause; natural theologians and natural theology; *Review of the Doctrine of a Vital Principle* (1829)
scientific medicine, 237, 345–46, 348–49
scientific method in psychiatry, 215–16, 251
the seed, 295
Select Committee on Aborigines, 376
Selmer, Harald, 240
Serres, Étienne, 439
Seyer, Samuel, 95–96
Shute, Thomas, 147
Six Ethnographical Maps, 423, 425
skeletons, call for national collection of, 400
skin color: in "Of the Varieties of the Human Race," 164; in *Physical History* and *Natural History*, 550n31; in *Physical History of Man* (1813), 172–73; in *Physical History of Mankind* (1826), 181, 182; of Ram Mohan Roy, 548n16. *See also* Black to white skin theory; white/light to Black skin theory

skull. *See* crania and craniology
slave trade, 8, 9, 154, 485n20
Slavonic nations, article on, 340, 341
sleepwalking, 227
Smith, Charles Hamilton, 435
Smith, Nathaniel, 147
Smith, Richard, 146, 207, 208
Smith, Samuel Stanhope, 158, 164, 431
social and political unrest, British, 273, 309, 310, 332, 368, 427, 477
social evolution: in *Physical History of Man* (1813), 168; in *Physical History of Mankind* (3rd ed.), 414, 415, 417–18; in Scottish Enlightenment thought, 157, 161–62, 168
social life. *See* Red Lodge
Société de Géographie de Paris, 393
Société des Observateurs de l'Homme, 381, 386
Société Ethnologique de Paris, 369–70, 386, 393
Society for the Diffusion of Useful Knowledge (SDUK), 421, 549n27
Society for the Extinction of the Slave Trade, 384
Society for the Publication of Ancient Welsh Manuscripts, 318
Society of Friends. *See* Friends, Society of
Socinianism and antitrinitarianism, 487n79
somatist theory, 238
Sömmerring, Samuel Thomas von, 158, 226
somnambulism, 227
Southey, Robert, 16, 290, 460
species as "permanent varieties" in *Physical History of Mankind* (3rd ed.), 416
Spurzheim, Johann, 242
ss *Great Britain*, 445
Starbuck, Daniel, 21
statistics and data: for fever, 191, 192, 193, 194; love of, 350; Lunacy Commission and, 466; psychiatric, 215–16; in scientific practice, 350; for social policies, 351. *See also* Bristol Statistical Society
Stewart, Dugald, 56, 73, 76, 162
Stock, John Edmonds, 133, 138, 144–45
Stock, Thomas, 134–35
St. Peter's Hospital, 120, 121, *121*, 122, 123, 124–25, 502n11, 534n116; appointment to, 122; cholera at, 328; duties at, 122; Lunacy Commission criticisms of, 466; lunatics at, 121, 122, 123, 124, 125, 212; resignation from, 328; typhus at, 189, 191
The Strange Case of Dr. Jekyll and Mr. Hyde (Stevenson), 250
St. Thomas's Hospital, London, 47, 49, 50
suicide, 472, 473. *See also* insanity; Prichard, Theodore Joseph ("The"; son)
Sumner, John Bird, 159
surgery, strides in, 276
Swayne, William, 143
Symonds, John Addington, 307–8, 360
Symons, Benjamin Parsons, 305

Temperance Movement, 335–36
Ten Hour Movement, 331–32
terminology, misleading and offensive, xxi, xxii, 541n14
terminology and neologisms, 320, 400, 419–20
Test Act, 57, 88, 98–99, 101
Thurnam, John, 406
Ticehurst Asylum, 457, 465–66
T. Kerslake's Catalogue, ix–x
Tory, 486n47
Tory allegiance, 105, 301, 327
Tothill, William, 46, 47, 199
Townsend, Joseph, 114
Tractarianism, 365
transformism. *See* evolution and evolutionary theory
transmutation. *See* evolution and evolutionary theory

traveling, cost of, 97–98
A Treatise on Diseases of the Nervous System (1822): brain and mind in, 216–17, 218–19, 221; influence of, 223–24; insanity in, 220–21, 222; nervous diseases and epilepsy in, 220, 222; reviews of, 222–23; vital principle in, 220. *See also* insanity
A Treatise on Insanity (1835): aims of, 230, 232; causes of insanity in, 233–34; definition and types of insanity in, 231–32, 233; influence of, 240, 241; jurisprudence of insanity in, 235–37; moral treatment in, 230, 234; research for, 229, 230, 237–38; reviews of, 238, 239, 240; therapeutics of insanity in, 234; translation of, 240. *See also* insanity
"Treatment of Some Diseases of the Brain" (1831), 348
Triangular Trade. *See* Bristol: and Triangular Trade
Trophonius, Cave of, 69, 493n45
tuberculosis, 272–73, 461, 471
Tuke, Samuel, 230, 234, 454
tutors and teachers, 3, 23, 484n5
Tweedie, Alexander, 225, 229, 478
Tylor, Edward Burnett, 174, 316, 428–29, 433, 441, 479, 552n52, 553n53
typhus and typhus epidemic, 189, 191, 192, 193, 194, 513n10; and "Cases of Typhus" (1817), 192, 193; fever hospital and, 191, 193–94; in *A History of the Epidemic Fever* (1820), 194, 195, 196, 197

Ueber die Sprache und Weisheit der Indier (Schlegel), 116
Unitarianism, 100, 101–2, 189–90, 290
unity of human species, xvii, 33, 153–54, 155, 163, 164, 179, 183–84, 417, 420, 425. *See also* polygenism and monogenism; race and race science
An Universal History, in Twenty-Four Books (1818), 199, 200–201

University of Edinburgh. *See* Edinburgh, University of
University of Oxford. *See* Oxford, University of

Vestiges, 368, 430
Villemarqué, T. C. H. Hersart de la, 318
Virey, Julien-Joseph, 154, 392
vitalism, 228. See also *Review of the Doctrine of a Vital Principle* (1829)
voting record (of Prichard), 499n52

Wagner, Rudolf, 297, 420
Wait, Daniel, 122, 131
Wales, traveling in, 21–22, 313
Walker, Isaac, 27
Walker, John, 27, 165
Wallace, Alfred Russel, 186
Wallis, George, 140, 145
Washington, John, 394, 395
Wells, William Charles, 49–50, 491n45
Welsh: ancestry, 25; and Edward Davies, 41; and Edward Williams, 115–16; English denigration of, 312, 313; love of, 312–13; revival of, 313–14. *See also* Abergavenny Eisteddfod; Celtic; *The Eastern Origin of the Celtic Nations* (1831)
Werner, Abraham Gottlob, 59
West of England Journal, 340–41
Whately, Richard, 369
Whewell, William, xvi, 350, 354, 355, 356
Whig, 486n47
White, Charles, 154, 158
white/light to Black skin theory, 160, 164. *See also* Black to white skin theory; race and race science; skin color
Wilde, William, 346, 400, 448
Wilkins, Ann (Prichard; aunt), 28, 338
Wilkins, Charlotte (cousin), 358
Wilkins, Mary (cousin), 338–39, 343
Williams, Edward, 115–16
Wilson, Daniel, 439–40
women and scholarship, 358

Worrall, Samuel "Devil," 198, 199

Yates, James, 272, 414
Young, Thomas, 204, 262, 339

Zodiac of Dendera, 116

In the Critical Studies in the History of Anthropology series

Invisible Genealogies: A History of Americanist Anthropology
Regna Darnell

The Shaping of American Ethnography: The Wilkes Exploring Expedition, 1838–1842
Barry Alan Joyce

Ruth Landes: A Life in Anthropology
Sally Cole

Melville J. Herskovits and the Racial Politics of Knowledge
Jerry Gershenhorn

Leslie A. White: Evolution and Revolution in Anthropology
William J. Peace

Rolling in Ditches with Shamans: Jaime de Angulo and the Professionalization of American Anthropology
Wendy Leeds-Hurwitz

Irregular Connections: A History of Anthropology and Sexuality
Andrew P. Lyons and Harriet D. Lyons

Ephraim George Squier and the Development of American Anthropology
Terry A. Barnhart

Ruth Benedict: Beyond Relativity, Beyond Pattern
Virginia Heyer Young

Looking through Taiwan: American Anthropologists' Collusion with Ethnic Domination
Keelung 'Hong and Stephen O. Murray

Visionary Observers: Anthropological Inquiry and Education
Jill B. R. Cherneff and Eve Hochwald
Foreword by Sydel Silverman

Anthropology Goes to the Fair: The 1904 Louisiana Purchase Exposition
Nancy J. Parezo and Don D. Fowler

The Meskwaki and Anthropologists: Action Anthropology Reconsidered
Judith M. Daubenmier

The 1904 Anthropology Days and Olympic Games: Sport, Race, and American Imperialism
Edited by Susan Brownell

Lev Shternberg: Anthropologist, Russian Socialist, Jewish Activist
Sergei Kan

Contributions to Ojibwe Studies: Essays, 1934–1972
A. Irving Hallowell
Edited and with introductions by Jennifer S. H. Brown and Susan Elaine Gray

Excavating Nauvoo: The Mormons and the Rise of Historical Archaeology in America
Benjamin C. Pykles
Foreword by Robert L. Schuyler

Cultural Negotiations: The Role of Women in the Founding of Americanist Archaeology
David L. Browman

Homo Imperii: A History of Physical Anthropology in Russia
Marina Mogilner

American Anthropology and Company: Historical Explorations
Stephen O. Murray

Racial Science in Hitler's New Europe, 1938–1945
Edited by Anton Weiss-Wendt and Rory Yeomans

Cora Du Bois: Anthropologist, Diplomat, Agent
Susan C. Seymour

Before Boas: The Genesis of Ethnography and Ethnology in the German Enlightenment
Han F. Vermeulen

American Antiquities: Revisiting the Origins of American Archaeology
Terry A. Barnhart

An Asian Frontier: American Anthropology and Korea, 1882–1945
Robert Oppenheim

Theodore E. White and the Development of Zooarchaeology in North America
R. Lee Lyman

Declared Defective: Native Americans, Eugenics, and the Myth of Nam Hollow
Robert Jarvenpa

Glory, Trouble, and Renaissance at the Robert S. Peabody Museum of Archaeology
Edited and with an introduction by Malinda Stafford Blustain and Ryan J. Wheeler

Race Experts: Sculpture, Anthropology, and the American Public in Malvina Hoffman's Races of Mankind
Linda Kim

The Enigma of Max Gluckman: The Ethnographic Life of a "Luckyman" in Africa
Robert J. Gordon

National Races: Transnational Power Struggles in the Sciences and Politics of Human Diversity, 1840–1945
Edited by Richard McMahon

Franz Boas: The Emergence of the Anthropologist
Rosemary Lévy Zumwalt

Maria Czaplicka: Gender, Shamanism, Race
Grażyna Kubica

Writing Anthropologists, Sounding Primitives: The Poetry and Scholarship of Edward Sapir, Margaret Mead, and Ruth Benedict
A. Elisabeth Reichel

The History of Anthropology: A Critical Window on the Discipline in North America
Regna Darnell

History of Theory and Method in Anthropology
Regna Darnell

Franz Boas: Shaping Anthropology and Working for Social Justice
Rosemary Lévy Zumwalt

A Maverick Boasian: The Life and Work of Alexander A. Goldenweiser
Sergei Kan

Hoarding New Guinea: Writing Colonial Ethnographic Collection Histories for Postcolonial Futures
Rainer F. Buschmann

Truth and Power in American Archaeology
Alice Beck Kehoe

Turning the Power: Indian Boarding Schools, Native American Anthropologists, and the Race to Preserve Indigenous Cultures
Nathan Sowry

James Cowles Prichard of the Red Lodge: A Life of Science during the Age of Improvement
Margaret M. Crump

Invisible Contrarian: Essays in Honor of Stephen O. Murray
Edited by Regna Darnell and Wendy Leeds-Hurwitz

To order or obtain more information on these or other University of Nebraska Press titles, visit nebraskapress.unl.edu.

www.ingramcontent.com/pod-product-compliance
Lightning Source LLC
Chambersburg PA
CBHW021358300426
44114CB00012B/1281